Regenerative Medicine: Clinical Aspects

Regenerative Medicine: Clinical Aspects

Editor: Cedric Pearson

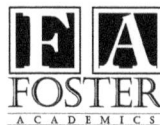

FA
FOSTER
ACADEMICS

www.fosteracademics.com

www.fosteracademics.com

Foster
ACADEMICS

Cataloging-in-Publication Data

Regenerative medicine : clinical aspects / edited by Cedric Pearson.
    p. cm.
Includes bibliographical references and index.
ISBN 978-1-63242-939-1
1. Regenerative medicine. 2. Stem cells--Therapeutic use. 3. Tissue engineering. I. Pearson, Cedric.
R857.T55 R44 2020
610.28--dc23

Foster Academics,
118-35 Queens Blvd., Suite 400,
Forest Hills, NY 11375, USA

ISBN 978-1-63242-939-1 (Hardback)

Contents

Preface

Every book is a source of knowledge and this one is no exception. The idea that led to the conceptualization of this book was the fact that the world is advancing rapidly; which makes it crucial to document the progress in every field. I am aware that a lot of data is already available, yet, there is a lot more to learn. Hence, I accepted the responsibility of editing this book and contributing my knowledge to the community.

Tissue repair after injury is a metabolically demanding and complex process. Depending on the regenerative capacity of tissues and the quality of the inflammatory response, the outcome is mostly imperfect, characterized by a degree of fibrosis. Inflammatory cells at a wound site facilitate wound debridement and produce metabolites, chemokines and growth factors. If this response becomes dysregulated, the wound becomes chronic or progressively fibrotic. This leads to impaired tissue function that may lead to organ failure. Regenerative medicine and inflammation research are intricately linked areas of research in the life sciences. Their significance in translational research has evolved considerably. This book explores all the important aspects of inflammation research and regenerative medicine in the present day scenario. The various studies that are constantly contributing towards advancing technologies and evolution of these fields are examined in detail. Coherent flow of topics, student-friendly language and extensive use of examples make this book an invaluable source of knowledge.

While editing this book, I had multiple visions for it. Then I finally narrowed down to make every chapter a sole standing text explaining a particular topic, so that they can be used independently. However, the umbrella subject sinews them into a common theme. This makes the book a unique platform of knowledge.

I would like to give the major credit of this book to the experts from every corner of the world, who took the time to share their expertise with us. Also, I owe the completion of this book to the never-ending support of my family, who supported me throughout the project.

Editor

Roles of renin-angiotensin system and Wnt pathway in aging-related phenotypes

Takehiro Kamo[1], Hiroshi Akazawa[1,3]*, Jun-ichi Suzuki[2] and Issei Komuro[1,3]

Abstract

The renin-angiotensin system (RAS) regulates diverse cellular responses and is crucial for normal organ development and function. On the other hand, RAS exerts deleterious effects promoting cardiovascular and multiple organ damage and contributes to promoting various aging-related diseases and aging-related decline in multiple organ functions. RAS blockade has been shown to prevent the progression of aging-related phenotypes and promote longevity. Wnt signaling pathway also plays a major role in the regulation of mammalian pathophysiology and is essential for organismal survival, and furthermore, it is substantially involved in the promotion of aging process. In this way, both RAS signaling and Wnt signaling have the functions of antagonistic pleiotropy during the process of growth and aging. Our recent study has demonstrated that an anti-aging effect of RAS blockade is associated with down-regulation of canonical Wnt signaling pathway, providing evidence for the hierarchical relationship between RAS signaling and Wnt signaling in promoting aging-related phenotypes. Here, we review how RAS signaling and Wnt signaling regulate the aging process and promote aging-related diseases.

Keywords: AT_1 receptor, ARB, Cardiovascular disease, Complement C1q, Skeletal muscle regeneration

Background

The renin-angiotensin system (RAS) plays pleiotropic roles in regulating mammalian pathophysiology. Angiotensin II (Ang II) is a key molecule of RAS and is produced as a result of sequential cleavage of angiotensinogen by renin and angiotensin-converting enzyme (ACE). Ang II exerts diverse pathophysiological effects on binding to Ang II type 1 (AT_1) receptor [1]. AT_1 receptor is a well-known member of the G protein-coupled receptor family, which shares the structure characterized by seven transmembrane-spanning α-helices. Mice have two AT_1 receptor isoforms (AT_{1a} and AT_{1b}) which are encoded by separate genes (*Agtr1a* and *Agtr1b*), whereas humans have a single AT_1 receptor isoform encoded by *AGTR1* gene. Mouse *Agtr1a* gene is a homolog to human *AGTR1* gene, and AT_{1a} receptor is the major AT_1 receptor isoform in mice. AT_1 receptor is activated by binding of Ang II or by mechanical stretch in the absence of Ang II [2, 3].

A decrease in extracellular volume caused by fluid loss or low salt intake stimulates secretion of renin, which leads to production of Ang II and thereby induces systemic vasoconstriction, salt and water retention, and sympathetic nervous activation. These responses restore blood pressure and electrolyte and water balance. In addition to regulation of hemodynamic homeostasis, RAS is essential for normal organ development. Mice deficient in angiotensinogen [4] or in both AT_{1a} and AT_{1b} receptor isoforms [5, 6] showed abnormal phenotypes in the kidney. The administration of ACE inhibitors or AT_1 receptor blockers (ARBs) is contraindicated during pregnancy due to an increased risk of fetal disorders [7]. Thus, RAS is crucial for both embryogenesis and maintaining homeostasis and apparently beneficial for survival.

On the other hand, RAS has detrimental effects on cardiovascular tissues. AT_1 receptor activation evokes diverse G protein-dependent and G protein-independent signaling pathways, leading to cell proliferation, hypertrophic responses, apoptosis, generation of reactive oxygen species (ROS), and tissue inflammation [8]. RAS has been shown to promote the pathophysiological processes of various aging-related disorders, including not only

* Correspondence: akazawah-tky@umin.ac.jp
[1]Department of Cardiovascular Medicine, Graduate School of Medicine, The University of Tokyo, 7-3-1 Hongo, Bunkyo-ku, Tokyo 113-8655, Japan
[3]AMED-CREST, Japan Agency for Medical Research and Development, Chiyoda-ku, Tokyo 100-0004, Japan
Full list of author information is available at the end of the article

cardiovascular diseases and heart failure but also diabetes, chronic kidney disease, dementia, osteoporosis, and cancer [9]. Recent studies have demonstrated that inhibition of RAS prolongs the physiological aging process and promotes longevity in rodents [10], suggesting the involvement of RAS in the aging process per se.

In addition to AT_1 receptor, Ang II type 2 (AT_2) receptor is also a functional receptor with high affinity for Ang II [1]. AT_2 receptor activation has vasodilatory, anti-proliferative, and anti-inflammatory effects, which counteract the effects of AT_1 receptor signaling [1]. Thus, AT_2 receptor signaling may provide cardiovascular protection and possibly prevent the progression of aging-related diseases. Ang II is cleaved by ACE2 to form another peptide Ang (1–7). This ACE2-Ang (1–7) axis, acting via another G protein-coupled receptor Mas, is also involved in vasodilatory, anti-fibrotic, and anti-inflammatory properties [11]. While the ACE-Ang II-AT_1 receptor axis has been extensively studied, research on the role of ACE2-Ang (1–7)-Mas receptor axis in the aging process has been limited.

Wnt signaling pathway also regulates diverse cellular responses during embryogenesis and is required for normal development and function of organs [12]. On the other hand, canonical Wnt/β-catenin signaling is also involved in the aging process and promotes aging-related phenotypes [13, 14]. Accordingly, both RAS and Wnt signaling pathway have antagonistic and pleiotropic effects in the physiological process of growth and aging because they are essential and beneficial early in life but deleterious later in life [9].

We have recently reported that RAS blockade prevented the aging-related functional decline in skeletal muscle and that this anti-aging effect of RAS blockade was associated with down-regulation of Wnt/β-catenin signaling pathway [15]. These findings suggest the relationship between RAS signaling and Wnt/β-catenin signaling in promoting aging-related phenotypes. This review focuses on how RAS and Wnt signaling pathway regulate the aging process and how they play roles as possible targets for preventing and treating aging-related diseases.

RAS in aging-related cardiovascular diseases and heart failure

Aging is usually defined as a progressive loss of multiple organ functions with advancing age. It is regulated by a wide variety of factors including genetic backgrounds and environmental stresses. Aging increases the risks of various cardiovascular diseases, such as hypertension, atherosclerotic vascular disease, cardiac remodeling, and congestive heart failure. RAS is widely recognized as a key factor contributing to the pathogenesis throughout the "cardiovascular continuum" [16].

RAS plays a fundamental role in the pathogenesis of hypertension even at an early stage. Sustained and excessive activation of RAS signaling induces continuous vasoconstriction and promotes vascular hypertrophy and endothelial dysfunction by direct as well as indirect hemodynamic effects, thereby contributing to the accelerated rise of blood pressure [17]. Indeed, the administration of an ARB reduced the development of hypertension in prehypertensive patients [18]. RAS blockade leads to a better outcome on survival in high-risk animals with hypertension. The treatment with an ACE inhibitor or ARB doubled the life span of stroke-prone spontaneously hypertensive rats to 30 months, which was comparable to that of normotensive rats [19, 20]. This life extension effect was associated with preservation of cardiac function as well as endothelial function by the treatment with an ACE inhibitor or ARB [19, 20].

RAS contributes to the promotion of atherosclerotic process. Ang II stimulates activity of nicotinamide adenine dinucleotide/nicotinamide adenine dinucleotide phosphate (NAD(P)H) oxidase which increased ROS formation [21]. Ang II also stimulates the release of proinflammatory cytokines and promotes the recruitment of macrophages and T cells through the generation of adhesion molecules and chemokines [22]. This increased oxidative stress and proinflammatory state leads to the development of endothelial dysfunction and vascular remodeling [23]. Furthermore, RAS promotes vasoconstriction, alters the composition of extracellular matrix, and enhances migration and proliferation of vascular smooth muscle cells [24]. Thus, RAS induces diverse cellular responses within the vascular wall, leading to the progression of atherosclerotic cascade.

Persistent and excessive activation of RAS plays a substantial role in pathological cardiac hypertrophy and cardiac remodeling. AT_1 receptor activation induces hypertrophic responses in cardiomyocytes and extracellular matrix protein synthesis in cardiac fibroblasts [25]. Ang II infusion induced cardiac hypertrophy independently of blood pressure elevation in rats [26], and cardiac-specific overexpression of AT_1 receptor induced cardiac hypertrophy, interstitial fibrosis, and contractile dysfunction in mice [27, 28]. RAS blockade is highly effective in preventing the progression of cardiac remodeling and heart failure. AT_{1a} receptor-deficient mice showed less severe cardiac dysfunction induced by myocardial infarction [29], administration of cardiotoxic agent doxorubicin [30], or genetic disruption of muscle LIM protein (MLP) [31]. A meta-analysis demonstrated that ARBs were the most effective among antihypertensive drugs for reducing left ventricular mass in patients with essential hypertension [32]. In addition, clinical trials have demonstrated that ACE inhibitors or ARBs reduce death and hospitalization in the broad spectrum of patients with heart failure [33].

RAS in other aging-related diseases

It has been demonstrated that RAS is involved in the pathophysiological processes of other aging-related disorders, such as diabetes, chronic kidney disease, dementia, osteoporosis, and cancer [9].

RAS contributes to the pathogenesis of insulin resistance, a notable feature of metabolic syndrome and type 2 diabetes mellitus [34]. Ang II-mediated activation of AT_1 receptor modulates the effects of insulin signaling [35]. For example, AT_1 receptor activation synergistically promotes the proliferative effects of insulin but inhibits its metabolic actions. Also, the direct effect of Ang II on islet contributes to impaired β cell function. Acute infusion of Ang II inhibited the early phase of insulin secretion in rats [36], and RAS blockade improved islet morphology and prevented islet fibrosis in diabetic rats [37]. Recent clinical trials have demonstrated that RAS blockade improves insulin sensitivity and reduces the incident risk of diabetes in high-risk patients [38].

RAS signaling plays a major role in promoting chronic kidney disease. Ang II induces vasoconstriction of the post-glomerular arterioles and increases the glomerular hydrostatic pressure and the ultrafiltration of plasma proteins, thereby contributing to the onset and progression of chronic renal damage [39]. In addition to hemodynamic effects, Ang II exerts non-hemodynamic effects promoting renal tissue injury, through increased generation of ROS, up-regulation of cytokines and adhesion molecules, activation and recruitment of macrophages, and increased synthesis of extracellular matrix proteins [40]. RAS inhibitors provide renal protection and reduce proteinuria and decline of glomerular filtration rate in patients with chronic kidney disease [41, 42].

Recent studies unraveled the possible involvement of RAS in neuropathology of Alzheimer's disease or bone metabolism. ARB treatment decreased the accumulation of β-amyloid proteins in the brain and attenuated the development of cognitive impairment in a mouse model of Alzheimer's disease [43]. In ovariectomized rats with hypertension, ARB treatment attenuated osteoporosis and suppressed an increase in osteoclast activity [44]. Clinical studies have suggested that antihypertensive treatment with ACE inhibitors was associated with high bone mineral density and reduced the risk of bone fractures [45].

Furthermore, RAS is associated with cancer-related signaling pathways. AT_1 receptor is expressed in several human cancer cell lines including pancreatic and prostate cancer cell lines [46, 47] and in a subpopulation of ER-positive, ERBB2-negative breast cancer cases [48], and ARB treatment suppressed AT_1 receptor-positive cancer cell proliferation and tumor growth. The growth of tumor cells engrafted in AT_{1a} receptor-deficient mice was reduced, accompanied by reduction in tumor-related angiogenesis [49]. Ang II induced the proliferation of myeloid progenitor cells in the spleen in a mouse model of lung adenocarcinoma, thereby supplying tumor-associated macrophages to promote tumor development [50]. These findings indicate that RAS signaling plays an important role in tumor growth and progression through inducing tumor cell proliferation, tumor-associated angiogenesis, and tumor-associated macrophage expansion.

RAS in physiological aging process

RAS blockade has been shown to suppress the deleterious effects during the physiological aging process in rodents. The administration of an ACE inhibitor or ARB to CF1 mice or Wistar rats led to a prolongation of life span, which was associated with a decrease in cardiac and renal fibrosis [51, 52]. CF1 mice treated with enalapril, but not with propranolol, nifedipine, or hydrochlorothiazide, revealed protection from organ damage associated with aging and prolonged life span, even though these drugs induced similar hypotensive effects [53]. Therefore, RAS inhibitor regulates life span independently of blood pressure-lowering effect. AT_{1a} receptor-deficient mice also exhibited a prolongation of life span, which was accompanied by less cardiac hypertrophy and fibrosis [10]. The accumulation of oxidative stress caused by ROS substantially contributes to the aging process [54]. The treatment with an ACE inhibitor was associated with a decrease in apoptosis and the suppression of aging-related decrease in mitochondrial number and mitochondrial superoxide dismutase in murine cardiomyocytes [51, 55]. AT_{1a} receptor-deficient mice showed less oxidative damage in the heart and kidney and prevention of aging-related loss of mitochondria in the kidney [10]. In addition, genetic disruption of AT_{1a} receptor induced an increase in expression levels of Nampt and Sirt3 in the kidneys of aging mice [10]. In a nutrient-deprived environment, increased expression of Nampt leads to the accumulation of its biosynthetic product nicotinamide adenine dinucleotide (NAD^+) in mitochondria, which in turn activates mitochondrial sirtuin 3 (SIRT3) [56]. SIRT3 is a NAD^+-dependent deacetylase that protects against stress-mediated cell death. These findings demonstrate that inhibition of RAS promotes longevity, possibly through attenuation of oxidative stress and up-regulation of prosurvival genes.

We have recently reported that AT_{1a} receptor-deficient mice showed less severe aging-related phenotypes in other tissues as well, such as functional decline in skeletal muscle [15]. RAS blockade can prevent aging-related sarcopenia. It has been demonstrated that elderly persons with hypertension taking ACE inhibitors had lower decline in muscle strength and larger muscle mass of the lower extremities than users of other antihypertensive drugs [57, 58]. In aged mice, ARB treatment protected against disuse atrophy of skeletal muscle [59]. One of the hallmarks of aging is a decline in the regenerative capacity of skeletal muscle following injury. ARB treatment led to histological improvement in skeletal muscle regeneration after laceration in mice [60]. ARB inhibited transforming growth factor-β (TGF-β) signaling and thereby attenuated TGF-β-mediated impairment of muscle regeneration in mice with myopathy [61]. In addition, Ang II may have direct anti-proliferative effects on satellite cells, which are crucial for skeletal muscle growth and regeneration, via AT_1 receptor [62]. We have shown that treatment with an ARB restored skeletal muscle function assessed by treadmill test after cryoinjury in mice [15]. ARB-treated mice showed an increase in satellite cell population, enhanced regeneration of myofibers, and decreased fibrosis in cryoinjured skeletal muscle. Taken together, RAS can be targeted to protect against deleterious effects associated with aging process and promote longevity.

Relationship between RAS and Wnt signaling in aging

Wnt proteins initiate signaling cascade on binding to Frizzled receptor and low-density lipoprotein receptor-related protein (LRP) 5/6 coreceptor, which leads to stabilization of cytosolic β-catenin [12, 63]. Then,

translocating to nucleus, β-catenin activates target gene transcription. It has been demonstrated that canonical Wnt/β-catenin signaling is also involved in the aging process. Wnt/β-catenin signaling activity was enhanced in multiple tissues of a klotho-deficient mouse model of accelerated aging [64]. Wnt treatment attenuated skeletal muscle regeneration in young mice, and inhibition of canonical Wnt signaling restored the impairment of muscle regeneration in aged mice [13]. Moreover, Wnt/β-catenin signaling was augmented in skeletal muscle satellite cells exposed to the serum of aged mice, indicating that components of aged serum contributed to the aging-related activation of Wnt signaling [13]. Complement C1q has recently been identified as an activator of Wnt/β-catenin signaling independently of Wnt [14]. C1q activates canonical Wnt/β-catenin signaling through binding to Frizzled receptor and inducing C1s-dependent cleavage of LRP6 coreceptor. Macrophages are major cells that secrete C1q [65]. Aging mice have increased serum and tissue levels of C1q and enhanced Wnt signaling activity [14]. C1q treatment stimulated fibroblast proliferation and collagen synthesis but suppressed satellite cell proliferation in skeletal muscle, and promoted aging-related impairment of skeletal muscle regeneration through activation of Wnt/β-catenin signaling [14]. C1q was secreted from macrophages recruited to the aorta in Ang II-infused mice, and C1q-mediated activation of Wnt/β-catenin signaling induced proliferation of vascular smooth muscle cells and promoted arterial remodeling [66].

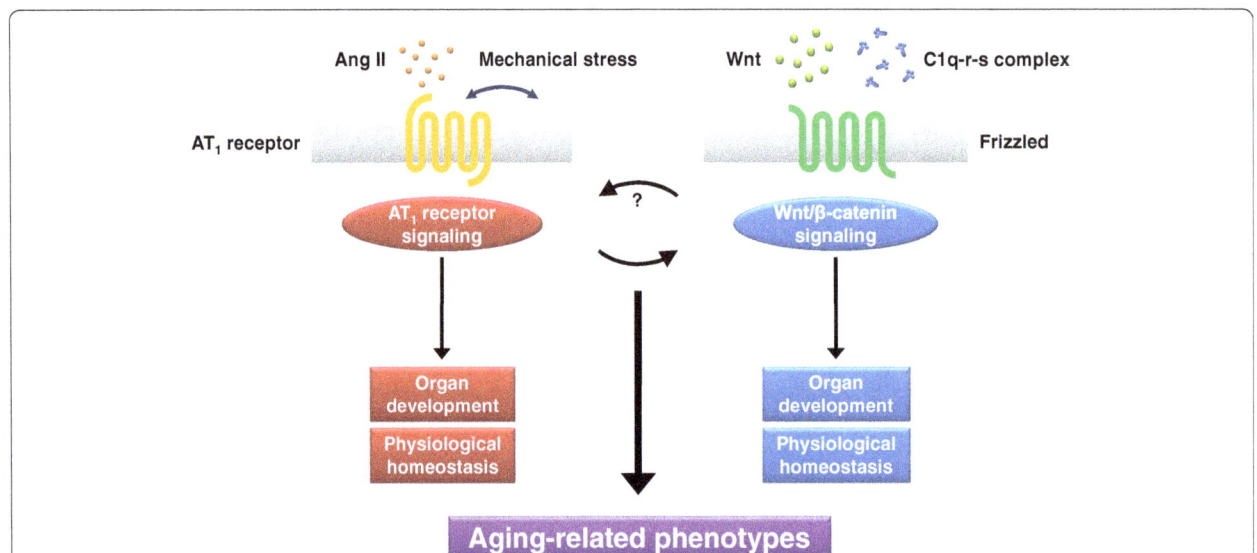

Fig. 1 RAS signaling and Wnt signaling in aging process. AT_1 receptor is activated upon stimulation by binding of Ang II or mechanical stress, and Wnt/β-catenin signaling cascade is initiated by binding of Wnt proteins or C1q-r-s complex to Frizzled receptor. Both AT_1 receptor signaling and Wnt/β-catenin signaling are essential for normal organ development and crucial for regulation of physiological homeostasis. On the other hand, AT_1 receptor signaling and Wnt/β-catenin signaling are involved in the aging process, and they are hierarchically related in promoting aging-related phenotypes. AT_1 receptor blockade protects against aging-related deleterious effects through down-regulation of aging-promoting C1q-Wnt/β-catenin signaling pathway

We have demonstrated that serum C1q concentration was increased, and C1q expression and Wnt/β-catenin signaling activity in skeletal muscle were augmented after cryoinjury in mice, but ARB treatment inhibited both the increase in serum C1q level and the activation of C1q-Wnt/β-catenin signaling in injured muscle [15]. C1q expression in macrophages was reduced by administration of ARB both in culture and in injured muscle. Moreover, these beneficial effects of ARB on skeletal muscle repair after injury were reversed by topical administration of C1q [15]. These findings suggest that RAS blockade prevents aging-related phenotypes through down-regulation of aging-promoting C1q-Wnt/β-catenin signaling pathway and that RAS signaling and Wnt/β-catenin signaling are hierarchically related in promoting the aging process (Fig. 1). We propose that RAS blockade reduces systemic and local levels of C1q through inhibiting C1q synthesis in infiltrated macrophages and thereby enhances proliferation and differentiation of satellite cells, leading to promotion of skeletal muscle repair. Besides selectively inhibiting Ang II-induced activation of AT_1 receptor, ARB may enhance Ang II-induced activation of AT_2 receptor [67]. Further studies will be required to elucidate whether AT_2 receptor activation contributes to down-regulation of C1q-Wnt/β-catenin signaling and protection against aging.

Conclusions

RAS is profoundly involved in the progression of various aging-related diseases and the promotion of the aging process. RAS blockade has been shown to protect against aging-related deleterious effects and promote longevity. We have recently shown that this anti-aging effect of RAS blockade was mediated by down-regulation of aging-promoting C1q-Wnt/β-catenin signaling pathway, suggesting the hierarchical relationship between RAS signaling and Wnt signaling in promoting aging-related phenotypes. It is a matter of interest whether blocking RAS signaling or C1q-Wnt/β-catenin signaling could prevent geriatric frailty and prolong life span in humans. It remains to be elucidated how RAS signaling induces C1q expression in macrophages during the aging process. Further investigations of the relationship between RAS signaling and C1q-Wnt/β-catenin signaling will provide insights into the mechanisms responsible for aging-related functional decline of multiple organs and open up a path toward the development of novel therapeutics against aging-related diseases.

Abbreviations
ACE, angiotensin-converting enzyme; Ang, angiotensin; ARB, angiotensin II type 1 receptor blocker; AT_1, angiotensin II type 1; LRP, low-density lipoprotein receptor-related protein; MLP, muscle LIM protein; NAD(P)H, nicotinamide adenine dinucleotide/nicotinamide adenine dinucleotide phosphate; NAD^+, nicotinamide adenine dinucleotide; RAS, renin-angiotensin system; ROS, reactive oxygen species; SIRT, sirtuin; TGF-β, transforming growth factor-β.

Funding
This work was supported in part by grants from the Japan Society for the Promotion of Science (KAKENHI 26670395 to HA and AMED-CREST, Japan Agency for Medical Research and Development to HA and IK) and Health and Labor Sciences Research Grants (to HA and IK).

Authors' contributions
TK and HA wrote the manuscript, and JS and IK helped to draft the manuscript. All authors read and approved the final manuscript.

Competing interests
HA has received trust research/joint research funding from Shionogi & Co., Ltd., and research funding from Takeda Pharmaceutical Co., Ltd., Daiichi Sankyo Co., Ltd., and Nippon Boehringer Ingelheim Co., Ltd. JS has received research funding from Nippon Boehringer Ingelheim Co., Ltd. IK has received research funding from Astellas Pharma Inc., Daiichi Sankyo Co., Ltd., Nippon Boehringer Ingelheim Co., Ltd., and Takeda Pharmaceutical Co., Ltd., and has affiliations with endowed department sponsored by Shionogi & Co., Ltd.

Author details
[1]Department of Cardiovascular Medicine, Graduate School of Medicine, The University of Tokyo, 7-3-1 Hongo, Bunkyo-ku, Tokyo 113-8655, Japan. [2]Department of Advanced Clinical Science and Therapeutics, Graduate School of Medicine, The University of Tokyo, Bunkyo-ku, Tokyo 113-8655, Japan. [3]AMED-CREST, Japan Agency for Medical Research and Development, Chiyoda-ku, Tokyo 100-0004, Japan.

References
1. Akazawa H, Yano M, Yabumoto C, Kudo-Sakamoto Y, Komuro I. Angiotensin II type 1 and type 2 receptor-induced cell signaling. Curr Pharm Des. 2013; 19:2988–95.
2. Zou Y, Akazawa H, Qin Y, Sano M, Takano H, Minamino T, et al. Mechanical stress activates angiotensin II type 1 receptor without the involvement of angiotensin II. Nat Cell Biol. 2004;6:499–506.
3. Yasuda N, Miura S, Akazawa H, Tanaka T, Qin Y, Kiya Y, et al. Conformational switch of angiotensin II type 1 receptor underlying mechanical stress-induced activation. EMBO Rep. 2008;9:179–86.
4. Niimura F, Labosky PA, Kakuchi J, Okubo S, Yoshida H, Oikawa T, et al. Gene targeting in mice reveals a requirement for angiotensin in the development and maintenance of kidney morphology and growth factor regulation. J Clin Invest. 1995;96:2947–54.
5. Oliverio MI, Kim HS, Ito M, Le T, Audoly L, Best CF, et al. Reduced growth, abnormal kidney structure, and type 2 (AT2) angiotensin receptor-mediated blood pressure regulation in mice lacking both AT1A and AT1B receptors for angiotensin II. Proc Natl Acad Sci USA. 1998;95:15496–501.
6. Tsuchida S, Matsusaka T, Chen X, Okubo S, Niimura F, Nishimura H, et al. Murine double nullizygotes of the angiotensin type 1A and 1B receptor genes duplicate severe abnormal phenotypes of angiotensinogen nullizygotes. J Clin Invest. 1998;101:755–60.
7. Cooper WO, Hernandez-Diaz S, Arbogast PG, Dudley JA, Dyer S, Gideon PS, et al. Major congenital malformations after first-trimester exposure to ACE inhibitors. N Engl J Med. 2006;354:2443–51.
8. Hunyady L, Catt KJ. Pleiotropic AT1 receptor signaling pathways mediating physiological and pathogenic actions of angiotensin II. Mol Endocrinol. 2006;20:953–70.
9. Kamo T, Akazawa H, Komuro I. Pleiotropic effects of angiotensin II receptor signaling in cardiovascular homeostasis and aging. Int Heart J. 2015;56:249–54.
10. Benigni A, Corna D, Zoja C, Sonzogni A, Latini R, Salio M, et al. Disruption of the Ang II type 1 receptor promotes longevity in mice. J Clin Invest. 2009; 119:524–30.
11. Jiang F, Yang J, Zhang Y, Dong M, Wang S, Zhang Q, et al. Angiotensin-converting enzyme 2 and angiotensin 1-7: novel therapeutic targets. Nat Rev Cardiol. 2014;11:413–26.
12. Clevers H. Wnt/β-catenin signaling in development and disease. Cell. 2006; 127:469–80.

13. Brack AS, Conboy MJ, Roy S, Lee M, Kuo CJ, Keller C, et al. Increased Wnt signaling during aging alters muscle stem cell fate and increases fibrosis. Science. 2007;317:807–10.

14. Naito AT, Sumida T, Nomura S, Liu ML, Higo T, Nakagawa A, et al. Complement C1q activates canonical Wnt signaling and promotes aging-related phenotypes. Cell. 2012;149:1298–313.

15. Yabumoto C, Akazawa H, Yamamoto R, Yano M, Kudo-Sakamoto Y, Sumida T, et al. Angiotensin II receptor blockade promotes repair of skeletal muscle through down-regulation of aging-promoting C1q expression. Sci Rep. 2015;5:14453.

16. Dzau V. The cardiovascular continuum and renin-angiotensin-aldosterone system blockade. J Hypertens Suppl. 2005;23:S9–17.

17. Folkow B. Physiological aspects of primary hypertension. Physiol Rev. 1982; 62:347–504.

18. Julius S, Nesbitt SD, Egan BM, Weber MA, Michelson EL, Kaciroti N, et al. Feasibility of treating prehypertension with an angiotensin-receptor blocker. N Engl J Med. 2006;354:1685–97.

19. Linz W, Jessen T, Becker RH, Schölkens BA, Wiemer G. Long-term ACE inhibition doubles lifespan of hypertensive rats. Circulation. 1997;96:3164–72.

20. Linz W, Heitsch H, Schölkens BA, Wiemer G. Long-term angiotensin II type 1 receptor blockade with fonsartan doubles lifespan of hypertensive rats. Hypertension. 2000;35:908–13.

21. Garrido AM, Griendling KK. NADPH oxidases and angiotensin II receptor signaling. Mol Cell Endocrinol. 2009;302:148–58.

22. Ferrario CM, Strawn WB. Role of the renin-angiotensin-aldosterone system and proinflammatory mediators in cardiovascular disease. Am J Cardiol. 2006;98: 121–8.

23. Koh KK, Oh PC, Quon MJ. Does reversal of oxidative stress and inflammation provide vascular protection? Cardiovasc Res. 2009;81:649–59.

24. Schmieder RE, Hilgers KF, Schlaich MP, Schmidt BM. Renin-angiotensin system and cardiovascular risk. Lancet. 2007;369:1208–19.

25. Kim S, Iwao H. Molecular and cellular mechanisms of angiotensin II-mediated cardiovascular and renal diseases. Pharmacol Rev. 2000;52:11–34.

26. Dostal DE, Baker KM. Angiotensin II stimulation of left ventricular hypertrophy in adult rat heart. Mediation by the AT1 receptor. Am J Hypertens. 1992;5:276–80.

27. Hein L, Stevens ME, Barsh GS, Pratt RE, Kobilka BK, Dzau VJ. Overexpression of angiotensin AT1 receptor transgene in the mouse myocardium produces a lethal phenotype associated with myocyte hyperplasia and heart block. Proc Natl Acad Sci USA. 1997;94:6391–6.

28. Paradis P, Dali-Youcef N, Paradis FW, Thibault G, Nemer M. Overexpression of angiotensin II type I receptor in cardiomyocytes induces cardiac hypertrophy and remodeling. Proc Natl Acad Sci USA. 2000;97:931–6.

29. Harada K, Sugaya T, Murakami K, Yazaki Y, Komuro I. Angiotensin II type 1A receptor knockout mice display less left ventricular remodeling and improved survival after myocardial infarction. Circulation. 1999;100:2093–9.

30. Toko H, Oka T, Zou Y, Sakamoto M, Mizukami M, Sano M, et al. Angiotensin II type 1a receptor mediates doxorubicin-induced cardiomyopathy. Hypertens Res. 2002;25:597–603.

31. Yamamoto R, Akazawa H, Ito K, Toko H, Sano M, Yasuda N, et al. Angiotensin II type 1a receptor signals are involved in the progression of heart failure in MLP-deficient mice. Circ J. 2007;71:1958–64.

32. Klingbeil AU, Schneider M, Martus P, Messerli FH, Schmieder RE. A meta-analysis of the effects of treatment on left ventricular mass in essential hypertension. Am J Med. 2003;115:41–6.

33. Mielniczuk L, Stevenson LW. Angiotensin-converting enzyme inhibitors and angiotensin II type I receptor blockers in the management of congestive heart failure patients: what have we learned from recent clinical trials? Curr Opin Cardiol. 2005;20:250–5.

34. Prasad A, Quyyumi AA. Renin-angiotensin system and angiotensin receptor blockers in the metabolic syndrome. Circulation. 2004;110:1507–12.

35. Velloso LA, Folli F, Sun XJ, White MF, Saad MJ, Kahn CR. Cross-talk between the insulin and angiotensin signaling systems. Proc Natl Acad Sci USA. 1996; 93:12490–5.

36. Carlsson PO, Berne C, Jansson L. Angiotensin II and the endocrine pancreas: effects on islet blood flow and insulin secretion in rats. Diabetologia. 1998; 41:127–33.

37. Tikellis C, Wookey PJ, Candido R, Andrikopoulos S, Thomas MC, Cooper ME. Improved islet morphology after blockade of the renin-angiotensin system in the ZDF rat. Diabetes. 2004;53:989–97.

38. Abuissa H, Jones PG, Marso SP, O'Keefe Jr JH. Angiotensin-converting enzyme inhibitors or angiotensin receptor blockers for prevention of type 2 diabetes: a meta-analysis of randomized clinical trials. J Am Coll Cardiol. 2005;46:821–6.

39. Remuzzi G, Bertani T. Pathophysiology of progressive nephropathies. N Engl J Med. 1998;339:1448–56.

40. Remuzzi G, Perico N, Macia M, Ruggenenti P. The role of renin-angiotensin-aldosterone system in the progression of chronic kidney disease. Kidney Int Suppl. 2005;68:S57–65.

41. Lewis EJ, Hunsicker LG, Clarke WR, Berl T, Pohl MA, Lewis JB, et al. Renoprotective effect of the angiotensin-receptor antagonist irbesartan in patients with nephropathy due to type 2 diabetes. N Engl J Med. 2001;345:851–60.

42. Brenner BM, Cooper ME, de Zeeuw D, Keane WF, Mitch WE, Parving HH, et al. Effects of losartan on renal and cardiovascular outcomes in patients with type 2 diabetes and nephropathy. N Engl J Med. 2001;345:861–9.

43. Wang J, Ho L, Chen L, Zhao Z, Zhao W, Qian X, et al. Valsartan lowers brain β-amyloid protein levels and improves spatial learning in a mouse model of Alzheimer disease. J Clin Invest. 2007;117:3393–402.

44. Shimizu H, Nakagami H, Osako MK, Hanayama R, Kunugiza Y, Kizawa T, et al. Angiotensin II accelerates osteoporosis by activating osteoclasts. FASEB J. 2008;22:2465–75.

45. Rejnmark L, Vestergaard P, Mosekilde L. Treatment with beta-blockers, ACE inhibitors, and calcium-channel blockers is associated with a reduced fracture risk: a nationwide case-control study. J Hypertens. 2006;24:581–9.

46. Fujimoto Y, Sasaki T, Tsuchida A, Chayama K. Angiotensin II type 1 receptor expression in human pancreatic cancer and growth inhibition by angiotensin II type 1 receptor antagonist. FEBS Lett. 2001;495:197–200.

47. Uemura H, Ishiguro H, Nakaigawa N, Nagashima Y, Miyoshi Y, Fujinami K, et al. Angiotensin II receptor blocker shows antiproliferative activity in prostate cancer cells: a possibility of tyrosine kinase inhibitor of growth factor. Mol Cancer Ther. 2003;2:1139–47.

48. Rhodes DR, Ateeq B, Cao Q, Tomlins SA, Mehra R, Laxman B, et al. AGTR1 overexpression defines a subset of breast cancer and confers sensitivity to losartan, an AGTR1 antagonist. Proc Natl Acad Sci USA. 2009;106:10284–9.

49. Egami K, Murohara T, Shimada T, Sasaki K, Shintani S, Sugaya T, et al. Role of host angiotensin II type 1 receptor in tumor angiogenesis and growth. J Clin Invest. 2003;112:67–75.

50. Cortez-Retamozo V, Etzrodt M, Newton A, Ryan R, Pucci F, Sio SW, et al. Angiotensin II drives the production of tumor-promoting macrophages. Immunity. 2013;38:296–308.

51. Ferder L, Inserra F, Romano L, Ercole L, Pszenny V. Effects of angiotensin-converting enzyme inhibition on mitochondrial number in the aging mouse. Am J Physiol. 1993;265:C15–8.

52. Basso N, Cini R, Pietrelli A, Ferder L, Terragno NA, Inserra F. Protective effect of long-term angiotensin II inhibition. Am J Physiol Heart Circ Physiol. 2007; 293:H1351–8.

53. Ferder LF, Inserra F, Basso N. Advances in our understanding of aging: role of the renin-angiotensin system. Curr Opin Pharmacol. 2002;2:189–94.

54. Finkel T, Holbrook NJ. Oxidants, oxidative stress and the biology of ageing. Nature. 2000;408:239–47.

55. Ferder L, Romano LA, Ercole LB, Stella I, Inserra F. Biomolecular changes in the aging myocardium: the effect of enalapril. Am J Hypertens. 1998;11: 1297–304.

56. Yang H, Yang T, Baur JA, Perez E, Matsui T, Carmona JJ, et al. Nutrient-sensitive mitochondrial NAD$^+$ levels dictate cell survival. Cell. 2007;130:1095–107.

57. Onder G, Penninx BW, Balkrishnan R, Fried LP, Chaves PH, Williamson J, et al. Relation between use of angiotensin-converting enzyme inhibitors and muscle strength and physical function in older women: an observational study. Lancet. 2002;359:926–30.

58. Di Bari M, van de Poll-Franse LV, Onder G, Kritchevsky SB, Newman A, Harris TB, et al. Antihypertensive medications and differences in muscle mass in older persons: the Health, Aging and Body Composition Study. J Am Geriatr Soc. 2004;52:961–6.

59. Burks TN, Andres-Mateos E, Marx R, Mejias R, Van Erp C, Simmers JL, et al. Losartan restores skeletal muscle remodeling and protects against disuse atrophy in sarcopenia. Sci Transl Med. 2011;3:82ra37.

60. Bedair HS, Karthikeyan T, Quintero A, Li Y, Huard J. Angiotensin II receptor blockade administered after injury improves muscle regeneration and decreases fibrosis in normal skeletal muscle. Am J Sports Med. 2008;36:1548–54.

61. Cohn RD, van Erp C, Habashi JP, Soleimani AA, Klein EC, Lisi MT, et al. Angiotensin II type 1 receptor blockade attenuates TGF-β-induced failure of muscle regeneration in multiple myopathic states. Nat Med. 2007;13:204–10.

62. Yoshida T, Galvez S, Tiwari S, Rezk BM, Semprun-Prieto L, Higashi Y, et al. Angiotensin II inhibits satellite cell proliferation and prevents skeletal muscle regeneration. J Biol Chem. 2013;288:23823–32.

63. MacDonald BT, Tamai K, He X. Wnt/β-catenin signaling: components, mechanisms, and diseases. Dev Cell. 2009;17:9–26.

64. Liu H, Fergusson MM, Castilho RM, Liu J, Cao L, Chen J, et al. Augmented Wnt signaling in a mammalian model of accelerated aging. Science. 2007; 317:803–6.

65. Petry F, Botto M, Holtappels R, Walport MJ, Loos M. Reconstitution of the complement function in C1q-deficient (C1qa-/-) mice with wild-type bone marrow cells. J Immunol. 2001;167:4033–7.

66. Sumida T, Naito AT, Nomura S, Nakagawa A, Higo T, Hashimoto A, et al. Complement C1q-induced activation of β-catenin signalling causes hypertensive arterial remodelling. Nat Commun. 2015;6:6241.

67. Wu L, Iwai M, Nakagami H, Li Z, Chen R, Suzuki J, et al. Roles of angiotensin II type 2 receptor stimulation associated with selective angiotensin II type 1 receptor blockade with valsartan in the improvement of inflammation-induced vascular injury. Circulation. 2001;104:2716–21.

2

Clinical trials using mesenchymal stem cells in liver diseases and inflammatory bowel diseases

Atsunori Tsuchiya[*], Yuichi Kojima, Shunzo Ikarashi, Satoshi Seino, Yusuke Watanabe, Yuzo Kawata and Shuji Terai

Abstract

Mesenchymal stem cell (MSC) therapies have been used in clinical trials in various fields. These cells are easily expanded, show low immunogenicity, can be acquired from medical waste, and have multiple functions, suggesting their potential applications in a variety of diseases, including liver disease and inflammatory bowel disease. MSCs help prepare the microenvironment, in response to inflammatory cytokines, by producing immunoregulatory factors that modulate the progression of inflammation by affecting dendritic cells, B cells, T cells, and macrophages. MSCs also produce a large amount of cytokines, chemokines, and growth factors, including exosomes that stimulate angiogenesis, prevent apoptosis, block oxidation reactions, promote remodeling of the extracellular matrix, and induce differentiation of tissue stem cells. According to ClinicalTrials.gov, more than 680 clinical trials using MSCs are registered for cell therapy of many fields including liver diseases (more than 40 trials) and inflammatory bowel diseases (more than 20 trials). In this report, we introduce background and clinical studies of MSCs in liver disease and inflammatory bowel diseases.

Keywords: Mesenchymal stem cell, Liver disease, Inflammatory bowel disease, Cell therapy

Background

The digestive system, which consists of the gastrointestinal tract, liver, pancreas, and biliary tree, functions in digestion, absorption, and metabolism and affects the basis of life. Various diseases, including cancer, inflammatory disease, infection, stones, and ulcers, are studied under the context of gastroenterology. While innovative drugs against *Helicobacter pylori* [1], hepatitis C virus [2], and inflammatory bowel disease (IBD) [3] have recently been developed, there are still unmet needs in this field, including in acute and chronic liver failure and refractory IBDs. Cell therapy may fulfill these unmet needs, and cell therapies using mesenchymal stem cells (MSCs) have become a major focus in many fields [4]. MSCs are reported to have multiple functions, especially anti-fibrosis and anti-inflammatory effects are focused in acute and chronic liver failure and refractory IBDs. Furthermore, MSCs have low immunogenicity, can expand easily, and can be obtained from medical waste, suggesting their potential to expand regenerative medicine for the treatment of liver diseases and IBDs.

In this paper, we review the current status of clinical trials using autologous/allogeneic MSCs in liver diseases and IBDs.

Characteristics of MSCs

MSCs have recently received attention as potential cell sources for cell therapy due to their ease of expansion and wide range of functions. MSCs can be obtained from not only bone marrow but also medical wastes, such as adipose tissue, umbilical tissue, and dental pulp. MSCs are positive for the common markers CD73, CD90, and CD105; however, they are negative for the endothelial marker CD31 and hematopoietic marker CD45 [4–7]. The expansion of MSCs in culture is relatively easy, and under appropriate conditions, MSCs have trilineage differentiation (osteogenic, chondrogenic, and adipogenic) potential. The effects of MSCs are broadly divided into two mechanisms: (1) recruited MSCs differentiate into functional cells to replace damaged cells, permitting the treatment of bone and cartilage damage; and (2) in response to inflammatory cytokines, MSCs help prepare the microenvironment by producing

* Correspondence: atsunori@med.niigata-u.ac.jp
Division of Gastroenterology and Hepatology, Graduate School of Medical and Dental Science, Niigata University, 1-757 Asahimachi-dori, Chuo-ku, Niigata 951-8510, Japan

immunoregulatory factors that modulate the progression of inflammation by affecting dendritic cells, B cells, T cells, and macrophages. MSCs also produce a large amount of cytokines, chemokines, and growth factors, including exosomes, which stimulate angiogenesis, prevent apoptosis, block oxidation reactions, promote remodeling of the extracellular matrix (ECM), and induce the differentiation of tissue stem cells [4, 7, 8]. These latter mechanisms can be applied for many diseases, including liver disease and IBSs. Some studies have reported that the effects of MSCs are determined by host conditions, such as inflammation stage and the use of immunosuppressants.

Although the behaviors of MSCs after administration have been analyzed, and some studies have shown that MSCs migrate to the injured site, MSC behaviors in humans have not been fully elucidated. Some studies have reported that MSCs disappear within a few weeks and do not remain long in the target tissue [5]. Recent studies have reported that only culture-conditioned medium or exosomes induce treatment effects, suggesting that the trophic effect is the most important effect of MSCs [9–11]. Another important characteristic of MSCs is that they generally have low immunogenicity. MSCs have no antigen-presenting properties and do not express major histocompatibility complex class II or costimulatory molecules; thus, injection of autologous or allogeneic MSCs has been employed in clinical studies. Allogeneic MSC therapy has the potential to expand MSC therapy to many patients [4, 7].

Clinical trials using MSCs

Since MSCs can be obtained relatively easily and have multiple functions, more than 680 clinical trials are ongoing according to ClinicalTrials.gov (https://clinicaltrials.gov/); most of these studies are phase I or II trials evaluating the use of MSCs in bone/cartilage, heart, neuron, immune/autoimmune, diabetes/kidney, lung, liver, and gastrointestinal fields. These studies aim to elucidate the safety/effectiveness of MSCs in the treatment of various diseases. In liver diseases, 40 trials are registered, most of which target liver cirrhosis or acute liver diseases (Table 1) [12–21]. The MSCs used in clinical trials of the liver are derived from the bone marrow (55%), umbilical cord tissue (35%), and adipose tissue (8%). Approximately 50% of MSCs are allogeneic. Additionally, while the major administration route is the peripheral blood, approximately 40% of cases are treated via the hepatic artery, reflecting the fact that hepatologists and radiologists often use catheters to treat hepatocellular carcinoma through the hepatic artery [22, 23] (Fig. 1).

In IBDs, 26 trials are registered (Table 2), 23 of which are investigating the use of MSCs in Crohn's disease (CD), and 3 of which are investigating the use of MSCs in ulcerative colitis (UC) [24–33]. More than 60% of trials are employing allogeneic MSCs, and in CD, more than 40% of the trials are evaluating intralesional injection into the fistula, which is the major and refractory complication of CD (Fig. 2).

Clinical trials in liver diseases
Background of liver diseases
Although the liver has high regenerative capacity, acute liver damage caused by viruses, drugs, alcohol, and autoimmune diseases, or chronic liver damage caused by hepatitis B or C virus, alcohol, non-alcoholic steatohepatitis (NASH), autoimmune hepatitis, and primary biliary cholangitis often cause liver failure [34]. The liver has a variety of functions, including metabolism of protein, sugar, and fat; detoxification; production of coagulation factors; and production of bile. Thus, during liver failure, several symptoms, including jaundice, edema, ascites, hepatic encephalopathy, and increased bleeding, can appear at the same time, resulting in life-threatening disease. In addition, during liver failure caused by chronic liver disease, accumulated liver fibrosis (i.e., liver cirrhosis) can cause portal hypertension, which often induces the varices, and long-term liver damage can cause gene abnormalities, leading to liver cancers. The ultimate therapy for liver failure is liver transplantation; however, only a small portion of patients with liver failure can receive liver transplantation due to the shortage of donor organs, invasiveness of operations, and economic reasons [35]. Revolutionary treatments, such as interferon-free treatment for hepatitis C and providing information regarding the importance of the daily lifestyle to prevent alcoholic liver disease and NASH, can potentially decrease the liver diseases; however, unmet needs to treat advanced liver failure will continue.

Advanced acute liver failure and chronic liver failure (liver cirrhosis) can be good targets for cell therapy. Since 2003, Terai et al. initiated autologous bone marrow cell infusion (ABMi) therapy against decompensated liver cirrhosis and confirmed the improvement of liver fibrosis and liver function [36–38]. However, due to the invasiveness of liver transplantation in patients with liver failure, minimally invasive procedures using specific cells, such as MSCs and macrophages [39–41], are now being developed, with a focus on MSCs. In the next section, we will describe recent reported results using MSCs registered at ClinicalTrials.gov.

Effects of MSC therapy in liver disease from published papers
Animal experiments have shown that MSCs can have antiapoptotic [42] and antioxidant effects in hepatocytes [43], and antifibrotic [44, 45], angiogenic [46], and immunosuppressive effects in T cells, macrophages, and dendritic cells [8]. In human clinical trials, all reports have shown that MSC injection is safe. Although the effects of cell therapy

Table 1 Clinical trials in liver diseases

No.	Start year	Cell source	Autologous/ allogeneic	Administration route	Number of cells infused	Etiology	Number of patients	Follow-up period	Phase	Study design	ClinicalTrials.gov identifier	Status	Result	References
1	2013	Bone marrow	Autologous	Peripheral vein	Unknown	LC	20	48 weeks	Phase 1–2	Non-randomized, single group assignment, open label	NCT01877759	Unknown		
2	2009	Bone marrow	Autologous	Hepatic artery	5 × 106 cells/ patient, 2 times	LC (alcohol)	11	24 weeks	Phase 2	Non-randomized, single group assignment, open label	NCT01741090	Unknown	Histological improvement. Improvement in Child- Pugh score. Decrease in TGFβ1, collagen type I, and α-SMA	13
3	2009	Bone marrow	Autologous	Peripheral vein	1.0 × 106/kg	LC	25	24 weeks	Unknown	Non-randomized, single group assignment, open label	NCT01499459	Unknown	Improvement in Alb and MELD scores.	
4	2014	Umbilical cord	Allogeneic	Peripheral vein	4.0 × 107/patient, 4 times	LC	320	144 weeks	Phase 1–2	Non-randomized, parallel assignment, open label	NCT01573923	Unknown		
5	2016	Adipose tissue	Autologous	Portal vein or hepatic artery	1.0 × 106/kg via peripheral vein, 3 times or 3.0 × 106/kg via hepatic artery, 3 times	LC (HCV)	5	48 weeks	Phase 1–2	Non-randomized, single group assignment, open label	NCT02705742	Recruiting		
6	2007	Bone marrow	Autologous	Peripheral or portal vein	30–50 × 106/patient	LC	8	24 weeks	Phase 1–2	Randomized, single group assignment, single blind	NCT00420134	Completed	Improvement in liver function and MELD scores.	14
7	2016	Bone marrow	Allogeneic	Peripheral vein	2.0 × 106/kg, 4 times	ACLF	30	96 weeks	Phase 1	Randomized, parallel assignment, double blind (subject, caregiver, investigator)	NCT02857010	Recruiting		
8	2009	Umbilical cord	Allogeneic	Peripheral vein	5.0 × 105/kg, 3 times	ACLF (HBV)	43	96 weeks	Phase 1–2	Randomized, parallel assignment, double blind (subject, caregiver)	NCT01218464	Unknown	Improvement in liver function and MELD scores.	15
9	2011	Bone marrow	Allogeneic	Peripheral vein	2.0 × 105/kg, 4 times or		120	48 weeks	Phase 2	Randomized, parallel	NCT01322906	Unknown		

Table 1 Clinical trials in liver diseases (Continued)

No.	Start year	Cell source	Autologous/ allogeneic	Administration route	Number of cells infused	Etiology	Number of patients	Follow-up period	Phase	Study design	ClinicalTrials.gov identifier	Status	Result	References
					1.0×10^6/kg, 4 times or 5.0×10^6/kg, 4 times	Liver failure (HBV)				assignment, open label				
10	2010	Umbilical cord	Allogeneic	Unknown	Unknown	LC	20	48 weeks	Phase 1–2	Randomized, parallel assignment, open label	NCT01342250	Completed		
11	2012	Bone marrow	Allogeneic	Hepatic artery	Unknown	LC (Alcohol)	40	96 weeks	Phase 2	Randomized, parallel assignment, open label	NCT01591200	Completed		
12	2012	Umbilical cord	Allogeneic	Peripheral vein	1.0×10^5/kg, 4 times	Liver failure (HBV)	120	48 weeks	Phase 1–2	Randomized, parallel assignment, open label	NCT01724398	Unknown		
13	2016	Bone marrow	Autologous	Portal vein	2.0×10^6/kg	LC	40	24 weeks	Phase 1–2	Non-randomized, parallel assignment, open label	NCT02943889	Not yet recruiting		
14	2009	Umbilical cord	Allogeneic	Portal vein or hepatic artery	Unknown	LC	200	48 weeks	Phase 1–2	Randomized, parallel assignment, single blind (subject)	NCT01233102	Suspended		
15	2009	Bone marrow	Autologous	Portal vein	Unknown	LC (HBV)	60	48 weeks	Phase 2	Non-randomized, parallel assignment, open label	NCT00993941	Unknown		
16	2010	Umbilical cord	Allogeneic	Hepatic artery	Unknown	LC	50	4 weeks	Phase 1–2	Randomized, parallel assignment, open label	NCT01224327	Unknown		
17	2013	Bone marrow	Autologous	Hepatic artery	1.0×10^6/kg	LC	30	12 weeks	Phase 3	Non-randomized, single group assignment, open label	NCT01854125	Enrolling by invitation		
18	2012	Umbilical cord	Allogeneic	Hepatic artery	1.0×10^6/kg	LC (HBV)	240	48 weeks	Phase 1–2	Randomized, parallel assignment, open label	NCT01728727	Unknown		
19	2013	Umbilical cord or	Allogeneic	Peripheral vein	1.0×10^5/kg, 1.0×10^6/kg		210	72 weeks	Phase 1–2	Randomized, parallel	NCT01844063	Recruiting		

Table 1 Clinical trials in liver diseases (*Continued*)

No.	Start year	Cell source	Autologous/ allogeneic	Administration route	Number of cells infused	Etiology	Number of patients	Follow-up period	Phase	Study design	ClinicalTrials.gov identifier	Status	Result	References
		bone marrow			or 1.0×10^7/kg, 8 times	Liver failure (HBV)				assignment, open label				
20	2016	Umbilical cord	Allogeneic	Peripheral vein	4 or 8 times	ACLF (HBV)	261	52 weeks	Phase 2	Randomized, parallel assignment, open label	NCT02812121	Not yet recruiting		
21	2010	Menstrual blood	Allogeneic	Peripheral vein	1.0×10^6/kg, 4 times	LC	50	48 weeks	Phase 1–2	Randomized, single group assignment, open label	NCT01483248	Enrolling by invitation		
22	2008	Bone marrow	Autologous	Hepatic artery	Unknown	LC	50	96 weeks	Phase 2	Randomized, parallel assignment, single blind (subject)	NCT00976287	Unknown		
23	2012	Bone marrow	Autologous	Hepatic artery	5×10^7/patient, 1 time or 2 times	LC (alcohol)	72	24 weeks	Phase 2	Randomized, parallel assignment, open label	NCT01875081	Completed	Histological improvement. Improvement in AST, ALT, ALP, γ-GTP, Child-Pugh score, and MELD score.	16
24	2014	Bone marrow	Autologous	Peripheral vein	Unknown	LC	10	24 weeks	Phase 1	Non-randomized, single group assignment, open label	NCT02237832	Recruiting		
25	2005	Bone marrow	Autologous	Hepatic artery	3.4×10^8/patient	Liver failure (HBV)	158	192 weeks	Phase 1–2	Case control, retrospective	NCT00956891	Completed	Improvement in Alb, T-Bil, PT, and MELD score.	
26	2009	Umbilical cord	Allogeneic	Peripheral vein	5.0×10^5/kg, 3 times	LC	45	48 weeks	Phase 1–2	Randomized, parallel assignment, open label	NCT01220492	Unknown	Improvement in Alb, T-Bil, and MELD score. Reduction of ascites.	17
27	2010	Bone marrow	Autologous	Portal vein	1.4–2.5×10^8/patient, 2 times	LC	2	48 weeks	Phase 1	Non-randomized, single group assignment, open label	NCT01454336	Completed	Transient improvement in MELD scores.	18
28	2007	Bone marrow	Autologous	Peripheral vein	$(1.2$–$2.95 \times 10^8)$ 1.95×10^8/patient	LC	27	48 weeks	Unknown	Randomized, parallel assignment, double	NCT00476060	Unknown	No beneficial effect.	19

Table 1 Clinical trials in liver diseases (*Continued*)

No.	Start year	Cell source	Autologous/ allogeneic	Administration route	Number of cells infused	Etiology	Number of patients	Follow-up period	Phase	Study design	ClinicalTrials.gov identifier	Status	Result	References
29	2011	Bone marrow	Allogeneic	Hepatic artery and peripheral artery	1.0 × 106/kg (5.0 × 107 cells via the hepatic artery and the remaining cells via the peripheral vein)	Wilson's disease	10	24 weeks	Unknown	Non-randomized, single group assignment, open label, blind (subject, outcomes assessor)	NCT01378182	Completed		
30	2016	Umbilical cord or bone marrow	Allogeneic	Portal vein or hepatic artery	2.0 × 107/patient, 4 times	LC	20	48 weeks	Phase 1	Non-randomized, single group assignment, open label	NCT02652351	Recruiting		
31	2016	Bone marrow	Autologous	Hepatic artery	5 × 107/patient, 1 time or 2 times	LC (alcohol)	50	144 weeks	Phase 2	Randomized, parallel assignment, open label	NCT02806011	Enrolling by invitation		
32	2011	Umbilical cord	Allogeneic	Peripheral vein	1.0 × 106/kg, 3 times	Liver failure (AIH)	100	96 weeks	Phase 1–2	Randomized, parallel assignment, open label	NCT01661842	Unknown		
33	2009	Adipose tissue	Autologous	Unknown	Unknown	LC	6	24 weeks	Phase 1	Non-randomized, single group assignment, open label	NCT00913289	Terminated		
34	2012	Adipose tissue	Autologous	Hepatic artery	Unknown	LC	4	4 weeks	Unknown	Non-randomized, single group assignment, open label	NCT01062750	Completed		
35	2016	Umbilical cord	Allogeneic	Lobe	5.0 × 108/patient	LC	40	96 weeks	Phase 1–2	Randomized, parallel assignment, double blind (subject, outcomes assessor)	NCT02786017	Recruiting		
36	2011	Bone marrow	Unknown	Peripheral vein	5.0–50 × 106/kg	LC (PBC)	20	96 weeks	Phase 1	Randomized, parallel assignment, open label	NCT01440309	Unknown		
37	2011	Umbilical cord	Allogeneic	Peripheral vein	5.0 ×105/kg, 3 times	LC (PBC)	7	48 weeks	Phase 1–2	Randomized, parallel	NCT01662973	Unknown	Improvement in Alb, T-Bil, and MELD score.	20

Table 1 Clinical trials in liver diseases *(Continued)*

No.	Start year	Cell source	Autologous/allogeneic	Administration route	Number of cells infused	Etiology	Number of patients	Follow-up period	Phase	Study design	ClinicalTrials.gov identifier	Status	Result	References
										assignment, open label			Reduction of ascites.	
38	2010	Bone marrow	Allogeneic	Portal vein or hepatic artery	Unknown	Liver failure (HBV)	60	48 weeks	Phase 2	Non-randomized, parallel assignment, open label	NCT01221454	Unknown		
39	2010	Bone marrow	Allogeneic	Portal vein or hepatic artery	Unknown	LC	60	48 weeks	Phase 2	Non-randomized, parallel assignment, open label	NCT01223664	Unknown		
40	2010	Bone marrow	Autologous	Hepatic artery	(0.25–1.25 × 106) 0.75 × 106/patient	LC (HBV)	39	24 weeks	Phase 2–3	Non-randomized, parallel assignment, open label	NCT01560845	Unknown	Decrease in Th-17 cells, RORγt, IL-17, TNF-α, and IL-6. Increase in Tregs and Foxp3.	21

LC liver cirrhosis, *ACLF* acute-on-chronic liver failure, *HBV* hepatitis B virus, *HCV* hepatitis C virus, *AIH* autoimmune hepatitis, *PBC* primary biliary cholangitis, *MELD* Model for End-Stage Liver Disease, *AST* aspartate transaminase, *ALT* alanine transaminase, *ALP* alkaline phosphatase, *γ-GTP* gamma-glutamyl transpeptidase, *Alb* albumin, *T-bil* total bilirubin, *PT* prothrombin time, *PC* protein C, *ROR* RAR-related orphan receptor, *Foxp3* forkhead box P3, IL interleukin, *Th* T helper, *SMA* smooth muscle actin, *TGF* transforming growth factor, *TNF* tumor necrosis factor

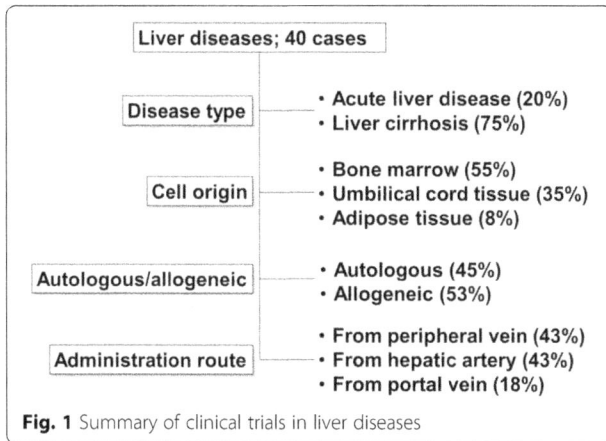

Fig. 1 Summary of clinical trials in liver diseases

are not uniform, the majority of therapies have some beneficial effects; in contrast, in a few reports, treatment effects were not observed. For example, Kantarcioglu et al. [13] and Mohamadnejad et al. [19] injected bone marrow-derived MSCs into patients with liver cirrhosis and did not observe treatment effects. However, Kharaziha et al. [14] reported phase I–II clinical trials using autologous bone marrow-derived MSCs against liver cirrhosis with a variety of etiologies, and improvement of liver function was confirmed. Jang et al. and Suk et al. [12, 16] reported a pilot study and a phase II study using autologous bone marrow-derived MSCs injected through the hepatic artery against alcoholic liver cirrhosis, and improvement of histological liver fibrosis and liver function was confirmed. Xu et al. [21] reported trials using autologous bone marrow-derived MSCs against hepatitis B virus-associated cirrhosis and confirmed the improvement of liver function, the decrease of Th17 cells, and the increase of regulatory T cells. Xhang et al. [17] and Wang et al. [20] reported trials using allogeneic umbilical cord-derived MSCs in patients with chronic hepatitis B having decompensated liver cirrhosis and primary biliary cirrhosis, respectively. They confirmed improvement of liver function, particularly reduced ascites and recovery of biliary enzymes, respectively. Shi et al. [15] reported a trial investigating acute or chronic liver failure associated with hepatitis B virus and confirmed that MSCs significantly increased survival rates. From these reports, MSCs appeared to improve liver function; however, additional trials are needed to confirm these effects and to elucidate the mechanisms in more detail.

Clinical trials in IBDs
Background of IBDs
IBDs are chronic inflammatory disorders, including UC and CD. The pathogenesis of IBD is thought to be highly complex due to several factors, such as environmental factors, genetic predisposition, and inflammatory abnormalities [47]. UC is characterized by inflammation of the mucosal membrane of the colon continued from the

rectum. Type 2 T helper cell (Th2) cytokine profile is associated with the pathogenesis of UC. In contrast, CD is a segmental, transluminal disorder that can arise within the entire gastrointestinal tract from the mouth to the anus. Th1 cells are associated with the pathogenesis of CD [48]. Furthermore, a recent report showed that Th17 cells are present in both UC and CD. Thus, mucosal CD4+ T cells are key mediators of the driving response [49]. Macrophages that produce tumor necrosis factor (TNF)-α have also been reported to be relevant in IBD. Imbalances in other cytokines, such as interleukin (IL)-1β, IL-6, IL-8, IL-10, IL-12, IL-17, IL-23, and transforming growth factor-β (TGF-β), are also detected during diseases [48]. Recent advancements in the development of drugs for IBD include drugs targeting TNF and new candidate drugs, such as antibodies against IL-6 [50] and IL-12/23 [51–53], small molecules including Janus kinase inhibitors [54], antisense oligonucleotides against SMAD7 mRNA [55], and inhibitors of leukocyte trafficking to intestinal sites of inflammation [56, 57]. However, some patients will fail to respond to current medical options, immunosuppressive agents, and anti-TNF biologicals. MSCs may be an effective option in these patients [9, 49]. In the next section, we will describe recently reported results using MSCs registered in ClinicalTrials.gov.

Effects of MSC therapy in IBD from published papers
Eight CD trials and one UC trial have been published in ClinicalTrials.gov. Six papers describing CD are on trials treating fistula, and two papers are trials for luminal CD. Molendijk et al. [25] reported improved healing of refractory perianal fistulas using allogeneic bone marrow-derived MSCs. They administered these allogeneic MSCs locally and concluded that injection of 3×10^7 MSCs appeared to promote the healing of perianal fistula. Panes et al. [31] reported a phase III randomized, double-blind, parallel-group, placebo-controlled study of complex perianal fistula using expanded allogeneic adipose-derived MSCs and confirmed the safety of the MSCs and the healing effects of MSCs on the fistula. Duijvestein et al. [32] reported a phase I study of refractory luminal CD using autologous bone marrow-derived MSCs and confirmed the safety and feasibility of MSC therapy. Forbes et al. [24] reported a phase II study using allogeneic bone marrow-derived MSCs for luminal CD refractory to biologic therapy. They administered 2×10^6 cells/kg weekly for 4 weeks and found that allogeneic MSCs reduced the CD activity index (CDAI) and CD endoscopic index of severity (CDEIS) scores in patients with luminal CD refractory to biologic therapy. Hu et al. [33] reported a phase I/II study for severe UC using umbilical cord-derived allogeneic MSCs by combination injection through the peripheral blood and superior mesenteric artery with a 7-day interval. They confirmed the safety of

Table 2 Clinical trials in inflammatory bowel diseases

No.	Start year	Cell source	Autologous/ allogeneic	Administration route	Number of cells infused	Diseases	Number of patients	Follow-up period	Phase	Study design	ClinicalTrials.gov identifier	Status	Result	References
1	2006	Bone marrow	Allogeneic	Peripheral vein	8×10^6 cells/kg, 2 times or 2×10^6 cells/kg, 2 times	Crohn's disease	10	4 weeks	Phase 2	Randomized, parallel assignment, open label	NCT00294112	Completed		
2	2007	Bone marrow	Allogeneic	Peripheral vein	Total of 6×10^8 cells/patient, 4 times or total of 12×10^8 cells/patient, 4 times	Crohn's disease	98	24 weeks	Phase 3	Randomized, parallel assignment, double blind	NCT00543374	Completed		
3	2010	Adipose tissue	Autologous	Unknown	Unknown	Fistulizing Crohn's disease	15	3 years	Phase 1–2	Non-randomized, single group assignment, open label	NCT01157650	Completed		
4	2015	Umbilical cord	Allogeneic	Peripheral vein	Unknown	Crohn's disease	32	1 year	Phase 1–2	Randomized, parallel assignment, open label	NCT02445547	Completed		
5	2012	Bone marrow	Allogeneic	Peripheral vein	2×10^8 cells/patient, more than 4 times	Crohn's disease	11	4 weeks	Phase 1–2	Non-randomized, single group assignment, open label	NCT01510431	Completed		
6	2010	Bone marrow	Allogeneic	Peripheral vein	2×10^6 cells/kg, 4 times	Crohn's disease	15	6 weeks	Phase 2	Non-randomized, single group assignment, open label	NCT01090817	Completed	Improvement in CDAI, AQoL score. Decrease in CRP. Endoscopic improvement	24
7	2012	Bone marrow	Autologous	Peripheral vein	2×10^6 cells/kg, 5×10^6 cells/kg, or 1×10^7 cells/kg	Crohn's disease	16	1 year	Phase 1	Non-randomized, single group assignment, open label	NCT01659762	Completed		
8	2010	Bone marrow	Allogeneic	Intralesional	1×10^7 cells/patient, 3×10^7 cells/patient, or 9×10^7 cells/patient	Fistulizing Crohn's disease	21	12 weeks	Phase 1–2	Randomized, parallel assignment, double blind	NCT01144962	Completed	Local treatment with MSCs showed promotion of fistula healing. Lower MSC dose seemed superior.	25
9	2009	Adipose tissue	Autologous	Intralesional	3×10^7 cells/patient (in the event of incomplete closure at 8 weeks, a second injection	Fistulizing Crohn's disease	43	8 weeks	Phase 1	Non-randomized, single group assignment, open label	NCT00992485	Completed	Local treatment with MSCs showed promotion of fistula healing.	26

Table 2 Clinical trials in inflammatory bowel diseases (*Continued*)

No.	Start year	Cell source	Autologous/ allogeneic	Administration route	Number of cells infused	Diseases	Number of patients	Follow-up period	Phase	Study design	ClinicalTrials.gov identifier	Status	Result	References
					was given that contained 1.5 times more cells than the f irst)									
10	2010	Adipose tissue	Allogeneic	Intralesional	2 × 107 cells/patient (in the event of incomplete closure at 12 weeks, an additional 4 × 107 cells were administered)	Fistulizing Crohn's disease	24	24 weeks	Phase 1–2	Non-randomized, single group assignment, open label	NCT01372969	Completed	Local treatment with MSCs showed promotion of fistula healing.	27
11	2009	Adipose tissue	Autologous	Intralesional	1 × 107 cells/patient, 2 × 107 cells/patient, or 4 × 107 cells/patient	Fistulizing Crohn's disease	10	4 weeks	Phase 1	Non-randomized, single group assignment, open label	NCT00992485	Completed	Local treatment with MSCs showed promotion of fistula healing. All patients with complete healing showed a sustained effect.	28
12	2009	Adipose tissue	Allogeneic	Intralesional	2 × 107 cells/patient (in the event of incomplete closure at 12 weeks, an additional 4 × 107 cells were administered)	Fistulizing Crohn's disease	10	12 weeks	Phase 1–2	Non-randomized, single group assignment, open label	NCT00999115	Completed	Local treatment with MSCs showed promotion of fistula healing; 60% of patients achieved complete healing.	29
13	2009	Adipose tissue	Autologous	Intralesional	1 × 107 cells/cm²	Fistulizing Crohn's disease	43	8 weeks	Phase 2	Non-randomized, single group assignment, open label	NCT01011244	Completed	In most cases, complete closure after initial treatment was well-sustained over a 24-month period.	30
14	2007	Bone marrow	Allogeneic	Peripheral vein	Total of 6 × 108 cells/patient, 4 times or total of 1.2 × 109 cells/patient, 4 times	Crohn's disease	330	4 weeks	Phase 3	Randomized, parallel assignment, double blind	NCT00482092	Active		
15	2012	Adipose tissue	Allogeneic	Intralesional	1.2 × 108 cells/patient	Fistulizing Crohn's disease	212	24 weeks	Phase 3	Randomized, parallel assignment, double blind	NCT01541579	Active	Local treatment with MSCs showed promotion of fistula healing.	31

Table 2 Clinical trials in inflammatory bowel diseases *(Continued)*

No.	Start year	Cell source	Autologous/allogeneic	Administration route	Number of cells infused	Diseases	Number of patients	Follow-up period	Phase	Study design	ClinicalTrials.gov identifier	Status	Result	References
16	2010	Bone marrow	Allogeneic	Peripheral vein	2×10^8 cells/patient, 3 times	Crohn's disease	120	180 days	Phase 3	Non-randomized, single group assignment, open label	NCT01233960	Active		
17	2015	Adipose tissue	Autologous	Intralesional	Unknown	Fistulizing Crohn's disease	10	62 weeks	Phase 2	Non-randomized, single group assignment, open label	NCT02403232	Recruiting		
18	2013	Bone marrow	Autologous	Intralesional	Unknown	Fistulizing Crohn's disease	10	16 weeks	Phase 1	Randomized, parallel assignment, single blind	NCT01874015	Recruiting		
19	2015	Adipose tissue	Allogeneic	Peripheral vein	5×10^7 cells/patient, 7.5×10^7 cells/patient, or 1×10^8 cells/patient	Crohn's disease	9	4 weeks	Phase 1	Non-randomized, single group assignment, open label	NCT02580617	Recruiting		
20	2013	Umbilical cord	Allogeneic	Peripheral vein	5×10^7 cells/patient or 1×10^8 cells/patient	Crohn's disease	24	12 weeks	Phase 1–2	Non-randomized, single group assignment, open label	NCT02000362	Recruiting		
21	2013	Adipose tissue	Autologous	Intralesional	2×10^7 cells/patient	Fistulizing Crohn's disease	20	2–24 months	Phase 1	Non-randomized, single group assignment, open label	NCT01915927	Recruiting		
22	Unknown	Bone marrow	Autologous	Peripheral vein	$1–2 \times 10^6$ cells/kg	Crohn's disease	10	6 weeks	Phase 1	Unknown	–	–	Three patients showed clinical response (decrease in CDAI). Three patients required surgery due to disease worsening.	32
23	2016	Bone marrow	Allogeneic	Intralesional	2×10^7 cells/patient	Fistulizing Crohn's disease	20	7, 10, 16 months	Phase 1	Non-randomized, single group assignment, open label	NCT02677350	Not yet recruiting		
24	2015	Umbilical cord	Allogeneic	Peripheral vein	1×10^6 cells/kg, 3 times	Ulcerative colitis	30	24 weeks	Phase 1–2	Randomized, parallel	NCT02442037	Recruiting		

Table 2 Clinical trials in inflammatory bowel diseases (*Continued*)

No.	Start year	Cell source	Autologous/ allogeneic	Administration route	Number of cells infused	Diseases	Number of patients	Follow-up period	Phase	Study design	ClinicalTrials.gov identifier	Status	Result	References
										assignment, single blind				
25	2015	Adipose tissue	Allogeneic	Through a colonoscope	6×10^7 cells/patient	Ulcerative colitis	8	12 weeks	Phase 1–2	Non-randomized, single group assignment, open label	NCT01914887	Unknown		
26	2015	Umbilical cord	Allogeneic	First: peripheral vein, second: superior mesenteric artery	First: $3.8 \pm 1.6 \times 10^7$ cells/ patient, second: 1.5×10^7 cells/patient	Ulcerative colitis	80	12 weeks	Phase 1–2	Non-randomized, single group assignment, open label	NCT01221428	Unknown	Decrease in the median Mayo score and histology score. Improvement in IBDQ scores.	33

CD Crohn's disease, *CDAI* Crohn's Disease Activity Index, *AQoL* The Assessment of Quality of Life, *CRP* C-reactive protein, *IBDQ* Inflammatory Bowel Disease Questionnaire

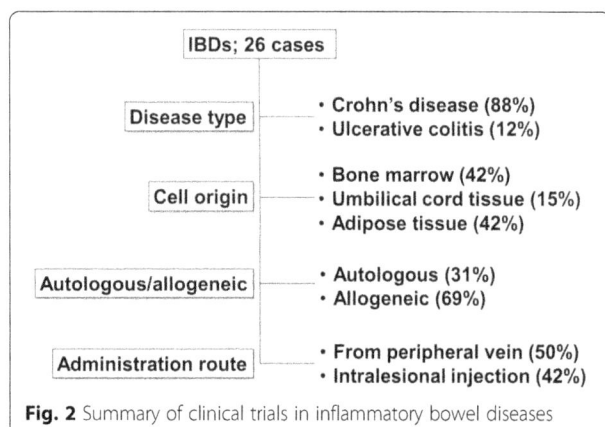

Fig. 2 Summary of clinical trials in inflammatory bowel diseases

matrix; GvHD: Graft-versus-host disease; IBD: Inflammatory bowel disease; IL: Interleukin; MSCs: Mesenchymal stem cells; NASH: Non-alcoholic steatohepatitis; TGF-β: Transforming growth factor; TNF: Tumor necrosis factor; UC: Ulcerative colitis

Acknowledgements
The authors thank Dr. Takayuki Watanabe and Dr. Suguru Takeuchi for their cooperation.

Funding
This work was supported by a Grant-in-Aid for Scientific Research (B) (26293175) from the Ministry of Education, Science, Technology, Sports, and Culture of Japan and by Highway Program for Realization of Regenerative Medicine from Japan Agency for Medical Research and Development, AMED.

Author's contributions
AT and ST wrote the paper. YK, SI, SS, YW, and YK prepared the data and made the tables. All authors read and approved the final manuscript.

Competing interests
The authors declare that they have no competing interests.

MSCs and alleviation of diffuse and deep ulcer formation and severe inflammatory mucosa by MSCs.

Safety of the MSC therapy
MSC therapy is associated with some concerns, such as adverse events related to infusion, tumor formation during the treatment of liver cirrhosis, and long-term observations of tumor formation. Regarding adverse events related to the infusion, Lalu et al. performed a meta-analysis of the safety of MSCs in clinical trials and showed that autologous and allogeneic MSC therapies were related to transient fever but not infusion toxicity, organ system complications, infection, death, and malignancies (Table 2) [5]. Regarding tumor formation during the treatment of liver cirrhosis, Peng et al. reported that no severe adverse events or no significant differences in tumor formation were detected compared with those in the control group during autologous bone marrow-derived MSC therapy for liver cirrhosis [58]. Regarding long-term observations of tumor formation derived from MSCs, Bahr et al. reported recent autopsy data from patients in a clinical trial of graft-versus-host disease (GvHD) who received MSC therapy between 2002 and 2007 and revealed no ectopic tissues, neoplasms, or donor-derived DNA [6].

Conclusions
Many clinical trials of autologous and allogeneic MSCs have aimed to elucidate the effects and mechanisms of MSCs. MSCs can expand easily and can be obtained from medical waste, suggesting their applications in regenerative medicine for the treatment of liver diseases and IBDs. Recently, limitations of MSCs have been reported. For example, therapeutic effects were not long term and were affected by inflammatory condition [59, 60]. Thus, the results of ongoing clinical studies will be expected to provide further insights.

Abbreviations
ABMi: Autologous bone marrow cell infusion; CD: Crohn's disease; CD CDEIS: Endoscopic index of severity; CDAI: CD activity index; ECM: Extracellular

References
1. Malfertheiner P, Megraud F, O'Morain CA, et al. Management of Helicobacter pylori infection-the Maastricht V/Florence Consensus Report. Gut. 2017;66:6–30.
2. Goldberg D, Ditah IC, Saeian K, et al. Changes in the prevalence of hepatitis C virus infection, non-alcoholic steatohepatitis, and alcoholic liver disease among patients with cirrhosis or liver failure on the waitlist for liver transplantation. Gastroenterology. 2017;152(5):1090-1099.e1.
3. Gecse KB, Lakatos PL. IBD in 2016: biologicals and biosimilars in IBD - the road to personalized treatment. Nat Rev Gastroenterol Hepatol. 2017;14(2): 74-76.
4. Trounson A, McDonald C. Stem cell therapies in clinical trials: progress and challenges. Cell Stem Cell. 2015;17:11–22.
5. Lalu MM, McIntyre L, Pugliese C, et al. Safety of cell therapy with mesenchymal stromal cells (SafeCell): a systematic review and meta-analysis of clinical trials. PLoS One. 2012;7:e47559.
6. Owen A, Newsome PN. Mesenchymal stromal cell therapy in liver disease: opportunities and lessons to be learnt? Am J Physiol Gastrointest Liver Physiol. 2015;309:G791–800.
7. Terai S, Tsuchiya A. Status of and candidates for cell therapy in liver cirrhosis: overcoming the "point of no return" in advanced liver cirrhosis. J Gastroenterol. 2017;52(2):129-40.
8. Wang Y, Chen X, Cao W, et al. Plasticity of mesenchymal stem cells in immunomodulation: pathological and therapeutic implications. Nat Immunol. 2014;15:1009–16.
9. Hawkey CJ, Hommes DW. Is stem cell therapy ready for prime time in treatment of inflammatory bowel diseases? Gastroenterology. 2017;152:389–97. e2.
10. Katsuda T, Kosaka N, Takeshita F, et al. The therapeutic potential of mesenchymal stem cell-derived extracellular vesicles. Proteomics. 2013;13:1637–53.
11. Li T, Yan Y, Wang B, et al. Exosomes derived from human umbilical cord mesenchymal stem cells alleviate liver fibrosis. Stem Cells Dev. 2013;22:845–54.
12. Jang YO, Kim YJ, Baik SK, et al. Histological improvement following administration of autologous bone marrow-derived mesenchymal stem cells for alcoholic cirrhosis: a pilot study. Liver Int. 2014;34:33–41.
13. Kantarcioglu M, Demirci H, Avcu F, et al. Efficacy of autologous mesenchymal stem cell transplantation in patients with liver cirrhosis. Turk J Gastroenterol. 2015;26:244–50.
14. Kharaziha P, Hellstrom PM, Noorinayer B, et al. Improvement of liver function in liver cirrhosis patients after autologous mesenchymal stem cell injection: a phase I-II clinical trial. Eur J Gastroenterol Hepatol. 2009;21:1199–205.

15. Shi M, Zhang Z, Xu R, et al. Human mesenchymal stem cell transfusion is safe and improves liver function in acute-on-chronic liver failure patients. Stem Cells Transl Med. 2012;1:725–31.

16. Suk KT, Yoon JH, Kim MY, et al. Transplantation with autologous bone marrow-derived mesenchymal stem cells for alcoholic cirrhosis: phase 2 trial. Hepatology. 2016;64(6):2185-97.

17. Zhang Z, Lin H, Shi M, et al. Human umbilical cord mesenchymal stem cells improve liver function and ascites in decompensated liver cirrhosis patients. J Gastroenterol Hepatol. 2012;27 Suppl 2:112–20.

18. Vosough M, Moossavi S, Mardpour S, et al. Repeated intraportal injection of mesenchymal stem cells in combination with pioglitazone in patients with compensated cirrhosis: a clinical report of two cases. Arch Iran Med. 2016;19:131–6.

19. Mohamadnejad M, Alimoghaddam K, Bagheri M, et al. Randomized placebo-controlled trial of mesenchymal stem cell transplantation in decompensated cirrhosis. Liver Int. 2013;33:1490–6.

20. Wang L, Li J, Liu H, et al. Pilot study of umbilical cord-derived mesenchymal stem cell transfusion in patients with primary biliary cirrhosis. J Gastroenterol Hepatol. 2013;28 Suppl 1:85–92.

21. Xu L, Gong Y, Wang B, et al. Randomized trial of autologous bone marrow mesenchymal stem cells transplantation for hepatitis B virus cirrhosis: regulation of Treg/Th17 cells. J Gastroenterol Hepatol. 2014;29:1620–8.

22. Tsuchiya A, Kubota T, Takizawa K, et al. Successful treatment in a case of massive hepatocellular carcinoma with paraneoplastic syndrome. Case Rep Gastroenterol. 2009;3:105–10.

23. Lencioni R, de Baere T, Soulen MC, et al. Lipiodol transarterial chemoembolization for hepatocellular carcinoma: a systematic review of efficacy and safety data. Hepatology. 2016;64:106–16.

24. Forbes GM, Sturm MJ, Leong RW, et al. A phase 2 study of allogeneic mesenchymal stromal cells for luminal Crohn's disease refractory to biologic therapy. Clin Gastroenterol Hepatol. 2014;12:64–71.

25. Molendijk I, Bonsing BA, Roelofs H, et al. Allogeneic bone marrow-derived mesenchymal stromal cells promote healing of refractory perianal fistulas in patients With Crohn's disease. Gastroenterology. 2015;149:918–27. e6.

26. Lee WY, Park KJ, Cho YB, et al. Autologous adipose tissue-derived stem cells treatment demonstrated favorable and sustainable therapeutic effect for Crohn's fistula. Stem Cells. 2013;31:2575–81.

27. de la Portilla F, Alba F, Garcia-Olmo D, et al. Expanded allogeneic adipose-derived stem cells (eASCs) for the treatment of complex perianal fistula in Crohn's disease: results from a multicenter phase I/IIa clinical trial. Int J Colorectal Dis. 2013;28:313–23.

28. Cho YB, Lee WY, Park KJ, et al. Autologous adipose tissue-derived stem cells for the treatment of Crohn's fistula: a phase I clinical study. Cell Transplant. 2013;22:279–85.

29. Garcia-Arranz M, Dolores Herreros M, Gonzalez-Gomez C, et al. Treatment of Crohn's-related rectovaginal fistula with allogeneic expanded-adipose derived stem cells: a phase I-IIa Clinical Trial. Stem Cells Transl Med. 2016; 5(11):1441-46.

30. Cho YB, Park KJ, Yoon SN, et al. Long-term results of adipose-derived stem cell therapy for the treatment of Crohn's fistula. Stem Cells Transl Med. 2015;4:532–7.

31. Panes J, Garcia-Olmo D, Van Assche G, et al. Expanded allogeneic adipose-derived mesenchymal stem cells (Cx601) for complex perianal fistulas in Crohn's disease: a phase 3 randomised, double-blind controlled trial. Lancet. 2016;388:1281–90.

32. Duijvestein M, Vos AC, Roelofs H, et al. Autologous bone marrow-derived mesenchymal stromal cell treatment for refractory luminal Crohn's disease: results of a phase I study. Gut. 2010;59:1662–9.

33. Hu J, Zhao G, Zhang L, et al. Safety and therapeutic effect of mesenchymal stem cell infusion on moderate to severe ulcerative colitis. Exp Ther Med. 2016;12:2983–9.

34. Tsuchiya A, Kamimura H, Takamura M, et al. Clinicopathological analysis of CD133 and NCAM human hepatic stem/progenitor cells in damaged livers and hepatocellular carcinomas. Hepatol Res. 2009;39:1080–90.

35. Fayek SA, Quintini C, Chavin KD, et al. The current state of liver transplantation in the United States: perspective from American Society of

Transplant Surgeons (ASTS) Scientific Studies Committee and Endorsed by ASTS Council. Am J Transplant. 2016;16:3093–104.

36. Terai S, Ishikawa T, Omori K, et al. Improved liver function in patients with liver cirrhosis after autologous bone marrow cell infusion therapy. Stem Cells. 2006;24:2292–8.

37. Kim JK, Park YN, Kim JS, et al. Autologous bone marrow infusion activates the progenitor cell compartment in patients with advanced liver cirrhosis. Cell Transplant. 2010;19:1237–46.

38. Saito T, Okumoto K, Haga H, et al. Potential therapeutic application of intravenous autologous bone marrow infusion in patients with alcoholic liver cirrhosis. Stem Cells Dev. 2011;20:1503–10.

39. Thomas JA, Pope C, Wojtacha D, et al. Macrophage therapy for murine liver fibrosis recruits host effector cells improving fibrosis, regeneration, and function. Hepatology. 2011;53:2003–15.

40. Forbes SJ, Rosenthal N. Preparing the ground for tissue regeneration: from mechanism to therapy. Nat Med. 2014;20:857–69.

41. Moore JK, Mackinnon AC, Wojtacha D, et al. Phenotypic and functional characterization of macrophages with therapeutic potential generated from human cirrhotic monocytes in a cohort study. Cytotherapy. 2015;17:1604–16.

42. Jin S, Li H, Han M, et al. Mesenchymal stem cells with enhanced Bcl-2 expression promote liver recovery in a rat model of hepatic cirrhosis. Cell Physiol Biochem. 2016;40:1117–28.

43. Quintanilha LF, Takami T, Hirose Y, et al. Canine mesenchymal stem cells show antioxidant properties against thioacetamide-induced liver injury in vitro and in vivo. Hepatol Res. 2014;44:E206–17.

44. Volarevic V, Nurkovic J, Arsenijevic N, et al. Concise review: therapeutic potential of mesenchymal stem cells for the treatment of acute liver failure and cirrhosis. Stem Cells. 2014;32:2818–23.

45. Dai LJ, Li HY, Guan LX, et al. The therapeutic potential of bone marrow-derived mesenchymal stem cells on hepatic cirrhosis. Stem Cell Res. 2009;2:16–25.

46. Xia X, Tao Q, Ma Q, et al. Growth hormone-releasing hormone and its analogues: significance for MSCs-mediated angiogenesis. Stem Cells Int. 2016;2016:8737589.

47. Nagaishi K, Arimura Y, Fujimiya M. Stem cell therapy for inflammatory bowel disease. J Gastroenterol. 2015;50:280–6.

48. Coskun M, Vermeire S, Nielsen OH. Novel targeted therapies for inflammatory bowel disease. Trends Pharmacol Sci. 2017;38(2):127-42.

49. Gregoire C, Lechanteur C, Briquet A, et al. Review article: mesenchymal stromal cell therapy for inflammatory bowel diseases. Aliment Pharmacol Ther. 2017;45:205–21.

50. Ito H, Takazoe M, Fukuda Y, et al. A pilot randomized trial of a human anti-interleukin-6 receptor monoclonal antibody in active Crohn's disease. Gastroenterology. 2004;126:989–96. discussion 947.

51. Sandborn WJ, Feagan BG, Fedorak RN, et al. A randomized trial of Ustekinumab, a human interleukin-12/23 monoclonal antibody, in patients with moderate-to-severe Crohn's disease. Gastroenterology. 2008;135:1130–41.

52. Sandborn WJ, Gasink C, Gao LL, et al. Ustekinumab induction and maintenance therapy in refractory Crohn's disease. N Engl J Med. 2012;367:1519–28.

53. Sandborn W, Gasink C, Blank M, et al. O-001 A multicenter, double-blind, placebo-controlled phase3 study of Ustekinumab, a human IL-12/23P40 mAB, in moderate-service Crohn's disease refractory to anti-TFNalpha: UNITI-1. Inflamm Bowel Dis. 2016;22 Suppl 1:S1.

54. Van Rompaey L, Galien R, van der Aar EM, et al. Preclinical characterization of GLPG0634, a selective inhibitor of JAK1, for the treatment of inflammatory diseases. J Immunol. 2013;191:3568–77.

55. Monteleone G, Neurath MF, Ardizzone S, et al. Mongersen, an oral SMAD7 antisense oligonucleotide, and Crohn's disease. N Engl J Med. 2015;372:1104–13.

56. Feagan BG, Rutgeerts P, Sands BE, et al. Vedolizumab as induction and maintenance therapy for ulcerative colitis. N Engl J Med. 2013;369:699–710.

57. Sandborn WJ, Feagan BG, Rutgeerts P, et al. Vedolizumab as induction and maintenance therapy for Crohn's disease. N Engl J Med. 2013;369:711–21.

58. Peng L, Xie DY, Lin BL, et al. Autologous bone marrow mesenchymal stem cell transplantation in liver failure patients caused by hepatitis B: short-term and long-term outcomes. Hepatology. 2011;54:820–8.

59. Dave M, Jaiswal P, Cominelli F. Mesenchymal stem/stromal cell therapy for inflammatory bowel disease: an updated review with maintenance of remission. Curr Opin Gastroenterol. 2017;33:59–68.

60. Kim N, Cho SG. New strategies for overcoming limitations of mesenchymal stem cell-based immune modulation. Int J Stem Cells. 2015;8:54–68.

3

Age-related sarcopenia and its pathophysiological bases

Sumito Ogawa*, Mitsutaka Yakabe and Masahiro Akishita

Abstract

Age-related loss of the skeletal muscle and its function is known as sarcopenia. Definition and diagnostic criteria for sarcopenia have been outlined as consensus statements from several study groups, including usual gait speed, grip strength, and skeletal muscle mass. Whereas underlying mechanisms and pathophysiology of sarcopenia remains to be clarified, recent studies have suggested that chronic inflammatory status as well as lifestyle-related factors in older individuals might contribute to the process and progress of sarcopenia.

Keywords: Aging, Sarcopenia, Inflammation, Frailty, Hormone

Background

Sarcopenia has been recently recognized as an age-related symptom which is characterized by low muscle mass, low muscle force, and low physical performance. In this review, we describe the recent progresses regarding the development of definition and diagnosis of sarcopenia, as well as its pathophysiology mainly related to age-related inflammatory processes.

Definition and diagnosis of sarcopenia

Recent clinical and studies have suggested the presence of age-related decline in skeletal muscle mass and muscle strength from approximately the fifth decade of life, called sarcopenia [1]. This debilitating process is known to associate with frailty, disability [2], and an increased risk of fall-related fractures [3], leading to higher mortality and morbidity in the older population [4, 5]. The number of older population with sarcopenia is expected to increase all over the world, and it is becoming one of the important public concerns and interests [6].

Sarcopenia (Greek "sarx" or flesh + "penia" or loss) was initially proposed by Rosenberg, representing age-related loss of muscle mass in its original concept [7]. Subsequently, the European Working Group on Sarcopenia in Older People (EWGSOP) defined sarcopenia in 2010 as a syndrome characterized by progressive and generalized loss of skeletal muscle mass and strength with the risk of adverse outcome such as physical disability, poor quality of life, and death [8]. The impact of sarcopenia on Asian regions including Japan is also estimated to be high, and the Asian Working Group for Sarcopenia (AWGS) agreed to describe sarcopenia as low muscle mass plus low muscle strength and/or low physical performance, further recommending its assessment in healthcare settings and in clinical practice [9] (Fig. 1). Thus, current approaches to the definition of sarcopenia are based on measurements of muscle mass, muscle strength, and functional capacity, and each indicator might be considered low when it is less than two standard deviations (2SD) away from the mean value of young male and female reference groups. The EWGSOP has developed a suggested algorithm based on gait speed measurement as the easiest and most reliable way to begin sarcopenia case finding or screening in practice.

As for the screening among community-dwelling people aged 65 years and older, the EWGSOP has developed a suggested algorithm based on (i) lower skeletal muscle mass plus (ii) lower gait speed and/or low grip strength for the diagnosis of sarcopenia [8]. AWGS also recommends using 60 or 65 years as the age for sarcopenia diagnosis according to the conditions of each country in Asia [9]. Operational sarcopenia definition by the International Working Group for Sarcopenia (IWGS) was targeted to individuals with functional decline, self-reported mobility-related difficulties, history of recurrent falls, recent unintentional body weight loss, post-hospitalization, and chronic conditions including metabolic diseases and

* Correspondence: suogawa-tky@umin.ac.jp
Department of Geriatric Medicine, Graduate School of Medicine, The University of Tokyo, Bunkyo-ku, Tokyo 113-8655, Japan

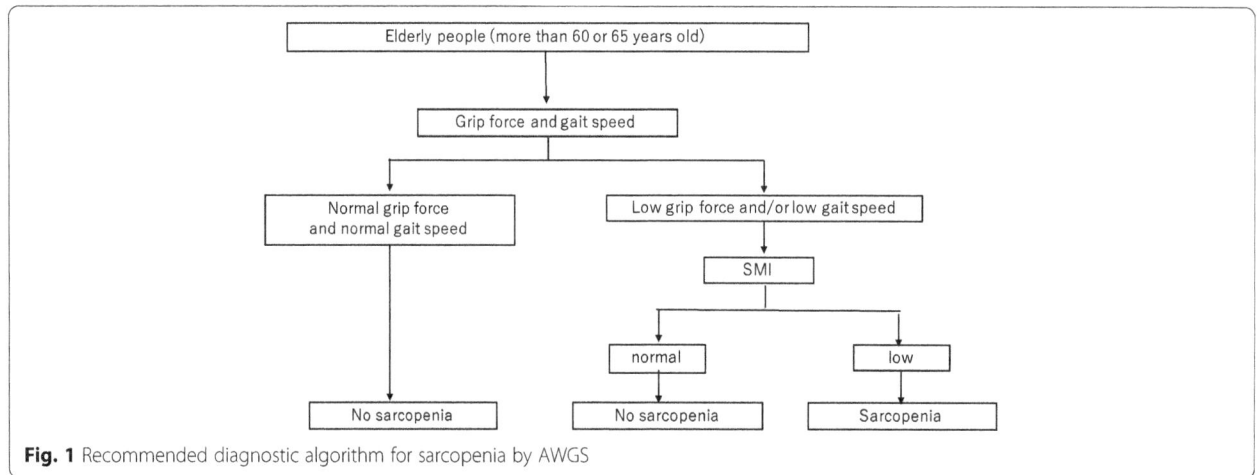

Fig. 1 Recommended diagnostic algorithm for sarcopenia by AWGS

cancer [10]. The Foundation for the National Institutes of Health (FNIH) used the data from nine sources of community-dwelling older population and proposed the cutoffs based on its analysis [11]. A comparison of definition/characteristics and cutoff values for sarcopenia in EWGSOP, AWGS, and IWGS criteria is shown in Table 1 [8–10].

It is proposed by the EWGSOP that sarcopenia is considered primary (or age-related) when no other cause is evident except aging itself, whereas it is considered secondary when one or more other causes are evident [8]. In practice, the etiology of sarcopenia is multi-factorial, and it might not be always possible to identify and characterize its single cause. EWGSOP also suggests a conceptual staging as severe sarcopenia, sarcopenia, and pre-sarcopenia. Severe sarcopenia is the stage when all three criteria (low muscle mass, low muscle strength, and low physical performance) are observed. The sarcopenia stage is defined as low muscle mass, accompanying either low muscle strength or low physical performance. The pre-sarcopenia stage is characterized by low muscle mass without low muscle strength or low physical performance. Evaluation of these sarcopenia stages might be helpful in light of setting appropriate recovery goals as well as selecting treatments and intervention.

In terms of epidemiology and prevalence of sarcopenia, Baumgartner et al., adopting a skeletal muscle mass index (SMI) cutoff of –2SDs below the mean of a young reference group, reported that the prevalence ranged from 13 to 24 % in persons aged 65 to 70 years old and was more than 50 % for those who were older than 80 years old [12]. Another study suggested that sarcopenia was prevalent in 10 % of men and 8 % of women older than 60 years old and that decrease in skeletal muscle was independently associated with functional impairment and disability, especially in older women [13]. The prevalence of sarcopenia in Japanese elderly men and women, based on the Asian diagnosis criteria, was 9.6 and 7.7 %, respectively [14]. The number of aged population over 60 years of age around the world was estimated to be 600 million in 2000 and is expected to rise to 2 billion by 2050. It is also estimated that sarcopenia will affect over 200 million people by the period, in contrast to the present estimation of about 50 million people [15].

Pathophysiology of sarcopenia related to chronic inflammatory state

It is suggested that significant changes in muscle mass and its quality are observed during aging process and that there is a decrease in muscle mass at an annual rate

Table 1 Comparison of definition/characteristics and cutoff values for sarcopenia by EWGSOP, AWGS, and IWGS criteria

	EWGSOP [8]	AWGS [9]	IWGS [10]
Definition/ characteristics	A syndrome characterized by progressive and generalized loss of skeletal muscle mass and strength with a risk of adverse outcomes	Age-related decline of skeletal muscle plus low muscle strength and/or physical performance	Age-associated loss of skeletal muscle mass and function
SMI	7.26 kg/m^2 for men and 5.5 kg/m^2 for women (by DXA). 8.87 kg/m^2 for men and 6.42 kg/m^2 for women (by BIA)	7.0 kg/m^2 for men and 5.4 kg/m^2 for women (by DXA). 7.0 kg/m^2 for men and 5.7 kg/m^2 for women (by BIA)	7.23 kg/m^2 for men and 5.67 kg/m^2 for women (by DXA)
Walking speed	<0.8 m/s	<0.8 m/s	<1.0 m/s
Grip force	<30 kg for men <20 kg for women	<26 kg for men <18 kg for women	Not specified

of 1 to 2 % after about 50 years old [16]. The decline in muscle strength is supposed to be more significant, reaching to 1.5 % per year in their sixth decade and to 3 % per year afterwards [17]. In average, age-related decreases in knee extensor strength are 20–40 % compared to that of young adult mean [18], and more significant losses have been observed for those in their ninth decades [19, 20]. Recent findings suggest that multiple factors including immobility, malnutrition, low protein intake, changes in hormones and metabolism, systemic inflammation, and neuromuscular aging are supposed to influence age-related sarcopenia [21, 22].

From a histological standpoint, the skeletal muscle consists of type I and type II fibers. Type II fast fibers possess a higher glycolytic potential, lower oxidative capacity, and faster response, whereas type I slow fibers are known as fatigue-resistant due to their characteristics such as greater density and content of mitochondria, capillaries, and myoglobin. And sarcopenia is characterized by the predominant atrophy of type II fibers together with smaller and fewer mitochondria [23, 24]. Although molecular and cellular mechanisms underlying sarcopenia still remain to be clarified, age-related low-grade inflammation has been suggested to be involved as described below.

In general, aging is associated with a significant rise in serum levels of inflammatory markers and its related factors [25]. Franceschi et al. described the state of chronic low-grade inflammatory state as "inflammaging" based on the related concept of immunosenescence [26, 27]. Inflammation can be beneficial as an acute, transient immune response to harmful conditions including tissue injury or pathogen invasion. During aging process, these acute inflammatory responses may be impaired, leading to increased susceptibility to infection. Inflammaging is characterized as low-grade, chronic, systemic inflammation in aging in the absence of infection, which results in responses that lead to tissue degeneration. Inflammaging is also suggested to be related to various age-related diseases represented by atherosclerosis, dementia, type 2 diabetes and osteoporosis and is a highly significant risk factor for both morbidity and mortality in the elderly people [26, 28] (Fig. 2). Inflammaging is supposed to be a consequence of a reduced immune response or lifetime exposure to antigenic stimuli [29, 30], leading to the production of reactive oxygen species and tissue damage with the release of cytokines mediated by innate and acquired immune system [31]. In practice, inflammaging is accompanied by age-related decline in the number of T and B cells together with an increase of natural killer cells [32], and tumor necrosis factor-α (TNF-α), interleukin-6 (IL-6), interleukin-1 (IL-1), and C-reactive protein (CRP) are mainly involved in this process [27, 33, 34]. These cytokines are suggested to lead to a predisposition to age-related sarcopenia subsequently through the activation of the ubiquitine-protease system [35, 36]. And this altered activation of cellular signaling pathway is considered to promote the inflammatory state regardless of tissue damage or antigenic exposure, further contributing to one of the pathogenetic bases underlying sarcopenia [37–39]. It is also suggested that cytokines may antagonize the anabolic effect mediated by insulin growth

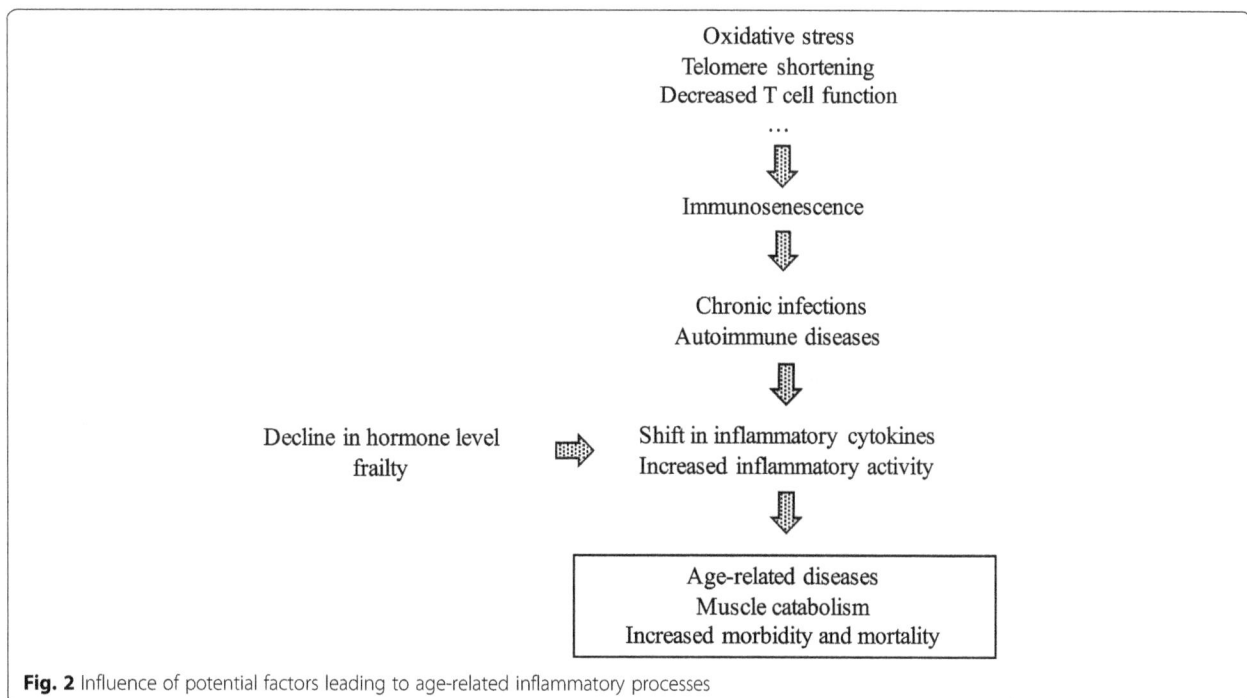

Oxidative stress
Telomere shortening
Decreased T cell function
...

⇩

Immunosenescence

⇩

Chronic infections
Autoimmune diseases

⇩

Decline in hormone level   ⇨   Shift in inflammatory cytokines
frailty   Increased inflammatory activity

⇩

Age-related diseases
Muscle catabolism
Increased morbidity and mortality

Fig. 2 Influence of potential factors leading to age-related inflammatory processes

factor-1 (IGF-1), involving in growth hormone resistance which limit IGF-I availability [40, 41]. Inflammaging also contributes to anabolic resistance, which is one of the main determinants of sarcopenia, implying that synthesis of skeletal muscle protein in response to physiologic stimuli is below the standard of muscle maintenance in the older population [42].

Possible cytokines involved in age-related sarcopenia

Recent findings suggest that some inflammatory cytokines including TNF-α and IL-6 are involved in pathophysiology of age-related sarcopenia.

TNF-α

Plasma TNF-α concentration preceded a significant decline in muscle strength at 4 years in study subjects aged 85 years [43] and in decline in muscle mass and its strength at 5 years in subjects aged 70 to 79 years at baseline [44]. Exposure of myoblasts to TNF-α causes inhibition of myogenic differentiation through increased proteolysis of MyoD by the ubiquitin-proteasome pathway in vitro [45]. TNF-α is also reported to suppress the Akt/mTOR pathway [41], promoting muscle catabolism, oxidative stress, and nitric acid production [46, 47]. Decrease of TNF-α level mediated by muscle training, for example, is suggested to cause muscle regeneration [48–50].

IL-6

Some clinical studies including a longitudinal study in the Netherlands reported that high levels of IL-6 and CRP are associated with lower physical performance, muscle strength, and muscle mass [38, 50–58]. In a 6-year cohort of community-dwelling elderly subjects, elevated serum concentrations of IL-6 and IL-1RA have been associated with decline in physical performance [58]. Hospitalized geriatric patients with inflammation represented significantly weaker muscle function, shoulder extension strength, and a worse fatigue resistance [59]. In a cross-sectional study carried out in community-dwelling women aged more than 65 years, serum IL-6 levels were associated with higher prevalence of frailty [60]. In older women, higher serum IL-6 levels were adversely associated with recovery of lower extremity function after hip fracture [61].

In an experimental study, IL-6 transgenic mice revealed decreased skeletal muscle mass, and anti-mouse IL-6R antibody inhibited the atrophy [62]. Another study suggested that IL-6 and serum amyloid A produced in the liver synergistically increased MuRF1 and atrogin-1 expression by inducing SOCS-3 expression and impairing its downstream insulin/IGF-1 signaling in the skeletal muscle [63]. On the other hand, IL-6 is a pleiotropic cytokine, acting both as an inflammatory cytokine and as a myokine. For example, acute exercise causes skeletal muscle contraction and promotes IL-6 release into the systemic circulation, which could be beneficial for muscle growth [64]. Further studies are needed to elucidate how IL-6 are involved in the pathogenesis of age-related sarcopenia.

Other cytokines and inflammatory substrates

A recent study suggested that IL-1 blocked differentiation of human myoblasts into myotubes by activating TGF-β-activated kinase (TAK)-1 in vitro [65] and might be involved in sarcopenia. In addition, several clinical studies imply the relationship between serum CRP concentration and sarcopenia. For example, high-sensitivity CRP levels were significantly associated with sarcopenic obesity in a Korean study [66]. Proinflammatory cytokines, such as IL-6 and TNF-α, induce the production of CRP in the liver, and it has not been clarified whether high CRP level directly affects sarcopenia.

Conclusions

Age-related sarcopenia is a phenomenon that results in significant mortality as well as morbidity in the older population and is becoming one of the major public health problems among aging society. Emerging evidences suggest underlying mechanisms and pathophysiology of age-related sarcopenia, in which the relationship between chronic inflammatory state, muscle strength, and muscle mass seems to possess a pathogenetic basis including the control of balance between protein synthesis and its catabolism. In terms of inflammaging, age-related changes in cytokines and hormones levels are also suggested to be important risk factors for muscular impairment. A better understanding and knowledge of risk factors for sarcopenia is important to promote multidimensional approach based on its pathophysiology, defining molecular targets for intervention toward successful prevention and treatment in the near future.

Abbreviations

CRP, C-reactive protein; IGF-1, insulin growth factor-1; IL-1, interleukin-1; IL-6, interleukin-6; SMI, skeletal muscle mass index; TNF, tumor necrosis factor

Acknowledgements

The authors thank H. Sasagawa for the cooperation and help for the manuscript preparation.

Funding

This study was supported by the Research Funding for Longevity Sciences from the National Center for Geriatrics and Gerontology (NCGG), Japan. This work was also supported by JSPS KAKENHI Grant Number 15K08898. The funders had no role in the study design, data collection and analysis, decision to publish, or preparation of the manuscript.

Authors' contributions

SO and MY drafted the review manuscript, and SO and MA conceived of the study and participated in its coordination. MA contributed to the writing of the manuscript. All authors read and approved the final manuscript.

Authors' information

None.

Competing interests

The authors declare that they have no competing interests.

References

1. Janssen I, Heymsfield SB, Wang ZM, Ross R. Skeletal muscle mass and distribution in 468 men and women aged 18–88 years. J Appl Physiol. 2000;89:81–8.
2. Morley JE. Sarcopenia in the elderly. Fam Pract. 2012;29 Suppl 1:i44–8.
3. Visser M, Schaap LA. Consequences of sarcopenia. Clin Geriatric Med. 2011;27:387–99.
4. Kemmler W, von Stengel S, Engelke K, Haberle L, Mayhew JL, Kalender WA. Exercise, body composition, and functional ability: a randomized controlled trial. Am J Prev Med. 2010;38:279–87.
5. Bunout D, de la Maza MP, Barrera G, Leiva L, Hirsch S. Association between sarcopenia and mortality in healthy older people. Australas J Ageing. 2011;30:89–92.
6. Kim TN, Choi KM. Sarcopenia: definition, epidemiology, and pathophysiology. J Bone Metab. 2013;20:1–10.
7. Rosenberg IH. Sarcopenia: origins and clinical relevance. J Nutr. 1997;127:990S–1.
8. Cruz-Jentoft AJ, Baeyens JP, Bauer JM, Boirie Y, Cederholm T, Landi F, Martin FC, Michel JP, Rolland Y, Schneider SM, Topinkova E, Vandewoude M, Zamboni M. Sarcopenia: European consensus on definition and diagnosis: Report of the European Working Group on Sarcopenia in Older People. Age Ageing. 2010;39:412–23.
9. Chen LK, Liu LK, Woo J, Assantachai P, Auyeung TW, Bahyah KS, Chou MY, Chen LY, Hsu PS, Krairit O, Lee JS, Lee WJ, Lee Y, Liang CK, Limpawattana P, Lin CS, Peng LN, Satake S, Suzuki T, Won CW, Wu CH, Wu SN, Zhang T, Zeng P, Akishita M, Arai H. Sarcopenia in Asia: consensus report of the Asian Working Group for Sarcopenia. J Am Med Dir Assoc. 2014;15:95–101.
10. Fielding RA, Vellas B, Evans WJ, Bhasin S, Morley JE, Newman AB, Abellan van Kan G, Andrieu S, Bauer J, Breuille D, Cederholm T, Chandler J, De Meynard C, Donini L, Harris T, Kannt A, Keime Guibert F, Onder G, Papanicolaou D, Rolland Y, Rooks D, Sieber C, Souhami E, Verlaan S, Zamboni M. Sarcopenia: an undiagnosed condition in older adults. Current consensus definition: prevalence, etiology, and consequences. International Working Group on Sarcopenia. J Am Med Dir Assoc. 2011;12:249–56.
11. Studenski SA, Peters KW, Alley DE, Cawthon PM, McLean RR, Harris TB, Ferrucci L, Guralnik JM, Fragala MS, Kenny AM, Kiel DP, Kritchevsky SB, Shardell MD, Dam TT, Vassileva MT. The FNIH sarcopenia project: rationale, study description, conference recommendations, and final estimates. J Gerontol A Biol Sci Med Sci. 2014;69:547–58.
12. Baumgartner RN, Koehler KM, Gallagher D, Romero L, Heymsfield SB, Ross RR, Garry PJ, Lindeman RD. Epidemiology of sarcopenia among the elderly in New Mexico. Am J Epidemiol. 1998;147:755–63.
13. Janssen I, Heymsfield SB, Ross R. Low relative skeletal muscle mass (sarcopenia) in older persons is associated with functional impairment and physical disability. J Am Geriatr Soc. 2002;50:889–96.
14. Yuki A, Ando F, Shimokata H. Transdisciplinary approach for sarcopenia. Sarcopenia: definition and the criteria for Asian elderly people. Clin Calcium. 2014;24:1441–8.
15. Santilli V, Bernetti A, Mangone M, Paoloni M. Clinical definition of sarcopenia. Clin Cases Miner Bone Metab. 2014;11:177–80.
16. Sehl ME, Yates FE. Kinetics of human aging: I. Rates of senescence between ages 30 and 70 years in healthy people. J Gerontol A Biol Sci Med Sci. 2001;56:198–208.
17. von Haehling S, Morley JE, Anker SD. An overview of sarcopenia: facts and numbers on prevalence and clinical impact. J Cachexia Sarcopenia Muscle. 2010;1:129–33.
18. Doherty TJ. Invited review: aging and sarcopenia. J Appl Physiol. 2003;95:1717–27.
19. Murray MP, Duthie Jr EH, Gambert SR, Sepic SB, Mollinger LA. Age-related differences in knee muscle strength in normal women. J Gerontol. 1985;40:275–80.
20. Murray MP, Gardner GM, Mollinger LA, Sepic SB. Strength of isometric and isokinetic contractions: knee muscles of men aged 20 to 86. Phys Ther. 1980;60:412–9.
21. Malafarina V, Uriz-Otano F, Iniesta R, Gil-Guerrero L. Sarcopenia in the elderly: diagnosis, physiopathology and treatment. Maturitas. 2012;71:109–14.
22. Yakabe M, Ogawa S, Akishita M. Clinical manifestations and pathophysiology of sarcopenia. RNA and Transcription. 2015;1:10–7.
23. Lang T, Streeper T, Cawthon P, Baldwin K, Taaffe DR, Harris TB. Sarcopenia: etiology, clinical consequences, intervention and assessment. Osteoporosis Int. 2010;21:543–59.
24. Evans WJ, Campbell WW. Sarcopenia and age-related changes in body composition and functional capacity. J Nutr. 1993;123:465–8.
25. Ferrucci L, Corsi A, Lauretani F, Bandinelli S, Bartali B, Taub DD, Guralnik JM, Longo DL. The origins of age-related proinflammatory state. Blood. 2005; 105:2294–9.
26. Franceschi C, Bonafe M, Valensin S, Olivieri F, De Luca M, Ottaviani E, De Benedictis G. Inflamm-aging. An evolutionary perspective on immunosenescence. Ann N Y Acad Sci. 2000;908:244–54.
27. Franceschi C, Campisi J. Chronic inflammation (inflammaging) and its potential contribution to age-associated diseases. J Gerontol A Biol Sci Med Sci. 2014;69:S4–9.
28. Castelo-Branco C, Soveral I. The immune system and aging: a review. Gynecol Endocrinol. 2014;30:16–22.
29. De Martinis M, Franceschi C, Monti D, Ginaldi L. Inflammageing and lifelong antigenic load as major determinants of ageing rate and longevity. FEBS Lett. 2005;579:2035–9.
30. Frasca D, Blomberg BB. Inflammaging decreases adaptive and innate immune responses in mice and humans. Biogerontology. 2016;17:7–19.
31. Cannizzo ES, Clement CC, Sahu R, Follo C, Santambrogio L. Oxidative stress, inflamm-aging and immunosenescence. J Proteomics. 2011;74:2313–23.
32. Sansoni P, Vescovini R, Fagnoni F, Biasini C, Zanni F, Zanlari L, Telera A, Lucchini G, Passeri G, Monti D, Franceschi C, Passeri M. The immune system in extreme longevity. Exp Gerontol. 2008;43:61–5.
33. Maggio M, Guralnik JM, Longo DL, Ferrucci L. Interleukin-6 in aging and chronic disease: a magnificent pathway. J Gerontol A Biol Sci Med Sci. 2006;6:575–84.
34. Thomas DR. Sarcopenia. Clin Geriatr Med. 2010;26:331–46.
35. Mitch WE, Goldberg AL. Mechanisms of muscle wasting. The role of the ubiquitin-proteasome pathway. N Eng J Med. 1996;335:1897–905.
36. Ferrucci L, Harris TB, Guralnik JM, Tracy RP, Corti MC, Cohen HJ, Penninx B, Pahor M, Wallace R, Havlik RJ. Serum IL-6 level and the development of disability in older persons. J Am Geriatr Soc. 1999;47:639–46.
37. Toth MJ, Ades PA, Tischler MD, Tracy RP, LeWinter MM. Immune activation is associated with reduced skeletal muscle mass and physical function in chronic heart failure. Int J Cardiol. 2006;109:179–87.
38. Visser M, Pahor M, Taaffe DR, Goodpaster BH, Simonsick EM, Newman AB, Nevitt M, Harris TB. Relationship of interleukin-6 and tumor necrosis factor-alpha with muscle mass and muscle strength in elderly men and women: the Health ABC study. J Gerontol. 2002;57A:M326–32.
39. Curtis E, Litwic A, Cooper C, Dennison E. Determinants of muscle and bone aging. J Cell Physiol. 2015;230:2618–25.
40. Lang CH, Frost RA, Vary TC. Regulation of muscle protein synthesis during sepsis and inflammation. Am J Physiol Endocrinol Metab. 2007;293:e453–9.
41. Frost RA, Lang CH. Protein kinase B/Akt: a nexus of growth factor and cytokine signalling determining muscle mass. J Appl Physiol. 2007;103:378–87.
42. Haran PH, Rivas DA, Fielding RA. Role and potential mechanisms of anabolic resistance in sarcopenia. J Cachexia Sarcopenia Muscle. 2012;3:157–62.
43. Taekema DG, Westendorp RG, Frölich M, Gussekloo J. High innate production capacity of tumor necrosis factor-alpha and decline of handgrip strength in old age. Mech Ageing Dev. 2007;128:517–21.
44. Schaap LA, Pluijm SM, Deeg DJ, Harris TB, Kritchevsky SB, Newman AB, Colbert LH, Pahor M, Rubin SM, Tylavsky FA, Visser M, Health ABC Study. Higher inflammatory marker levels in older persons: associations with 5-year change in muscle mass and muscle strength. J Gerontol A Biol Sci Med Sci. 2009;64:1183–9.
45. Langen RC, Van Der Velden JL, Schols AM, Kelders MC, Wouters EF, Janssen-Heininger YM. Tumor necrosis factor-alpha inhibits myogenic differentiation through MyoD protein destabilization. FASEB J. 2004;18:227–37.

46. Reid MB, Li YP. Tumor necrosis factor-alpha and muscle wasting: a cellular perspective. Respir Res. 2001;2:269–72.

47. Reid MB, Lännergren J, Westerblad H. Respiratory and limb muscle weakness induced by tumor necrosis factor-alpha: involvement of muscle myofilaments. Am J Respir Crit Care Med. 2002;166:479–84.

48. Mourkioti F, Kratsios P, Luedde T, Song YH, Delafontaine P, Adami R, Parente V, Bottinelli R, Pasparakis M, Rosenthal N. Targeted ablation of IKK2 improves skeletal muscle strength, maintains mass, and promotes regeneration. J Clin Invest. 2006;116:2945–54.

49. Starkie R, Ostrowski SR, Jauffred S, Febbraio M, Pedersen BK. Exercise and IL-6 infusion inhibit endotoxin-induced TNF-alpha production in humans. FASEB J. 2003;17:884–6.

50. Greiwe JS, Cheng B, Rubin DC, Yarasheski KE, Semenkovich CF. Resistance exercise decreases skeletal muscle tumor necrosis factor alpha in frail elderly humans. FASEB J. 2001;15:475–82.

51. Schaap L, Pluijim SMF, Deeg DJH, Visser M. Inflammatory markers and loss of muscle mass (sarcopenia) and strength. Am J Med. 2006;119:526. e9–526.e17.

52. Cesari M, Penninx BW, Pahor M, Lauretani F, Corsi AM, Rhys Williams G, Guralnik JM, Ferrucci L. Inflammatory markers and physical performance in older persons: the InCHIANTI study. J Gerontol A Biol Sci Med Sci. 2004;59:242–8.

53. Schaap LA, Pluijm SM, Deeg DJ, Harris TB, Kritchevsky SB, Newman AB, Colbert LH, Pahor M, Rubin SM, Tylavsky FA, Visser M, Health ABC Study. Higher inflammatory markers levels in older persons: association with 5-year change in muscle mass and strength. J Gerontol A Bio Sci Med Sci. 2009;64A:1183–9.

54. Pedersen M, Bruunsgaard H, Weis N, Hendel HW, Andreassen BU, Eldrup E, Dela F, Pedersen BK. Circulating levels of TNF-alpha and IL-6-relation to truncal fat mass and muscle mass in healthy elderly individuals and in patients with type-2 diabetes. Mech Ageing Dev. 2003;124:495–502.

55. Barbieri M, Ferrucci L, Ragno E, Corsi A, Bandinelli S, Bonafè M, Olivieri F, Giovagnetti S, Franceschi C, Guralnik JM, Paolisso G. Chronic inflammation and the effect of IGF-I on muscle strength and power in older persons. Am J Physiol Endocrinol Metab. 2003;284:E481–7.

56. Norman K, Stobaus N, Kulka K, Schulzke J. Effect of inflammation on handgrip strength in the non-critically ill is independent from age, gender and body composition. European J Clin Nutrition. 2014;68:155–8.

57. Ferrucci L, Penninx BW, Volpato S, Harris TB, Bandeen-Roche K, Balfour J, Leveille SG, Fried LP, Md JM. Change in muscle strength explains accelerated decline of physical function in older women with high interleukin-6 serum levels. J Am Geriatr Soc. 2002;50:1947–54.

58. Stenholm S, Maggio M, Lauretani F, Bandinelli S, Ceda GP, Di Iorio A, Giallauria F, Guralnik JM, Ferrucci L. Anabolic and catabolic biomarkers as predictors of muscle strength decline: the InCHIANTI study. Rejuvenation Res. 2010;13:3–11.

59. Bautmans I, Njemini R, Lambert M, Demanet C, Mets T. Circulating acute phase mediators and skeletal muscle performance in hospitalized geriatric patients. J Gerontol. 2005;60A:361–7.

60. Leng SX, Xue QL, Tian J, Walston JD, Fried LP. Inflammation and frailty in older women. J Am Geriatr Soc. 2007;55:864–71.

61. Miller RR, Cappola AR, Shardell MD, Hawkes WG, Yu-Yahiro JA, Hebel JR, Magaziner J. Persistent changes in interleukin-6 and lower extremity function following hip fracture. J Gerontol A Biol Sci Med Sci. 2006;61:1053–8.

62. Tsujinaka T, Fujita J, Ebisui C, Yano M, Kominami E, Suzuki K, Tanaka K, Katsume A, Ohsugi Y, Shiozaki H, Monden M. Interleukin 6 receptor antibody inhibits muscle atrophy and modulates proteolytic systems in interleukin 6 transgenic mice. J Clin Invest. 1996;97:244–9.

63. Zhang L, Du J, Hu Z, Han G, Delafontaine P, Garcia G, Mitch WE. IL-6 and serum amyloid A synergy mediates angiotensin II-induced muscle wasting. J Am Soc Nephrol. 2009;20:604–12.

64. Fischer CP. Interleukin-6 in acute exercise and training: what is the biological relevance? Exerc Immunol Rev. 2006;12:6–33.

65. Trendelenburg AU, Meyer A, Jacobi C, Feige JN, Glass DJ. TAK-1/p38/nNFkB signaling inhibits myoblast differentiation by increasing levels of Activin A. Skelet Muscle. 2012;2:3.

66. Kim TN, Park MS, Lim KI, Choi HY, Yang SJ, Yoo HJ, Kang HJ, Song W, Choi H, Baik SH, Choi DS, Choi KM. Relationships between sarcopenic obesity and insulin resistance, inflammation, and vitamin D status: the Korean Sarcopenic Obesity Study. Clin Endocrinol (Oxf). 2013;78:525–32.

4

Organ dysfunction as a new standard for defining sepsis

Seitaro Fujishima

Abstract

Despite advances in intensive care and the widespread use of standardized care included in the Surviving Sepsis Campaign Guidelines, sepsis remains a leading cause of death, and the prevalence of sepsis increases concurrent with the aging process. The diagnosis of sepsis was originally based on the evidence of persistent bacteremia (septicemia) but was modified in 1992 to incorporate systemic inflammatory response syndrome (SIRS). Since then, SIRS has become the gold standard for the diagnosis of sepsis. In 2016, the Society of Critical Care Medicine and the European Society of Intensive Care Medicine published a new clinical definition of sepsis that is called Sepsis-3. In contrast to previous definitions, Sepsis-3 is based on organ dysfunctions and uses a sequential organ failure (SOFA) score as an index. Thus, patients diagnosed with respect to Sepsis-3 will inevitably represent a different population than those previously diagnosed. We assume that this drastic change in clinical definition will affect not only clinical practice but also the viewpoint and focus of basic research. This review intends to summarize the pathophysiology of sepsis and organ dysfunction and discusses potential directions for future research.

Keywords: Sepsis-3, Sequential organ failure assessment score, Acute respiratory distress syndrome, Acute kidney injury, Disseminated intravascular coagulation

Background

There have been significant advances in intensive care and the widespread use of standardized care in the Surviving Sepsis Campaign Guidelines. However, sepsis remains a leading cause of death and its prevalence increases concurrent with the aging process. In 2016, the Society of Critical Care Medicine and the European Society of Intensive Care Medicine published a new clinical definition of sepsis that is termed as Sepsis-3. This new definition was subsequently endorsed by a range of affiliated societies, including the Japanese Society of Intensive Care Medicine and the Japanese Association for Acute Medicine (JAAM). The consensus of opinion indicates that Sepsis-3 will lead to significant changes in the concept of sepsis [1].

The diagnosis of sepsis was historically based on the evidence of persistent bacteremia (septicemia). However, in accordance with the progress in our understanding of the pathophysiology of sepsis, the definition was greatly modified in 1992 to exclude bacteremia and to incorporate

parameters related to systemic inflammation (Sepsis-1), namely the systemic inflammatory response syndrome (SIRS) [2] (Fig. 1). At the same time, two severe subgroups of sepsis were defined as severe sepsis and septic shock. Although the definition of sepsis was reevaluated and modified to include a wider range of parameters in 2003 (Sepsis-2), SIRS continues to be widely used for diagnosing sepsis in various clinical settings [3]. However, the inadequate specificity and sensitivity of the SIRS criteria were recognized as a significant limitation and, thus, were omitted from Sepsis-3 [4]. In contrast to previous definitions, Sepsis-3 is based on organ dysfunctions and sepsis is diagnosed when there is an increase of more than 2 points in the total sequential organ failure assessment (SOFA) score; thus, patients diagnosed with respect to Sepsis-3 will inevitably represent a different population from those diagnosed with respect to Sepsis-1 or Sepsis-2. Therefore, we assumed that this drastic change in clinical definition will not only affect clinical practice, especially the evaluation of patients with suspected infection, but also lead to changes in the focus of basic research. In this review, we intend to provide an overview of the pathophysiology of sepsis-induced organ dysfunction

Correspondence: fujishim@keio.jp
Center for General Medicine Education, Keio University School of Medicine, Tokyo, Japan

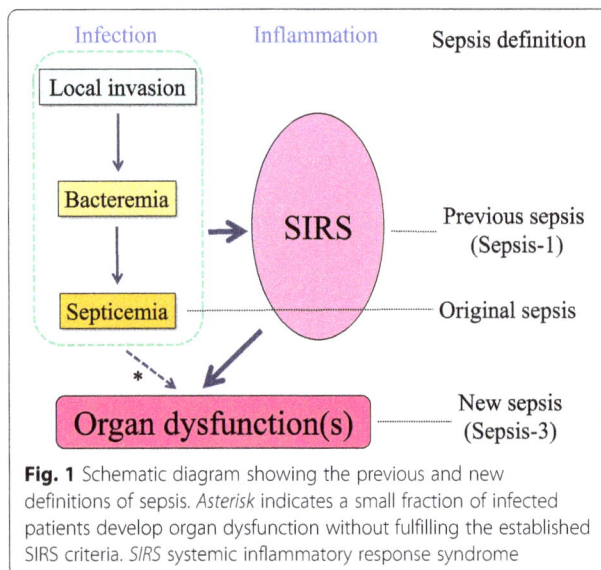

Fig. 1 Schematic diagram showing the previous and new definitions of sepsis. *Asterisk* indicates a small fraction of infected patients develop organ dysfunction without fulfilling the established SIRS criteria. *SIRS* systemic inflammatory response syndrome

and elucidate the present unresolved questions for indicating the direction of the research in this field.

Pathophysiology of sepsis

Infection is initiated by the local invasion of microorganisms into a living body. When the host's immune system is healthy and the quantity and virulence of the microorganisms involved are below a tolerance limit, infection is restricted and spontaneously cures. However, if microorganisms overcome a host's immunological self-defense system, they can locally extend or spread to distant tissues and organs via the blood stream. In response to the systemic invasion of microorganisms, the body triggers the production of inflammatory mediators and characteristic signs and symptoms, such as fever or hypothermia, tachycardia, tachypnea, and an increase or decrease in peripheral white blood cell counts develop, all of which are essential components of the SIRS criteria. It was at this stage that the diagnosis of sepsis was made with respect to the former definition, which often predisposed the failure of vital organs, currently referred to as multiple organ dysfunction syndrome (MODS). Thus, sepsis diagnosed with respect to the Sepsis-3 definition, namely infection-induced single or multiple organ dysfunctions, is more advanced and manifests with more severe conditions than that diagnosed by previous definitions.

Pathogen-derived substances with immunological properties, notably lipopolysaccharide (LPS), are referred to as pathogen-associated molecular patterns (PAMPs) and have been shown to induce sepsis-like conditions in vivo and activate immune cells in vitro [5]. Injured tissues also release a set of molecules with similar properties, including high-mobility group box 1 (HMGB-1)

and histones, collectively referred to as damage (danger)-associated molecular patterns (DAMPs) [6]. Under septic conditions, PAMPs and DAMPs bind to specific cell-surface or cytosolic proteins that are called pattern recognition receptors, which are located on monocytes/macrophages, vascular endothelial cells, and other stromal cells, and that trigger the activation of intracellular signaling cascades [7]. Activated cells release various humoral mediators, particularly cytokines, which accelerate local and systemic inflammations.

Cytokines are classified as pro-inflammatory and anti-inflammatory, and the time course of their expressions vary. Pro-inflammatory cytokines play major roles in inducing systemic inflammation and in the development of MODS. Among the pro-inflammatory cytokines, tumor necrosis factor alpha (TNFα) and interleukin 1beta (IL-1β) are detected in the blood of patients with sepsis and are known to induce septic shock-like conditions when administered to animals in vivo, thus suggesting their key pathogenic roles in sepsis [8, 9]. In contrast, anti-inflammatory cytokines contribute to the regulation and resolution of acute inflammation, while also contributing to the immunosuppression and hypersensitivity to infection that is observed during the later phase of sepsis.

Sepsis-associated lung dysfunction: ARDS

Lung dysfunction, referred to as acute respiratory distress syndrome (ARDS) or acute lung injury (ALI), is frequently associated with sepsis. In our recent epidemiological analysis, ALI was complicated in 40.2 % of patients with severe sepsis or septic shock and had a significantly poor outcome [10]. A previous report revealed that sepsis-related ARDS was associated with a poorer outcome than non-sepsis-related ARDS [11]. An increase in microvascular permeability, resulting from the dysregulation of cell-to-cell interaction or tissue destruction, is the fundamental pathophysiology underlying ARDS. Extensive investigation has revealed the prominent contribution of neutrophils, which are major terminal effector cells in innate immunity, to tissue injury in ARDS [12, 13]. Neutrophils have also been shown to play a role in the dysfunction of other organs. Neutrophils release granular enzymes, reactive oxygen metabolites, bioactive lipids, and cytokines [14] and can induce the formation of neutrophil extracellular traps [15], most of which can either directly or indirectly injure tissues, leading to an increase in microvascular permeability and resulting in pulmonary edema. Interleukin 8 (also called CXCL8), a potent neutrophil chemotactic chemokine, also plays important roles in the pathophysiology of ARDS, along with TNFα and IL-1β, which represent major players in septic shock [16]. In addition, some DAMPs have been recently recognized as mediators or cytokines with respect to their regulated production and immune-regulating functions. A pathogenic role of

HMGB-1, a molecule originally identified as a nuclear binding protein, was initially reported in sepsis [17] and later in sepsis-associated ARDS [18]. Mitochondrial DAMPs can stimulate PMNs and induce a sepsis-like state and ALI [19]. Along with neutrophil-mediated tissue injury, apoptosis and autophagy are also involved in sepsis-induced tissue injuries that are associated with ARDS [20, 21]. However, these findings did not lead to the development of appropriate clinical therapeutics.

Dysfunction of other organs in sepsis

As mentioned in the above section, sepsis is often complicated with organ dysfunctions other than ARDS. Table 1 summarizes the pathophysiology, clinical features, SOFA score indices, and available treatments for individual organ dysfunctions. The type of failure or dysfunction observed in each organ is relatively stereotyped and most are associated with poor outcomes [22, 23]. Sepsis-derived systemic shock and resultant tissue hypoperfusion commonly contribute to the development of most organ dysfunctions, which is supported by the findings that early goal-directed therapy (EGDT), a protocol-based therapeutic intervention involving fluid resuscitation, improved the MODS score and outcome [24]. Furthermore, plasma pro-inflammatory cytokine levels were significantly reduced in an EGDT group compared with a control group, suggesting that global tissue ischemia is an important contributor to the early inflammatory response in sepsis [25]. However, as the mere recovery of systemic circulation by fluid resuscitation and inotropic agents is insufficient to completely restore organ function, other injurious mechanisms are most certainly involved.

During infection, the liver plays critical roles in modulating host defense and regulating inflammation, mostly via the clearance of pathogens and PAMPs, and in producing acute phase proteins such as C-reactive protein and serum amyloid A [26, 27]. A previous study revealed through a multivariate analysis that liver cirrhosis was associated with a 2.4-fold increase in sepsis mortality [28]. Our analysis and that of other groups showed that 10–17 % of patients with severe sepsis were complicated with hepatic dysfunction [22, 23], which was shown to be associated with a poorer clinical outcome in a large observational study [23]. Sepsis-associated hepatic dysfunction is clinically recognized by jaundice or cholestasis and is caused by various underlying mechanisms such as the impairment of energy-dependent bile and bile acid transport by hypoxia, hypoperfusion, and overproduced cytokines. No treatments are currently established for such conditions.

The kidneys are the main controllers of water and electrolyte metabolism under normal physiological conditions, and the roles of the kidneys become even more important during sepsis for maintaining vital organ circulation and cellular electrolyte balance and for protecting the lungs from life-threatening pulmonary edema.

Table 1 Organ dysfunction in sepsis

Target organ	Pathophysiology	Clinical features	SOFA score indices (other beneficial indices)	Available treatments
Lung (ARDS)	Vascular hyper-permeability, neutrophil accumulation	Impaired oxygenation	PaO_2/FIO_2 <400 (bilateral infiltration on CXR)	Mechanical ventilation with low tidal volume and PEEP
Liver	Disturbed intracellular and extracellular bile salt transport	Jaundice, cholestasis	Serum bilirubin ≥1.2 mg/dl	Not established
Kidney (AKI)	Tubular epithelial cell injury, dysfunction or adaptive response of tubular epithelial cells	Reduced GFR, reduced urine volume	Serum creatinine ≥1.2 Urine output <500 ml/day	Hemodialysis
Cardiovascular system	Myocardial depression, impaired intracellular calcium homeostasis, disrupted high energy phosphate production.	Ventricular dilatation, reduced ejection fraction, reduced contractility	Mean arterial pressure <70 mmHg	Inotropic agents, beta-blocker
Gastrointestinal tract	Epithelial hyper-permeability, altered microbiome	Mucosal bleeding, paralytic ileus	Not included	Proton pump inhibitor, early enteral nutrition, probiotics, SDD
Central nervous system (SAE)	Direct cellular damage, mitochondrial and endothelial dysfunction, neurotransmission disturbances, calcium dyshomeostasis	Altered mental status	GCS <15	Light sedation, early rehabilitation
Blood coagulation system (DIC)	Intravascular coagulation, microvascular damage, systemic thrombin generation, endothelial injury	Bleeding diathesis, microthrombi and tissue ischemia	Platelets <150 × 10^3/μl (prolonged prothrombin time, increased FDP)	Antithrombin, recombinant thrombomodulin, concentrated platelet preparation

SOFA sequential organ failure assessment, *ARDS* acute respiratory distress syndrome, *CXR* chest X-ray, *PEEP* positive end-expiratory pressure, *AKI* acute kidney injury, *GFR* glomerular filtration ratio, *SDD* selective digestive decontamination, *SAE* sepsis-associated encephalopathy, *GCS* Glasgow coma scale, *DIC* disseminated intravascular coagulation, *FDP* fibrin degradation product

Acute dysfunction of the kidneys is referred to as acute kidney injury (AKI) and was observed in 37–40 % of cases with severe sepsis [22, 23]. AKI is clinically detected as an increase in serum creatinine level or a decrease in urine volume and is associated with poorer clinical outcomes [22, 23, 28]. Renal tubular epithelial cell injury, which is because of disturbed microcirculation and hypoxia, as well as the dysfunction or adaptive response of tubular epithelial cells, including the downregulation of metabolism and cell cycle arrest, is induced by excessive inflammation and represents a key feature of AKI [29]. Although hemodialysis has been established as a clinical therapy for AKI, no strategy to prevent AKI or to help patients recover from AKI has been developed.

Blood coagulation and fibrinolysis systems contribute in the maintenance of systemic and organ circulation against various injuries to the living body. Under the condition of sepsis, these systems tend to dysfunction, a condition referred to as disseminated intravascular coagulation (DIC), which induces organ dysfunction and is closely associated with higher mortality. The major pathophysiology of DIC includes the generalized activation of intravascular coagulation, microvascular damage, systemic thrombin generation, and endothelial injury [30]. There are several diagnostic criteria for DIC, such as those by JAAM, the International Society on Thrombosis and Haemostasis (ISTH), and the Japanese Ministry of Health, Labour and Welfare, with increasingly reduced levels of sensitivity in this order. The SOFA score used in the new Sepsis-3 definition includes platelet counts as a parameter for DIC. In retrospective and prospective studies, DIC was observed in 18–41 % by ISTH and 47 % by the JAAM criteria [31–33]. Although several potentially effective drugs have been clinically used, such as antithrombin III and recombinant thrombomodulin, their efficacy in terms of survival and protection against MODS remains to be clarified.

In addition to the abovementioned organs, it is known that the functions of the cardiovascular system, gastrointestinal tract, and central nervous system are often impaired during sepsis and are crucial for patient outcome. Although some therapies, including beta-blockers for the cardiovascular system, early enteral nutrition for the gastrointestinal tract, and light sedation/ early rehabilitation for the central nervous system, are potentially effective, their efficacy is limited. Consequently, new organ-specific strategies based on a novel insight into the pathophysiology should be explored.

Future directions for sepsis research

Previous research in both animal models and patients revealed that sepsis is inevitably associated with excessive inflammation. However, anti-inflammatory strategies have failed to demonstrate clear benefit in terms of patient outcome. To begin a new era of clinical practice for sepsis, it is important to consider the appropriate direction for future research. The introduction of new clinical definition may provide us a favorable opportunity to change our emphasis with regard to research. Although the true causal relationship between individual organ dysfunction and clinical outcome remains unresolved, the extent of organ dysfunction and the total number of dysfunctional organs involved are both associated with increased mortality, rendering attempts to protect or recover from organ dysfunction as a promising approach for sepsis research. Although the lungs will continue to be the main target, all vital organs could be possible targets for research.

In most preclinical experiments on sepsis, LPS or pathogens were administered to small animals, and the post-mortem characteristics of single organs and survival rates were evaluated. However, the function of multiple organs would usually be impaired in such models and additively or synergistically affect the outcome, in a manner similar to real human patients. Consequently, in future research, simultaneous evaluation of dysfunction in more than two vital organs will be mandatory in such sepsis models. Additionally, the pathophysiology and therapeutic strategy for individual organ dysfunction should be more extensively examined using existing or newly developed single organ dysfunction models, including the septic ARDS model via the intratracheal administration of pathogens or PAMPs.

For such investigations, it is important to develop novel techniques to sequentially monitor organ function hopefully in vivo. To begin with, such research would be significantly enhanced by developing small-scale apparatus to monitor the partial pressure or saturation of arterial blood oxygen and arterial blood pressure. In addition, it would be important to incorporate measurements of serum bilirubin, creatinine, and urea nitrogen for in vivo monitoring across a range of animal models. In contrast, novel strategies need to be developed to enable the evaluation of species-specific parameters such as blood cells and proteins involved in the coagulation and fibrinolysis systems.

Conclusions

Excessive inflammation has been established as the key feature of sepsis pathophysiology and therefore a prime target of intervention. This understanding led us to the concept of SIRS, and sepsis was defined as the infection-induced SIRS. However, anti-inflammatory strategies have failed to improve clinical outcome in patients with sepsis. As described earlier, the definition of sepsis was drastically modified in 2016 so as not to include SIRS criteria and inflammatory variables. Instead, sepsis is now clinically defined by an increase in SOFA score. Thus, patients diagnosed with Sepsis-3 will inevitably represent a population different from that previously diagnosed. We assume that this drastic change in clinical definition will affect not only clinical practice but also the direction of future basic research.

Simultaneously evaluating multiple organ dysfunction in animal models of sepsis or investigating single organ dysfunction models will enable the development of potential organ-protective treatments in a robust experimental manner. Such organ-targeted investigations will certainly strengthen our understanding of the pathophysiology of sepsis and may help to develop truly effective therapies to protect or recover from organ dysfunction in sepsis.

Abbreviations
AKI: Acute kidney injury; ALI: Acute lung injury; ARDS: Acute respiratory distress syndrome; DAMPs: Damage (danger)-associated molecular patterns; DIC: Disseminated intravascular coagulation; HMGB-1: High-mobility group box 1; IL-1β: Interleukin 1beta; ISTH: International Society on Thrombosis and Haemostasis; JAAM: Japanese Association for Acute Medicine; LPS: Lipopolysaccharide; MODS: Multiple organ dysfunction syndrome; PAMPs: Pathogen-associated molecular patterns; SIRS: Systemic inflammatory response syndrome; SOFA: Sequential organ failure assessment; TNFα: Tumor necrosis factor alpha

Acknowledgements
None.

Funding
This study was funded by JSPS KAKENHI Grant Number 26462767.

Authors' contributions
SF drafted and completed the manuscript.

Competing interests
S. Fujishima is a task force member of the "Surviving Sepsis Guidelines 2016," the "Japanese Guidelines for the Management of Sepsis," and "Clinical Practice Guidelines" for Acute Respiratory Distress Syndrome.

References
1. Singer M, Deutschman CS, Seymour CW, Shankar-Hari M, Annane D, Bauer M, et al. The third international consensus definitions for sepsis and septic shock (sepsis-3). JAMA. 2016;315(8):801–10.
2. Bone RC, Balk RA, Cerra FB, Dellinger RP, Fein AM, Knaus WA, et al. Definitions for sepsis and organ failure and guidelines for the use of innovative therapies in sepsis. The ACCP/SCCM Consensus Conference Committee. American College of Chest Physicians/Society of Critical Care Medicine. Chest. 1992;101(6):1644–55.
3. Levy MM, Fink MP, Marshall JC, Abraham E, Angus D, Cook D, et al. 2001 SCCM/ESICM/ACCP/ATS/SIS international sepsis definitions conference. Crit Care Med. 2003;31(4):1250–6.
4. Kaukonen KM, Bailey M, Pilcher D, Cooper DJ, Bellomo R. Systemic inflammatory response syndrome criteria in defining severe sepsis. N Engl J Med. 2015;372(17):1629–38.
5. Hayashi T, Nakamura T, Takaoka A. Pattern recognition receptors. Jpn J Clin Immunol. 2011;34:329–45.
6. Schaefer L. Complexity of danger: the diverse nature of damage-associated molecular patterns. J Biol Chem. 2014;289(51):35237–45.
7. Opitz B, van Laak V, Eitel J, Suttorp N. Innate immune recognition in infectious and noninfectious diseases of the lung. Am J Respir Crit Care Med. 2010;181(12):1294–309.
8. Okusawa S, Gelfand JA, Ikejima T, Connolly RJ, Dinarello CA. Interleukin 1 induces a shock-like state in rabbits. Synergism with tumor necrosis factor and the effect of cyclooxygenase inhibition. J Clin Invest. 1988;81(4):1162–72.
9. Tracey KJ, Beutler B, Lowry SF, Merryweather J, Wolpe S, Milsark IW, et al. Shock and tissue injury induced by recombinant human cachectin. Science. 1986;234(4775):470–4.
10. Fujishima S, Gando S, Daizoh S, Kushimoto S, Ogura H, Mayumi T, et al. Infection site is predictive of outcome in acute lung injury associated with severe sepsis and septic shock. Respirology. 2016;21(5):898–904.
11. Sheu CC, Gong MN, Zhai R, Chen F, Bajwa EK, Clardy PF, et al. Clinical characteristics and outcomes of sepsis-related vs non-sepsis-related ARDS. Chest. 2010;138(3):559–67.
12. Mallick AA, Ishizaka A, Stephens KE, Hatherill JR, Tazelaar HD, Raffin TA. Multiple organ damage caused by tumor necrosis factor and prevented by prior neutrophil depletion. Chest. 1989;95(5):1114–20.
13. Stephens KE, Ishizaka A, Wu ZH, Larrick JW, Raffin TA. Granulocyte depletion prevents tumor necrosis factor-mediated acute lung injury in guinea pigs. Am Rev Respir Dis. 1988;138(5):1300–7.
14. Fujishima S, Aikawa N. Neutrophil-mediated tissue injury and its modulation. Intensive Care Med. 1995;21(3):277–85.
15. Luo L, Zhang S, Wang Y, Rahman M, Syk I, Zhang E, et al. Proinflammatory role of neutrophil extracellular traps in abdominal sepsis. Am J Physiol Lung Cell Mol Physiol. 2014;307(7):L586–96.
16. Fujishima S. A prominent role of IL-8 in various inflammatory lung diseases and multiple organ dysfunction syndrome. Jpn J Inflamm. 1998;18(6):433–7.
17. Wang H, Bloom O, Zhang M, Vishnubhakat JM, Ombrellino M, Che J, et al. HMG-1 as a late mediator of endotoxin lethality in mice. Science. 1999; 285(5425):248–51.
18. Ueno H, Matsuda T, Hashimoto S, Amaya F, Kitamura Y, Tanaka M, et al. Contributions of high mobility group box protein in experimental and clinical acute lung injury. Am J Respir Crit Care Med. 2004;170(12):1310–6.
19. Zhang Q, Raoof M, Chen Y, Sumi Y, Sursal T, Junger W, et al. Circulating mitochondrial DAMPs cause inflammatory responses to injury. Nature. 2010; 464(7285):104–7.
20. Figueiredo N, Chora A, Raquel H, Pejanovic N, Pereira P, Hartleben B, et al. Anthracyclines induce DNA damage response-mediated protection against severe sepsis. Immunity. 2013;39(5):874–84.
21. Hashimoto S, Kobayashi A, Kooguchi K, Kitamura Y, Onodera H, Nakajima H. Upregulation of two death pathways of perforin/granzyme and FasL/Fas in septic acute respiratory distress syndrome. Am J Respir Crit Care Med. 2000;161(1):237–43.
22. Fujishima S, Gando S, Saitoh D, Mayumi T, Kushimoto S, Shiraishi S, et al. A multicenter, prospective evaluation of quality of care and mortality in Japan based on the Surviving Sepsis Campaign guidelines. J Infect Chemother. 2014;20(2):115–20.
23. Levy MM, Dellinger RP, Townsend SR, Linde-Zwirble WT, Marshall JC, Bion J, et al. The Surviving Sepsis Campaign: results of an international guideline-based performance improvement program targeting severe sepsis. Crit Care Med. 2010;38(2):367–74.
24. Rivers E, Nguyen B, Havstad S, Ressler J, Muzzin A, Knoblich B, et al. Early goal-directed therapy in the treatment of severe sepsis and septic shock. N Engl J Med. 2001;345(19):1368–77.
25. Rivers EP, Kruse JA, Jacobsen G, Shah K, Loomba M, Otero R, et al. The influence of early hemodynamic optimization on biomarker patterns of severe sepsis and septic shock. Crit Care Med. 2007;35(9):2016–24.
26. Nesseler N, Launey Y, Aninat C, Morel F, Malledant Y, Seguin P. Clinical review: the liver in sepsis. Crit Care. 2012;16(5):235.
27. Gabay C, Kushner I. Acute-phase proteins and other systemic responses to inflammation. N Engl J Med. 1999;340(6):448–54.

28. Vincent JL, Sakr Y, Sprung CL, Ranieri VM, Reinhart K, Gerlach H, et al. Sepsis in European intensive care units: results of the SOAP study. Crit Care Med. 2006;34(2):344–53.

29. Zarbock A, Gomez H, Kellum JA. Sepsis-induced acute kidney injury revisited: pathophysiology, prevention and future therapies. Curr Opin Crit Care. 2014;20(6):588–95.

30. Gando S, Levi M, Toh CH. Disseminated intravascular coagulation. Nat Rev Dis Primers. 2016;2:16037.

31. Gando S, Saitoh D, Ogura H, Fujishima S, Mayumi T, Araki T, et al. A multicenter, prospective validation study of the Japanese Association for Acute Medicine disseminated intravascular coagulation scoring system in patients with severe sepsis. Crit Care. 2013;17(3):R111.

32. Kienast J, Juers M, Wiedermann CJ, Hoffmann JN, Ostermann H, Strauss R, et al. Treatment effects of high-dose antithrombin without concomitant heparin in patients with severe sepsis with or without disseminated intravascular coagulation. J Thromb Haemost. 2006;4(1):90–7.

33. Dhainaut JF, Yan SB, Joyce DE, Pettila V, Basson B, Brandt JT, et al. Treatment effects of drotrecogin alfa (activated) in patients with severe sepsis with or without overt disseminated intravascular coagulation. J Thromb Haemost. 2004;2(11):1924–33.

5

Regulation of blood vascular permeability in the skin

Sachiko Ono[1], Gyohei Egawa[1] and Kenji Kabashima[1,2,3*]

Abstract

Regulation of blood vessel permeability is essential for the homeostasis of peripheral tissues. This regulation controls the trafficking of plasma contents, including water, vitamins, ions, hormones, cytokines, amyloids, lipoproteins, carrier proteins, and immunoglobulins. The properties of blood vessels vary among tissues based on their structural differences: continuous, fenestrated, or sinusoidal. These three types of blood vessels have different charge and size barrier properties. The anionic luminal glycocalyx layer on endothelial cells establishes the "charge barrier" that repels the attachment of negatively charged blood cells and plasma molecules. In contrast, the "size barrier" of blood vessels largely relies on the interendothelial junctions (IEJs) between endothelial cells, which define the paracellular permeability. As in most peripheral tissues, blood capillaries in the skin are composed of continuous and/or fenestrated blood vessels that have relatively tighter IEJs compared to those in the internal organs. Small vesicles in the capillary endothelium were discovered in the 1950s, and studies have since confirmed that blood endothelial cells transport the plasma contents by endocytosis and subsequent transcytosis and exocytosis—this process is called transcellular permeability. The permeability of blood vessels is highly variable as a result of intrinsic and extrinsic factors. It is significantly elevated upon tissue inflammations as a result of disabled IEJs and increased paracellular permeability due to inflammatory mediators. An increase in transcellular permeability during inflammation has also been postulated. Here, we provide an overview of the general properties of vascular permeability based on our recent observations of murine skin inflammation models, and we discuss its physiological significance in peripheral homeostasis.

Keywords: Blood vessel, Permeability, Interendothelial junctions, Paracellular, Transcellular, Skin, Inflammation, Immunoglobulin

Background

Blood vessels, especially those of microvessels, serve as a semipermeable barrier between blood contents and the tissue, which is much more permeable than epithelial systems. Acting as canals, blood vessels carry cargos with different sizes and charges in plasma to their proper destinations (Fig. 1).

The permeability of blood vessels is composed of two distinct barriers: the charge barrier and the size barrier (reviewed in [1–3]). The luminal glycocalyx layer on endothelial cells establishes the anionic "charge barrier," with some additional roles have been postulated to date

(discussed later). The paracellular permeability between the interendothelial junctions (IEJs) is often responsible for the size barrier, which is regulated by the presence or absence of adherens junctions (AJs) and/or tight junctions (TJs) in the IEJs (reviewed in [1, 4]). However, IEJs are not solely responsible for defining the size barrier; there appears to be a large contribution of basement membranes, fenestrae, and diaphragms [3] (Table 1). In addition to endothelial organization, non-cellular and cellular components surrounding blood endothelial cells, the extracellular matrix ([5], reviewed in [6]), pericytes [7], and immune cells such as perivascular mast cells, may participate in regulating the permeability of blood vessels [8] (Fig. 2). Furthermore, in terms of vesicular transportation through endothelial cells, the transcellular pathway may dominate the paracellular pathway in determining the vascular permeability of selective molecules, especially in vessels with tight IEJs.

* Correspondence: kaba@kuhp.kyoto-u.ac.jp
[1]Department of Dermatology, Kyoto University Graduate School of Medicine, 54 Shogoin-Kawahara, Sakyo, Kyoto 606-8507, Japan
[2]Singapore Immunology Network (SIgN) and Institute of Medical Biology, Agency for Science, Technology and Research (A*STAR), Biopolis, Singapore
Full list of author information is available at the end of the article

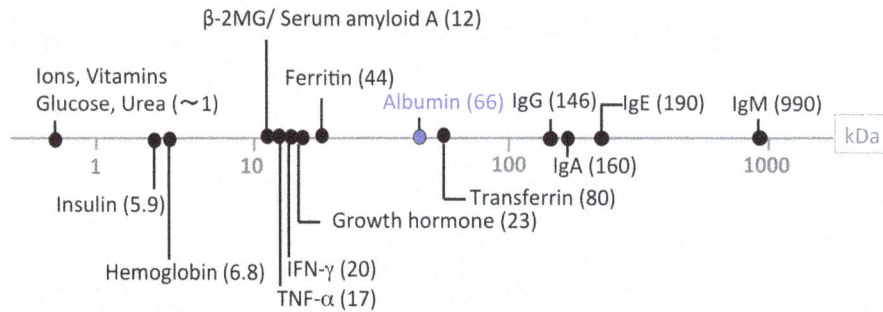

Fig. 1 The molecular weights of representative plasma molecules. *β-2MG* beta-2 microglobulin, *IFN-γ* interferon-γ, *TNF-α* tumor necrosis-α (Modification from a figure in [14]). The background colors discriminate plasma molecules that may (*gray*) or may not (*blue*) extravasate via paracellular pathway of the cutaneous blood vessels

Here, we provide an overview of the current knowledge of the permeability of blood vessels. We then cut into the dynamic regulation of blood vascular permeability especially upon inflammation. We also focus on the extravasation of immunoglobulins (Igs), the representative macromolecules in plasma, to the skin, because they may be essential for the homeostasis of cutaneous immune systems not only in terms of host protection but also for the pathogenesis of allergic and autoimmune skin disorders.

Types of blood vessels and their size barriers determine paracellular permeability

The human body has three types of blood vessels based on their structural differences: continuous (non-fenestrated), fenestrated, and sinusoidal (reviewed in [2]). In brief, blood vessels can first be classified into sinusoidal (discontinuous) or non-sinusoidal by the presence or absence of continuous basement membranes beneath endothelial cells. Non-sinusoidal blood vessels can be

Table 1 Types of blood vessels in various organs with different permeability

A. Charge barrier [17–23]

Glycocalyx layer	Anionic mesh-like layer with regular spacing of <20 nm for continuous and fenestrated vessels (irregularly found on sinusoidal vessels), on both the surface of IEJ clefts and endothelial cells.

B. Size barrier (reviewed in [2])

Types of blood vessels		Types of endothelial cells	Interendothelial junctions (IEJs)	Representative organs	Estimated upper limit for paracellular transportation [4]
Continuous (non-fenestrated)	Continuous basement membrane	No fenestrae	Tight junctions and adherens junctions	Retina [2] brain, spinal cord [66] thymus [67]	Determined by IEJs (TJs) <1 nm
			Adherens junctions with limited contribution of tight junctions	skin [12, 13] muscle, heart [68, 69] adipose tissue [70] lung [71, 72]	Determined by IEJs (AJs) <5 nm
Fenestrated		Fenestrated (with diaphragm)		skin [12, 13] exocrine glands [73] kidney (peritubular) [74] endocrine glands [73, 75, 76] intestinal mucosa [77, 78] lymph node [79, 80]	Determined by diaphragm <6–12 nm [81]
		Fenestrated (open pores without diaphragm)		Kidney (glomerulus) [82, 83]	Determined by glycocalyx <15 nm [2, 19]
Sinusoidal (discontinuous)	Discontinuous basement membrane	Fenestrated (with and/or without diaphragm)		Liver [84–86] spleen [87]	<50–280 nm, largely differ among species <3–5 μm

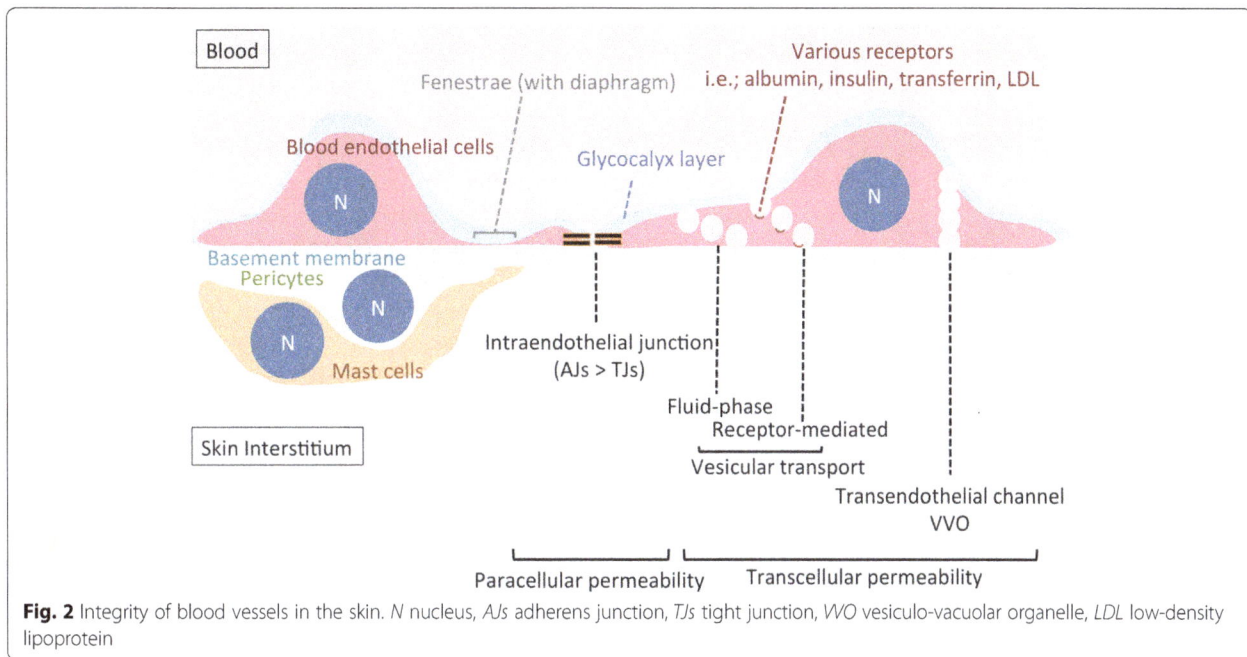

Fig. 2 Integrity of blood vessels in the skin. *N* nucleus, *AJs* adherens junction, *TJs* tight junction, *VVO* vesiculo-vacuolar organelle, *LDL* low-density lipoprotein

termed as continuous blood vessels in a broad sense and can be further classified into fenestrated and non-fenestrated (continuous blood vessels in a narrow sense), based on their endothelial types with or without fenestrations. Fenestrated blood vessels can further be subclassified by the existence of a diaphragm [9] (Table 1).

IEJs, the structures connecting adjacent blood endothelial cells, are composed of AJs and TJs. AJs are composed of vascular endothelial (VE)-cadherin complexes with catenin; and TJs are composed of claudins, occludins, and junctional adhesion molecules [1, 4, 10]. In human umbilical vein endothelial cells, TJs represent only approximately 20% of the total junctional complexes [11]. Therefore, it is generally accepted that IEJs are primary established by AJs in most peripheral blood vessels (reviewed in [4]). In specific continuous vessels, blood endothelial cells are much more firmly adhered to each other with enriched TJs to serve as specialized interfaces such as the blood-brain barrier or the blood-retinal barrier, bringing about low accessibility of plasma contents to these tissues.

The blood vessels in the skin are reportedly composed of continuous (non-fenestrated) and fenestrated blood vessels [12, 13], limiting passive diffusion of albumin, which has the molecular size of 66 kDa (approximately 7 nm in a diameter), and of dextrans larger than 70 kDa (as discussed later) [14]. This is consistent with the previous studies on other continuous vessels [2, 15]. Taken together, cutaneous blood vessels may act as the size barrier around 70 kDa, presumably allowing the passive diffusion of small molecules, including ions, glucose, urea, amino acids, insulin, cytokines, amyloids, and some

hormones via the paracellular pathway in the steady state but not of albumin, transferrin, and Igs (Fig. 1). Of note, the size barrier only reflects one aspect of overall vascular permeability because the extravasation of each plasma molecule may be induced by the transcellular and paracellular permeability with variable dependency (Fig. 2).

The charge barrier

Glycocalyx is a negatively charged continuous coat of proteoglycans, glycosaminoglycans, and absorbed plasma proteins, on the luminal surface of blood endothelial cells [4, 16, 17] (Fig. 2). Its thickness has been reported to range between 20 and 3000 nm depending on the detection method, vessel types, and the tissues [17–20]. Glycocalyx acts as a primary charge barrier for the transportation of plasma molecules. Several studies using enzymatic procedures that induce shedding or disruption of the glycocalyx layer or neutralize its negative charge have demonstrated the increased vascular permeability to water without affecting the IEJs [20–23].

Glycocalyx can also act as the primary size barrier in fenestrated blood vessels. In these vessels, the diameter of endothelial fenestrations is around 60 nm irrespective of the presence of a diaphragm, but the physiologically estimated upper limit of the size barrier is smaller than 15 nm [2] (Table 1). It is assumed that this discrepancy may be due to glycolcalyx occupying the fenestrations [18]. These observations lead to the "fiber matrix" theory, the idea that glycocalyx's fiber mesh-like structure with regular spacing of 20 nm may regulate vascular permeability [19]. Glycocalyx may modulate the permeability of plasma molecules, and in turn, plasma proteins can be an intrinsic part of glycocalyx [3, 24]. In this context, it is interesting to consider that plasma molecules can indirectly regulate the vascular permeability of other plasma molecules. Glycolcalyx can also sense a fluid shear stress and induce endothelial nitric oxide synthesis within endothelial cells to stabilize the barrier function of blood vessels [25].

The drastic increase in vascular permeability upon various cutaneous inflammations

Both the size and the charge barriers of blood vessels are largely affected by the physiological state of the surrounding tissue interstitium. These changes in permeability were conventionally assessed by an in vitro transwell assay system that measured the flux of variable molecules through the endothelial cell monolayer cultured in transwell chambers under various stimulus agents [26–29]. Despite the utility of the assay, it has frequently been pointed out that this assay system might not reconstitute the actual vascular integrity and permeability in vivo (discussed in [27]). Alternatively, the Miles assay has been widely used to assess vascular permeability in mice [30]. Intravenously administered tracers (such as Evan's blue) bind to albumin, and the accumulation of the tracer in the skin is evaluated after the local administration of stimulants to evoke vascular hyperpermeability. The Miles assay is useful in evaluating gross changes in vascular permeability in vivo but lacks anatomical information, i.e., the site of hyperpermeability in the net of blood vessels or the interaction of endothelial cells with perivascular cells. Furthermore, the subtle extravasation of tracers in the steady state is under the detection limit in the Miles assay.

In addition to these conventional methods, a new intravital evaluation system for vascular permeability in mice using two-photon microscopy has revealed in a more detailed manner how the blood vascular permeability is dynamically regulated in vivo in the skin [14]. By the intravenous administration of different sizes of fluorescein-conjugated dextrans (20 to 2000 kDa), it was clearly visualized that the passive diffusion, which may reflect the paracellular transportation, occurs only when dextrans are smaller than 70 kDa. When fluorescein-conjugated bovine albumin (molecule size 66 kDa) was administered intravenously, the majority seemed to be retained in the blood. A gradual extravasation was, however, observed within 1 h after an injection of albumin but not for 70 kDa dextrans. This may reflect the different regulation of the transcellular transportation of albumin and dextran with similar size. The same in vivo system also clarified the site of vascular hyperpermeability induced in both type I and type IV allergic cutaneous inflammation. Upon inflammation, the size limitation for plasma molecules was abolished, allowing the immediate

leakage of up to 2000 kDa dextrans to the skin interstitium. This leakage was selectively induced in the postcapillary venules. This corresponded to the previous assumption that postcapillary venules are the specific site of vascular leakage in inflammation. The physiological barrier of the postcapillary venules seems intrinsically sensitive and vulnerable to inflammation, due to abundant receptors for chemical mediators such as histamine and bradykinin [31, 32], less-abundant TJs [33], and low coverage rate by pericytes of these vessels [34]. Numerous chemical mediators, which are released upon inflammation, can lead to diminishment of AJs and the contraction of blood endothelial cells that lead to the formation of IEJ gaps in postcapillary venules. The molecular detail of underlying mechanism for the dysregulation of paracellular permeability is discussed in other reviews [4]. In addition to vascular leakage, postcapillary venules can also serve as the specific site of leukocyte infiltration and inflammatory cell gathering, which is essential for immune responses in the skin [35–38].

As discussed later, the transcellular pathway might play a central role in the extravasation of plasma macromolecules in the steady state. It is of note that the increase in the transcellular transportation of albumin due to increased caveolae function has also been demonstrated in inflammation [39]. Furthermore, the regularity of glycocalyx is disrupted upon inflammation, resulting in irregular thickened layers and gaps between them. Clustering of glycocalyx induced by inflammation can also activate intracellular signals and provoke cytoskeletal reorganization that leads to barrier dysfunction. This change in glycocalyx structures may also contribute to the elevation of permeability, although this appears to be ignored in recent studies. Overall, the changes in the paracellular permeability, the transcellular permeability, and the charge barrier can all participate in gross increase in vascular permeability upon inflammation.

The increase in immunoglobulin G extravasation to the skin upon inflammation

As mentioned in the previous sections, the drastic increase in vascular permeability might allow the extravasation of plasma contents, including macromolecules. Among them, here, we focus on the regulation of IgG and IgE extravasation in the skin because they may play important roles in the terms of protective and pathological immune reactions in the skin.

Historically, IgG kinetics has mostly been studied in the intestinal epithelia or the placenta in view of maternal-to-neonatal/fetal IgG passage. The necessity of the neonatal Fcγ receptor in epithelial cells and trophoblasts has well been established; however, few studies have examined IgG kinetics at the blood vessel walls [40–45]. The molecular weight of IgG is approximately

150 kDa (Fig. 1). It was thus presumed that the extravasation of IgGs is tightly regulated in the steady state.

Recent observation using a murine pemphigus model, which is a representative model for autoantibody-related disorders in the skin, revealed that variable local inflammation, such as ultraviolet B irradiation or the topical application of irritants to the skin, enhanced autoantibody deposition in the skin [36]. This increase in autoantibody deposition in the skin leads to exacerbated skin manifestation in the murine pemphigus model. The human body is frequently exposed to external stimuli such as frictions, heat, and the sunlight, which can elicit minor local inflammation. Therefore, IgG distribution in the periphery might be largely influenced by external circumstances. Indeed, it is well known that IgG deposition in the epidermal basement membrane is more frequently detected in sun-exposed sites in patients with systemic lupus erythematosus. In view of host protection, enhanced IgG recruitment into the inflammatory site would be important for neutralization of invading pathogens.

Despite the strict regulation, constitutive IgG extravasation to the tissue parenchyma in the steady state appeared to exist [36], and the same observation was made for albumin. This homeostatic extravasation of plasma macromolecules may rely on transcellular permeability (Table 2).

Importance of transcellular permeability

Conventionally, it is considered that there are two different types of transcellular pathway: receptor-mediated transcytosis and non receptor-mediated bulk-phase transcytosis (often called "fluid-phase" transcytosis) [27, 46]

(Fig. 2). In this review, we do not discuss the transendothelial channels or vesiculo-vacuolar organelles [47, 48]. Plasma molecules those are smaller than the size barrier of the blood vessels (<70 kDa), like insulin, might be able to extravasate in both paracellular and transcellular pathways. However, the transporting efficiency is reportedly much higher in paracellular transportation [49, 50]. Plasma macromolecules that are larger than the size barrier of the blood vessels (>70 kDa) might extravasate by either fluid-phase or receptor-mediated transcytosis; however, its balance in vivo for most macromolecules has not been elucidated.

The transcellular permeability of albumin has extensively been studied and found to be largely dependent on the receptor-mediated transcytosis via gp60 in caveolae [51–53]. Even for albumin, to what extent fluid-phase transcytosis contributes to the overall albumin extravasation remains undefined. Furthermore, in fluid-phase transcytosis, it is believed that the selectivity of molecules might exist, due to their size and charge. Collectively, the mechanism of transcellular transportation remains to be elucidated for most plasma molecules. The proposed routes for the extravasation of plasma molecules are shown in Table 2.

In epithelial cells, the transcellular pathway is initiated by endocytosis [27]. Therefore, it might also be important to define the way of endocytosis of each molecule to understand the mechanism of transcytosis in blood endothelial cells. Endocytosis can define the destinations of the contents, i.e., to lysosomal degradation, to recycling, or to the transcellular pathway [40–42, 54, 55]

Table 2 Transportation of plasma contents in the steady state

Routes	Molecules		
Paracellular pathway	Water molecules <3 nm molecular radius (i.e., urea, amino acids, glucose, ions)		
Transcellular pathway	Aquaporin channels		Water (up to 40% of total hydraulic pathway)
	Fluid-phase	Caveolae	Albumin [27, 46] intact native, acetylated and oxidized LDL [88, 89] IgG [44] transferrin and iron [90]
		Undetermined	IgG (bound to FcRn in endosomes after fluid-phase endocytosis [40, 41, 43, 49])
	Receptor-mediated	Caveolae	Albumin (via gp60 receptor) [50–52] insulin (via unknown receptor) [49]
		Clathrin	Insulin [91] transferrin and iron (via transferrin receptor [92, 93]) gonadotrophin (via gonadotropin receptor [94])
		Undetermined carrier vesicle	IgG (via FcRn or FcγR2b [45, 95, 96]) LDL (via LDL receptor [97]) insulin (via insulin receptor [98])
	Transendothelial channels		
	Vesiculo-vacuolar organelles		
Direct probing by non-endothelial cells over blood vessels	IgE (via FcεRI by mast cells) [58]		

(discussed in [51]). Various forms of endocytosis by eukaryotic cells have been found to date, including phagocytosis, macropinocytosis, clathrin-mediated endocytosis, clathrin-independent caveolae-mediated endocytosis, and newly defined clathrin-independent non-caveolar endocytosis [56, 57]. Because caveolae are abundantly observed in blood endothelial cells [50], it is sometimes oversimply stated that both fluid-phase transcytosis and receptor-mediated transcytosis is mediated by caveolae. However, the abundance of caveolae can vary widely among blood vessels in different tissues [27, 46]. Some studies have suggested the possibility of endocytic pathways other than caveolae in blood endothelial cells (Table 2), but we believe that the actual contribution of various endocytic vesicles on transcellular transportation should be more rigorously explored. In addition to investigating the transcellular route for each macromolecule, their relation to intracellular membrane organelles, such as early endosomes, sorting endosomes, or lysosomes, is also essential in order to understand their final destination. Transcellular permeability is a key issue that requires further research to improve our understanding of vascular homeostasis.

Another unique style of molecular extravasation in the skin—immunoglobulin E

A unique extravasation mechanism of IgE in the skin has recently been demonstrated using an in vivo imaging technique [58]. Mast cells are abundantly located in the skin along the blood vessels [8]. Mast cells are best known as the effector cells of IgE-mediated allergic responses, such as allergic dermatitis and urticaria. Under crosslinking of high-affinity IgE receptors on their surface by specific antigens, mast cells are activated and release proinflammatory molecules, including histamine, leading to vascular hyperpermeability. Intriguingly, recent studies have demonstrated that perivascular mast cells capture blood-circulating IgE by extending their processes across the vessel wall in the steady state [58]. Because the plasma concentration of IgE is significantly lower compared to other Igs and proteins, the way in which mast cells probe and capture IgE by their surface high-affinity IgE receptor (FcεRI) appears to be strategic.

No studies have properly assessed the transcellular transportion of IgE, IgA, and IgM via blood endothelial cells. In addition, low-affinity IgE receptors (CD23) or polymeric Ig receptors in epithelial cells have been reported responsible for the transcellular transportation of IgE or IgA and IgM [59–63]. Discriminating the difference between endothelial systems and epithelial systems would reveal the characteristic nature of the blood-tissue interface.

Conclusions

The regulation of blood vessel permeability is important for tissue homeostasis and has attracted the attention of vascular biologists for decades. Considering that nanoparticles [64], antibody-based biologics, or immune checkpoint inhibitors [65] are globally accepted as promising therapeutic tools for autoimmune disorders and various cancers, the basic insight into the kinetics of micro- and macromolecules at the blood-tissue interface would provide a practical clinical information. By employing accumulated knowledge and well-established conventional methods, the in vivo techniques introduced in this review to finely evaluate blood vascular permeability would enable an enhanced understanding of this physical process.

Abbreviations
AJs: Adherens junctions; IEJs: Interendothelial junctions; Ig: Immunoglobulin; TJs: Tight junctions

Acknowledgements
None.

Funding
This work was supported by the JSPS KAKENHI (263395), Grants-in-Aid for Scientific Research 15H05790, 15H1155, 15K15417, Japan Science and Technology Agency, Precursory Research for Embryonic Science and Technology (PRESTO) (16021031300), and Japan Agency for Medical Research and Development (AMED) (16ek0410011h0003, 16he0902003h0002).

Authors' contributions
OS and GE drafted the manuscript. KK completed the manuscript. All authors read and approved the final manuscript.

Competing interests
The authors declare that they have no competing interests.

Author details
[1]Department of Dermatology, Kyoto University Graduate School of Medicine, 54 Shogoin-Kawahara, Sakyo, Kyoto 606-8507, Japan. [2]Singapore Immunology Network (SIgN) and Institute of Medical Biology, Agency for Science, Technology and Research (A*STAR), Biopolis, Singapore. [3]PRESTO, Japan Science and Technology Agency, Saitama, Japan.

References
1. Mehta D, Malik AB. Signaling mechanisms regulating endothelial permeability. Physiol Rev. 2006;86:279–367.
2. Sarin H. Physiologic upper limits of pore size of different blood capillary types and another perspective on the dual pore theory of microvascular permeability. J Angiogenes Res. 2010;2:14.

3. Squire JM, Chew M, Nneji G, Neal C, Barry J, Michel C. Quasi-periodic substructure in the microvessel endothelial glycocalyx: a possible explanation for molecular filtering? J Struct Biol. 2001;136:239–55.

4. Komarova Y, Malik AB. Regulation of endothelial permeability via paracellular and transcellular transport pathways. Annu Rev Physiol. 2010;72:463–93.

5. Qiao RL, Wang HS, Yan W, Odekon LE, Del Vecchio PJ, Smith TJ, et al. Extracellular matrix hyaluronan is a determinant of the endothelial barrier. Am J Physiol. 1995;269:C103–109.

6. Kalluri R. Basement membranes: structure, assembly and role in tumour angiogenesis. Nat Rev Cancer. 2003;3:422–33.

7. Armulik A, Genove G, Mae M, Nisancioglu MH, Wallgard E, Niaudet C, et al. Pericytes regulate the blood-brain barrier. Nature. 2010;468:557–61.

8. Dudeck A, Dudeck J, Scholten J, Petzold A, Surianarayanan S, Kohler A, et al. Mast cells are key promoters of contact allergy that mediate the adjuvant effects of haptens. Immunity. 2011;34:973–94.

9. Stan RV. Endothelial stomatal and fenestral diaphragms in normal vessels and angiogenesis. J Cell Mol Med. 2007;11:621–43.

10. González-Mariscal L, Betanzos A, Nava P, Jaramillo BE. Tight junction proteins. Prog Biophys Mol Biol. 2003;81:1–44.

11. Wojciak-Stothard B, Potempa S, Eichholtz T, Ridley AJ. Rho and Rac but not Cdc42 regulate endothelial cell permeability. J Cell Sci. 2001;114:1343–55.

12. Takada M, Hattori S. Presence of fenestrated capillaries in the skin. Anat Rec. 1972;173:213–9.

13. Imayama S. Scanning and transmission electron microscope study on the terminal blood vessels of the rat skin. J Invest Dermatol. 1981;76:151–7.

14. Egawa G, Nakamizo S, Natsuaki Y, Doi H, Miyachi Y, Kabashima K. Intravital analysis of vascular permeability in mice using two-photon microscopy. Sci Rep. 2013;3:1932.

15. Predescu D, Vogel SM, Malik AB. Functional and morphological studies of protein transcytosis in continuous endothelia. Am J Physiol Lung Cell Mol Physiol. 2004;287:L895–901.

16. Vink H, Duling BR. Capillary endothelial surface layer selectively reduces plasma solute distribution volume. Am J Physiol Heart Circ Physiol. 2000; 278:H285–289.

17. Pries AR, Secomb TW, Gaehtgens P. The endothelial surface layer. Pflugers Arch. 2000;440:653–66.

18. Luft JH. Fine structures of capillary and endocapillary layer as revealed by ruthenium red. Fed Proc. 1966;25:1773–83.

19. Haldenby KA, Chappell DC, Winlove CP, Parker KH, Firth JA. Focal and regional variations in the composition of the glycocalyx of large vessel endothelium. J Vasc Res. 1994;31:2–9.

20. Huxley VH, Williams DA. Role of a glycocalyx on coronary arteriole permeability to proteins: evidence from enzyme treatments. Am J Physiol Heart Circ Physiol. 2000;278:H1177–1185.

21. Lum H, Malik AB. Regulation of vascular endothelial barrier function. Am J Physiol. 1994;267:L223–241.

22. Desjardins C, Duling BR. Heparinase treatment suggests a role for the endothelial cell glycocalyx in regulation of capillary hematocrit. Am J Physiol. 1990;258:H647–654.

23. Sunnergren KP, Fairman RP, deBlois GG, Glauser FL. Effects of protamine, heparinase, and hyaluronidase on endothelial permeability and surface charge. J Appl Physiol (1985). 1987;63:1987–92.

24. Schneeberger EE, Mccormack JA, Hamelin M. Interaction of circulating proteins with pulmonary endothelial glycocalyx and its effect on endothelial permeability. J Cell Biol. 1983;97:A476–6.

25. Florian JA, Kosky JR, Ainslie K, Pang ZY, Dull RO, Tarbell JM. Heparan sulfate proteoglycan is a mechanosensor on endothelial cells. Circ Res. 2003;93:E136–42.

26. Albelda SM, Sampson PM, Haselton FR, McNiff JM, Mueller SN, Williams SK, et al. Permeability characteristics of cultured endothelial cell monolayers. J Appl Physiol (1985). 1988;64:308–22.

27. Tuma P, Hubbard AL. Transcytosis: crossing cellular barriers. Physiol Rev. 2003;83:871–932.

28. Cooper JA, Del Vecchio PJ, Minnear FL, Burhop KE, Selig WM, Garcia JG, et al. Measurement of albumin permeability across endothelial monolayers in vitro. J Appl Physiol (1985). 1987;62:1076–83.

29. Kluger MS, Clark PR, Tellides G, Gerke V, Pober JS. Claudin-5 controls intercellular barriers of human dermal microvascular but not human umbilical vein endothelial cells. Arterioscler Thromb Vasc Biol. 2013;33:489–500.

30. Nagy JA, Benjamin L, Zeng HY, Dvorak AM, Dvorak HF. Vascular permeability, vascular hyperpermeability and angiogenesis. Angiogenesis. 2008;11:109–19.

31. Heltianu C, Simionescu M, Simionescu N. Histamine receptors of the microvascular endothelium revealed in situ with a histamine-ferritin conjugate: characteristic high-affinity binding sites in venules. J Cell Biol. 1982;93:357–64.

32. Simionescu N, Heltianu C, Antohe F, Simionescu M. Endothelial cell receptors for histamine. Ann N Y Acad Sci. 1982;401:132–49.

33. Bazzoni G, Dejana E. Endothelial cell-to-cell junctions: molecular organization and role in vascular homeostasis. Physiol Rev. 2004;84:869–901.

34. Armulik A, Genove G, Betsholtz C. Pericytes: developmental, physiological, and pathological perspectives, problems, and promises. Dev Cell. 2011;21: 193–215.

35. Natsuaki Y, Egawa G, Nakamizo S, Ono S, Hanakawa S, Okada T, et al. Perivascular leukocyte clusters are essential for efficient activation of effector T cells in the skin. Nat Immunol. 2014;15:1064–9.

36. Ono S, Egawa G, Kitoh A, Dainichi T, Otsuka A, Nakajima S, et al. Local inflammation exacerbates cutaneous manifestations in a murine autoimmune pemphigus model. J Allergy Clin Immunol. 2017. [in press].

37. Ono S, Kabashima K. Proposal of inducible skin-associated lymphoid tissue (iSALT). Exp Dermatol. 2015;24:630–1.

38. Ono S, Kabashima K. Novel insights into the role of immune cells in skin and inducible skin-associated lymphoid tissue (iSALT). Allergo J. 2015;24:18–27.

39. Hu G, Vogel SM, Schwartz DE, Malik AB, Minshall RD. Intercellular adhesion molecule-1-dependent neutrophil adhesion to endothelial cells induces caveolae-mediated pulmonary vascular hyperpermeability. Circ Res. 2008; 102:e120–131.

40. Ober RJ, Martinez C, Lai X, Zhou J, Ward ES. Exocytosis of IgG as mediated by the receptor. FcRn: an analysis at the single-molecule level. Proc Natl Acad Sci U S A. 2004;101:11076–81.

41. Ober RJ, Martinez C, Vaccaro C, Zhou J, Ward ES. Visualizing the site and dynamics of IgG salvage by the MHC class I-related receptor, FcRn. J Immunol. 2004;172:2021–9.

42. Ward ES, Zhou J, Ghetie V, Ober RJ. Evidence to support the cellular mechanism involved in serum IgG homeostasis in humans. Int Immunol. 2003;15:187–5.

43. Antohe F, Radulescu L, Gafencu A, Ghetie V, Simionescu M. Expression of functionally active FcRn and the differentiated bidirectional transport of IgG in human placental endothelial cells. Hum Immunol. 2001;62:93–105.

44. Leach L, Eaton BM, Firth JA, Contractor SF. Uptake and intracellular routing of peroxidase-conjugated immunoglobulin-G by the perfused human placenta. Cell Tissue Res. 1990;261:383–8.

45. Gafencu A, Heltianu C, Burlacu A, Hunziker W, Simionescu M. Investigation of IgG receptors expressed on the surface of human placental endothelial cells. Placenta. 2003;24:664–76.

46. Simionescu N. Cellular aspects of transcapillary exchange. Physiol Rev. 1983; 63:1536–79.

47. Feng D, Nagy JA, Hipp J, Dvorak HF, Dvorak AM. Vesiculo-vacuolar organelles and the regulation of venule permeability to macromolecules by vascular permeability factor, histamine, and serotonin. J Exp Med. 1996;183:1981–6.

48. Kohn S, Nagy JA, Dvorak HF, Dvorak AM. Pathways of macromolecular tracer transport across venules and small veins—structural basis for the hyperpermeability of tumor blood-vessels. Lab Invest. 1992;67:596–607.

49. Bendayan M, Rasio EA. Transport of insulin and albumin by the microvascular endothelium of the rete mirabile. J Cell Sci. 1996;109:1857–64.

50. Bendayan M. Morphological and cytochemical aspects of capillary permeability. Microsc Res Tech. 2002;57:327–49.

51. Ghitescu L, Fixman A, Simionescu M, Simionescu N. Specific binding sites for albumin restricted to plasmalemmal vesicles of continuous capillary endothelium: receptor-mediated transcytosis. J Cell Biol. 1986;102:1304–11.

52. Milici AJ, Watrous NE, Stukenbrok H, Palade GE. Transcytosis of albumin in capillary endothelium. J Cell Biol. 1987;105:2603–12.

53. Minshall RD, Tiruppathi C, Vogel SM, Niles WD, Gilchrist A, Hamm HE, et al. Endothelial cell-surface gp60 activates vesicle formation and trafficking via G(i)-coupled Src kinase signaling pathway. J Cell Biol. 2000;150:1057–70.

54. Schnitzer JE, Bravo J. High affinity binding, endocytosis, and degradation of conformationally modified albumins. Potential role of gp30 and gp18 as novel scavenger receptors. J Biol Chem. 1993;268:7562–70.

55. Kim MJ, Dawes J, Jessup W. Transendothelial transport of modified low-density lipoproteins. Atherosclerosis. 1994;108:5–17.

56. Howes MT, Kirkham M, Riches J, Cortese K, Walser PJ, Simpson F, et al. Clathrin-independent carriers form a high capacity endocytic sorting system at the leading edge of migrating cells. J Cell Biol. 2010;190:675–91.

57. Conner SD, Schmid SL. Regulated portals of entry into the cell. Nature. 2003; 422:37–44.

58. Cheng LE, Hartmann K, Roers A, Krummel MF, Locksley RM. Perivascular mast cells dynamically probe cutaneous blood vessels to capture immunoglobulin E. Immunity. 2013;38:166–75.

59. Li H, Nowak-Wegrzyn A, Charlop-Powers Z, Shreffler W, Chehade M, Thomas S, et al. Transcytosis of IgE-antigen complexes by CD23a in human intestinal epithelial cells and its role in food allergy. Gastroenterology. 2006;131:47–58.

60. Palaniyandi S, Liu X, Periasamy S, Ma A, Tang J, Jenkins M, et al. Inhibition of CD23-mediated IgE transcytosis suppresses the initiation and development of allergic airway inflammation. Mucosal Immunol. 2015;8:1262–74.

61. Brown WR, Isobe K, Nakane PK, Pacini B. Studies on translocation of immunoglobulins across intestinal epithelium. IV. Evidence for binding of IgA and IgM to secretory component in intestinal epithelium. Gastroenterology. 1977;73:1333–9.

62. Richardson JM, Kaushic C, Wira CR. Polymeric immunoglobin (Ig) receptor production and IgA transcytosis in polarized primary cultures of mature rat uterine epithelial cells. Biol Reprod. 1995;53:488–98.

63. Stadtmueller BM, Huey-Tubman KE, Lopez CJ, Yang Z, Hubbell WL, Bjorkman PJ. The structure and dynamics of secretory component and its interactions with polymeric immunoglobulins. Elife. 2016;5:e10640.

64. Davis ME, Chen ZG, Shin DM. Nanoparticle therapeutics: an emerging treatment modality for cancer. Nat Rev Drug Discov. 2008;7:771–82.

65. Pardoll DM. The blockade of immune checkpoints in cancer immunotherapy. Nat Rev Cancer. 2012;12:252–64.

66. Abbott NJ, Ronnback L, Hansson E. Astrocyte-endothelial interactions at the blood-brain barrier. Nat Rev Neurosci. 2006;7:41–53.

67. Raviola E, Karnovsky MJ. Evidence for a blood-thymus barrier using electron-opaque tracers. J Exp Med. 1972;136: 466- + .

68. Ward BJ, Bauman KF, Firth JA. Interendothelial junctions of cardiac capillaries in rats—their structure and permeability properties. Cell Tissue Res. 1988;252:57–66.

69. Aird WC. Phenotypic heterogeneity of the endothelium I. Structure, function, and mechanisms. Circ Res. 2007;100:158–73.

70. Williamson JR. Adipose tissue—morphological changes associated with lipid mobilization. J Cell Biol. 1964;20: 57-&.

71. Schneeberger EE. The permeability of the alveolar-capillary membrane to ultrastructural protein tracers. Ann N Y Acad Sci. 1974;221:238–43.

72. Stevens T, Phan S, Frid MG, Alvarez D, Herzog E, Stenmark KR. Lung vascular cell heterogeneity: endothelium, smooth muscle, and fibroblasts. Proc Am Thorac Soc. 2008;5:783–91.

73. Henderson JR, Moss MC. A morphometric study of the endocrine and exocrine capillaries of the pancreas. Q J Exp Physiol. 1985;70:347–56.

74. Deen WM, Ueki IF, Brenner BM. Permeability of renal peritubular capillaries to neutral dextrans dextrans and endogenous albumin. Am J Physiol. 1976; 231:283–91.

75. Farquhar MG. Fine structure and function in capillaries of the anterior pituitary gland. Angiology. 1961;12:270–92.

76. Ekholm R, Sjostrand FS. The ultrastructural organization of the mouse thyroid gland. J Ultrastruct Res. 1957;1:178–99.

77. Milici AJ, Bankston PW. Fetal and neonatal rat intestinal capillaries: permeability to carbon, ferritin, hemoglobin, and myoglobin. Am J Anat. 1982;165:165–86.

78. Milici AJ, Bankston PW. Fetal and neonatal rat intestinal capillaries: a TEM study of changes in the mural structure. Am J Anat. 1981;160:435–48.

79. Gretz JE, Norbury CC, Anderson AO, Proudfoot AEI, Shaw S. Lymph-borne chemokines and other low molecular weight molecules reach high endothelial venules via specialized conduits while a functional barrier limits access to the lymphocyte microenvironments in lymph node cortex. J Exp Med. 2000;192:1425–39.

80. Rantakari P, Auvinen K, Jappinen N, Kapraali M, Valtonen J, Karikoski M, et al. The endothelial protein PLVAP in lymphatics controls the entry of lymphocytes and antigens into lymph nodes (vol 16, pg 386, 2015). Nat Immunol. 2015;16:544–4.

81. Stan RV, Tse D, Deharvengt SJ, Smits NC, Xu Y, Luciano MR, et al. The diaphragms of fenestrated endothelia: gatekeepers of vascular permeability and blood composition. Dev Cell. 2012;23:1203–18.

82. Caulfield JP, Farquhar MG. The permeability of glomerular capillaries to graded dextrans. Identification of the basement membrane as the primary filtration barrier. J Cell Biol. 1974;63:883–903.

83. Avasthi PS, Koshy V. The anionic matrix at the rat glomerular endothelial surface. Anat Rec. 1988;220:258–66.

84. Snoeys J, Lievens J, Wisse E, Jacobs F, Duimel H, Collen D, et al. Species differences in transgene DNA uptake in hepatocytes after adenoviral transfer correlate with the size of endothelial fenestrae. Gene Ther. 2007;14:604–12.

85. Wisse E, Jacobs F, Topal B, Frederik P, De Geest B. The size of endothelial fenestrae in human liver sinusoids: implications for hepatocyte-directed gene transfer. Gene Ther. 2008;15:1193–9.

86. Naito M, Wisse E. Filtration effect of endothelial fenestrations on chylomicron transport in neonatal rat liver sinusoids. Cell Tissue Res. 1978;190:371–82.

87. Chen LT. Microcirculation of spleen—open or closed circulation. Science. 1978;201:157–9.

88. Sun SW, Zu XY, Tuo QH, Chen LX, Lei XY, Li K, et al. Caveolae and caveolin-1 mediate endocytosis and transcytosis of oxidized low density lipoprotein in endothelial cells. Acta Pharmacol Sin. 2010;31:1336–42.

89. Vasile E, Simionescu M, Simionescu N. Visualization of the binding, endocytosis, and transcytosis of low-density lipoprotein in the arterial endothelium in situ. J Cell Biol. 1983;96:1677–89.

90. Holash JA, Harik SI, Perry G, Stewart PA. Barrier properties of testis microvessels. Proc Natl Acad Sci U S A. 1993;90:11069–73.

91. Azizi PM, Zyla RE, Guan S, Wang C, Liu J, Bolz SS, et al. Clathrin-dependent entry and vesicle-mediated exocytosis define insulin transcytosis across microvascular endothelial cells. Mol Biol Cell. 2015;26:740–50.

92. Crowe A, Morgan EH. Iron and transferrin uptake by brain and cerebrospinal fluid in the rat. Brain Res. 1992;592:8–16.

93. Roberts R, Sandra A, Siek GC, Lucas JJ, Fine RE. Studies of the mechanism of iron transport across the blood-brain barrier. Ann Neurol. 1992;32(Suppl): S43–50.

94. Ghinea N, Milgrom E. A new function for the LH/CG receptor: transcytosis of hormone across the endothelial barrier in target organs. Semin Reprod Med. 2001;19:97–101.

95. Takizawa T, Anderson CL, Robinson JM. A novel Fc gamma R-defined. IgG-containing organelle in placental endothelium. J Immunol. 2005;175:2331–9.

96. Borvak J, Richardson J, Medesan C, Antohe F, Radu C, Simionescu M, et al. Functional expression of the MHC class I-related receptor, FcRn, in endothelial cells of mice. Int Immunol. 1998;10:1289–98.

97. Dehouck B, Fenart L, Dehouck MP, Pierce A, Torpier G, Cecchelli R. A new function for the LDL receptor: transcytosis of LDL across the blood-brain barrier. J Cell Biol. 1997;138:877–89.

98. Pardridge WM, Kang YS, Buciak JL, Yang J. Human insulin receptor monoclonal antibody undergoes high affinity binding to human brain capillaries in vitro and rapid transcytosis through the blood-brain barrier in vivo in the primate. Pharm Res. 1995;12:807–16.

6

Inflammatory predisposition predicts disease phenotypes in muscular dystrophy

Yuko Nitahara-Kasahara[1,2], Shin'ichi Takeda[2] and Takashi Okada[1,2]*

Abstract

Duchenne muscular dystrophy is an incurable genetic disease that presents with skeletal muscle weakness and chronic inflammation and is associated with early mortality. Indeed, immune cell infiltration into the skeletal muscle is a notable feature of the disease pathophysiology and is strongly associated with disease severity. Interleukin (IL)-10 regulates inflammatory immune responses by reducing both M1 macrophage activation and the production of pro-inflammatory cytokines, thereby promoting the activation of the M2 macrophage phenotype. We previously reported that genetic ablation of IL-10 in dystrophic mice resulted in more severe phenotypes, in regard to heart and respiratory function, as evidenced by increased macrophage infiltration, high levels of inflammatory factors in the muscle, and progressive cardiorespiratory dysfunction. These data therefore indicate that IL-10 comprises an essential immune-modulator within dystrophic muscles. In this review, we highlight the pivotal role of the immune system in the pathogenesis of muscular dystrophy and discuss how an increased understanding of the pathogenesis of this disease may lead to novel therapeutic strategies.

Keywords: IL-10, Anti-inflammation, Muscular dystrophy, Animal model

Background

Muscular disorders are a heterogeneous group of genetic diseases caused by mutations in genes encoding sarcolemmal, sarcomeric, and cytosolic muscle proteins. Deficiency or loss of function in any of these proteins leads to varying degrees of progressive loss of motor control. In particular, contraction of dystrophin-deficient myofibers produces severe damage and generates cycles of muscle fiber necrosis and regeneration.

In muscular dystrophy, dystrophin and the associated glycoprotein complex proteins are absent from the sarcolemmal membrane, resulting in altered mechanical and signaling functions and subsequently leading to immune cell infiltration, progressive muscle wasting, necrosis, and membrane fragility [1]. Indeed, the infiltration of inflammatory cells into the skeletal muscle is a notable characteristic of disease pathophysiology. Moreover, recent reports have demonstrated that inflammatory responses disrupt muscle homeostasis and inhibit processes that

promote muscle repair and regeneration and that cytokines and chemokines produced by these inflammatory cells regulate the skeletal muscle inflammation observed in muscular dystrophy [2–5]. These findings therefore indicate that the degree of inflammatory cell infiltration is strongly associated with disease severity in muscular dystrophy patients.

This review points out inflammatory predisposition and immune-mediated mechanisms that regulate the disease severity of muscular dystrophy. We also discuss how the application of this knowledge could lead to novel therapeutic strategies.

Characteristics of the inflammation involved in muscle diseases

In muscle diseases associated with chronic inflammation, the infiltration of muscle tissues by a variety of activated immune cells is typically heavily dependent on the presence of multiple cytokines [6]. Key cellular sources of these cytokines include $CD4^+$ and $CD8^+$ T cells, dendritic cells, B cells, neutrophils, and macrophages of both the pro-inflammatory M1 and the tissue regeneration-focused M2 phenotype. In particular, $CD8^+$ T cells trigger muscle fiber death, and $CD4^+$ T cells contribute to this process by

* Correspondence: t-okada@nms.ac.jp
[1]Department of Biochemistry and Molecular Biology, Nippon Medical School, Bunkyo-ku, Tokyo, Japan
[2]Department of Molecular Therapy, National Institute of Neuroscience, National Center of Neurology and Psychiatry, Kodaira, Tokyo, Japan

providing inflammatory cytokines to $CD8^+$ T cells and other immune cells [7, 8]. Meanwhile, macrophages perform a variety of important immunoregulatory and inflammatory functions and lyse muscle fibers through the production of nitric oxide, resulting in the release of high concentrations of cytolytic and cytotoxic molecules [9–11]. The high levels of tumor necrosis factor (TNF), interferon (IFN)-γ, and interleukin (IL)-12 observed in the blood and muscle tissues of patients with various types of myositis have implicated the T helper type 1 (Th1) response as a key mediator of the pathogenesis of these diseases [12]. Necrotizing myofibers are attacked by inflammatory cells at the endomysial, perimysial, and perivascular areas. Furthermore, a number of cytokines, including IL-1α and IL-17, can exert direct effects on the muscle tissue [13, 14] via the activation of signaling pathways, such as the nuclear factor NF-kB pathway, which further enhances the inflammatory response through up-regulation of cytokine/chemokine production. Notably, depending on their concentrations, these cytokines also display anti-inflammatory properties and exhibit duality of function [15]. Satellite cell-mediated regeneration is also mediated by several cytokines, as well as myofiber degeneration [16]. Thus, a tightly regulated, transient inflammatory response is required for normal muscle regeneration. The satellite cells which are muscle-resident stem cells get activated and start to proliferate as myoblasts upon muscle injury, then fuse and differentiate into myotubes that later grow, replacing damaged muscle [17, 18]. Dysregulated expression of cytokines such as TNF-α, TGF-β, or Il-1β leads to aberrant repair by chronic inflammation [19]. The prolonged inflammation is observed in severe myopathies such as Duchenne muscular dystrophy [20].

Muscular dystrophy

Duchenne muscular dystrophy (DMD) is a severe X-linked muscular disease characterized by mutations in the gene encoding the cytoskeletal protein dystrophin that result in chronic inflammation, fibrosis, fat infiltration, and impaired vasoregulation, which manifests as muscle weakness and eventually leads to skeletal and cardiac muscle atrophy [21, 22]. Although mechanical injury and membrane defects are crucial factors that promote dystrophic disease pathology [23, 24], inflammation plays a large role in the muscle pathology of DMD. As an anti-inflammatory therapy, glucocorticoids, specifically prednisone and deflazacort, are widely used to improve muscle strength in DMD patients [25–27]; however, the beneficial effects of this therapy vary from patient to patient, and administration of these compounds sometimes result in negative side effects. Furthermore, it is currently unclear whether the efficacy of glucocorticoid therapy is dependent on the anti-inflammatory activity of these compounds, as glucocorticoids might also act

directly on muscle fibers by stabilizing the sarcolemma [28, 29]. To develop new and improved therapeutic approaches for the treatment of DMD, it is essential to characterize the effects of chronic inflammation on disease progression.

Inflammation in muscular dystrophy

In the pathogenesis of DMD, large numbers of inflammatory cells influence muscle pathology [7, 9, 30] [31–33]. However, the formation of muscle lesions is associated with immune cell infiltration that is clearly distinct from that which occurs during inflammatory responses to muscle injury in DMD patients and mouse models of muscular dystrophy [7, 9, 31, 32, 34]. The infiltrating mononuclear cells in the muscle tissues of DMD patients between 2 and 8 years of age are predominantly comprised of macrophages and T cells, while B cell infiltration is minimal [35, 36]. Meanwhile, in the muscles of *mdx* mice, the most widely used animal model for pathological analysis and evaluation of therapeutic approaches for DMD, the largest numbers of infiltrating immune cells were observed at 2–4 weeks of age. This infiltration, which was comprised of macrophages, T cells, and neutrophils, subsequently decreased in severity by 3 months of age [33].

Previous studies have observed the expression of pro-inflammatory factors (e.g., TNF-α, IFN-γ, IL-1, TGF-β, and MCP-1) prior to the onset of muscle degeneration in both DMD patients and *mdx* mice [37–39]. These factors also damage signals that have a profound impact on satellite cell behavior during the repair process. In an inflamed muscle of DMD, a persistently altered and reorganizing extracellular matrix (ECM) promotes damage and dysfunction. Exacerbated deposition of fibrin within the ECM promotes inflammation-mediated muscle degeneration and regeneration via $\alpha_M\beta_2$ integrin engagement on macrophages, which eventually could lead to fibrosis development and loss of normal muscle architecture [18, 40]. M1 macrophages induce the expression of pro-inflammatory cytokines, IL-1β, TNF-α, and IL-6, which in turn may negatively regulate satellite cell functions [18].

Notably, depleting or inhibiting the expression of pro-inflammatory factors has resulted in significant improvements in dystrophic muscle pathology [30, 31, 41]. For example, TNF-α-deficient *mdx* mice exhibited improved pathological progression within the diaphragm and limb muscles compared to those of *mdx* mice expressing TNF-α [38]. IFN-γ expression is elevated in *mdx* muscles during the stage of the disease when macrophage-mediated muscle damage is rampant and numbers of M1 macrophages are greatly elevated [10]. Ablation of IFN-γ reduced muscle damage in *mdx* mice, showing the significantly lower pathological markers such as macrophage/neutrophil infiltration and necrosis of myofibers [42].

As a result, these pro-inflammatory cytokines are considered key factors in mediating the muscle damage caused by M1 macrophages [37]. In addition, the expression level of IL-10, which plays a particularly important role in mediating the switch from the M1 to the M2 phenotype through suppression of pro-inflammatory responses in dystrophic muscles, was observed to increase concurrently with those of TNF-α and IFN-γ during the acute stage of DMD (8- to 15-fold higher compared to that observed in wild-type muscles), thereby promoting muscle repair [10, 42].

Immune-mediated regulation in DMD pathogenesis

IL-10 prevents the production of Th1-associated cytokines such as IFN-γ, TNF-α, IL-1β, and IL-6 in inflamed tissues [43]. As such, even low levels of IL-10 expression might affect the severity of inflammatory diseases and the immunopathology that results from high concentrations of pro-inflammatory cytokines. Indeed, IL-10-deficient mice display several features of the inflammatory bowel disease and Crohn's disease [44], as well as increased susceptibility to *Helicobacter hepaticus*-induced colitis [45]. Moreover, IL-10 null mice did not exhibited severely reduced muscle strength due to severe inflammation [46], while older IL-10-deficient *mdx* mice presented with abnormal cardiac function that shared several characteristics with DMD-associated cardiomyopathy [47–49]. Notably, this change in cardiac function is paralleled by an increase in myocardial fibrosis and the occurrence of foci of myocardial necrosis and inflammation [50–53]. However, it remains unclear whether inflammation in the dystrophic muscle affects cardiac and respiratory dysfunction.

To study the effects of inflammatory predisposition on the severity of DMD, we previously generated mice lacking both dystrophin and IL-10 (*IL-10⁻/⁻/mdx* mice) and subsequently demonstrated that these mice exhibit a phenotype that closely approximates that of DMD, as characterized by progressive muscle dysfunction associated with severe inflammation [54]. Indeed, compared to *mdx* mice, *IL-10⁻/⁻/mdx* mice exhibited severe cardiac muscle degeneration and extensive myofiber loss with increased immune cell infiltration. Specifically, higher levels of CD68⁺ macrophage infiltration were detected in the diaphragms and heart muscles of *IL-10⁻/⁻/mdx* mice than in those of *mdx* mice. Moreover, the cellular infiltration observed in *IL-10⁻/⁻/mdx* mice increased with age, without the alternative activation of M2 (CD207⁺) phenotypes observed in *mdx* mice. We also showed that ablation of IL-10 in dystrophic muscles results in increased levels of macrophage infiltration and continuously distributed activation of M1 phenotype.

We detected increased levels of IL-1α, IL-1β, IL-1ra, IL-16, RANTES, M-CSF, MIG, JE/MCP-1, and TIMP-1 in the diaphragm and/or heart tissues of aged *IL-10⁻/⁻/mdx* mice. NF-kB activity is thought to contribute to this up-regulation of pro-inflammatory factors, as the activity of this transcription factor is inhibited by IL-10 but not by other factors such as IL-6 and AP-1, or even by NF-kB itself [55]. Meanwhile, similar to IL-1 and the IL-1 receptor, increased production of IL-16, a potent chemoattractant for several immune cells, including monocytes and CD4⁺T cells [56], likely promotes further immune cell infiltration and activation within damaged muscles. Since IL-1β and IL-1ra are produced by M1 macrophages, our results suggest that there is strong activation of M1 macrophages in IL-10-deficient dystrophic muscles. We also demonstrated that elevated TGF-β signaling and type-I collagen expression resulted in widespread fibrosis within the diaphragm and heart tissues of *IL-10⁻/⁻/mdx* mice but not in those of *mdx* mice.

IL-10⁻/⁻/mdx mice had a smaller average body mass at the juvenile stage and a significantly shorter life span than *mdx* mice; however, the diaphragms of both *mdx* and *IL-10⁻/⁻/mdx* mice showed severe muscle degeneration and extensive myofiber loss with cell infiltration. Transient apnea was sporadically detected in *IL-10⁻/⁻/mdx* mice, and juvenile *IL-10⁻/⁻/mdx* mice displayed similar levels of fibrosis as aged *mdx* mice (8 months old). In association with the development of age-dependent heart failure, there was significantly increased cardiac fibrosis in the *IL-10⁻/⁻/mdx* compared to the aged *mdx* mice. Lastly, echocardiographic analysis detected decreased fractional shortening (FS) percentage and ejection fraction percent (EF%) values in *IL-10⁻/⁻/mdx* mice, indicating decreased left ventricular function with left and right ventricular dilatation (Fig. 1).

In summary, via pathophysiological analysis of *IL-10⁻/⁻/mdx* mice, we confirmed that a predisposition to inflammation results in both chronic inflammation and more severe cardiorespiratory dysfunction. As such, these mice should comprise a useful DMD model for long-term observation of disease phenotypes under various therapeutic conditions.

Therapeutic options

A number of anti-inflammatory therapies have been reported to have beneficial effects on DMD phenotypes [37]. For example, several anti-cytokine drugs that are currently available for use in human patients are capable of improving dystrophic muscle pathology [30, 57]. Meanwhile, the TNF-α blockers infliximab and etanercept and the IL-1 receptor antagonist anakinra, which have already been used for treatment of patients with rheumatoid arthritis and/or other inflammatory diseases [58, 59], could potentially be utilized in *mdx* mice [30, 57] and DMD patients. The proteasome inhibitor bortezomib has been shown to block NF-kB

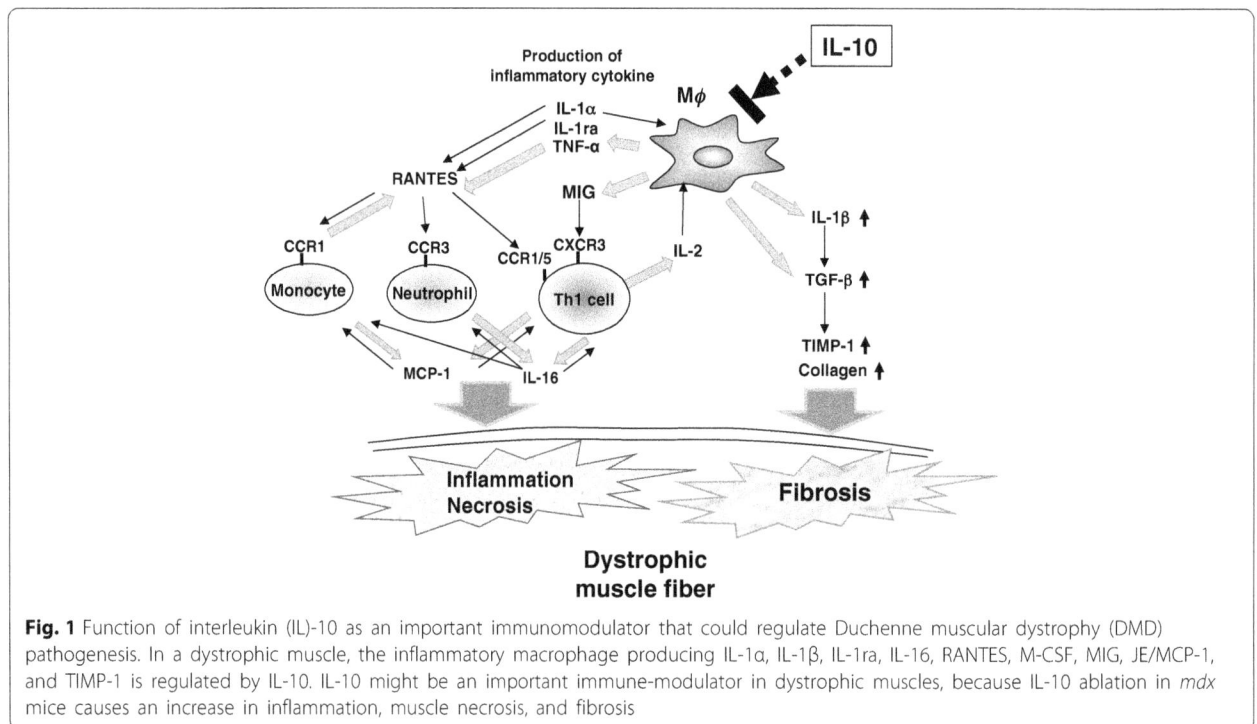

Fig. 1 Function of interleukin (IL)-10 as an important immunomodulator that could regulate Duchenne muscular dystrophy (DMD) pathogenesis. In a dystrophic muscle, the inflammatory macrophage producing IL-1α, IL-1β, IL-1ra, IL-16, RANTES, M-CSF, MIG, JE/MCP-1, and TIMP-1 is regulated by IL-10. IL-10 might be an important immune-modulator in dystrophic muscles, because IL-10 ablation in *mdx* mice causes an increase in inflammation, muscle necrosis, and fibrosis

activation, thereby improving the appearance of DMD dog (GRMD) muscle fibers and reducing both connective tissue deposition and inflammatory cell infiltration [60]. Moreover, treatment with an adeno-associated virus vector encoding a short hairpin RNA (shRNA) that specifically targets NF-kB ameliorated muscle pathologies in *mdx* mice [61].

The clinical interest in the therapeutic application of mesenchymal stromal cells (MSCs) is based on the anti-inflammatory properties of these cells and their ability to release cytokines into the surrounding environment, thereby modifying the developmental fate of neighboring cells. Combinatorial application of the immunosuppressive and/or anti-inflammatory effects and myogenic differentiation of MSCs comprises a promising therapeutic approach for treating muscle diseases.

Conclusions
In this review, we introduced immune-mediated systems that regulate the time course of disease progression in muscular dystrophy. We also suggested that IL-10 comprises an important immunomodulator that could be utilized to regulate the pathogenesis of this disease. Indeed, IL-10-based strategies would be promising for the treatment of cardiac and respiratory dysfunction in DMD. These findings are important for the development of effective therapies using anti-inflammatory drugs and/ or immunomodulatory stem cells, such as MSCs, to improve muscle and cardiorespiratory dysfunction.

Abbreviations
DMD, Duchenne muscular dystrophy; IFN, interferon; IL, interleukin; MHC, myosin heavy chain; MSCs, mesenchymal stem cells; Th1, T helper type 1; TNF, tumor necrosis factor

Acknowledgements
We thank our colleagues, laboratory members, and collaborators for their excellent experimental assistance and discussions.

Funding
Funding was received from a Grant-in-Aid for Scientific Research (KAKENHI) and a grant from the National Center for Child Health and Development (24-1).

Authors' contribution
All authors have read and approved the final manuscript.

Competing interests
We received research support from JCR Pharmaceuticals Co., Ltd., and TaKaRa Bio, Inc.

References
1. Spence HJ, Chen YJ, Winder SJ. Muscular dystrophies, the cytoskeleton and cell adhesion. Bioessays. 2002;24(6):542–52.
2. McDouall RM, Dunn MJ, Dubowitz V. Nature of the mononuclear infiltrate and the mechanism of muscle damage in juvenile dermatomyositis and Duchenne muscular dystrophy. J Neurol Sci. 1990;99(2-3):199–217.
3. Morrison J et al. T-cell-dependent fibrosis in the mdx dystrophic mouse. Lab Invest. 2000;80(6):881–91.
4. Morrison J et al. Effects of T-lymphocyte depletion on muscle fibrosis in the mdx mouse. Am J Pathol. 2005;166(6):1701–10.
5. Morrison J, Partridge T, Bou-Gharios G. Nude mutation influences limb skeletal muscle development. Matrix Biol. 2005;23(8):535–42.
6. Moran EM, Mastaglia FL. Cytokines in immune-mediated inflammatory myopathies: cellular sources, multiple actions and therapeutic implications. Clin Exp Immunol. 2014;178(3):405–15.

7. Spencer MJ et al. Helper (CD4(+)) and cytotoxic (CD8(+)) T cells promote the pathology of dystrophin-deficient muscle. Clin Immunol. 2001;98(2):235–43.

8. Spencer MJ, Tidball JG. Do immune cells promote the pathology of dystrophin-deficient myopathies? Neuromuscul Disord. 2001;11(6-7):556–64.

9. Wehling M, Spencer MJ, Tidball JG. A nitric oxide synthase transgene ameliorates muscular dystrophy in mdx mice. J Cell Biol. 2001;155(1):123–31.

10. Villalta SA et al. Shifts in macrophage phenotypes and macrophage competition for arginine metabolism affect the severity of muscle pathology in muscular dystrophy. Hum Mol Genet. 2009;18(3):482–96.

11. Tiidus PM. Radical species in inflammation and overtraining. Can J Physiol Pharmacol. 1998;76(5):533–8.

12. Allenbach Y et al. Th1 response and systemic treg deficiency in inclusion body myositis. PLoS One. 2014;9(3):e88788.

13. Moran EM, Mastaglia FL. The role of interleukin-17 in immune-mediated inflammatory myopathies and possible therapeutic implications. Neuromuscul Disord. 2014;24(11):943–52.

14. Tournadre A, Miossec P. A critical role for immature muscle precursors in myositis. Nat Rev Rheumatol. 2013;9(7):438–42.

15. Shachar I, Karin N. The dual roles of inflammatory cytokines and chemokines in the regulation of autoimmune diseases and their clinical implications. J Leukoc Biol. 2013;93(1):51–61.

16. Collins RA, Grounds MD. The role of tumor necrosis factor-alpha (TNF-alpha) in skeletal muscle regeneration. Studies in TNF-alpha(-/-) and TNF-alpha(-/-)/LT-alpha(-/-) mice. J Histochem Cytochem. 2001;49(8):989–1001.

17. Tidball JG, Villalta SA. Regulatory interactions between muscle and the immune system during muscle regeneration. Am J Physiol Regul Integr Comp Physiol. 2010;298(5):R1173–1187.

18. Kharraz Y et al. Macrophage plasticity and the role of inflammation in skeletal muscle repair. Mediators Inflamm. 2013;2013:491497.

19. Lagrota-Candido J et al. Characteristic pattern of skeletal muscle remodelling in different mouse strains. Int J Exp Pathol. 2010;91(6):522–9.

20. Segawa M et al. Suppression of macrophage functions impairs skeletal muscle regeneration with severe fibrosis. Exp Cell Res. 2008;314(17):3232–44.

21. Campbell KP. Three muscular dystrophies: loss of cytoskeleton-extracellular matrix linkage. Cell. 1995;80(5):675–9.

22. Ervasti JM et al. Deficiency of a glycoprotein component of the dystrophin complex in dystrophic muscle. Nature. 1990;345(6273):315–9.

23. Pasternak C, Wong S, Elson EL. Mechanical function of dystrophin in muscle cells. J Cell Biol. 1995;128(3):355–61.

24. Petrof BJ et al. Dystrophin protects the sarcolemma from stresses developed during muscle contraction. Proc Natl Acad Sci U S A. 1993;90(8):3710–4.

25. Manzur, A.Y., et al. Glucocorticoid corticosteroids for Duchenne muscular dystrophy. Cochrane Database Syst Rev. 2008: (1); CD003725.

26. Mantovani A et al. The chemokine system in diverse forms of macrophage activation and polarization. Trends Immunol. 2004;25(12):677–86.

27. Moxley 3rd RT et al. Practice parameter: corticosteroid treatment of Duchenne dystrophy: report of the Quality Standards Subcommittee of the American Academy of Neurology and the Practice Committee of the Child Neurology Society. Neurology. 2005;64(1):13–20.

28. Jacobs SC et al. Prednisone can protect against exercise-induced muscle damage. J Neurol. 1996;243(5):410–6.

29. Serra F et al. Inflammation in muscular dystrophy and the beneficial effects of non-steroidal anti-inflammatory drugs. Muscle Nerve. 2012; 46(5):773–84.

30. Hodgetts S et al. Reduced necrosis of dystrophic muscle by depletion of host neutrophils, or blocking TNF alpha function with etanercept in mdx mice. Neuromuscul Disord. 2006;16(9-10):591–602.

31. Cai B et al. Eosinophilia of dystrophin-deficient muscle is promoted by perforin-mediated cytotoxicity by T cell effectors. Am J Pathol. 2000;156(5): 1789–96.

32. Gorospe JR et al. A role for mast cells in the progression of Duchenne muscular dystrophy? Correlations in dystrophin-deficient humans, dogs, and mice. J Neurol Sci. 1994;122(1):44–56.

33. Spencer MJ et al. Myonuclear apoptosis in dystrophic mdx muscle occurs by perforin-mediated cytotoxicity. J Clin Invest. 1997;99(11):2745–51.

34. Gorospe JR et al. Dystrophin-deficient myofibers are vulnerable to mast cell granule-induced necrosis. Neuromuscul Disord. 1994;4(4):325–33.

35. Arahata K, Engel AG. Monoclonal antibody analysis of mononuclear cells in myopathies. I: quantitation of subsets according to diagnosis and sites of accumulation and demonstration and counts of muscle fibers invaded by T cells. Ann Neurol. 1984;16(2):193–208.

36. Engel AG, Arahata K. Mononuclear cells in myopathies: quantitation of functionally distinct subsets, recognition of antigen-specific cell-mediated cytotoxicity in some diseases, and implications for the pathogenesis of the different inflammatory myopathies. Hum Pathol. 1986;17(7):704–21.

37. Evans NP et al. Immune-mediated mechanisms potentially regulate the disease time-course of Duchenne muscular dystrophy and provide targets for therapeutic intervention. PM R. 2009;1(8):755–68.

38. Spencer MJ, Marino MW, Winckler WM. Altered pathological progression of diaphragm and quadriceps muscle in TNF-deficient, dystrophin-deficient mice. Neuromuscul Disord. 2000;10(8):612–9.

39. Pescatori M et al. Gene expression profiling in the early phases of DMD: a constant molecular signature characterizes DMD muscle from early postnatal life throughout disease progression. FASEB J. 2007;21(4):1210–26.

40. Serrano AL et al. Cellular and molecular mechanisms regulating fibrosis in skeletal muscle repair and disease. Curr Top Dev Biol. 2011;96:167–201.

41. Radley HG, Grounds MD. Cromolyn administration (to block mast cell degranulation) reduces necrosis of dystrophic muscle in mdx mice. Neurobiol Dis. 2006;23(2):387–97.

42. Villalta SA et al. IFN-gamma promotes muscle damage in the mdx mouse model of Duchenne muscular dystrophy by suppressing M2 macrophage activation and inhibiting muscle cell proliferation. J Immunol. 2011;187(10):5419–28.

43. Fiorentino DF et al. IL-10 inhibits cytokine production by activated macrophages. J Immunol. 1991;147(11):3815–22.

44. Tso VK et al. Metabolomic profiles are gender, disease and time specific in the interleukin-10 gene-deficient mouse model of inflammatory bowel disease. PLoS One. 2013;8(7):e67654.

45. Yang I et al. Intestinal microbiota composition of interleukin-10 deficient C57BL/6J mice and susceptibility to Helicobacter hepaticus-induced colitis. PLoS One. 2013;8(8):e70783.

46. Villalta SA et al. Interleukin-10 reduces the pathology of mdx muscular dystrophy by deactivating M1 macrophages and modulating macrophage phenotype. Hum Mol Genet. 2011;20(4):790–805.

47. Bia BL et al. Decreased myocardial nNOS, increased iNOS and abnormal ECGs in mouse models of Duchenne muscular dystrophy. J Mol Cell Cardiol. 1999;31(10):1857–62.

48. Wehling-Henricks M et al. Cardiomyopathy in dystrophin-deficient hearts is prevented by expression of a neuronal nitric oxide synthase transgene in the myocardium. Hum Mol Genet. 2005;14(14):1921–33.

49. Spurney CF et al. Dystrophin-deficient cardiomyopathy in mouse: expression of Nox4 and Lox are associated with fibrosis and altered functional parameters in the heart. Neuromuscul Disord. 2008;18(5):371–81.

50. Quinlan JG et al. Evolution of the mdx mouse cardiomyopathy: physiological and morphological findings. Neuromuscul Disord. 2004;14(8-9):491–6.

51. Van Erp C, Irwin NG, Hoey AJ. Long-term administration of pirfenidone improves cardiac function in mdx mice. Muscle Nerve. 2006;34(3):327–34.

52. Cohn RD et al. Myostatin does not regulate cardiac hypertrophy or fibrosis. Neuromuscul Disord. 2007;17(4):290–6.

53. Buyse GM et al. Long-term blinded placebo-controlled study of SNT-MC17/ idebenone in the dystrophin deficient mdx mouse: cardiac protection and improved exercise performance. Eur Heart J. 2009;30(1):116–24.

54. Nitahara-Kasahara Y et al. Dystrophic mdx mice develop severe cardiac and respiratory dysfunction following genetic ablation of the anti-inflammatory cytokine IL-10. Hum Mol Genet. 2014;23(15):3990–4000.

55. Wang P et al. Interleukin (IL)-10 inhibits nuclear factor kappa B (NF kappa B) activation in human monocytes. IL-10 and IL-4 suppress cytokine synthesis by different mechanisms. J Biol Chem. 1995;270(16):9558–63.

56. Cruikshank WW, Kornfeld H, Center DM. Interleukin-16. J Leukoc Biol. 2000;67(6):757–66.

57. Grounds MD, Torrisi J. Anti-TNF alpha (Remicade) therapy protects dystrophic skeletal muscle from necrosis. FASEB J. 2004;18(6):676–82.

58. Radley HG et al. Duchenne muscular dystrophy: focus on pharmaceutical and nutritional interventions. Int J Biochem Cell Biol. 2007;39(3):469–77.

59. Kalliolias GD, Liossis SN. The future of the IL-1 receptor antagonist anakinra: from rheumatoid arthritis to adult-onset Still's disease and systemic-onset juvenile idiopathic arthritis. Expert Opin Investig Drugs. 2008;17(3):349–59.

60. Araujo KP et al. Bortezomib (PS-341) treatment decreases inflammation and partially rescues the expression of the dystrophin-glycoprotein complex in GRMD dogs. PLoS One. 2013;8(4):e61367.

61. Yang Q et al. AAV-based shRNA silencing of NF-kappaB ameliorates muscle pathologies in mdx mice. Gene Ther. 2012;19(12):1196–204.

7

Pathophysiology and therapeutic potential of cardiac fibrosis

Hironori Hara, Norifumi Takeda[*] and Issei Komuro

Abstract

Inflammatory and fibrotic responses to myocardial damage are essential for cardiac repair; however, these responses often result in extensive fibrotic remodeling with impaired systolic function. Recent reports have suggested that such acute phase responses provide a favorable environment for endogenous cardiac regeneration, which is mainly driven by the division of pre-existing cardiomyocytes (CMs). Existing CMs in mammals can re-acquire proliferative activity after substantial cardiac damage, and elements other than CMs in the physiological and/or pathological environment, such as hypoxia, angiogenesis, and the polarity of infiltrating macrophages, have been reported to regulate replication. Cardiac fibroblasts comprise the largest cell population in terms of cell number in the myocardium, and they play crucial roles in the proliferation and protection of CMs. The in vivo direct reprogramming of functional CMs has been investigated in cardiac regeneration. Currently, growth factors, transcription factors, microRNAs, and small molecules promoting the regeneration and protection of these CMs have also been actively researched. Here, we summarize and discuss current studies on the relationship between cardiac inflammation and fibrosis, and cardiac regeneration and protection, which would be useful for the development of therapeutic strategies to treat and prevent advanced heart failure.

Keywords: Cardiomyocytes, Cardiac fibroblasts, Cardiac regeneration, Direct reprogramming, Angiogenesis

Background

The number of deaths from cardiovascular diseases is increasing globally, and cardiac dysfunction is closely associated with increased myocardial fibrosis and loss of cardiomyocytes (CMs). Although cardiac fibrosis plays an essential role in the response to pressure overload and/or cardiac injury such as myocardial infarction (MI), its excessive and prolonged reaction can lead to cardiac diastolic and systolic dysfunction. Therefore, the regulation of inflammation and fibrosis at the appropriate timing and duration is crucial for the preservation or recovery of cardiovascular homeostasis. Currently, the inhibition of the renin–angiotensin system (RAS) using angiotensin-converting enzyme (ACE) inhibitors and angiotensin receptor blockers (ARBs) is the most validated clinical strategy for treating patients with advanced heart failure [1].

Cardiac fibroblasts comprise the largest cell population in the myocardium [2], in terms of cell number, and they play a major role in fibrosis by producing the extracellular matrix (ECM) [3]. Cardiac fibroblasts interact with not only CMs but also with non-CMs, including vascular endothelial cells, smooth muscle cells, and immune cells, via direct and indirect cellular communications in an autocrine or paracrine manner [4] (Fig. 1). Recently, cardiac inflammation and fibrosis have been reported to be associated with the cardiac regenerative ability, which is mainly driven by the division of pre-existing CMs [5]; therefore, the modulation of the function of non-MCs for cardiac protection and regeneration has been actively investigated.

Here, we summarize and discuss current studies on the relationship between cardiac inflammation and fibrosis, and cardiac regeneration and protection, which would be useful for the development of therapeutic strategies for treating patients with advanced heart failure.

Main text

Types of cardiac fibrosis

Cardiac fibrosis is classified into two types: reactive fibrosis and reparative (replacement) fibrosis. Reactive fibrosis, which is characterized by the excessive deposition of ECM

* Correspondence: notakeda-tky@umin.ac.jp
Department of Cardiovascular Medicine, The University of Tokyo Hospital,
7-3-1 Hongo, Bunkyo-ku, Tokyo 113-8655, Japan

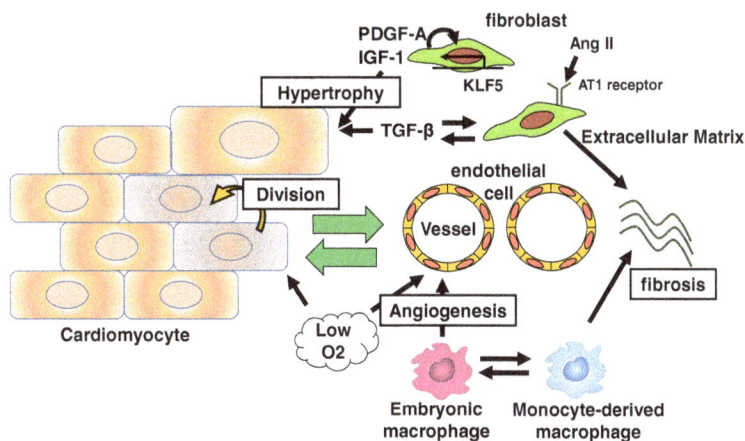

Fig. 1 Interactions among cardiac cells. Most types of cardiac cells, including CMs, cardiac fibroblasts, macrophages, and endothelial cells, regulate cardiac fibrosis and regeneration in a coordinated manner. Some paracrine factors from fibroblasts, including TGF-β and IGF-1, are known to promote the hypertrophic responses of CMs. The regulation of hypoxic environment and macrophage polarization is a key factor for enhancing crucial angiogenic responses involved in cardiac repair and regeneration

in the interstitial or perivascular spaces, is triggered by hemodynamic stress, such as pressure overload, and it is not directly associated with CM death [6, 7]. Reactive fibrosis is considered an adaptive response aimed at normalizing the increased wall stress and preserving the cardiac output. However, excessive fibrosis in interstitial spaces may cause mechanical stiffness, resulting in cardiac diastolic dysfunction, and impairment in electric conduction by forming a barrier between CMs, leading to cardiac systolic dysfunction. In addition, excessive fibrosis in perivascular areas decreases the flow of oxygen and nutrients, leading to an energy-starved condition in the myocardium [3]. Therefore, reactive cardiac fibrosis is closely associated with physiological and pathological cardiac conditions. Reparative fibrosis, which occurs in response to the loss of viable myocardium and forms a scar, maintains the structural integrity of the ventricles. A balance between reactive and reparative fibrosis is important for the prevention of excessive and inappropriate cardiac dysfunction, particularly after CM death due to cardiac injury, such as MI [8].

Cardiac fibroblasts

Cardiac fibroblasts are flat, spindle-shaped cells located in the myocardium, with multiple processes originating from the cell body, and lack a basement membrane [3]. They play a major role in cardiac fibrosis by producing the ECM [3], and recent studies have demonstrated that mouse cardiac resident fibroblasts derived from the cells of the embryonic proepicardial organ (PEO) [9, 10] are major cell type producing the fibrotic ECM in a pressure overload model [11, 12]. However, other cell types have also been reported as origins of cardiac fibroblasts such as embryonic endothelium, which undergo endothelial-to-mesenchymal transition (EndMT) [13], circulating bone

marrow cells [14], pericytes, and endothelial cells [15]. Because these cardiac fibroblasts lack a specific marker [11, 16, 17], investigating their regulation remains a challenging task.

Paracrine factors associated with cardiac fibrosis

Transforming growth factor-beta (TGF-β) and angiotensin II (Ang II) are major factors that regulate cardiac fibrosis (Fig. 1). The expression of the Ang II type 1 (AT1) receptor is greater in fibroblasts than in CMs [18]. The activation of the AT1 receptor in fibroblasts by Ang II leads to the secretion of TGF-β, which stimulates fibroblast proliferation and ECM protein synthesis in an autocrine manner [19, 20] and induces CM hypertrophy in a paracrine manner [18]. The infusion of a subpressor dose of Ang II into mice induces both cardiac hypertrophy and fibrosis [21]. Clinical studies have demonstrated that the blockade of RAS signaling by an ACE inhibitor or ARB effectively reduces cardiac fibrosis and remodeling and that this is independent of the blood pressure-lowering effect [22]. However, the concomitant use of aliskiren, the direct renin inhibitor, with an ACE inhibitor or ARB in post-MI patients with reduced left ventricular (LV) ejection fraction does not further attenuate LV remodeling but is instead associated with more adverse effects [23]. The effect of blocking RAS signaling for cardiac fibrosis may eventually reach a plateau, with an excessive RAS blockade increasing adverse effects. Therefore, the appropriate regulation of RAS signaling is important for the prevention of cardiac fibrosis without any adverse effects.

TGF-β plays an essential role in cardiac fibrosis. Treatment with a subpressor dose of Ang II does not induce cardiac hypertrophy or fibrosis in *Tgfb1*-deficient mice [24]. Therefore, Ang II-induced cardiac fibrosis is believed to be mediated, at least in part, by TGF-β. Although cardiac hypertrophy and fibrosis induced by TGF-β signaling are adaptive responses to acute stress [3], the inhibition of TGF-β signaling may be useful for treating cardiac fibrosis. Therapies targeting TGF-β signaling have already been investigated in various mammalian models. An intraperitoneal injection of a TGF-β neutralizing antibody into rats subjected to pressure overload not only inhibits fibroblast activation and cardiac fibrosis but also prevents diastolic dysfunction [25]. In contrast, in a mouse aortic banding-induced pressure overload model, an orally active, small molecule inhibitor of the TGF-β type I receptor (TGFBR1, also known as activin receptor-like kinase 5), SM16, attenuates the development of cardiac fibrosis but causes death because of rupture at the site of aortic banding [26]. Further studies using other models of hypertension-induced cardiac fibrosis, which are independent of aortic banding, should be conducted. An MI model has been used to evaluate the effects on cardiac fibrosis and function. The treatment of rats with GW788388, another orally active TGFBR1 inhibitor, 1 week after MI, significantly reduces TGF-β signaling and attenuates LV remodeling and systolic dysfunction [27]. However, an intraperitoneal injection of a TGF-β neutralizing antibody started either 1 week before or 5 days after MI increases mortality and exacerbates LV dilatation and contractile dysfunction in mice [28]. These results indicate that the consequences of inhibiting TGF-β are variable, depending on the disease model and the timing of inhibition, presumably because TGF-β signaling in the heart during stress plays different roles during the early and late phases of cardiovascular disease.

Cardiac hypertrophy induced by cardiac fibroblasts

Some paracrine factors from cardiac fibroblasts induce CM proliferation and/or hypertrophy. Embryonic, but not adult, cardiac fibroblasts secrete high levels of fibronectin, collagen III, and heparin-binding EGF-like growth factor

in mice. These embryonic cardiac fibroblast-specific factors collaboratively interact and promote embryonic CM proliferation (Fig. 2) [29]. On the other hand, in adult mice, various paracrine factors secreted by cardiac fibroblasts, including TGF-β, induce CM hypertrophy but not proliferation; the Krüppel-like factor 5 (KLF5) transcription factor expressed in adult cardiac fibroblasts promotes CM hypertrophy and cardiac protection (Fig. 1). KLF5 transactivates the expression of platelet-derived growth factor A (PDGF-A), which leads to the migration and proliferation of fibroblasts in an autocrine manner. Further, KLF5 transactivates insulin-like growth factor-1 (IGF-1) to promote CM hypertrophy in a paracrine manner. The cardiac fibroblast-specific deletion of *Klf5* ameliorates cardiac hypertrophy and fibrosis elicited by a moderate-intensity pressure overload [30]. On the other hand, a high-intensity pressure overload causes severe heart failure and early death in these mice. Furthermore, in wild-type mice, the administration of a peptide inhibitor of IGF-1 severely exacerbates heart failure induced by a high-intensity pressure overload. These results demonstrate that cardiac fibroblasts play pivotal roles in cardiac adaptive responses to pressure overload, which are, at least in part, regulated by IGF-1.

Cellular sources of cardiac regeneration

The regenerative capacity greatly differs in adult mammalian organs, and organ-specific stem cells have been shown to contribute to regeneration in certain organs, such as the intestines, lungs, taste buds, and hair follicles [31–34]. In the mammalian heart, CMs rapidly proliferate during embryonic development; however, CMs exit the cell cycle, with the number of binucleated CMs increasing soon after birth [35]. One-day-old mice retain an adequate CM proliferative capacity and can completely regenerate CMs after cardiac injury, such as

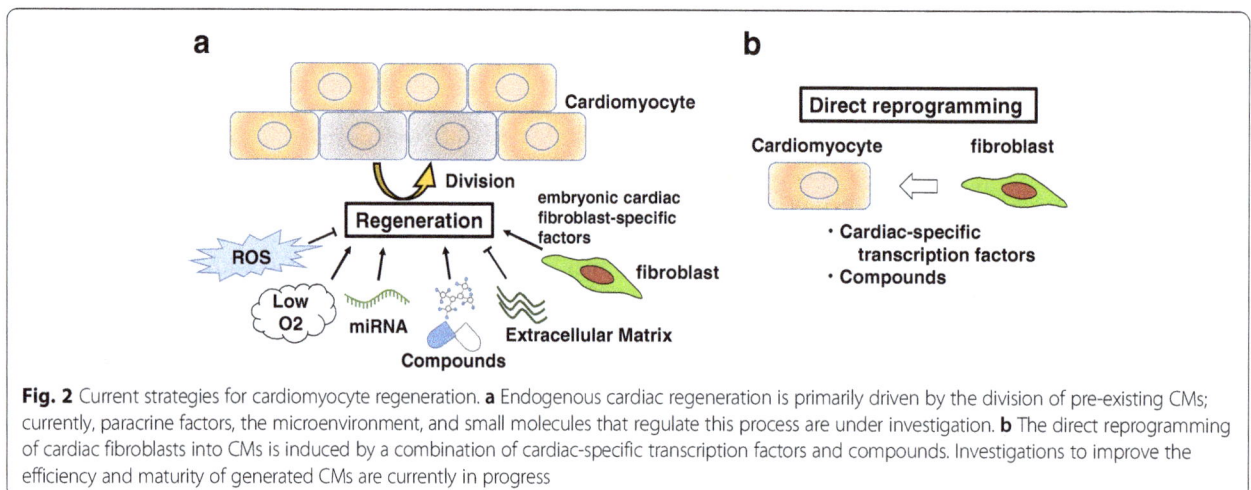

Fig. 2 Current strategies for cardiomyocyte regeneration. **a** Endogenous cardiac regeneration is primarily driven by the division of pre-existing CMs; currently, paracrine factors, the microenvironment, and small molecules that regulate this process are under investigation. **b** The direct reprogramming of cardiac fibroblasts into CMs is induced by a combination of cardiac-specific transcription factors and compounds. Investigations to improve the efficiency and maturity of generated CMs are currently in progress

apical resection and MI. In response to cardiac injury, inflammation causes the proliferation of myofibroblasts and increases fibrosis in the regenerative area, but the myocardium is finally regenerated without fibrosis. Therefore, cardiac fibroblast-rich scar tissue may be an important component of cardiac repair in neonatal mice [17]. However, this efficient regenerative potential is lost within the first week of postnatal life [36, 37]; adult mice do not regenerate CMs adequately to compensate for the impaired cardiac function, inducing reparative fibrosis after injury instead. On the other hand, in certain lower vertebrates, such as teleost fish and urodele amphibians, adult CMs have sufficient regenerative capacity, and the myocardium can completely regenerate after injury without forming scar tissue [38, 39]. It is not known what causes these differences in the regenerative capacity of CMs between adult mammals and lower vertebrates. The fact that CMs in lower vertebrates are mononucleated and smaller in size with fewer myofibrils than those in adult mammals may be responsible for the differences observed in the CM regenerative capacity between these groups [40].

Recently, it has been shown that new CMs in adult humans are generated throughout life at a low rate (0.5–1% per year) [41]. Additional lines of evidence support the fact that the regeneration of adult mammalian CMs occurs at a low rate, decreasing with age but increasing with injury [42]. Various cell sources of endogenously regenerated CMs, such as pre-existing CMs, cardiac progenitor cells (CPCs), and cardiac fibroblasts, have been proposed, and lineage-tracing analyses (fate map) and/or cell transplantation studies have been used to determine the cellular source of regenerated CMs [5, 43–50]. Cardiac stem cells, such as c-kit-positive CPCs, islet 1-positive CPCs, stem cell antigen-1-

positive CPCs, and cardiosphere-derived cells, have attracted considerable attention as cellular sources of regenerated CMs in the 2000s [44–47]; further, clinical trials using cardiac stem cells in patients with LV dysfunction have been conducted (Table 1). In the prospective, randomized CArdiosphere-Derived aUtologous stem CElls to reverse ventricUlar dySfunction (CADU-CEUS) trial, an intracoronary infusion of cardiosphere-derived cells 1.5–3 months after MI reduced cardiac scar size; however, it did not improve LV systolic function after 1 year [51, 52]. In the Stem Cell Infusion in Patients with Ischemic cardiOmyopathy (SCIPIO) trial, post-MI patients with LV dysfunction who underwent coronary artery bypass grafting (CABG) were assigned to receive treatment with an intracoronary infusion of autologous c-kit-positive CPCs 4 ± 1 months after CABG. An intracoronary infusion of c-kit-positive CPCs effectively improved the LV systolic function and reduced the infarct size in these patients [53]. However, it is unclear whether c-kit-positive CPCs efficiently transdifferentiated into functional CMs [44, 54, 55]. To examine this possibility, Molkentin et al. performed lineage-tracing analysis after the labeling of c-kit-expressing cells in adult mice and demonstrated that the number of c-kit-positive cells that transdifferentiated into new CMs was low (<0.03%) even after cardiac injury, indicating that c-kit-positive CPCs are not a major source of newly generated CMs [56].

Recent genetic fate-mapping experiments revealed that the regeneration of CMs occurs by the division of pre-existing CMs during normal aging at a low rate and that this process is enhanced in response to cardiac injury [5]. Therefore, it is accepted that new CMs are primarily derived from the division of pre-existing CMs. However, it

Table 1 Clinical trials using cardiac stem cells

Trial			CADUCEUS	SCIPIO
Inclusion criteria	Patient characteristics		Previous MI	Previous MI and CABG
	EF (%)		25–45	≤40
No. of patients	Total		25	23
	Cell therapy group		17	16
	Control group		8	7
Cell therapy	Type of cardiac stem cells		Cardiosphere-derived cells	c-kit-positive CPCs
	Dose of injected cells		12.5–25 million	0.5–1 million
	Delivery method		Intracoronary infusion	Intracoronary infusion
	Timing of delivery		1.5–3 months after MI	4 ± 1 months after CABG
Outcomes	EF (%); baseline/follow-up	Cell therapy	42.4/48.2 (1 year)	30.3/38.5 (4 months)
		Control	42.5/48.1 (1 year)	30.1/30.2 (4 months)
	Scar size (%LV or g); baseline/follow-up	Cell therapy	23.8/12.9 (1 year) (%LV)	32.6/22.8 (1 year) (g)
		Control	22.4/20.3 (1 year) (%LV)	N/A
References			[51, 52]	[53]

CABG coronary artery bypass grafting;, *CPCs* cardiac progenitor cells, *EF* ejection fraction, *LV* left ventricular, *MI* myocardial infarction, *N/A* not available

remains unclear what prevents cell division in adult mammalian CMs whose endogenous regenerative capacity is insufficient to restore cardiac function after substantial damage. Therefore, growth factors, transcription factors, microRNAs, and small molecules that stimulate CM replication have been actively studied (Table 2) [37, 57–67]. Furthermore, the roles of the physiological and pathological environments of the heart in the regulation of cardiac regeneration have been studied with great detail (Fig. 1).

Impact of reactive oxygen species on CM regeneration

Recently, considerable attention has been given to the impact of reactive oxygen species (ROS) on cardiovascular diseases. Cardiac injury has been shown to increase the amount of ROS in the heart, which induces CM cell cycle arrest via the activation of responses to DNA damage (Fig. 2) [68, 69]. The inhibition of ROS by pretreatment with N-acetyl-L-cysteine has been shown to promote CM regeneration after ischemia–reperfusion injury even in 21-day-old mice [69]. In addition, the presence of oxygen in the environment has been reported to influence the production or scavenging of ROS and regeneration of CMs. Hyperoxic (100% oxygen) and hypoxic (15% oxygen) environments have been found to diminish and enhance CM proliferation, respectively, in neonatal mice with adequate CM regenerative capacities (Fig. 2) [69]. Furthermore, in adult mice, gradual exposure to severe hypoxia after MI, in which inspired oxygen is gradually decreased by 1% beginning 1 week after MI for 2 weeks, and then maintained at 7% for another 2 weeks, has been found to induce CM regeneration and coronary angiogenesis, resulting in improvements in the LV systolic function [70]. To evaluate the proliferation of hypoxic CMs in the adult heart, hypoxic CMs in αMHC-$creERT2$-ODD; $R26R$/$tdTomato$ mice were genetically labeled at 2 months of age and fate mapped for 1 month under normal conditions; the results of this study demonstrated that labeled hypoxic CMs have a higher proliferative capacity than unlabeled CMs and can be a source of newly generated CMs [71].

Role of macrophages in cardiac regeneration

One-day-old mice can completely regenerate their hearts after MI injury. However, 14-day-old mice do not retain sufficient capacity for cardiac regeneration and cause fibrosis in response to cardiac injury. Clodronate liposome-mediated depletion of monocytes/macrophages in 1-day-old mice after MI reduces the angiogenic response, blocks the cardiac regenerative capacity, and induces cardiac fibrosis and dysfunction [72]. To identify the role of cardiac monocytes/macrophages in cardiac regeneration, immunophenotyping and gene expression profiling of cardiac monocytes/macrophages from 1-day-old and 14-day-old mice were isolated and compared

after MI [72]. Regenerative macrophages from 1-day-old mice displayed both M1- and M2-associated gene transcription patterns and expressed more chemokines, proangiogenic factors, and oxidative stress responders, which may facilitate the formation of new myocardium than macrophages from 14-day-old mice.

Embryonic-derived resident cardiac macrophages (MHC-II^{low}CCR2$^-$) and two types of resident cardiac macrophages (MHC-II^{low}CCR2$^-$ and MHC-II^{high}CCR2$^-$) are the major populations of monocytes/macrophages in neonatal and adult mouse hearts, respectively; monocytes (MHC-II^{low}CCR2$^+$) and monocyte-derived macrophages (MHC-II^{high}CCR2$^+$) are not abundant in either neonatal or adult hearts under normal physiological conditions [73]. To elucidate essential cardiac monocyte/macrophage subsets involved in cardiac regeneration, Lavine et al. used a diphtheria toxin receptor-mediated CM ablation mouse model [73], in which cardiac injury was induced without concomitant systemic inflammation. In response to diphtheria toxin receptor-mediated cardiac injury, the neonatal heart selectively expanded the population of embryonic-derived resident cardiac macrophages and cardiac dysfunction recovered to baseline. In contrast, in adult mice, the heart recruits CCR2$^+$ pro-inflammatory monocytes and monocyte-derived macrophages and loses CCR2$^-$ resident cardiac macrophages after cardiac injury; cardiac function recovery was not observed. However, the administration of selective CCR2 inhibitors in adult mice after cardiac injury inhibited CCR2$^+$ monocyte recruitment to the heart and preserved CCR2$^-$ resident cardiac macrophages, resulting in reduced inflammation and enhanced angiogenesis. Collectively, embryonic-derived resident cardiac macrophages are key mediators of angiogenesis, leading to cardiac regeneration in response to cardiac injury (Fig. 3).

Interactions between endothelial cells and fibroblasts

EndMT is a fundamental cellular mechanism that regulates embryonic development and fibrotic diseases. During the embryonic development of the heart, the endocardium undergoes EndMT and forms an atrioventricular cushion: the primordial valves and septa of the adult heart [74]. Zeisberg et al. demonstrated that Tie1-expressing endothelial cells in the adult heart underwent EndMT and differentiated into fibroblasts during cardiac fibrosis in response to pressure overload [15]. Endothelial cells undergoing EndMT lost tight junctions that hold neighboring cells, gained the ability to move, and contributed to the total pool of cardiac fibroblasts. Although endothelial cells are not major origins of cardiac fibroblasts under normal conditions, inflammation induces EndMT of endothelial cells. As a result, approximately one-third of all cardiac fibroblasts originated from endothelial cells in the fibrotic heart in response to pressure overload. During this process, TGF-β1

Table 2 Growth factors, transcription factors, microRNAs, and small molecules that stimulate CM replication

		Models/treatments		Species	Age or weight/cells	Follow-up	Markers of proliferation	Functional improvements comments	References
Factors	Neuregulin 1	In vitro		Rat	ARCM		BrdU, Aurora B		[57]
		In vivo	IP injection	Mouse	12 weeks	9 days	BrdU, pH3, Aurora B		
		MI	IP injection after MI	Mouse	8 weeks	14 weeks	BrdU, pH3, Aurora B	EF, scar size	
	Periostin	In vitro		Rat	ARCM		BrdU, Aurora B		[58]
		In vivo	Injection into the myocardium	Rat	300 g	7 days	BrdU, Aurora B		
		MI	Gelfoam patches to epicardial after MI	Rat	300 g	12 weeks	BrdU, Aurora B (1 and 12 weeks)	EF, FS, scar size	
	Oncostatin M	In vitro		Rat	NRCM		EdU		[59]
		MI	IP injection after MI	Mouse	12 weeks	21 days		survival, EF	
	Salvador (Salv)	In vivo	NKX 2.5-Cre; Salv flox/flox (Salv CKO)	Mouse	E12.5, P2		pH3 (E12.5)	Thickened ventricular walls, enlarged ventricular chambers	[60]
	Yes-associated protein (Yap)	In vivo	αMHC-YapS112A	Mouse	P28	21 days	pH3, Aurora B (7 days)	FS, scar size (21 days)	[61]
	Yes-associated protein (Yap)	In vivo	αMHC-rtTA; Yap, induction by doxycycline	Mouse	8 weeks	5 weeks	EdU, pH3	EF, scar size	[62]
		In vivo	AAV9-cTnT-hYap injection into the myocardium	Mouse	10–12 weeks	23 weeks	EdU (5 days)	FS (4 weeks), survival (23 weeks)	
miRNAs	miR-15 family	In vivo	anti-miR-15/16 s.c. injection	Mouse	P2	10 days	pH3		[63]
	miR-15 family	I/R	anti-miR-15 s.c. injection before I/R	Mouse	P21	21 days	pH3 (7 days)	FS (21 days)	[37]
	miR-590, miR-199a	In vitro	Transfection	Rat/Mouse	ARCM, NRCM, NMCM		Ki67, EdU, pH3, Aurora B		[64]
		In vivo	hsa-miR-590-3p or hsa-miR-199a-3p injection into the myocardium	Rat	P0	4 days	EdU		
		In vivo	AAV9-miR-590 or AAV9-miR-199a IP injection	Mouse	P0	12 days	pH3		
		MI	AAV9-miR-590 or AAV9-miR-199a IP injection after MI	Mouse	8–12 weeks	60 days	EdU	EF, FS, scar size	
	miR-222	In vitro	Transfection	Rat	NRCM		Ki67, EdU		[65]
		I/R	αMHC-tTA; miR-222 induction by doxycycline deprivation before I/R	Mouse	10–12 weeks	6 weeks	EdU. pH3	FS, scar size	
	miR-17-92 family	In vitro	Transfection	Rat	NRCM		EdU, Aurora B		[66]
		In vivo	NKX 2.5-Cre; miR-17–92	Mouse	E16.5, P4		pH3		
		In vivo	αMHC-Cre; miR-17–92	Mouse	P15		EdU, pH3, Aurora B		
		MI	αMHC-MerCreMer; miR-17–92 induction by tamoxifen after MI	Mouse	2 months	4 months	EdU	FS, scar size	
Small molecule	BIO	In vitro		Rat	NRCM		BrdU, pH3		[67]

AAV adeno-associated virus, ARCM adult rat cardiomyocytes, BrdU 5-bromo-2'-deoxyuridine, EdU 5-ethynyl-2'-deoxyuridine, EF ejection fraction, FS fractional shortening, IP intraperitoneal, I/R Ischemia/reperfusion, MI myocardial infarction, NMCM neonatal mouse cardiomyocytes, NRCM neonatal rat cardiomyocytes, pH3 Phospho-Histone H3; s.c. subcutaneous

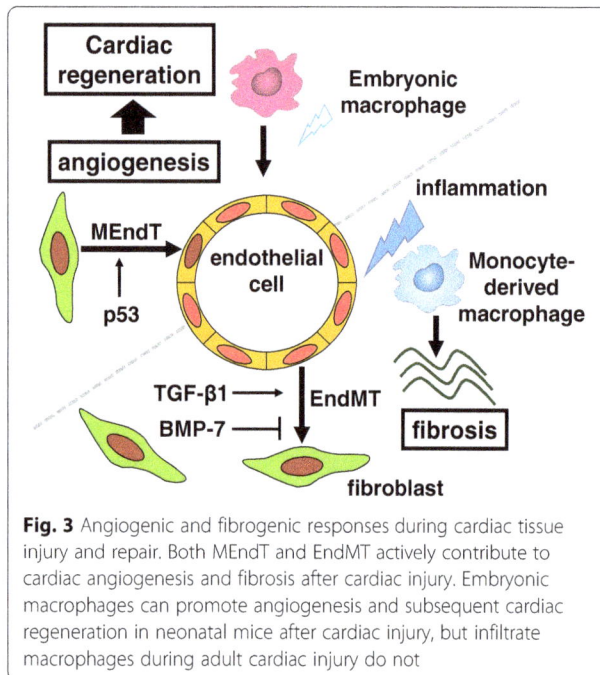

Fig. 3 Angiogenic and fibrogenic responses during cardiac tissue injury and repair. Both MEndT and EndMT actively contribute to cardiac angiogenesis and fibrosis after cardiac injury. Embryonic macrophages can promote angiogenesis and subsequent cardiac regeneration in neonatal mice after cardiac injury, but infiltrate macrophages during adult cardiac injury do not

induces EndMT, whereas bone morphogenic protein 7 (BMP-7) prevents EndMT and preserves the endothelial phenotype [15]. Therefore, the anti-fibrotic effects of recombinant human BMP-7 have been investigated. An intraperitoneal injection of recombinant human BMP-7 inhibited EndMT and the progression of cardiac fibrosis and improved diastolic cardiac function in a moderate-intensity pressure overload model. Furthermore, the inhibition of EndMT and cardiac fibrosis by recombinant human BMP-7 has been observed in a mouse model of chronic heart rejection caused by heterotopic heart transplantation with a class II major histocompatibility mismatch between donor and recipient [15].

Cardiac fibroblasts can undergo mesenchymal-to-endothelial transition (MEndT) immediately after ischemic cardiac injury [75]. Approximately 30% of fibroblasts in the injury zone undergo MEndT, and fibroblast-derived endothelial cells exhibit anatomical and functional characteristics of native endothelial cells and contribute to angiogenesis of the injured heart. p53, a transcription factor, regulates MEndT in cardiac fibroblasts [75]. The loss of p53 in Col1a2-expressing fibroblasts severely decreases the formation of fibroblast-derived endothelial cells, reduces the post-MI vascular area, and worsens cardiac function. Conversely, the stimulation of the p53 pathway after ischemic cardiac injury by an intraperitoneal injection of the small molecule: reactivation of p53 and induction of tumor cell apoptosis (RITA), which inhibits ubiquitin-mediated p53 degradation, augments MEndT, enhances angiogenesis, and improves cardiac function. However, although

cardiac fibroblasts cultured in vitro under serum-free conditions have been found to form tubular structures resembling the endothelial cell architecture and express endothelial markers, cardiac fibroblasts cultured under serum-fed conditions fail to generate tubular structures, even when p53 is artificially overexpressed. This result suggests that p53 expression alone is insufficient to induce MEndT and that the microenvironment, growth factors, and other signals are involved in this process. Collectively, these close interactions between endothelial cells and fibroblasts regulate cardiac fibrosis and angiogenesis (Fig. 3), and the regulation of both EndMT and MEndT is a potential therapeutic target for enhancing cardiac repair.

Direct reprogramming of cardiac fibroblasts into CMs

In 2006, Takahashi and Yamanaka generated induced pluripotent stem (iPS) cells from mouse fibroblasts by introducing four factors: Oct3/4, Sox2, c-Myc, and Klf4 [76]. Subsequently, the direct reprogramming of fibroblasts by lineage-specific transcription factors into the primary functional cells of each organ, such as neurons, hepatocytes, and renal tubular epithelial cells, was accomplished [77–80]. Further, the direct reprogramming of mouse cardiac fibroblasts into CMs is induced by a combination of cardiac-specific transcription factors (Gata4, Mef2c, and Tbx5) in vitro [81]. Furthermore, endogenous cardiac fibroblasts were directly reprogrammed into CMs by the retrovirus-mediated delivery of cardiac-specific transcription factors in vivo, with such newly generated CMs reducing scar formation and cardiac dysfunction after MI [49, 50]. Several laboratories demonstrated that in vivo reprogramming yields higher quality of CMs than in vitro reprogramming. These results suggest that factors within the native microenvironment, such as the ECM, growth factors, local signals, and mechanical forces, enhance the maturity of CMs in the heart.

Although the direct reprogramming of cardiac fibroblasts into CMs in vivo can be a new cardiac regenerative therapy (Fig. 2), the efficiency of reprogramming is currently low to adequately improve cardiac function, and the mechanisms of reprogramming and properties of newly generated CMs have not yet been fully defined [82]. Therefore, the modification of transcription factors and induction of microRNAs have been studied, with the goal of improving the quality of cardiac reprogramming [50, 83]; the addition of factors that regulate the native microenvironment may enhance the efficacy of cardiac direct reprogramming.

Conclusions

Most types of cardiac cells, including cardiac fibroblasts, CMs, macrophages, and endothelial cells, regulate cardiac fibrosis in a coordinated manner; therefore, various elements and signals could be therapeutic targets for cardiac protection and the prevention of cardiac fibrosis. We commonly use ACE inhibitors or ARBs to block RAS signaling and inhibit cardiac fibrosis in patients with hypertension and cardiac diseases; however, there are few effective therapies that target other pathways involved in the prevention of cardiac fibrosis. Although targeting TGF-β signaling is a promising strategy, optimizing the appropriate timing and duration of treatment remains a challenging task.

Recently, it has been revealed that inflammatory and fibrotic responses to myocardial damage are essential for cardiac repair as well as cardiac regeneration; paracrine factors, the microenvironment, and small molecules that regulate these processes are all currently under investigation. Non-CMs, including macrophages, fibroblasts, and endothelial cells, cooperate with CMs to promote cardiac repair and regeneration. The regulation of the hypoxic environment and macrophage polarization may enhance crucial angiogenic responses involved in these processes. Further, the direct reprogramming of cardiac fibroblasts into functional CMs is an attractive strategy, and currently, investigations to improve the efficiency and maturity of generated CMs are in progress. Further research to unravel the regulatory mechanisms underlying cardiac fibrosis and regeneration will aid the development of therapeutic strategies to treat and prevent advanced heart failure.

Abbreviations
AAV: Adeno-associated virus; ACE: Angiotensin-converting enzyme; Ang II: Angiotensin II; ARB: Angiotensin receptor blocker; ARCM: Adult rat cardiomyocytes; AT1: Ang II type 1; BMP-7: Bone morphogenic protein 7; BrdU: 5-bromo-2'-deoxyuridine; CABG: Coronary artery bypass grafting; CM: Cardiomyocyte; CPCs: Cardiac progenitor cells; ECM: Extracellular matrix; EdU: 5-ethynyl-2'- deoxyuridine; EF: Ejection fraction; EndMT: Endothelial-to-mesenchymal transition; FS: Fractional shortening; I/R: Ischemia/reperfusion; IGF-1: Insulin-like growth factor-1; IP: Intraperitoneal; KLF5: Krüppel-like factor 5; LV: Left ventricular; MEndT: Mesenchymal-to-endothelial transition; MI: Myocardial infarction; N/A: Not available; NMCM: Neonatal mouse cardiomyocytes; NRCM: Neonatal rat cardiomyocytes; PDGF-A: Platelet-derived growth factor-A; PEO: Proepicardial organ; pH3: Phospho-Histone H3; RAS: Renin–angiotensin system; RITA: Reactivation of p53 and induction of tumor cell apoptosis; ROS: Reactive oxygen species; s.c.: Subcutaneous; TGFBR1: TGF-β type I receptor; TGF-β: Transforming growth factor-beta

Acknowledgements
We would like to express our sincere gratitude to all the researchers, collaborators, technical assistants, and secretaries for contributing to the studies cited in this review article. We also thank the grants supporting our research work.

Funding
There is no funding support for this review article.

Authors' contributions
HH drafted the manuscript, and HH, NT, and IK revised it. All authors read and approved the final manuscript.

Competing interests
The authors declare that they have no competing interests.

References
1. Akazawa H, Yabumoto C, Yano M, Kudo-Sakamoto Y, Komuro I. ARB and cardioprotection. Cardiovasc Drugs Ther. 2013;27:155–60.
2. Banerjee I, Fuseler JJW, Price RL, Borg TK, Baudino T, Jw F, et al. Determination of cell types and numbers during cardiac development in the neonatal and adult rat and mouse. Am Physiol. 2007;293:1883–91.
3. Takeda N, Manabe I. Cellular interplay between cardiomyocytes and nonmyocytes in cardiac remodeling. Int J Inflam. 2011;2011:535241.
4. Pellman J, Zhang J, Sheikh F. Myocyte-fibroblast communication in cardiac fibrosis and arrhythmias: mechanisms and model systems. J Mol Cell Cardiol. 2016;94:22–31.
5. Senyo SE, Steinhauser ML, Pizzimenti CL, Yang VK, Cai L, Wang M, et al. Mammalian heart renewal by pre-existing cardiomyocytes. Nature. 2013;493:433–6.
6. Anderson KR, Sutton MG, Lie JT. Histopathological types of cardiac fibrosis in myocardial disease. J Pathol. 1979;128:79–85.
7. Weber KT. Cardiac interstitium in health and disease: the fibrillar collagen network. J Am Coll Cardiol. 1989;13:1637–52.
8. Ramos G, Hofmann U, Frantz S. Myocardial fibrosis seen through the lenses of T-cell biology. J Mol Cell Cardiol. 2016;92:41–5.
9. Mikawa T, Gourdie RG. Pericardial mesoderm generates a population of coronary smooth muscle cells migrating into the heart along with ingrowth of the epicardial organ. Dev Biol. 1996;174:221–32.
10. Cai C-L, Martin JC, Sun Y, Cui L, Wang L, Ouyang K, et al. A myocardial lineage derives from Tbx18 epicardial cells. Nature. 2008;454:104–8.
11. Moore-Morris T, Guimarães-Camboa N, Banerjee I, Zambon AC, Kisseleva T, Velayoudon A, et al. Resident fibroblast lineages mediate pressure overload-induced cardiac fibrosis. J Clin Invest. 2014;124:2921–34.
12. Ali SR, Ranjbarvaziri S, Talkhabi M, Zhao P, Subat A, Hojjat A, et al. Developmental heterogeneity of cardiac fibroblasts does not predict pathological proliferation and activation. Circ Res. 2014;115:625–35.
13. Moore-morris T, Guimarães-camboa N, Banerjee I, Zambon AC, Kisseleva T, Velayoudon A, et al. Resident fibroblast lineages mediate pressure overload–induced cardiac fibrosis. J Clin Invest. 2014;124:1–14.
14. Van Amerongen MJ, Bou-Gharios G, Popa ER, Van Ark J, Petersen AH, Van Dam GM, et al. Bone marrow-derived myofibroblasts contribute functionally to scar formation after myocardial infarction. J Pathol. 2008;214:377–86.
15. Zeisberg EM, Tarnavski O, Zeisberg M, Dorfman AL, McMullen JR, Gustafsson E, et al. Endothelial-to-mesenchymal transition contributes to cardiac fibrosis. Nat Med. 2007;13:952–61.
16. Travers JG, Kamal FA, Robbins J, Yutzey KE, Blaxall BC. Cardiac fibrosis: the fibroblast awakens. Circ Res. 2016;118:1021–40.
17. Moore-Morris T, Cattaneo P, Puceat M, Evans SM. Origins of cardiac fibroblasts. J Mol Cell Cardiol. 2016;91:1–5.
18. Gray MO, Long CS, Kalinyak JE, Li HT, Karliner JS. Angiotensin II stimulates cardiac myocyte hypertrophy via paracrine release of TGF-β1 and endothelin-1 from fibroblasts. Cardiovasc Res. 1998;40:352–63.
19. Villarreal FJ, Kim NN, Ungab GD, Printz MP, Dillmann WH. Identification of functional angiotensin II receptors on rat cardiac fibroblasts. Circulation. 1993;88:2849–61.
20. Rosenkranz S. TGF-β1 and angiotensin networking in cardiac remodeling. Cardiovasc Res. 2004;63:423–32.
21. Harada K, Komuro I, Shiojima I, Hayashi D, Kudoh S, Mizuno T, et al. Pressure overload induces cardiac hypertrophy in angiotensin II type 1A receptor knockout mice. Circulation. 1998;97:1952–9.

22. Hoogwerf BJ. Renin-angiotensin system blockade and cardiovascular and renal protection. Am J Cardiol. 2010;105:30A–5A.

23. Solomon SD, Hee Shin S, Shah A, Skali H, Desai A, Kober L, et al. Effect of the direct renin inhibitor aliskiren on left ventricular remodelling following myocardial infarction with systolic dysfunction. Eur Heart J. 2011;32:1227–34.

24. Schultz JEJ, Witt SA, Glascock BJ, Nieman ML, Reiser PJ, Nix SL, et al. TGF-β1 mediates the hypertrophic cardiomyocyte growth induced by angiotensin II. J Clin Invest. 2002;109:787–96.

25. Kuwahara F, Kai H, Tokuda K, Kai M, Takeshita A, Egashira K, et al. Transforming growth factor-β function blocking prevents myocardial fibrosis and diastolic dysfunction in pressure-overloaded rats. Circulation. 2002;106:130–5.

26. Engebretsen KVT, Skårdal K, Bjørnstad S, Marstein HS, Skrbic B, Sjaastad I, et al. Attenuated development of cardiac fibrosis in left ventricular pressure overload by SM16, an orally active inhibitor of ALK5. J Mol Cell Cardiol. 2014;76:148–57.

27. Tan SM, Zhang Y, Connelly K, Gilbert RE, Kelly DJ. Targeted inhibition of activin receptor-like kinase 5 signaling attenuates cardiac dysfunction following myocardial infarction. Am J Physiol Heart Circ Physiol. 2010;298:H1415–25.

28. Frantz S, Hu K, Adamek A, Wolf J, Sallam A, Maier SKG, et al. Transforming growth factor beta inhibition increases mortality and left ventricular dilatation after myocardial infarction. Basic Res Cardiol. 2008;103:485–92.

29. Ieda M, Tsuchihashi T, Ivey KN, Ross RS, Hong TT, Shaw RM, et al. Cardiac fibroblasts regulate myocardial proliferation through β1 integrin signaling. Dev Cell. 2009;16:233–44.

30. Takeda N, Manabe I, Uchino Y, Eguchi K, Matsumoto S, Nishimura S, et al. Cardiac fibroblasts are essential for the adaptive response of the murine heart to pressure overload. J Clin Invest. 2010;120:254–65.

31. Takeda N, Jain R, LeBoeuf MR, Wang Q, Lu MM, Epstein J. Interconversion between intestinal stem cell populations in distinct niches. Science. 2011;334:1420–4.

32. Takeda N, Jain R, Leboeuf MR, Padmanabhan A, Wang Q, Li L, et al. Hopx expression defines a subset of multipotent hair follicle stem cells and a progenitor population primed to give rise to K6+ niche cells. Development. 2013;140:1655–64.

33. Takeda N, Jain R, Li D, Li L, Lu MM, Epstein J. Lgr5 identifies progenitor cells capable of taste bud regeneration after injury. PLoS ONE. 2013;8:1.

34. Jain R, Barkauskas CE, Takeda N, Bowie EJ, Aghajanian H, Wang Q, et al. Plasticity of Hopx(+) type I alveolar cells to regenerate type II cells in the lung. Nat Commun. 2015;6:6727.

35. Soonpaa MH, Kim KK, Pajak L, Franklin M, Field LJ. Cardiomyocyte DNA synthesis and binucleation during murine development. Am J Physiol. 1996;271:H2183–9.

36. Porrello ER, Mahmoud AI, Simpson E, Hill J, Richardson J, Olson EN, et al. Transient regenerative potential of the neonatal mouse heart. Science. 2011;331:1078–80.

37. Porrello ER, Mahmoud AI, Simpson E, Johnson B, Grinsfelder D, Canseco D, et al. Regulation of neonatal and adult mammalian heart regeneration by the miR-15 family. Proc Natl Acad Sci U S A. 2013;110:187–92.

38. Poss KD, Wilson LG, Keating MT. Heart regeneration in zebrafish. Science. 2002;298:2188–90.

39. Witman N, Murtuza B, Davis B, Arner A, Morrison JI. Recapitulation of developmental cardiogenesis governs the morphological and functional regeneration of adult newt hearts following injury. Dev Biol. 2011;354:67–76.

40. Kikuchi K, Poss KD. Cardiac regenerative capacity and mechanisms. Annu Rev Cell Dev Biol. 2012;28:719–41.

41. Bergmann O, Bhardwaj RD, Bernard S, Zdunek S, Barnabé-Heider F, Walsh S, et al. Evidence for cardiomyocyte renewal in humans. Science. 2009;324:98–102.

42. Garbern JC, Lee RT. Cardiac stem cell therapy and the promise of heart regeneration. Cell Stem Cell. 2013;12:689–98.

43. Van Berlo JH, Molkentin JD. An emerging consensus on cardiac regeneration. Nat Med. 2014;20:1386–93.

44. Beltrami AP, Barlucchi L, Torella D, Baker M, Limana F, Chimenti S, et al. Adult cardiac stem cells are multipotent and support myocardial regeneration. Cell. 2003;114:763–76.

45. Laugwitz K-L, Moretti A, Lam J, Gruber P, Chen Y, Woodard S, et al. Postnatal isl1+ cardioblasts enter fully differentiated cardiomyocyte lineages. Nature. 2005;433:647–53.

46. Oh H, Bradfute SB, Gallardo TD, Nakamura T, Gaussin V, Mishina Y, et al. Cardiac progenitor cells from adult myocardium: homing, differentiation, and fusion after infarction. Proc Natl Acad Sci U S A. 2003;100:12313–8.

47. Messina E, De Angelis L, Frati G, Morrone S, Chimenti S, Fiordaliso F, et al. Isolation and expansion of adult cardiac stem cells from human and murine heart. Circ Res. 2004;95:911–21.

48. Anversa P, Kajstura J, Rota M, Leri A. Regenerating new heart with stem cells. J Clin Invest. 2013;123:62–70.

49. Qian L, Huang Y, Spencer CI, Foley A, Vedantham V, Liu L, et al. In vivo reprogramming of murine cardiac fibroblasts into induced cardiomyocytes. Nature. 2012;485:593–8.

50. Song K, Nam Y-J, Luo X, Qi X, Tan W, Huang GN, et al. Heart repair by reprogramming non-myocytes with cardiac transcription factors. Nature. 2012;485:599–604.

51. Makkar RR, Smith RR, Cheng K, Malliaras K, Thomson LEJ, Berman D, et al. Intracoronary cardiosphere-derived cells for heart regeneration after myocardial infarction (CADUCEUS): a prospective, randomised phase 1 trial. Lancet. 2012;379:895–904.

52. Malliaras K, Makkar RR, Smith RR, Cheng K, Wu E, Bonow RO, et al. Intracoronary cardiosphere-derived cells after myocardial infarction: evidence of therapeutic regeneration in the final 1-year results of the CADUCEUS trial (CArdiosphere-derived aUtologous stem CElls to reverse ventricular dysfunction). J Am Coll Cardiol. 2014;63:110–22.

53. Bolli R, Chugh AR, D'Amario D, Loughran JH, Stoddard MF, Ikram S, et al. Cardiac stem cells in patients with ischaemic cardiomyopathy (SCIPIO): initial results of a randomised phase 1 trial. Lancet. 2011;378:1847–57.

54. Zaruba MM, Soonpaa M, Reuter S, Field LJ. Cardiomyogenic potential of C-kit + -expressing cells derived from neonatal and adult mouse hearts. Circulation. 2010;121:1992–2000.

55. Jesty SA, Steffey MA, Lee FK, Breitbach M, Hesse M, Reining S, et al. c-kit + precursors support postinfarction myogenesis in the neonatal, but not adult, heart. Proc Natl Acad Sci U S A. 2012;109:13380–5.

56. Van Berlo JH, Kanisicak O, Maillet M, Vagnozzi RJ, Karch J, Lin S-CJ, et al. C-kit + cells minimally contribute cardiomyocytes to the heart. Nature. 2014;509:337–41.

57. Bersell K, Arab S, Haring B, Kühn B. Neuregulin1/ErbB4 signaling induces cardiomyocyte proliferation and repair of heart injury. Cell. 2009;138:257–70.

58. Kühn B, Del Monte F, Hajjar RJ, Chang Y-S, Lebeche D, Arab S, et al. Periostin induces proliferation of differentiated cardiomyocytes and promotes cardiac repair. Nat Med. 2007;13:962–9.

59. Kubin T, Pöling J, Kostin S, Gajawada P, Hein S, Rees W, et al. Oncostatin M is a major mediator of cardiomyocyte dedifferentiation and remodeling. Cell Stem Cell. 2011;9:420–32.

60. Heallen T, Zhang M, Wang J, Bonilla-Claudio M, Klysik E, Johnson RL, et al. Hippo pathway inhibits Wnt signaling to restrain cardiomyocyte proliferation and heart size. Science. 2011;332:458–61.

61. Xin M, Kim Y, Sutherland LB, Murakami M, Qi X, McAnally J, et al. Hippo pathway effector Yap promotes cardiac regeneration. Proc Natl Acad Sci U S A. 2013;110:13839–44.

62. Lin Z, Von Gise A, Zhou P, Gu F, Ma Q, Jiang J, et al. Cardiac-specific YAP activation improves cardiac function and survival in an experimental murine MI model. Circ Res. 2014;115:354–63.

63. Porrello ER, Johnson B, Aurora AB, Simpson E, Nam YJ, Matkovich SJ, et al. MiR-15 family regulates postnatal mitotic arrest of cardiomyocytes. Circ Res. 2011;109:670–9.

64. Eulalio A, Mano M, Dal Ferro M, Zentilin L, Sinagra G, Zacchigna S, et al. Functional screening identifies miRNAs inducing cardiac regeneration. Nature. 2012;492:376–81.

65. Liu X, Xiao J, Zhu H, Wei X, Platt C, Damilano F, et al. miR-222 is necessary for exercise-induced cardiac growth and protects against pathological cardiac remodeling. Cell Metab. 2015;21:584–95.

66. Chen J, Huang ZP, Seok HY, Ding J, Kataoka M, Zhang Z, et al. Mir-17-92 cluster is required for and sufficient to induce cardiomyocyte proliferation in postnatal and adult hearts. Circ Res. 2013;112:1557–66.

67. Tseng AS, Engel FB, Keating MT. The GSK-3 inhibitor BIO promotes proliferation in mammalian cardiomyocytes. Chem Biol. 2006;13:957–63.

68. Tao G, Kahr PC, Morikawa Y, Zhang M, Rahmani M, Heallen TR, et al. Pitx2 promotes heart repair by activating the antioxidant response after cardiac injury. Nature. 2016;534:119–23.

69. Puente BN, Kimura W, Muralidhar S, Moon J, Amatruda JF, Phelps KL, et al. The oxygen-rich postnatal environment induces cardiomyocyte cell-cycle arrest through DNA damage response. Cell. 2014;157:565–79.

70. Nakada Y, Canseco DC, Thet S, Abdisalaam S, Asaithamby A, Santos CX, et al. Hypoxia induces heart regeneration in adult mice. Nature. 2017;541:222–7.
71. Kimura W, Xiao F, Canseco DC, Muralidhar S, Thet S, Zhang HM, et al. Hypoxia fate mapping identifies cycling cardiomyocytes in the adult heart. Nature. 2015;523:226–30.
72. Aurora AB, Porrello ER, Tan W, Mahmoud AI, Hill J, Bassel-Duby R, et al. Macrophages are required for neonatal heart regeneration. J Clin Invest. 2014;124:1382–92.
73. Lavine KJ, Epelman S, Uchida K, Weber KJ, Nichols CG, Schilling JD, et al. Distinct macrophage lineages contribute to disparate patterns of cardiac recovery and remodeling in the neonatal and adult heart. Proc Natl Acad Sci. 2014;111:16029–34.
74. Eisenberg LM, Markwald RR. Molecular regulation of atrioventricular valvuloseptal morphogenesis. Circ Res. 1995;77:1–6.
75. Ubil E, Duan J, Pillai ICL, Rosa-Garrido M, Wu Y, Bargiacchi F, et al. Mesenchymal-endothelial transition contributes to cardiac neovascularization. Nature. 2014;514:585–90.
76. Takahashi K, Yamanaka S. Induction of pluripotent stem cells from mouse embryonic and adult fibroblast cultures by defined factors. Cell. 2006;126: 663–76.
77. Kalani MYS, Martirosyan N. Direct conversion of fibroblasts to functional neurons. World Neurosurg. 2012;77:7–8.
78. Sekiya S, Suzuki A. Direct conversion of mouse fibroblasts to hepatocyte-like cells by defined factors. Nature. 2011;475:1–6.
79. Huang P, He Z, Ji S, Sun H, Xiang D, Liu C, et al. Induction of functional hepatocyte-like cells from mouse fibroblasts by defined factors. Nature. 2011;475:386–9.
80. Kaminski MM, Tosic J, Kresbach C, Engel H, Klockenbusch J, Müller A-L, et al. Direct reprogramming of fibroblasts into renal tubular epithelial cells by defined transcription factors. Nat Cell Biol. 2016;18:1269–80.
81. Ieda M, Fu JD, Delgado-Olguin P, Vedantham V, Hayashi Y, Bruneau BG, et al. Direct reprogramming of fibroblasts into functional cardiomyocytes by defined factors. Cell. 2010;142:375–86.
82. Sadahiro T, Yamanaka S, Ieda M. Direct cardiac reprogramming: progress and challenges in basic biology and clinical applications. Circ Res. 2015;116:1378–91.
83. Jayawardena TM, Finch EA, Zhang L, Zhang H, Hodgkinson CP, Pratt RE, et al. MicroRNA induced cardiac reprogramming in vivo evidence for mature cardiac myocytes and improved cardiac function. Circ Res. 2015;116:418–24.

8

Epithelial stem cell culture: modeling human disease and applications for regenerative medicine

Yusuke Yamamoto[*] and Takahiro Ochiya

Abstract

The inability to maintain the immaturity of stem cell populations in vitro restricts the long-term expansion of various types of human epithelial stem cells. However, recent technical advances in epithelial stem cell culture have led to the development of novel in vitro strategies for regenerating epithelial tissues and for closely mimicking human diseases such as cancer and inflammation. Specifically, improvements in culture conditions provided by small molecules in combination with three-dimensional (3D) culture approaches have facilitated the establishment of in vitro systems that recapitulate biological properties in epithelial organs, and these systems may be used to model disease. In this review article, we describe the biological significance of technical improvements in the development of these methods, focusing on human epithelial cells, including stratified and columnar epithelial cells. We also discuss the potential and future perspectives of this technology, which is only beginning to be explored.

Keywords: Epithelial stem cells, Feeder cells, Small molecules, 3D culture

Background

The isolation and long-term expansion of primary cells, particularly stem/progenitor populations, are fundamental and important basic techniques in various biological fields, including developmental biology and stem cell biology, and medical science. Cells in stratified and columnar epithelial tissues are highly regenerative and disproportionately accountable for many human cancers; however, cloning adult stem cells is limited by difficulties in maintaining these cells in an immature state. In recent years, technical innovations have resulted in rapid and dramatic progress in stem cell biology, such as the use of small molecules and growth factors to mimic tissue niche environments and facilitating "Organoid culture" [1].

In 1975, Rheinwald and Green established the first successful example of human adult stem cell culture using human keratinocytes [2]. Specifically, they maintained human keratinocytes long-term in combination with a sublethally irradiated mouse fibroblast cell line, 3T3-J2. Although they did not use the term "stem cells" for cloned keratinocytes grown on 3T3 cells, Green and colleagues found colonies with the remarkable capacity to divide and form new colonies after passage, which they termed "Holoclones" [3]. These holoclones consists of small, immature cells that all exhibited intense nuclear staining with p63, a master regulator of stemness, in stratified epithelial cells [4]. In the stratified epithelium, including skin, lung bronchia, mammary gland, and bladder urothelium, the stem cell population was mainly localized in the basal layer, and immature cells were stained with p63, consistent with the in vitro studies [5]. Significantly, isolated and expanded human keratinocytes from autologous skin have been successfully grafted to burn patients and regenerated a permanent epidermis resembling that result from split-thickness skin grafts [6, 7]. Notably, the same procedure has been applied to isolate and expand human corneal epithelial cells for transplantation [8–10]. Although this technology was limited to stem cells in the epidermis and cornea at that time, Green and colleagues created the foundation for cloning human adult stem cells in the fields of basic biology and regenerative medicine.

In this review article, we provide an overview of recent research progress and accumulating evidence of a cell culture system that has led to technical breakthroughs in epithelial cell technologies. Novel culture strategies for

* Correspondence: yuyamamo@ncc.go.jp
Division of Molecular and Cellular Medicine, National Cancer Center Research Institute, 5-1-1, Tsukiji, Chuo-ku, Tokyo 104-0045, Japan

both stratified epithelial cells and columnar epithelial cells have enabled human epithelial development to be recapitulated and can be used to generate a human disease model in vitro. We also discuss the potential and possible applications of normal epithelial cell culture technologies for regenerative medicine and highlight a cancer cell culture system that reproduces individual patient phenotypes.

Stratified epithelial cell culture

In stratified epithelial tissues, including glandular and pseudostratified epithelium, p63+ cells, which are localized on the basement membrane, can self-renew to maintain stem/progenitor populations and give rise to progeny that form functional tissues [4, 5]. As mentioned above, the cloning and expansion of epithelial stem cells, such as skin keratinocytes and corneal epithelial cells, have been well-established in co-culture systems with irradiated mouse 3T3-J2 fibroblasts. However, this standard protocol has largely been limited to the long-term culture of keratinocytes and corneal cells. Nevertheless, cloned stem cells from thymic epithelia have been reported, as has the isolation of thymic epithelial stem cells from diverse species, including human cells, cultured with a 3T3 feeder system [4, 11, 12]. Furthermore, Frey and colleagues recently applied the 3T3 feeder method to isolate urothelial stem cells that expressed sonic hedgehog and resided in the basal layer of the bladder urothelium [13]. These urothelial stem

cells from isolated human and porcine tissue were stably grown on a 3T3 feeder layer and were able to give rise to multiple cell lineages, including p63+ basal cells and Uroplakin 2+ and 3+ urothelial cells, after renal capsule transplantation in nude mice. In 2011, Pooja et al. exploited the 3T3 culture system to isolate three types of human airway epithelial stem cells, i.e., nasal, tracheal and distal airway stem cells, and found that these airway epithelial stem cells exhibited distinct cellular phenotypes after in vitro differentiation, although the immature stem cell clones appeared to be morphologically indistinguishable (Fig. 1) [14]. In a follow-up study, the transplantation of mouse tracheal and distal airway epithelial stem cells demonstrated that distal airway stem cells were readily incorporated into H1N1 influenza-damaged lung tissue and differentiated into multiple epithelial cell types, i.e., bronchioles and alveoli, whereas transplanted tracheal stem cells were localized only in major airways [15]. Clonogenic stem cells were also isolated from human esophagus endoscopic biopsy samples, and these cells were able to form well differentiated, stratified squamous epithelia-like structures in an air liquid interface (ALI) culture system [16].

Schlegel and colleagues reported that a Rho-associated protein kinase (ROCK) inhibitor in combination with 3T3 feeder cells significantly increased the proliferative capacity of epithelial stem cells, including human keratinocytes, prostate cells, and mammary gland cells, and they termed this phenomenon "conditional reprogramming"

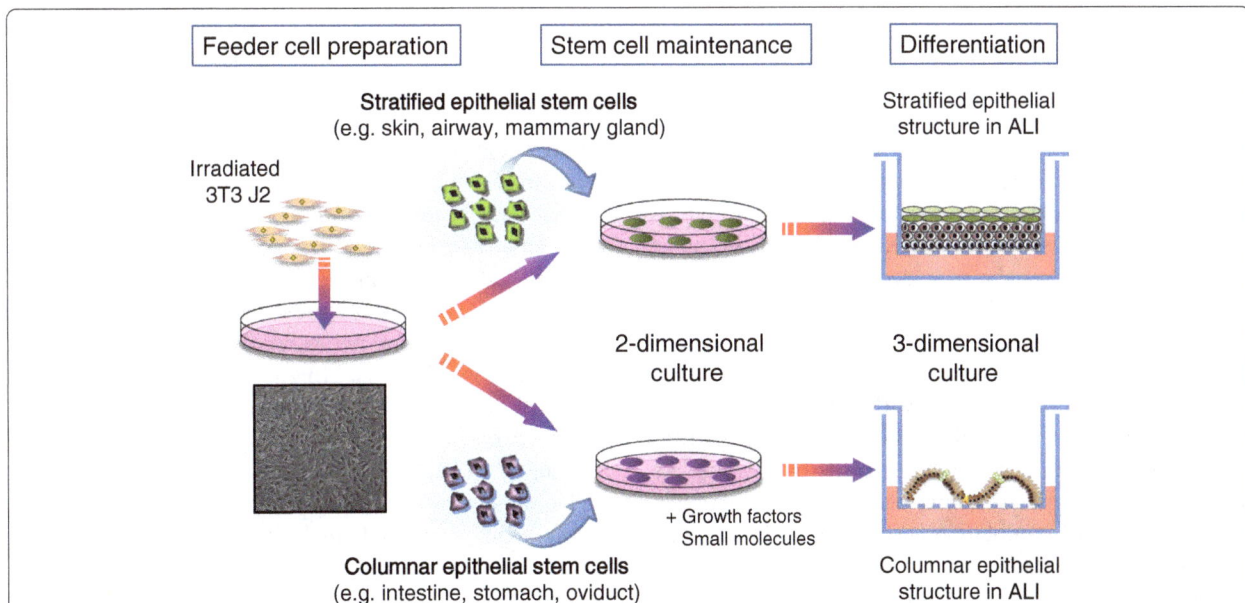

Fig. 1 Schematic of the cell culture process for human stratified and columnar epithelial stem cells on a 3T3 mouse feeder layer. For stratified epithelial stem cells, they are isolated from biopsy or surgical specimens are plated on a 3T3 layer for a long-term culture. For columnar epithelial stem cells, they are plated on a 3T3 layer with defined factors which are essential for stem cell growth and maintenance. Morphologically immature colonies (packed colonies with small cells) of epithelial stem cells are mechanically picked-up for further homogeneous expansion. In the ALI culture, the cells undergo differentiation into mature cell types in a Transwell

[17, 18]. The ability to efficiently generate epithelial stem cell cultures from patients provides critical and valuable insights into cell-based diagnostics and therapeutics [19]. More recently, Rajagopal and colleagues showed that the TGFβ/BMP/SMAD signaling pathway is important in various epithelial tissues, including ectoderm-derived skin and mammary gland tissue, endoderm-derived esophagus and prostate tissue, and mesoderm-derived epididymis. They discovered that the dual inhibition of SMAD signaling (the BMP signal was blocked by DMH-1 and the TGFβ signal was inhibited by A-83-01) facilitated the stable propagation of human and mouse epithelial basal cell populations. Surprisingly, dual TGFβ/BMP inhibition enabled the robust expansion of epithelial stem cells without the need for mouse 3T3 feeder cells.

Collectively, these technical advances, in combination with small molecules and feeder cells, can be used to continuously and efficiently expand stratified epithelial stem/progenitor populations in vitro. Another breakthrough in stratified epithelial culture, organoid culture, has been utilized to expand both basal and luminal human prostate progenitors. These human luminal progenitors were multipotent and formed prostate gland-like structures in vitro [20]. However, generating three-dimensional structures consisting of stratified or pseudostratified epithelia to recapitulate authentic in vivo architecture remains challenging, although many researchers have reported spheroid and organoid cultures. This problem may be solved by establishing a method to facilitate self-organization, as performed in pluripotent stem cell-derived tissues [21, 22].

Columnar epithelial cell culture

Although intestinal stem cells possess the remarkable capacity to proliferate at a high turnover rate to maintain intestinal epithelia, and hepatocytes are highly regenerative in response to damage, the ability to clone stem cell populations from columnar epithelial cells is severely limited, presumably due to a lack of tissue niche signals in vitro. Over the past decade, Clevers and colleagues discovered LGR5 (leucine-rich repeat-containing G-protein coupled receptor 5), an intestinal stem cell marker, in a sophisticated mouse model (Lgr5-EGFP-ires-CreERT2 mice crossed with the Cre-activated Rosa26 LacZ reporter) and established a mouse intestinal organoid culture method that consists of villus-like structures and crypt-like zones with multiple intestinal cell types [23]. In combination with growth factors and small-molecule cocktails, an isolated LGR5+ stem cell fraction was suspended in Matrigel and cultured long-term [24]. Modifying the culture condition with the use of nicotinamide, a p38 and TGFβ receptor inhibitor, human epithelial cells isolated from the small intestine and colon were able to infinitely expand long-term

in vitro [25, 26]. This technique is applicable to culture other types of cells, such as pancreatic duct cells [27] and hepatocytes [28], and facilitated revolutionary advances in columnar epithelial cell culture.

Organoid culture employs a Matrigel-based 3D culture platform and can be extensively used to stably culture diverse types of adult epithelial cells, including stratified epithelial cells, with stem/progenitor cell populations [1]. However, the ability to rapidly and efficiently propagate a fraction of uniform stem cells in vitro is also useful and important for the detailed study of self-renewal and fate specification in tissue stem cells and possible future applications of cell transplantation for regenerative medicine. Xian and colleagues recently developed a novel culture system for the homogeneous expansion of human fetal intestinal stem cells, including small intestine and colon cells. This system employed a 3T3 mouse feeder layer in combination with growth factors and signal pathway inhibitors to robustly expand human columnar epithelial stem cells (Fig. 1) [29, 30]. Moreover, more than 50% of intestinal stem cells grown on 3T3 fibroblasts were able to form colonies. In the mammalian intestine, defined niche factors, such as Wnt and Notch signals, are essential for governing the stemness of intestinal stem cells at the crypt base. Furthermore, Paneth cells, which are also located at the crypt base, arise from stem cells and act as the stem cell niche by providing essential factors in a paracrine manner. Because organoid cultures consist of stem cells and various derivatives, such as Paneth cells, niche factors are autonomously supplied [31]. By contrast, because a pure population of intestinal stem cells is grown on a 3T3 feeder layer, the cells cannot secrete niche factors. Therefore, extrinsic factors resembling niche factors need to be supplemented. In addition to the stem cell maintenance protocol, a differentiation protocol has been established in an ALI culture model to give rise to at least four types of major intestinal cells, i.e., Paneth cells, entero-endocrine cells, goblet cells, and enterocytes (intestinal absorptive cells) [29]. The formation of intestinal villus-like structures was observed according to the original tissue types, such small intestine and colon tissues (Fig. 1). In a different ALI culture approach, Kuo and colleagues robustly cultured small pieces of mouse neonatal intestine with a stromal element long-term [32].

The same strategy was also applied to clone human gastric stem cells obtained from endoscopic biopsy. Specifically, clonogenic gastric cells were stably expanded on a 3T3 feeder layer in combination with growth factors and small molecules and differentiated into gastric epithelial lineages typically found in the stomach, such as pepsinogen-expressing chief cells [16]. In addition to cloned digestive organ stem cells, oviduct progenitor cells from the distal uterus tube were also able to infinitely propagate on a 3T3 feeder layer in the presence of niche factors [33]. The distal oviduct, fimbria epithelium, is a simple columnar epithelium layer that consists of the following two types of cells: ciliated cells, which enhance the transport of gametes, and secretory cells, which secrete mucus. Using a slight modification of the differentiation protocol for intestinal stem cells, long-term ALI-cultured oviductal stem cells gave rise to a 3D architecture, containing both ciliated and secretory cells, that was reminiscent of the in vivo epithelium structure [34]. The ability to produce epithelial lineages with proper cell types from a stem cell population could be a useful tool to study physiological epithelial development and homeostasis and develop acute and chronic disease models in vitro.

Cancer cell culture

Since the first cancer cell line, the HeLa cell line, was established from a cervical cancer patient in 1951 [35], cancer cell lines established from a wide variety of cancer types have been widely used to study the pathobiology of cancer and provided opportunities to generate in vivo xenograft models and test anti-cancer drugs in vitro and in vivo. Although tremendous advances have been made in cancer biology using cancer cell lines, the results obtained using these cells may not sufficiently reflect the complexity of the disease as originally expected because cancer exhibits interpatient and intratumor heterogeneity, as revealed by recent advances in next-generation sequencing [36]. To more precisely reflect cancer phenotypes, including the patient's gene mutation status and pathology, Welm and colleagues developed patient-derived xenograft (PDX) models of breast cancer in nonobese diabetic severe combined immunodeficiency (NOD-SCID) mice that maintained the essential features of the original tumors and exhibited metastatic capacity to specific sites [37]. In addition to the breast cancer model, the establishment of various types of solid tumors demonstrated the feasibility of PDX models [38], which are anticipated to accelerate the preclinical testing of new cancer therapies and help realize the goal of "personalized medicine".

Culture methods for adult stem cells, such as organoid and feeder systems, are also applicable to different approaches that use patient-derived cancer cells. Specifically, Clevers and colleagues reported that organoid culture can be used to model pancreas [39], prostate [40], and colorectal cancer [41] and showed that the original cancer traits, including genetic heterogeneity and drug sensitivity, can be recapitulated. Therefore, they termed this system a "living organoid biobank". These technologies could also be used to isolate a stem cell population from a precancerous lesion, such as Barrett's esophagus, a precursor of human esophageal adenocarcinoma [16, 25].

Isolated and expanded Barrett's esophagus stem cells were transformed by introducing SV40 large T antigen, hTERT, and c-myc and xenografted into immunocompromised NSG (NOD.Cg-Prkdcscid Il2rgtm1Wjl/SzJ) mice [16]. As expected, Barrett's esophagus stem cells transformed into esophageal adenocarcinoma-like tumors in mice. A similar approach demonstrated that human oviductal stem cells were the cell of origin in high-grade serous ovarian epithelial cancer [34]. This finding corroborates recent human pathology and the transgenic mouse model evidence, which indicated that the distal oviductal epithelium is the tissue of origin for this cancer [42, 43]. In combination with the CRISPR/Cas9 system, normal colon stem cells were sequentially transformed by introducing the driver mutations that are frequently detected in colorectal cancer [44, 45]. The resultant cells were allowed to form xenografts in the kidney capsule and exhibited progressive transformation into adenocarcinoma-like phenotypes characterized by invasive and metastatic properties. Overall, the ability to isolate and culture cells from tumor- and patient-matched normal epithelial tissues facilitates the production of a platform that not only complements classic in vivo animal work in the field of cancer biology but also facilitates patient-specific genetics and genomics approaches in vitro.

Modeling inflammation disease with adult stem cells

Modeling human disease is hindered by the limited accessibility of human diseased tissues. Nevertheless, advances in adult stem cell cultivation have allowed us to reproduce disease phenotypes in vitro by expanding stem cells and deriving mature cell types from small human biopsy samples. Because 3D culture methods, such as ALI and organoid culture, provide structures that consist of multiple cell types and resemble the epithelium architecture observed in vivo, they should be suitable for studying inflammatory diseases, including infectious and hereditary diseases. Specifically, reproducing the disease phenotype is simple when the pathogen (or main cause) and targeted cell type are known.

Pseudomembranous colitis (PMC) is caused by a disproportionally increased population of Clostridium difficile (C. difficile) after antibiotics treatment. C. difficile is a Gram-positive, spore-forming bacterium, and produces the high-molecular-weight toxins TcdA and TcdB, which induce fluid secretion, inflammation, and colonic tissue damage. Colonic epithelial cells differentiated from clonogenic colonic stem cells in ALI culture were challenged with these toxins, which caused devastating epithelial damage in a time- and dose-dependent manner. This result indicated that the 3D culture model may be used to represent C. difficile pathology [29]. Similarly, the effect of Helicobacter pylori (H. pylori) infection, which causes chronic gastritis, gastric ulcers and cancer, was studied by microinjecting H. pylori into organoid cultures. Bacteria-infected organoid cultures exhibited increased inflammation, such as NF-kB activation and IL8 induction, and IL8 expression was significantly higher in gland-type organoid cultures than in pit-type organoid cultures [46].

Adult stem cells have also been used to model hereditary disease. Beekman and colleagues reported an intestinal organoid culture derived from cystic fibrosis (CF) patients. CF is caused by mutations in the cystic fibrosis transmembrane conductance regulator (CFTR), which is normally expressed in the epithelial cells of many organs, such as lung and digestive tissues. Although normal intestinal organoid cultures exhibited robust swelling in response to Forskolin, the swelling response was not observed in CF organoid cultures [47]. Moreover, when the mutated CFTR locus was corrected using the CRISPR/Cas9 technology in intestinal organoids of CF patients, the corrected genes were shown to functionally work [48]. Therefore, in vitro differentiation of adult stem cells, resembling in vivo phenotypes with multiple cell types in combination with gene editing technologies, provides powerful means for treating human disease and may provide direct insight into human pathology.

Application of epithelial stem cells for regenerative medicine

Despite promising strategies that use human embryonic stem (ES) cells and induced pluripotent stem (iPS) cells for applications in regenerative medicine, few clinical trials of these strategies are ongoing, which is in part due to difficulties in lineage specification and the possibility of tumorigenesis. Because adult stem cells are essentially committed to specific tissue types, producing intended cell types is relatively easy, and the potential risk for tumorigenesis is low. Thus, therapeutic approaches are aiming to use adult stem cells as the cell source for transplantation. Although Green and colleagues established the human keratinocyte culture method in 1975 and the cultured cells were transplantable into patients with burns or chemical injuries, the long-term cultivation of other types of adult stem cells was subject to significant technical barriers. As described above, recent technical advances overcame this limitation for diverse types of epithelial cells. Hence, the ability to rapidly and efficiently expand stem cell populations is valuable for their use in regenerative medicine.

For example, mouse Lgr5+ colonic stem cells have been expanded in organoid culture and transplanted into the damaged mouse colon, and engrafted cells that were able to self-renew and differentiated were detected even after 25 weeks [49]. In a different approach, Zhang K and colleagues harnessed engineered adult stem cells for a transplantation study. First, they successfully cultured corneal epithelial cells in a dish without feeder cells and then found that Pax6 is a key transcription factor that differentiates corneal stem cells (CSCs) from skin keratinocytes. Surprisingly, Pax6-overexpression in keratinocytes induced limbal stem cell-like cells, and these cells could be transplanted into the injured corneas of rabbits [50]. Because keratinocytes are more readily accessible than CSCs, this method may be applicable for the treatment of human eye disease. More recently, Liu et al. reported an attractive approach for tissue repair and regeneration that used endogenous stem cells. In their study, lens epithelial stem cells (LECs) that expressed Pax6 and Bmi1 were characterized and exhibited regenerative potential in vivo. A surgical cataract removal method that preserves endogenous LECs was employed, and these LECs contributed to the spontaneous regeneration of lenses with visual function in rabbits, macaques, and human infants. This method could be a therapeutic breakthrough for cataract treatment and potentially replace artificial intraocular lens implantation [51].

Because of the high turnover rates of many epithelial cells, transplanting stem cell populations is essential for long-term tissue maintenance. Theoretically, a single stem cell can reconstitute whole tissues, and several research groups empirically demonstrated this notion [52, 53]. Despite the potential of pluripotent stem cells (PSCs), which can give rise to all cell types, PSC-derived tissue stem cells likely cannot be maintained in the immature state in vitro. Therefore, the use of adult stem cells for regenerative medicine presents a significant advantage.

Conclusions

In recent years, remarkable progress has been made in the development of in vitro culture system for epithelial stem cells. The realization of the long-term culture of epithelial stem cells allows us not only to reproduce physiological events in vitro but also enables the development of therapeutic platforms based on cell transplantation. An increasing number of studies of epithelial stem cells clearly indicated that understanding the basic biology of these cells will be closely linked with clinical studies of human disease pathology, such as cancer and inflammation. The interactions of biological networks during tissue development and disease progression are complex at the cellular and molecular levels. Building an in vitro epithelial structure model can simplify this complexity and provide comprehensive views of epithelial physiology and pathophysiology. Moreover, in vitro epithelial models can easily be combined with genomic and epigenetic approaches and single-cell analyses. In addition, genome editing, e.g., the CRISPR-Cas9 system, can also be readily incorporated into the model. One drawback of in vitro epithelial structure models derived from the stem cells is that epithelial structures lack stromal populations. Although a simplified system provides direct insight into epithelial physiology in most cases, the interaction between different cell types is important for reproducing a genuine phenotype because all tissues consist of multiple cell types, such as epithelial cells, endothelial cells, mesothelial cells, fibroblasts, and hematopoietic cells. One possible solution to this problem is a self-organizing method, in which several cell types are mixed in vitro and spontaneously form actual organ-like structures. Although improvements are required to recapitulate the in vivo behavior of human organs, the ability to expand epithelial stem cells and generate a 3D structure model holds great promise for both basic and clinical research.

Abbreviations
3D: Three-dimentional; ALI: Air-liquid interface; C. difficile: Clostridium difficile; CF: Cystic fibrosis; CFTR: Cystic fibrosis transmembrane conductance regulator; CSC: Corneal stem cell; ES: Embryonic stem; H. pylori: Helicobacter pylori; iPS: Induced pluripotent stem; LEC: Lens epithelial stem cell; LGR5: Leucine-rich repeat-containing G-protein coupled receptor 5; NOD-SCID: Nonobese diabetic severe combined immunodeficiency; PDX: Patient-derived xenograft; PMC: Pseudomembranous colitis; PSC: Pluripotent stem cell; ROCK: Rho-associated protein kinase

Acknowledgements
The authors thank A. Inoue for the kind assistance of the manuscript preparation.

Funding
This work was supported in part by Japan Agency for Medical Research and Development (AMED) and the New Energy and Industrial Technology Development Organization (NEDO).

Authors' contributions
YY and TO wrote this review. Both authors read and approved the final manuscript.

Competing interests
The authors declare that they have no competing interests.

References
1. Clevers H. Modeling Development and Disease with Organoids. Cell. 2016; 165:1586–97.
2. Rheinwald JG, Green H. Serial cultivation of strains of human epidermal keratinocytes: the formation of keratinizing colonies from single cells. Cell. 1975;6:331–43.
3. Barrandon Y, Green H. Three clonal types of keratinocyte with different capacities for multiplication. Proc Natl Acad Sci U S A. 1987;84:2302–6.
4. Senoo M, Pinto F, Crum CP, McKeon F. p63 Is essential for the proliferative potential of stem cells in stratified epithelia. Cell. 2007;129:523–36.
5. Yang A, Schweitzer R, Sun D, Kaghad M, Walker N, Bronson RT, et al. p63 is essential for regenerative proliferation in limb, craniofacial and epithelial development. Nature. 1999;398:714–8.
6. O'Connor NE, Mulliken JB, Banks-Schlegel S, Kehinde O, Green H. Grafting of burns with cultured epithelium prepared from autologous epidermal cells. Lancet. 1981;317:75–8.
7. Gallico 3rd GG, O'Connor NE, Compton CC, Kehinde O, Green H. Permanent coverage of large burn wounds with autologous cultured human epithelium. N Engl J Med. 1984;311:448–51.
8. Pellegrini G, Traverso CE, Franzi AT, Zingirian M, Cancedda R, De Luca M. Long-term restoration of damaged corneal surfaces with autologous cultivated corneal epithelium. Lancet. 1997;349:990–3.
9. Pellegrini G, Dellambra E, Golisano O, Martinelli E, Fantozzi I, Bondanza S, et al. p63 identifies keratinocyte stem cells. Proc Natl Acad Sci U S A. 2001;98:3156–61.
10. Rama P, Matuska S, Paganoni G, Spinelli A, De Luca M, Pellegrini G. Limbal stem-cell therapy and long-term corneal regeneration. N Engl J Med. 2010;363:147–55.
11. Bonfanti P, Claudinot S, Amici AW, Farley A, Blackburn CC, Barrandon Y. Microenvironmental reprogramming of thymic epithelial cells to skin multipotent stem cells. Nature. 2010;466:978–82.
12. Sun TT, Bonitz P, Burns WH. Cell culture of mammalian thymic epithelial cells: growth, structural, and antigenic properties. Cell Immunol. 1984;83:1–13.
13. Larsson HM, Gorostidi F, Hubbell JA, Barrandon Y, Frey P. Clonal, self-renewing and differentiating human and porcine urothelial cells, a novel stem cell population. PLoS One. 2014;9:e90006.
14. Kumar PA, Hu Y, Yamamoto Y, Hoe NB, Wei TS, Mu D, et al. Distal airway stem cells yield alveoli in vitro and during lung regeneration following H1N1 influenza infection. Cell. 2011;147:525–38.
15. Zuo W, Zhang T, Wu DZ, Guan SP, Liew AA, Yamamoto Y, et al. p63(+)Krt5(+) distal airway stem cells are essential for lung regeneration. Nature. 2015;517:616–20.
16. Yamamoto Y, Wang X, Bertrand D, Kern F, Zhang T, Duleba M, et al. Mutational spectrum of Barrett's stem cells suggests paths to initiation of a precancerous lesion. Nat Commun. 2016;7:10380.
17. Liu X, Ory V, Chapman S, Yuan H, Albanese C, Kallakury B, et al. ROCK inhibitor and feeder cells induce the conditional reprogramming of epithelial cells. Am J Pathol. 2012;180:599–607.
18. Chapman S, Liu X, Meyers C, Schlegel R, McBride AA. Human keratinocytes are efficiently immortalized by a Rho kinase inhibitor. J Clin Invest. 2010; 120:2619–26.
19. Yuan H, Myers S, Wang J, Zhou D, Woo JA, Kallakury B, et al. Use of reprogrammed cells to identify therapy for respiratory papillomatosis. N Engl J Med. 2012;367:1220–7.
20. Karthaus WR, Iaquinta PJ, Drost J, Gracanin A, van Boxtel R, Wongvipat J, et al. Identification of multipotent luminal progenitor cells in human prostate organoid cultures. Cell. 2014;159:163–75.
21. Eiraku M, Takata N, Ishibashi H, Kawada M, Sakakura E, Okuda S, et al. Self-organizing optic-cup morphogenesis in three-dimensional culture. Nature. 2011;472:51–6.
22. Takebe T, Sekine K, Enomura M, Koike H, Kimura M, Ogaeri T, et al. Vascularized and functional human liver from an iPSC-derived organ bud transplant. Nature. 2013;499:481–4.
23. Barker N, van Es JH, Kuipers J, Kujala P, van den Born M, Cozijnsen M, et al. Identification of stem cells in small intestine and colon by marker gene Lgr5. Nature. 2007;449:1003–7.
24. Sato T, Vries RG, Snippert HJ, van de Wetering M, Barker N, Stange DE, et al. Single Lgr5 stem cells build crypt-villus structures in vitro without a mesenchymal niche. Nature. 2009;459:262–5.
25. Sato T, Stange DE, Ferrante M, Vries RG, Van Es JH, Van den Brink S, et al. Long-term expansion of epithelial organoids from human colon, adenoma, adenocarcinoma, and Barrett's epithelium. Gastroenterology. 2011;141:1762–72.
26. Jung P, Sato T, Merlos-Suárez A, Barriga FM, Iglesias M, Rossell D, et al. Isolation and in vitro expansion of human colonic stem cells. Nat Med. 2011;17:1225–7.
27. Huch M, Bonfanti P, Boj SF, Sato T, Loomans CJ, van de Wetering M, et al. Unlimited in vitro expansion of adult bi-potent pancreas progenitors through the Lgr5/R-spondin axis. EMBO J. 2013;32:2708–21.
28. Huch M, Gehart H, van Boxtel R, Hamer K, Blokzijl F, Verstegen MM, et al. Long-term culture of genome-stable bipotent stem cells from adult human liver. Cell. 2015;160:299–312.
29. Wang X, Yamamoto Y, Wilson LH, Zhang T, Howitt BE, Farrow MA, et al. Cloning and variation of ground state intestinal stem cells. Nature. 2015;522:173–8.
30. Shimokawa M, Sato T. Back to 2D Culture for Ground State of Intestinal Stem Cells. Cell Stem Cell. 2015;17:5–7.

31. Sato T, van Es JH, Snippert HJ, Stange DE, Vries RG, van den Born M, et al. Paneth cells constitute the niche for Lgr5 stem cells in intestinal crypts. Nature. 2011;469:415–8.

32. Ootani A, Li X, Sangiorgi E, Ho QT, Ueno H, Toda S, et al. Sustained in vitro intestinal epithelial culture within a Wnt-dependent stem cell niche. Nat Med. 2009;15:701–6.

33. Ning G, Bijron JG, Yamamoto Y, Wang X, Howitt BE, Herfs M, et al. The PAX2-null immunophenotype defines multiple lineages with common expression signatures in benign and neoplastic oviductal epithelium. J Pathol. 2014;234:478–87.

34. Yamamoto Y, Ning G, Howitt BE, Mehra K, Wu L, Wang X, et al. In vitro and in vivo correlates of physiological and neoplastic human Fallopian tube stem cells. J Pathol. 2016;238:519–30.

35. Scherer WF, Syverton JT, Gey GO. Studies on the propagation in vitro of poliomyelitis viruses. IV. Viral multiplication in a stable strain of human malignant epithelial cells (strain HeLa) derived from an epidermoid carcinoma of the cervix. J Exp Med. 1953;97:695–710.

36. McGranahan N, Swanton C. Biological and therapeutic impact of intratumor heterogeneity in cancer evolution. Cancer Cell. 2015;27:15–26.

37. DeRose YS, Wang G, Lin YC, Bernard PS, Buys SS, Ebbert MT, et al. Tumor grafts derived from women with breast cancer authentically reflect tumor pathology, growth, metastasis and disease outcomes. Nat Med. 2011;17:1514–20.

38. Liu ET, Bult CJ, Shultz LD. Patient-derived tumor xenografts: why now? JAMA Oncol. 2016;2:567–8.

39. Boj SF, Hwang CI, Baker LA, Chio II, Engle DD, Corbo V, et al. Organoid models of human and mouse ductal pancreatic cancer. Cell. 2015;160:324–38.

40. Gao D, Vela I, Sboner A, Iaquinta PJ, Karthaus WR, Gopalan A, et al. Organoid cultures derived from patients with advanced prostate cancer. Cell. 2014;159:176–87.

41. van de Wetering M, Francies HE, Francis JM, Bounova G, Iorio F, Pronk A, et al. Prospective derivation of a living organoid biobank of colorectal cancer patients. Cell. 2015;161:933–45.

42. Carlson JW, Miron A, Jarboe EA, Parast MM, Hirsch MS, Lee Y, et al. Serous tubal intraepithelial carcinoma: its potential role in primary peritoneal serous carcinoma and serous cancer prevention. J Clin Oncol. 2008;26:4160–5.

43. Perets R, Wyant GA, Muto KW, Bijron JG, Poole BB, Chin KT, et al. Transformation of the fallopian tube secretory epithelium leads to high-grade serous ovarian cancer in Brca;Tp53;Pten models. Cancer Cell. 2013;24:751–65.

44. Matano M, Date S, Shimokawa M, Takano A, Fujii M, Ohta Y, et al. Modeling colorectal cancer using CRISPR-Cas9-mediated engineering of human intestinal organoids. Nat Med. 2015;21:256–62.

45. Drost J, van Jaarsveld RH, Ponsioen B, Zimberlin C, van Boxtel R, Buijs A, et al. Sequential cancer mutations in cultured human intestinal stem cells. Nature. 2015;521:43–7.

46. Bartfeld S, Bayram T, van de Wetering M, Huch M, Begthel H, Kujala P, et al. In vitro expansion of human gastric epithelial stem cells and their responses to bacterial infection. Gastroenterology. 2015;148:126–36.

47. Dekkers JF, Wiegerinck CL, de Jonge HR, Bronsveld I, Janssens HM, de Winter-de Groot KM, et al. A functional CFTR assay using primary cystic fibrosis intestinal organoids. Nat Med. 2013;19:939–45.

48. Schwank G, Koo BK, Sasselli V, Dekkers JF, Heo I, Demircan T, et al. Functional repair of CFTR by CRISPR/Cas9 in intestinal stem cell organoids of cystic fibrosis patients. Cell Stem Cell. 2013;13:653–8.

49. Yui S, Nakamura T, Sato T, Nemoto Y, Mizutani T, Zheng X, et al. Functional engraftment of colon epithelium expanded in vitro from a single adult Lgr5 + stem cell. Nat Med. 2012;18:618–23.

50. Ouyang H, Xue Y, Lin Y, Zhang X, Xi L, Patel S, et al. WNT7A and PAX6 define corneal epithelium homeostasis and pathogenesis. Nature. 2014; 511:358–61.

51. Lin H, Ouyang H, Zhu J, Huang S, Liu Z, Chen S, et al. Lens regeneration using endogenous stem cells with gain of visual function. Nature. 2016; 531:323–8.

52. Notta F, Doulatov S, Laurenti E, Poeppl A, Jurisica I, Dick JE. Isolation of single human hematopoietic stem cells capable of long-term multilineage engraftment. Science. 2011;333:218–21.

53. Leong KG, Wang BE, Johnson L, Gao WQ. Generation of a prostate from a single adult stem cell. Nature. 2008;456:804–8.

9

Resident fibroblasts in the kidney: a major driver of fibrosis and inflammation

Yuki Sato[1,2] and Motoko Yanagita[2*]

Abstract

Background: Chronic kidney disease (CKD) is a leading cause of end stage renal disease (ESRD) and cardiovascular morbidity and mortality worldwide, resulting in a growing social and economic burden. The prevalence and burden of CKD is anticipated to further increase over the next decades as a result of aging.

Main body of abstract: In the pathogenesis of CKD, irrespective of the etiology, resident fibroblasts are key players and have been demonstrated to play crucial roles for disease initiation and progression. In response to injury, resident fibroblasts transdifferentiate into myofibroblasts that express alpha smooth muscle actin (αSMA) and have an increased capacity to produce large amounts of extracellular matrix (ECM) proteins, leading to renal fibrosis. In addition to this fundamental role of fibroblasts as drivers for renal fibrosis, growing amounts of evidence have shown that resident fibroblasts are also actively involved in initiating and promoting inflammation during kidney injury. During the myofibroblastic transition described above, resident fibroblasts activate NF-κB signaling and produce pro-inflammatory cytokines and chemokines, promoting inflammation. Furthermore, under aging milieu, resident fibroblasts transdifferentiate into several distinct phenotypic fibroblasts, including CXCL13/CCL19-producing fibroblasts, retinoic acid-producing fibroblasts, and follicular dendritic cells, in response to injury and orchestrate tertiary lymphoid tissue (TLT) formation, which results in uncontrolled aberrant inflammation and retards tissue repair. Anti-inflammatory agents can improve myofibroblastic transdifferentiation and abolish TLT formation, suggesting that targeting these inflammatory fibroblasts can potentially ameliorate kidney disease.

Short conclusion: Beyond its conventional role as an executor of fibrosis, resident fibroblasts display more pro-inflammatory phenotypes and contribute actively to driving inflammation during kidney injury.

Keywords: Fibroblast, Inflammation, Myofibroblast, Chronic kidney disease, Erythropoietin, Heterogeneity, Tertiary lymphoid tissue, CXCL13

Background

Fibroblasts reside in virtually all tissues in our body and provide three-dimensional architecture and mechanical strength to the tissues. Emerging evidence suggests that they also have tissue-specific physiologic functions and participate actively in pathogenesis during injury. In the kidney, resident fibroblasts produce erythropoietin (EPO) in response to hypoxic insults to maintain homeostasis under physiologic condition, whereas, under pathologic conditions, resident fibroblasts trans-

* Correspondence: motoy@kuhp.kyoto-u.ac.jp
[2]Department of Nephrology, Graduate School of Medicine, Kyoto University, Kyoto, Japan
Full list of author information is available at the end of the article

differentiate into myofibroblasts, which execute renal fibrosis by producing large amounts of extracellular matrix proteins, at the cost of EPO production [1, 2]. Recently, the role and phenotype of resident fibroblasts in the kidney during injury have been demonstrated to be more diverse and crucial for disease initiation and progression. Under the aging milieu, for example, resident fibroblasts further gain a variety of distinct phenotypes in response to injury and orchestrate tertiary lymphoid tissue formation, which results in uncontrolled inflammation and retards tissue repair [3]. In this review, we provide the current state of knowledge of the renal fibroblasts as a driver of fibrosis and inflammation, and consider a novel therapeutic strategy to treat patients with kidney disease.

Resident fibroblasts as sentinels in the kidney

The kidney plays a central role in body fluid homeostasis and metabolic waste elimination. Each human kidney is composed of about 1 million nephrons, which are functional units of the kidney that comprise the glomerulus and the tubules. The glomerulus is a capillary loop that is specialized for plasma filtration. The glomeruli receive blood supply from the renal artery, and the glomerular filtrate subsequently travels through renal tubules, where metabolic exchange, and reabsorption and secretion occur. Resident fibroblasts are spindle-shaped mesenchymal cells that reside in the renal interstitium [4], which is the extracellular compartment between tubules and peritubular capillaries [5]. Several pathological studies have shown that the magnitude of renal impairment correlates better with interstitial changes than the glomerular changes in most forms of chronic kidney disease (CKD), suggesting that renal function is critically dependent on the environment in this compartment.

The kidney interstitium contains two cellular components: resident fibroblasts and resident renal mononuclear phagocytes (rMoPh) [6, 7]. Although these two types of cells reside in virtually all tissues, they are versatile cell types with strong organ-specific modifications. The kidney is continually exposed to various kinds of endogenous and exogenous substances, which must be monitored and possibly eliminated, and most of the reabsorbed substances have to traverse the interstitium before entering the capillaries. Fibroblasts and rMoPh are strategically positioned at the interstitium to sense these circulating substances and environmental changes [5]. Indeed, with the progression of kidney disease, many kinds of uremic toxins have accumulated in the body and have various effects on these renal cells. For instance, indoxyl sulfate (IS), a typical uremic toxin derived from indole, suppresses EPO production in resident fibroblasts in the kidney [8], which may partly explain the relative deficiency of EPO production in CKD patients described in the next chapter.

The readiness to respond to diverse environmental cues has been well described for rMoPh, and these cells have been considered to be sentinels in the kidney [6]. However, it has recently been demonstrated that fibroblasts also express most immune receptors, including pattern recognition receptors such as Toll-like receptors (TLRs), and that they are also highly sensitive to local tissue injury. Leaf et al. demonstrated that, although various types of cell are likely to become activated through TLRs, fibroblasts respond to damage-associated molecular patterns (DAMPs) more sensitively than other cell types including epithelial cells, endothelial cells, and even monocyte-derived macrophage in the context of sterile inflammation, and they produce higher amount of pro-inflammatory cytokine, participating actively in the initiation of renal inflammation [9]. Macrophages, on the other hand, have a higher sensitivity to pathogen ligands, suggesting that these two cell types may collaborate together and serve as a sophisticated network that senses both intrinsic and extrinsic substances under physiologic and pathologic conditions.

Pericytes, which are defined as mesenchymal cells wrapping around the microvessels, also reside in interstitium and are positive for CD73 and PDGFRβ, both of which are also utilized as markers for resident fibroblasts [10]. Overlapping definitions of resident fibroblasts and pericytes have generated confusion and controversy, although it is becoming increasingly clear that they are overlapping populations in the kidney [11]. Recent studies of the lineage relationships demonstrated that almost all fibroblasts in the renal cortex and outer medulla, including EPO-producing cells, are derived from cells that are lineage-labeled with *myelin protein zero (P0)-Cre* [12], which labels migrating neural crest cells and neural crest-derived Schwann cells [13], whereas almost all pericytes are derived from *Foxd1-Cre* lineage-labeled stromal cells [14]. *P0-Cre* lineage-labeled cells transiently express FoxD1 during development, whereas FoxD1 is expressed in the migrating neural crest, indicating that these two populations are overlapping [11].

Role of resident fibroblasts during kidney injury

Fibrosis is a common pathologic feature in CKD patients, and myofibroblasts are major drivers of fibrosis. Myofibroblasts are not present under physiologic conditions, but emerge de novo in injured tissues. The origin of myofibroblasts has been controversial for a long time, and various precursor cells of myofibroblasts in fibrotic kidneys have been reported [1]. Over the last 5 years, comprehensive cell fate mapping experiments using various Cre mouse lines have been conducted by several groups and the origin of myofibroblasts has been reconsidered. We also demonstrated that *P0-Cre* lineage-labeled resident fibroblasts transdifferentiate αSMA-positive myofibroblasts in response to kidney injury [12]. Together with the results from other groups, it is currently believed that resident fibroblasts or pericytes seem to be the most important precursor of myofibroblasts, which is consistent with recent studies in liver [15], lung [16, 17], and skin fibrosis [18, 19], all of which concluded that myofibroblasts are derived from resident fibroblasts. Interestingly, Kramman et al. recently identified the myofibroblast progenitor, which represents a small fraction of renal pericytes in the healthy kidney, and they were lineage-labeled with Gli1 [20]. Gli1-positive pericytes fulfill the criteria of mesenchymal stem cells, having tri-lineage differentiation potential and colony-forming capability in vitro. The blood vessel wall was shown to be a niche for mesenchymal stem cells in multiple human organs including the skeletal muscle, pancreas, adipose tissue, placenta, and kidney [21, 22].

In CKD patients, fibrosis progresses for decades. This clinical course suggests that epigenetic changes, which can persist long after the removal of initial trigger, have been involved and played an important role in this process. A recent genome-wide methylation scan of fibroblasts in the kidney identified epigenetic silencing of RASAL1, a suppressor of the Ras oncoprotein, as the cause of spontaneous proliferation of fibroblasts [23], providing a new molecular explanation for a sustained activation of fibroblasts in the injured kidneys.

In parallel with renal fibrosis, as the severity of kidney disease progresses, renal anemia increases in prevalence. Renal anemia is driven predominantly by a relative deficiency in the production of EPO, a principal regulatory hormone of red blood cell production [2], which is produced by renal resident fibroblasts in response to hypoxia [24]. We have previously demonstrated that, during kidney injury, EPO-producing cells transdifferentiate into myofibroblasts, same as other resident fibroblasts in the kidney, at the cost of EPO production [12]. EPO production is mainly regulated by hypoxia-inducible factors (HIFs) in healthy kidney. However, in injured kidneys, despite their hypoxic conditions, most of the HIF target gene expression is insufficient to counteract hypoxia [25]. Notably, we also showed that these transdifferentiated myofibroblasts regain their EPO production ability after the induction of severe anemia or the administration of neuroprotective agents such as neurotrophin and selective estrogen receptor modulator (SERM) [12]. These results indicate that resident fibroblasts possess functional plasticity and myofibroblasts still have the potential to produce EPO in response to hypoxic insults, which is consistent with epidemiological evidence indicating the presence of hypoxia-driven EPO regulation even in the patients with ESRD who require hemodialysis [26].

What triggers this phenotypic change in fibroblast in the kidney? In the previous study, we have demonstrated that proximal tubule injury alone can drive this phenotypic change and lead to renal fibrosis and deficiency in EPO production [27]. This phenomenon has been supported by the evidences from other groups, which demonstrate that TGF-β derived from injured tubules promotes the transdifferentiation from fibroblast into myofibroblast [28]. In addition to this, the pathways regulating this phenotypic change, including PDGFR pathway and hedgehog pathway, have been already identified and considered as targets of novel therapeutic approaches [11]. Interestingly, during this phenotypic transition, fibroblasts also become both extracellular

matrix (ECM)-producing cells and inflammatory effector cells [29, 30]. In response to injury, renal fibroblasts have been shown to activate NF-κB signaling, which leads to the production of pro-inflammatory cytokines and chemokines. The pro-inflammatory cytokines such as IL-1 and TNFα activate GATA-2 and NF-κB, both of which inhibit EPO transcription by binding the EPO promoter [29, 31], leading to relative EPO deficiency in CKD patients. Together with the findings that anti-inflammatory agents such as dexamethasone can restore the myofibroblast phenotype [12, 29], the inflammatory phenotypes of fibroblasts can be a promising therapeutic target and require more characterization in future studies.

In addition, various types of cells in the kidney, including fibroblasts, produce prostaglandins (PGs), which have also been recognized as a mediator of inflammatory responses [32]. Growing amounts of evidence have shown that PGs are involved in tissue fibrosis and inflammation. PGE2 is the most abundant PG in the kidney, and it plays a suppressive role in renal fibrosis via its receptor EP4 [33], although specific EP4 depletion in podocytes, which are a critical component of the filtration barrier in the glomerulus, results in milder glomerular injury [34]. These potential confounding features suggest that the PG cellular source and function are highly variable depending on the conditions and the cell type. PG signaling is considered to be a promising therapeutic target because PGs have been shown to amplify cytokine signaling and induce chemokine expression in other organs [32].

Heterogeneity of resident fibroblasts involved in tertiary lymphoid tissue formation in aged injured kidney

Several phenotypically novel heterogeneous fibroblasts in the injured kidney have been identified recently, and they were characterized in both the rodent and human kidneys, which are involved in tertiary lymphoid tissue (TLT) formation [3]. TLTs are inducible ectopic lymphoid tissues that are composed of a hematopoietic compartment, which comprises mostly T cells and B cells, and stromal components, which include fibroblasts in particular (Fig. 1) [35]. TLTs can propagate local antigen-specific immune responses within non-lymphoid tissues, although their roles are context dependent and can be either beneficial or detrimental [36]. In chronic inflammatory disorders, for instance, TLTs are generally considered to be perpetuators of aberrant immune responses and detrimental to the host [37], whereas, during infections, TLTs generate robust immune responses to pathogens and play protective roles for the host [38]. Besides anatomical and functional similarities, TLT and secondary lymphoid organs, such as lymph nodes, both depend on related mechanisms and molecules for their development [39, 40]. In lymph nodes, homeostatic

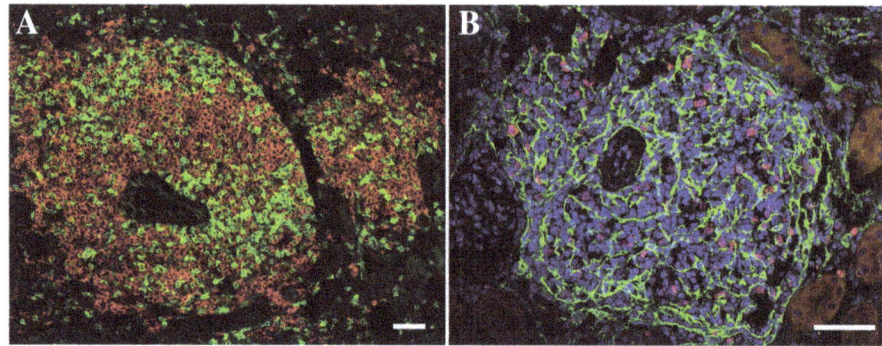

Fig. 1 Tertiary lymphoid tissues in aged injured mouse kidney. Tertiary lymphoid tissues are mainly composed of T cells and B cells, some of which are proliferating. p75NTR-positive fibroblasts extend their projections and form a structural backbone within TLTs. **a** *green*: CD3ε, *red*: B220. **b** *green*: p75NTR, *red*: Ki67. *Scale bar* (**a**, **b**) 50 μm

chemokines, including CXCL13, CCL19, and CCL21, play essential roles in their development, maturation, and homeostasis [39, 40]. The homeostatic chemokine is a powerful driving force for recruiting lymphocytes and is also sufficient to drive TLTs in non-lymphoid tissue, as transgenic expression of homeostatic chemokines in non-lymphoid organs induce the development of functional TLTs [41, 42].

Recent studies have increasingly highlighted the potential roles for TLTs in regulating local immune responses in various pathological conditions. We showed that aged mice, but not young mice, developed multiple TLTs in the kidney after acute kidney injury (AKI) (Fig. 2). This unique response program in aged injured kidneys might explain why aged kidneys fail to repair themselves after kidney injury and progress to ESRD [43], since aberrant chronic inflammation hinders normal tissue repair and results in worse remodeling and dysfunction [44, 45]. Administration of anti-CD4 monoclonal antibody and dexamethasone abolished TLT formation and improved renal outcomes. Thus, the molecular mechanisms that govern the development and maintenance of TLT identity are of great interest, having implications for the

prevention of TLT formation and the subsequent aberrant inflammation [46].

In aged injured kidneys, resident fibroblasts transdifferentiate into myofibroblasts and also into several distinct phenotypic fibroblasts, which are involved in TLT formation (Fig. 3). After kidney injury, some resident fibroblasts acquire the ability to produce retinoic acid, which induces the neural crest marker p75NTR. Some p75NTR-positive fibroblasts in aged injured kidneys produce CXCL13 and CCL19, resulting in TLT formation [3]. Additionally, in the later phase of TLT formation, some of the p75NTR-positive fibroblasts appear to lose their p75NTR expression and mature into follicular dendritic cells (FDCs). FDCs express high amounts of CD21, complement receptors-2, and CXCL13, resulting in forming B cell areas and supporting germinal center response [47]. Lineage tracing demonstrated that *P0-Cre* lineage-labeled resident fibroblasts diversified into fibroblasts with these several distinct phenotypes essential for TLT formation (Fig. 3). These findings in renal TLT are consistent with the results of lineage-tracing studies in stromal cells in secondary lymphoid organs [48, 49], indicating that FDCs in the spleen are lineage-labeled with

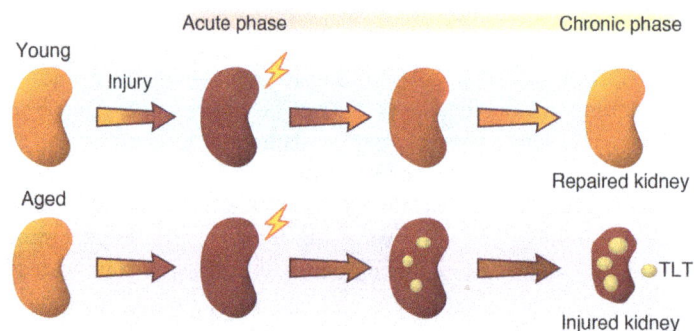

Fig. 2 The distinct injury response in young and aged mice. Aged mice, but not young mice, developed multiple tertiary lymphoid tissues (TLTs) in the kidney after acute kidney injury (AKI). TLTs sustain and amplify inflammation and retard regeneration, resulting a poor renal outcome in aged mice

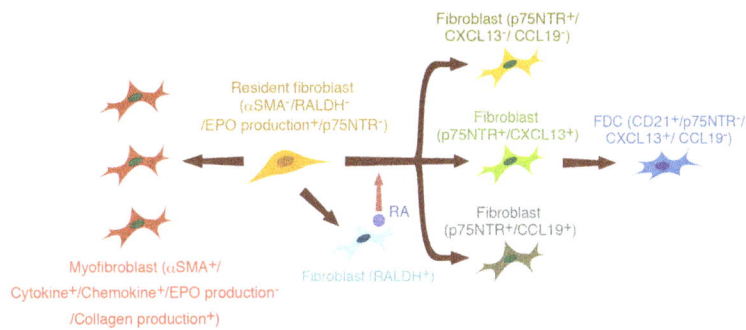

Fig. 3 Fibroblasts have two jobs during CKD: fibrosis and inflammation. Resident fibroblasts critically contribute to fibrosis and the persistence of inflammation in the injured kidney [3]. Upon injury, resident fibroblasts transdifferentiate into myofibroblasts, which produce a large amount of ECM protein and pro-inflammatory cytokines/chemokines, at the cost of EPO production. Moreover, in the aging milieu, resident fibroblasts also transdifferentiate into several distinct phenotypic fibroblasts, which orchestrate TLT formation. In response to injury, resident fibroblasts differentiate into RALDH-positive fibroblasts, which induce transdifferentiation of other fibroblasts into p75NTR-positive fibroblasts with three phenotypes, which include CXCL13- and CCL19-producing fibroblasts. In the later phase of TLT formation, some of these p75NTR-positive fibroblasts lose this expression and mature into CD21/CXCL13-positive FDCs

PDGFRβ-Cre, whereas FDCs in lymph nodes are lineage-labeled with *Wnt1-Cre*, which is another Cre line which labels neural crest-derived cells. Collectively, our results confirm and extend the concept that resident fibroblasts in the kidney exhibit striking plasticity and functional diversity depending on their residing microenvironments. One important remaining question to be addressed is "why the renal environment is prone to TLT formation with aging." One possibility is the contribution of hematopoietic cell aging, especially CD4 positive T cells, because depletion of CD4 positive cells abolished TLTs [3]. Because of thymic involution, T cells undergo a global phenotype shift from naïve to memory T cells with aging, and unique age-dependent memory CD4 positive T cell subpopulation has been identified [50]. Another possibility is the contribution of aging in stromal cells, especially resident fibroblasts in the kidney. Further studies will be required to determine which cell aging is critical for the TLT formation.

The developmental mechanism of age-dependent TLTs in the kidney and inducible bronchus-associated lymphoid tissue (iBALT) in the lung is similar in that both TLTs are driven by CXCL13 and CCL19 [3, 51]. Although lymphoid tissue is normally absent in the lung, iBALT develops following to various kinds of infection and inflammatory diseases [52]. iBALT has separated T and B cell areas, some of which contain FDCs and germinal centers, and generate immune responses. Although various types of cells, such as monocyte-lineage cells and fibroblasts, have been reported as to be a source of CXCL13 in the lung, bone marrow chimera experiments have demonstrated that the majority of CXCL13 producing cells are non-hematopoietic cells in iBALT [53]. Rangel et al. have showed that wild type mice reconstituted with CXCL13-deficient bone marrow exhibited nearly identical lung expression of CXCL13

compared with wild type controls [53]. Furthermore, the same group has also demonstrated that interleukin-17 produced by CD4-positive T cells triggers the expression of CXCL13 and CCL19, but not CCL21, in pulmonary fibroblasts, which results in iBALT formation [51]. Altogether, these results suggested that resident fibroblasts have the potential to become homeostatic chemokine-producing cells in various organs. Though monocyte lineage cells have also been reported as CXCL13-producing cells in murine lupus models in the kidney [54, 55], the expression of CXCL13 in fibroblasts was not examined in these studies, and the relative contribution of hematopoietic cells and non-hematopoietic cells to overall CXCL13 expression in the kidney has yet to be determined in this model. Further studies are required to determine the main cellular source of renal CXCL13 in this model.

It is difficult to determine whether TLT is beneficial, harmful, or neutral for the host. This is partly because it is technically challenging to deplete TLTs specifically at any time without affecting the immune system systemically. Another way to determine whether TLTs play pathogenic roles is to determine whether TLTs produce autoantibodies. Given that TLTs lead to the production of tissue-specific autoantibodies, targeting TLT formation could be beneficial. Indeed, this idea has been already tested. Lehmann-Horn et al. demonstrated that in experimental autoimmune encephalomyelitis (EAE), autoantibodies with modified affinity for myelin self-antigens are generated within TLT in the meninges of central nerve system [56], suggesting the pathological roles of TLT in this context. In addition to the conventional roles of TLT as an amplifier of inflammation, recent studies have shown that, in some pathological conditions, TLTs can function as niches for tumor progenitor cells [57] and pathogenic memory T cells [58], which might represent new therapeutic targets for cancer and chronic inflammatory diseases. The role of TLTs may be variable and be influenced by the stage of the disease, site of formation, and various environmental factors, all of which determine the impact of TLTs on disease progression. Further studies are required to determine the precise roles of TLTs in various pathologic conditions.

Conclusions

Dysfunction of resident fibroblasts leads to a series of clinically relevant pathological conditions that are common in CKD, indicating their importance in maintaining homeostasis under normal conditions. Beyond its conventional role as an executor of fibrosis, resident fibroblasts display more pro-inflammatory phenotypes and contribute actively to driving inflammation during kidney injury (Fig. 3), and intervention with anti-inflammatory agents has the potential to ameliorate kidney injury. Further studies are required to create novel therapeutic approaches, which may emerge as a consequence of a better understanding of the behavior of fibroblast under physiologic and pathologic conditions.

Abbreviations

AKI: Acute kidney injury; CKD: Chronic kidney disease; DAMPs: Damage-associated molecular patterns; ECM: Extracellular matrix; EPO: Erythropoietin; ESRD: End stage renal disease; FDC: Follicular dendritic cell; iBALT: Inducible bronchus-associated lymphoid tissue; P0: Myelin protein zero; PG: Prostaglandin; rMoPh: Resident renal mononuclear phagocytes; TLR: Toll-like receptor; TLT: Tertiary lymphoid tissue; αSMA: Alpha smooth muscle actin

Acknowledgements
The authors would like to express sincere appreciation to Prof. Hideyuki Okano and Prof. Masataka Kuwano for giving us the opportunity to write this review article, to Dr. Hirosuke Nakata for drawing the illustrations, and to all lab members and collaborators.

Funding
YS receives funding from Mitsubishi Tanabe Pharma Corporation. MY receives research grants from Astellas, Chugai, Daiichi Sankyo, Fujiyakuhin, Kyowa Hakko Kirin, Mitsubishi Tanabe Pharma Corporation, MSD, Nippon Boehringer Ingelheim, and Torii.

,

Authors contributions
YS drafted the manuscript, and MY revised it. Both authors read and approved the final manuscript.

Competing interests
YS is employed by the TMK project. MY is on the advisory board of Astellas.

Ethics approval
Not applicable.

Author details
[1]Medical Innovation Center, TMK project, Graduate School of Medicine, Kyoto University, Kyoto, Japan. [2]Department of Nephrology, Graduate School of Medicine, Kyoto University, Kyoto, Japan.

References
1. Mack M, Yanagita M. Origin of myofibroblasts and cellular events triggering fibrosis. Kidney Int. 2015;87(2):297–307.
2. Sato Y, Yanagita M. Renal anemia: from incurable to curable. Am J Physiol Renal Physiol. 2013;305(9):F1239–48.
3. Sato Y, Mii A, Hamazaki Y, Fujita H, Nakata H, Masuda K, Nishiyama S, Shibuya S, Haga H, Ogawa O, et al. Heterogeneous fibroblasts underlie age-dependent tertiary lymphoid tissues in the kidney. JCI Insight. 2016; 1(11), e87680.
4. Boor P, Floege J. The renal (myo-)fibroblast: a heterogeneous group of cells. Nephrol Dial Transplant. 2012;27(8):3027–36.
5. Kaissling B, Le Hir M. The renal cortical interstitium: morphological and functional aspects. Histochem Cell Biol. 2008;130(2):247–62.
6. Nelson PJ, Rees AJ, Griffin MD, Hughes J, Kurts C, Duffield J. The renal mononuclear phagocytic system. J Am Soc Nephrol. 2012;23(2):194–203.
7. Weisheit CK, Engel DR, Kurts C. Dendritic cells and macrophages: sentinels in the kidney. Clin J Am Soc Nephrol. 2015;10(10):1841–51.
8. Chiang CK, Tanaka T, Inagi R, Fujita T, Nangaku M. Indoxyl sulfate, a representative uremic toxin, suppresses erythropoietin production in a HIF-dependent manner. Lab Invest. 2011;91(11):1564–71.
9. Leaf IA, Nakagawa S, Johnson BG, Cha JJ, Mittelsteadt K, Guckian KM, Gomez IG, Altemeier WA, Duffield JS. Pericyte MyD88 and IRAK4 control inflammatory and fibrotic responses to tissue injury. J Clin Invest. 2017; 127(1):321–34.
10. Armulik A, Genove G, Betsholtz C. Pericytes: developmental, physiological, and pathological perspectives, problems, and promises. Dev Cell. 2011;21(2): 193–215.
11. Duffield JS. Cellular and molecular mechanisms in kidney fibrosis. J Clin Invest. 2014;124(6):2299–306.
12. Asada N, Takase M, Nakamura J, Oguchi A, Asada M, Suzuki N, Yamamura K, Nagoshi N, Shibata S, Rao TN, et al. Dysfunction of fibroblasts of extrarenal origin underlies renal fibrosis and renal anemia in mice. J Clin Invest. 2011;121(10):3981–90.
13. Yamauchi Y, Abe K, Mantani A, Hitoshi Y, Suzuki M, Osuzu F, Kuratani S, Yamamura K. A novel transgenic technique that allows specific marking of the neural crest cell lineage in mice. Dev Biol. 1999;212(1):191–203.
14. Humphreys BD, Lin SL, Kobayashi A, Hudson TE, Nowlin BT, Bonventre JV, Valerius MT, McMahon AP, Duffield JS. Fate tracing reveals the pericyte and not epithelial origin of myofibroblasts in kidney fibrosis. Am J Pathol. 2010; 176(1):85–97.
15. Iwaisako K, Jiang C, Zhang M, Cong M, Moore-Morris TJ, Park TJ, Liu X, Xu J, Wang P, Paik YH, et al. Origin of myofibroblasts in the fibrotic liver in mice. Proc Natl Acad Sci U S A. 2014;111(32):E3297–305.
16. Hung C, Linn G, Chow YH, Kobayashi A, Mittelsteadt K, Altemeier WA, Gharib SA, Schnapp LM, Duffield JS. Role of lung pericytes and resident fibroblasts in the pathogenesis of pulmonary fibrosis. Am J Respir Crit Care Med. 2013;188(7):820–30.
17. Xie T, Liang J, Liu N, Huan C, Zhang Y, Liu W, Kumar M, Xiao R, D'Armiento J, Metzger D, et al. Transcription factor TBX4 regulates myofibroblast accumulation and lung fibrosis. J Clin Invest. 2016;126(8):3063–79.
18. Dulauroy S, Di Carlo SE, Langa F, Eberl G, Peduto L. Lineage tracing and genetic ablation of ADAM12(+) perivascular cells identify a major source of profibrotic cells during acute tissue injury. Nat Med. 2012;18(8):1262–70.
19. Rinkevich Y, Walmsley GG, Hu MS, Maan ZN, Newman AM, Drukker M, Januszyk M, Krampitz GW, Gurtner GC, Lorenz HP, et al. Skin fibrosis. Identification and isolation of a dermal lineage with intrinsic fibrogenic potential. Science. 2015;348(6232):aaa2151.
20. Kramann R, Schneider RK, DiRocco DP, Machado F, Fleig S, Bondzie PA, Henderson JM, Ebert BL, Humphreys BD. Perivascular Gli1+ progenitors are key contributors to injury-induced organ fibrosis. Cell Stem Cell. 2015;16(1):51–66.
21. Crisan M, Yap S, Casteilla L, Chen CW, Corselli M, Park TS, Andriolo G, Sun B, Zheng B, Zhang L, et al. A perivascular origin for mesenchymal stem cells in multiple human organs. Cell Stem Cell. 2008;3(3):301–13.

22. Stefanska A, Kenyon C, Christian HC, Buckley C, Shaw I, Mullins JJ, Peault B. Human kidney pericytes produce renin. Kidney Int. 2016;90(6):1251–61.

23. Bechtel W, McGoohan S, Zeisberg EM, Muller GA, Kalbacher H, Salant DJ, Muller CA, Kalluri R, Zeisberg M. Methylation determines fibroblast activation and fibrogenesis in the kidney. Nat Med. 2010;16(5):544–50.

24. Obara N, Suzuki N, Kim K, Nagasawa T, Imagawa S, Yamamoto M. Repression via the GATA box is essential for tissue-specific erythropoietin gene expression. Blood. 2008;111(10):5223–32.

25. Souma T, Yamazaki S, Moriguchi T, Suzuki N, Hirano I, Pan X, Minegishi N, Abe M, Kiyomoto H, Ito S, et al. Plasticity of renal erythropoietin-producing cells governs fibrosis. J Am Soc Nephrol. 2013;24(10):1599–616.

26. Brookhart MA, Schneeweiss S, Avorn J, Bradbury BD, Rothman KJ, Fischer M, Mehta J, Winkelmayer WC. The effect of altitude on dosing and response to erythropoietin in ESRD. J Am Soc Nephrol. 2008;19(7):1389–95.

27. Takaori K, Nakamura J, Yamamoto S, Nakata H, Sato Y, Takase M, Nameta M, Yamamoto T, Economides AN, Kohno K, et al. Severity and frequency of proximal tubule injury determines renal prognosis. J Am Soc Nephrol. 2016; 27(8):2393–406.

28. Yang L, Besschetnova TY, Brooks CR, Shah JV, Bonventre JV. Epithelial cell cycle arrest in G2/M mediates kidney fibrosis after injury. Nat Med. 2010; 16(5):535–43. 1p following 143.

29. Souma T, Yamazaki S, Moriguchi T, Suzuki N, Hirano I, Pan X, Minegishi N, Abe M, Kiyomoto H, Ito S, et al. Plasticity of renal erythropoietin-producing cells governs fibrosis. Journal of the American Society of Nephrology : JASN. 2013;24(10):1599–616.

30. Campanholle G, Ligresti G, Gharib SA, Duffield JS. Cellular mechanisms of tissue fibrosis. 3. Novel mechanisms of kidney fibrosis. Am J Physiol Cell Physiol. 2013;304(7):C591–603.

31. Tanaka T, Nangaku M. Recent advances and clinical application of erythropoietin and erythropoiesis-stimulating agents. Exp Cell Res. 2012; 318(9):1068–73.

32. Aoki T, Narumiya S. Prostaglandins and chronic inflammation. Trends Pharmacol Sci. 2012;33(6):304–11.

33. Nakagawa N, Yuhki K, Kawabe J, Fujino T, Takahata O, Kabara M, Abe K, Kojima F, Kashiwagi H, Hasebe N, et al. The intrinsic prostaglandin E2-EP4 system of the renal tubular epithelium limits the development of tubulointerstitial fibrosis in mice. Kidney Int. 2012;82(2):158–71.

34. Stitt-Cavanagh EM, Faour WH, Takami K, Carter A, Vanderhyden B, Guan Y, Schneider A, Breyer MD, Kennedy CR. A maladaptive role for EP4 receptors in podocytes. J Am Soc Nephrol. 2010;21(10):1678–90.

35. Neyt K, Perros F, GeurtsvanKessel CH, Hammad H, Lambrecht BN. Tertiary lymphoid organs in infection and autoimmunity. Trends Immunol. 2012; 33(6):297–305.

36. Aloisi F, Pujol-Borrell R. Lymphoid neogenesis in chronic inflammatory diseases. Nat Rev Immunol. 2006;6(3):205–17.

37. Wu Q, Salomon B, Chen M, Wang Y, Hoffman LM, Bluestone JA, Fu YX. Reversal of spontaneous autoimmune insulitis in nonobese diabetic mice by soluble lymphotoxin receptor. J Exp Med. 2001;193(11):1327–32.

38. Moyron-Quiroz JE, Rangel-Moreno J, Kusser K, Hartson L, Sprague F, Goodrich S, Woodland DL, Lund FE, Randall TD. Role of inducible bronchus associated lymphoid tissue (iBALT) in respiratory immunity. Nat Med. 2004;10(9):927–34.

39. Drayton DL, Liao S, Mounzer RH, Ruddle NH. Lymphoid organ development: from ontogeny to neogenesis. Nat Immunol. 2006;7(4):344–53.

40. Jones GW, Hill DG, Jones SA. Understanding immune cells in tertiary lymphoid organ development: it is all starting to come together. Front Immunol. 2016;7(401). doi:10.3389/fimmu.2016.00401.

41. Luther SA, Lopez T, Bai W, Hanahan D, Cyster JG. BLC expression in pancreatic islets causes B cell recruitment and lymphotoxin-dependent lymphoid neogenesis. Immunity. 2000;12(5):471–81.

42. Luther SA, Bidgol A, Hargreaves DC, Schmidt A, Xu Y, Paniyadi J, Matloubian M, Cyster JG. Differing activities of homeostatic chemokines CCL19, CCL21, and CXCL12 in lymphocyte and dendritic cell recruitment and lymphoid neogenesis. J Immunol. 2002;169(1):424–33.

43. Ishani A, Xue JL, Himmelfarb J, Eggers PW, Kimmel PL, Molitoris BA, Collins AJ. Acute kidney injury increases risk of ESRD among elderly. J Am Soc Nephrol. 2009;20(1):223–8.

44. Medzhitov R. Origin and physiological roles of inflammation. Nature. 2008; 454(7203):428–35.

45. Frangogiannis NG. Regulation of the inflammatory response in cardiac repair. Circ Res. 2012;110(1):159–73.

46. Barone F, Gardner DH, Nayar S, Steinthal N, Buckley CD, Luther SA. Stromal fibroblasts in tertiary lymphoid structures: a novel target in chronic inflammation. Front Immunol. 2016;7(477). doi:10.3389/fimmu.2016.00477.

47. Heesters BA, Myers RC, Carroll MC. Follicular dendritic cells: dynamic antigen libraries. Nat Rev Immunol. 2014;14(7):495–504.

48. Krautler NJ, Kana V, Kranich J, Tian Y, Perera D, Lemm D, Schwarz P, Armulik A, Browning JL, Tallquist M, et al. Follicular dendritic cells emerge from ubiquitous perivascular precursors. Cell. 2012;150(1):194–206.

49. Jarjour M, Jorquera A, Mondor I, Wienert S, Narang P, Coles MC, Klauschen F, Bajenoff M. Fate mapping reveals origin and dynamics of lymph node follicular dendritic cells. J Exp Med. 2014;211(6):1109–22.

50. Shimatani K, Nakashima Y, Hattori M, Hamazaki Y, Minato N. PD-1+ memory phenotype CD4+ T cells expressing C/EBPalpha underlie T cell immunodepression in senescence and leukemia. Proc Natl Acad Sci U S A. 2009;106(37):15807–12.

51. Hwang JY, Randall TD, Silva-Sanchez A. Inducible bronchus-associated lymphoid tissue: taming inflammation in the lung. Front Immunol. 2016; 7(258). doi:10.3389/fimmu.2016.00258.

52. Rangel-Moreno J, Carragher DM, de la Luz Garcia-Hernandez M, Hwang JY, Kusser K, Hartson L, Kolls JK, Khader SA, Randall TD. The development of inducible bronchus-associated lymphoid tissue depends on IL-17. Nat Immunol. 2011;12(7):639–46.

53. Rangel-Moreno J, Moyron-Quiroz JE, Hartson L, Kusser K, Randall TD. Pulmonary expression of CXC chemokine ligand 13, CC chemokine ligand 19, and CC chemokine ligand 21 is essential for local immunity to influenza. Proc Natl Acad Sci U S A. 2007;104(25):10577–82.

54. Ishikawa S, Sato T, Abe M, Nagai S, Onai N, Yoneyama H, Zhang Y, Suzuki T, Hashimoto S, Shirai T, et al. Aberrant high expression of B lymphocyte chemokine (BLC/CXCL13) by C11b+ CD11c+ dendritic cells in murine lupus and preferential chemotaxis of B1 cells towards BLC. J Exp Med. 2001; 193(12):1393–402.

55. Moreth K, Brodbeck R, Babelova A, Gretz N, Spieker T, Zeng-Brouwers J, Pfeilschifter J, Young MF, Schaefer RM, Schaefer L. The proteoglycan biglycan regulates expression of the B cell chemoattractant CXCL13 and aggravates murine lupus nephritis. J Clin Invest. 2010;120(12):4251–72.

56. Lehmann-Horn K, Wang SZ, Sagan SA, Zamvil SS, von Budingen HC. B cell repertoire expansion occurs in meningeal ectopic lymphoid tissue. JCI Insight. 2016;1(20), e87234.

57. Finkin S, Yuan D, Stein I, Taniguchi K, Weber A, Unger K, Browning JL, Goossens N, Nakagawa S, Gunasekaran G, et al. Ectopic lymphoid structures function as microniches for tumor progenitor cells in hepatocellular carcinoma. Nat Immunol. 2015;16(12):1235–44.

58. Shinoda K, Hirahara K, Iinuma T, Ichikawa T, Suzuki AS, Sugaya K, Tumes DJ, Yamamoto H, Hara T, Tani-Ichi S, et al. Thy1 + IL-7+ lymphatic endothelial cells in iBALT provide a survival niche for memory T-helper cells in allergic airway inflammation. Proc Natl Acad Sci U S A. 2016;113(20):E2842–51.

10

Receptor-associated prorenin system contributes to development of inflammation and angiogenesis in proliferative diabetic retinopathy

Atsuhiro Kanda[*] (iD) and Susumu Ishida

Abstract

The renin-angiotensin system (RAS) plays a potential role in the development of end-organ damage, and tissue RAS activation has been suggested as a risk factor of several diseases including diabetes. So far, using animal disease models, we have shown molecular mechanisms, in which tissue RAS stimulates retinal angiogenesis, and the critical roles of (pro)renin receptor [(P)RR] in retinal RAS activation and its concurrent intracellular signal transduction, referred to as the receptor-associated prorenin system (RAPS). Moreover, we recently reported that the protein levels of prorenin and soluble (P)RR increased in the vitreous fluids obtained from patients with proliferative diabetic retinopathy (PDR), suggesting the association of (P)RR with vascular endothelial growth factor (VEGF)-driven angiogenic activity in human PDR, and also showed a close relationship between the vitreous renin activity and VEGF-induced pathogenesis of diabetic retinopathy. Our data using animal disease models and human clinical samples suggest that both vitreous RAS and retinal RAPS play critical roles in the molecular pathogenesis of diabetic retinopathy.

Keywords: Receptor-associated prorenin system, Renin-angiotensin system, Angiotensin II type 1 receptor, (Pro) renin receptor

Abbreviations: (P)RR, (Pro)renin receptor; ACE, Angiotensin-converting enzyme; AGT, Angiotensinogen; Ang, Angiotensin; AT1R, Angiotensin II type 1 receptor; DR, Diabetic retinopathy; ERK, Extracellular signal-regulated kinase; NF-kB, Nuclear factor-kB; PDR, Proliferative diabetic retinopathy; RAPS, Receptor-associated prorenin system; RAS, Renin-angiotensin system; VEGF, Vascular endothelial growth factor

Background

Diabetic retinopathy (DR) is one of the severe complications of diabetes and leading cause of severe vision loss and blindness when it progresses to the stage of proliferative DR (PDR) characterized by fibrovascular proliferation. Fibrovascular tissue develops by the extension of retinal angiogenesis into the vitreous cavity, and formation of the fibrovascular tissue results in severe complications, such as tractional retinal detachment and vitreous hemorrhage. Several growth factors and cytokines are involved in the molecular pathogenesis of diabetic retinopathy; however, vascular endothelial growth factor (VEGF) has been considered as the major angiogenic and proinflammatory factor in PDR [1–3]. VEGF plays important roles in normal physiology such as in embryogenesis, endometrial maturation, and wound healing. However, it also causes profound pathogenesis complicating diabetes and cancer. Tumor growth requires new vessel formation, which is driven predominantly by VEGF, the most potent angiogenic factor and the principal target for anti-angiogenic therapy [4]. We previously revealed a significant contribution of VEGF165 isoform to angiogenic activity in PDR, showing that fibrovascular tissues co-expressing VEGF receptor (VEGFR)-2 and neuropilin (NRP) 1, the specific receptor for VEGF165, were highly vascularized [5–7].

* Correspondence: kanda@med.hokudai.ac.jp
Laboratory of Ocular Cell Biology and Visual Science, Department of Ophthalmology, Hokkaido University Graduate School of Medicine, N-15, W-7, Kita-ku, Sapporo, Hokkaido 060-8638, Japan

VEGF165 were shown to increase the expression of adhesion molecules and subsequently stimulates leukocyte infiltration leading to the development of retinal angiogenesis [5–7].

The renin-angiotensin system (RAS), a known important controller of systemic blood pressure (circulatory RAS), plays distinct roles in inflammation and pathological vascular conditions in organs including the brain, eye, heart, liver, and kidney (tissue RAS) [8]. Tissue RAS acts in a paracrine fashion and regulates various biological and pathological events such as cell signaling, apoptosis, proliferation, angiogenesis, immune responses, and extracellular matrix formation [9–11]. In this review, we focus on the relationship between diabetic retinopathy and tissue RAS and suggest a novel concept for the molecular pathogenesis of tissue RAS in the vitreous, referred to as "vitreous RAS."

Vitreous renin-angiotensin system and retinal receptor-associated prorenin system in diabetic retinopathy

Several types of organ damage are known to result from activation of tissue RAS. As concerns its relationship with the eye, pharmacological blockade of angiotensin-converting enzyme (ACE) or angiotensin II type 1 receptor (AT1R) resulted in beneficial effects on the incidence and progression of DR in several clinical trials including the EUCLID study, DIRECT-Prevent 1, DIRECT-Protect 1, DIRECT-Protect 2, and the RAS study [12–15]. We unraveled the molecular mechanisms in which tissue RAS causes retinal inflammation and angiogenesis in the murine model of endotoxin-induced uveitis, strepotozotocin-induced diabetes, and laser-induced choroidal neovascularization [16–18] and the critical role of (pro)renin receptor [(P)RR] in retinal RAS activation [19–22]. Tissue RAS is initiated by prorenin binding with (P)RR to acquire renin activity, which also causes RAS-independent signal transduction in cells bearing (P)RR. Prorenin binding to (P)RR causes renin activity through the conformational change of prorenin (non-proteolytic activation of prorenin causing tissue RAS) instead of the conventional proteolysis of the prorenin prosegment by processing enzymes (proteolytic activation of prorenin causing circulatory RAS). In addition to tissue RAS activation, prorenin binding to (P)RR activates RAS-independent signal transduction via mitogen-activated protein kinases including extracellular signal-regulated kinase (ERK) 1/2 pathway, which has been shown to contribute to organ damage. (P)RR can bind to both prorenin and renin, but the binding affinity of prorenin is much higher than that of renin [23]. The (P)RR-mediated dual activation of tissue RAS and RAS-independent signaling pathways, referred to as the receptor-associated prorenin system (RAPS), was shown to be involved in the molecular pathogenesis of ocular disorders including retinal inflammation and choroidal

neovascularization [20, 21, 24], both of which are due to the upregulated expression of VEGF in the downstream of retinal and choroidal RAPS, respectively.

Remarkably, (P)RR was reported to undergo cleavage by proteases to generate a soluble form of (P)RR [s(P)RR], whereas it still has a capability for non-proteolytic activation of prorenin, causing the conversion of angiotensinogen (AGT) to angiotensin I (Ang I) in vitro [25]. We have shown that s(P)RR, prorenin, activated prorenin, and VEGF protein levels together with renin activity levels in vitreous fluids were significantly higher in PDR eyes compared to non-diabetic controls [26, 27]. Increased protein levels of s(P)RR in PDR eyes, released from neovascular endothelial cells in fibrovascular tissues, were significantly correlated with vitreous prorenin, activated prorenin, and VEGF protein levels and the vascular density of fibrovascular tissues [26]. Interestingly, renin activity levels also significantly correlated with the vitreous protein levels of s(P)RR, prorenin, activated prorenin, and VEGF [27]. These data indicate that the vitreous renin activity stems from s(P)RR-mediated non-proteolytic activation of prorenin, suggesting the significant role of (P)RR in the pathogenesis of PDR. Indeed, (P)RR and RAS components were expressed in diabetic fibrovascular tissues, human retinal cell lines, and normal ocular tissues [26, 28–30], and the vitreous levels of prorenin and angiotensin II (Ang II) were shown to be elevated in PDR eyes [31–34]. Furthermore, a close link between the vitreous renin activity and VEGF protein levels validates our concept of vitreous RAS that contributes to the angiogenic activity of DR. Consequently, in concert with vitreous RAS due to s(P)RR (Fig. 1a) [27], retinal RAPS due to membrane-type (i.e., full-length) (P)RR [26] (Fig. 1b) is thought to regulate VEGF expression in DR. Moreover, we have recently shown that RAPS is involved in the molecular pathogenesis of organ damage, such as inflammation, angiogenesis, and fibrosis, including conjunctival lymphoma [28] and other ocular disorders (under review).

Although we have shown the significant role of (P)RR signaling via ERK [21, 26] as well as AT1R signaling via nuclear factor (NF)-kB [16] in the upregulation of VEGF expression, it is difficult to determine the ratio of involvement with the angiogenic activity in human PDR. Cleavage enzymes for processing full-length (P)RR to s(P)RR include the proprotein convertase furin [35] and ADAM (a disintegrin and metalloproteinase) 19 [36], both of which proved to be present in endothelial cells in the fibrovascular tissue in PDR [26]. Gene expression and enzymatic activity of these proteases in the neovascular endothelial cells are likely to define the contribution ratio between vitreous RAS and retinal RAPS. Investigation into the biochemical regulation of furin and ADAM19 is required in the future to further elucidate (P)RR-related molecular pathogenesis of diabetic retinopathy.

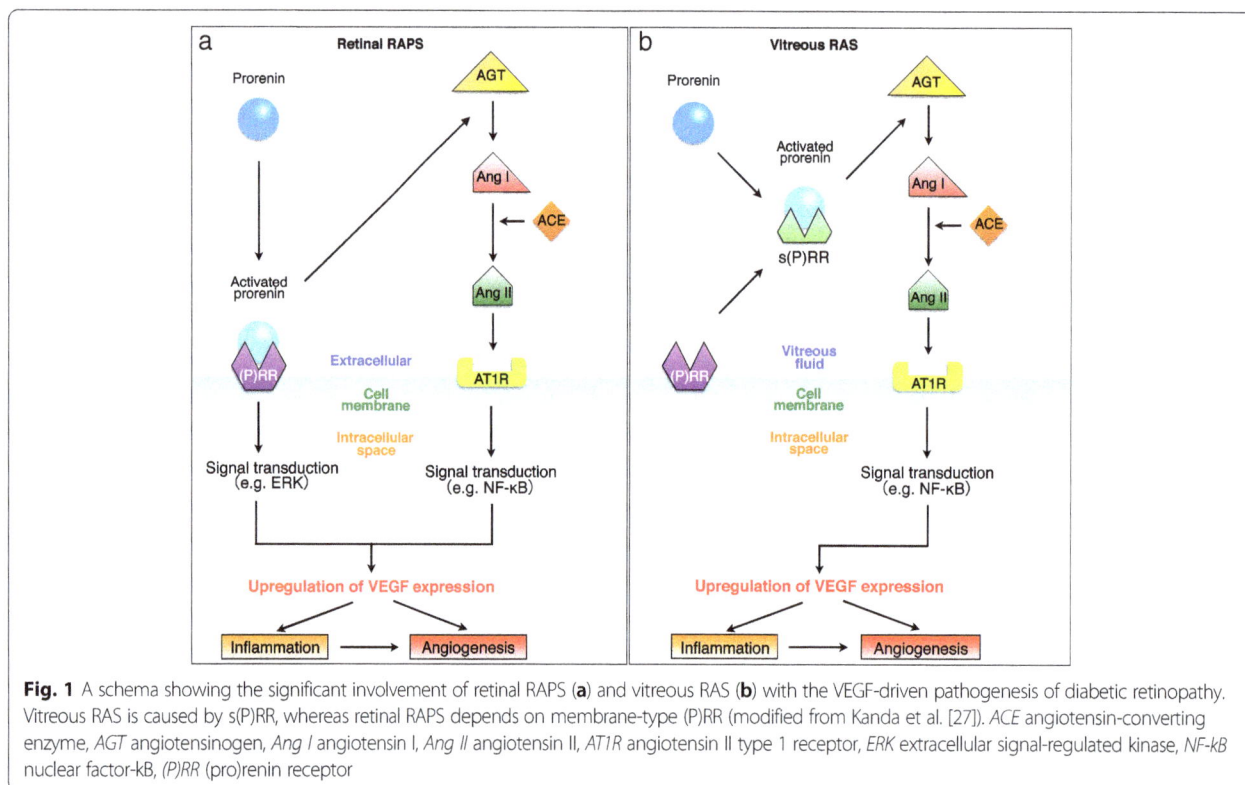

Fig. 1 A schema showing the significant involvement of retinal RAPS (**a**) and vitreous RAS (**b**) with the VEGF-driven pathogenesis of diabetic retinopathy. Vitreous RAS is caused by s(P)RR, whereas retinal RAPS depends on membrane-type (P)RR (modified from Kanda et al. [27]). *ACE* angiotensin-converting enzyme, *AGT* angiotensinogen, *Ang I* angiotensin I, *Ang II* angiotensin II, *AT1R* angiotensin II type 1 receptor, *ERK* extracellular signal-regulated kinase, *NF-kB* nuclear factor-kB, *(P)RR* (pro)renin receptor

The significance of the pathogenic system vitreous RAS may be attributed in part to a possibility of revising the current surgical indication and concept of vitrectomy for DR. In clinical setting, retinal surgeons remove the vitreous from PDR eyes because of (1) vitreous hemorrhage from newly formed vessels disturbing the visual axis and (2) tractional retinal detachment in which the retina is elevated by the vitreous that functions as the scaffold of the fibrovascular proliferative tissue originating from retinal vessels. These two major classic indications to the advanced stage have long been applied in terms of a mechanical or physical cue. In contrast, our data on vitreous renin activity indicate the possibility of the vitreous per se as the amplifier of the molecular pathogenesis of PDR. Retinal surgeons frequently encounter surgical cases where diabetic macular edema, a consequence of VEGF-induced vascular hyperpermeabiliy, is diminished soon after vitrectomy. This is explained at least in part by the pathological concept of vitreous RAS, the driving force of the downstream AT1R/nuclear factor-kB (NF-kB)/VEGF axis responsible for the pathogenesis of diabetic retinopathy (Fig. 1). It is reasonable, therefore, to think that the vitreous is not just the reservoir of detrimental cytokines but the factory of pathogenic RAS components. In this sense, vitrectomy procedure harbors a biochemical implication, which may expand the current surgical strategy to earlier intervention for broader indications to reduce the vitreous RAS-derived capability of producing VEGF and other several cytokines.

Conclusions

Our findings may not only lead to a new understanding of the molecular pathogenesis that implies a close link among the vitreous RAS, retinal RAPS, and VEGF-induced pathogenesis of diabetic retinopathy but also activate the clinical research in the surgical as well as medical point of view, thus contributing to further improvement of visual prognosis in patients with DR.

Acknowledgements
We thank Ikuyo Hirose (Hokkaido University) for their skillful technical assistance.

Funding
This work was supported in part by the Matching Program for Innovations in Future Drug Discovery and Medical Care, Takeda Science Foundation, and a grant-in-aid from the Ministry of Education, Science and Culture of Japan KAKENHI to A.K. (24791823, 16K11279) and S.I. (16H05484).

Authors' contributions
The authors equally contributed to the preparation of this review. All authors read and approved the final manuscript.

Competing interests
The authors declare that they have no competing interests.

References

1. Adamis AP, Miller JW, Bernal MT, D'Amico DJ, Folkman J, Yeo TK, Yeo KT. Increased vascular endothelial growth factor levels in the vitreous of eyes with proliferative diabetic retinopathy. Am J Ophthalmol. 1994;118:445–50.
2. Aiello LP, Avery RL, Arrigg PG, Keyt BA, Jampel HD, Shah ST, Pasquale LR, Thieme H, Iwamoto MA, Park JE, et al. Vascular endothelial growth factor in ocular fluid of patients with diabetic retinopathy and other retinal disorders. N Engl J Med. 1994;331:1480–7.
3. Malecaze F, Clamens S, Simorre-Pinatel V, Mathis A, Chollet P, Favard C, Bayard F, Plouet J. Detection of vascular endothelial growth factor messenger RNA and vascular endothelial growth factor-like activity in proliferative diabetic retinopathy. Arch Ophthalmol. 1994;112:1476–82.
4. Hurwitz H, Fehrenbacher L, Novotny W, Cartwright T, Hainsworth J, Heim W, Berlin J, Baron A, Griffing S, Holmgren E, et al. Bevacizumab plus irinotecan, fluorouracil, and leucovorin for metastatic colorectal cancer. N Engl J Med. 2004;350:2335–42.
5. Ishida S, Usui T, Yamashiro K, Kaji Y, Ahmed E, Carrasquillo KG, Amano S, Hida T, Oguchi Y, Adamis AP. VEGF164 is proinflammatory in the diabetic retina. Invest Ophthalmol Vis Sci. 2003;44:2155–62.
6. Ishida S, Usui T, Yamashiro K, Kaji Y, Amano S, Ogura Y, Hida T, Oguchi Y, Ambati J, Miller JW, et al. VEGF164-mediated inflammation is required for pathological, but not physiological, ischemia-induced retinal neovascularization. J Exp Med. 2003;198:483–9.
7. Usui T, Ishida S, Yamashiro K, Kaji Y, Poulaki V, Moore J, Moore T, Amano S, Horikawa Y, Dartt D, et al. VEGF164(165) as the pathological isoform: differential leukocyte and endothelial responses through VEGFR1 and VEGFR2. Invest Ophthalmol Vis Sci. 2004;45:368–74.
8. Paul M, Poyan Mehr A, Kreutz R. Physiology of local renin-angiotensin systems. Physiol Rev. 2006;86:747–803.
9. Ager EI, Neo J, Christophi C. The renin-angiotensin system and malignancy. Carcinogenesis. 2008;29:1675–84.
10. Ramalho FS, Ramalho LN, Castro-e-Silva Junior O, Zucoloto S, Correa FM. Effect of angiotensin-converting enzyme inhibitors on liver regeneration in rats. Hepatogastroenterology. 2002;49:1347–51.
11. Yayama K, Miyagi R, Sugiyama K, Sugaya T, Fukamizu A, Okamoto H. Angiotensin II regulates liver regeneration via type 1 receptor following partial hepatectomy in mice. Biol Pharm Bull. 2008;31:1356–61.
12. Chaturvedi N, Sjolie AK, Stephenson JM, Abrahamian H, Keipes M, Castellarin A, Rogulja-Pepeonik Z, Fuller JH. Effect of lisinopril on progression of retinopathy in normotensive people with type 1 diabetes. The EUCLID study group. EURODIAB controlled trial of lisinopril in insulin-dependent diabetes mellitus. Lancet. 1998;351:28–31.
13. Chaturvedi N, Porta M, Klein R, Orchard T, Fuller J, Parving HH, Bilous R, Sjolie AK. Effect of candesartan on prevention (DIRECT-Prevent 1) and progression (DIRECT-Protect 1) of retinopathy in type 1 diabetes: randomised, placebo-controlled trials. Lancet. 2008;372:1394–402.
14. Sjolie AK, Klein R, Porta M, Orchard T, Fuller J, Parving HH, Bilous R, Chaturvedi N. Effect of candesartan on progression and regression of retinopathy in type 2 diabetes (DIRECT-Protect 2): a randomised placebo-controlled trial. Lancet. 2008;372:1385–93.
15. Mauer M, Zinman B, Gardiner R, Suissa S, Sinaiko A, Strand T, Drummond K, Donnelly S, Goodyer P, Gubler MC, Klein R. Renal and retinal effects of enalapril and losartan in type 1 diabetes. N Engl J Med. 2009;361:40–51.
16. Nagai N, Izumi-Nagai K, Oike Y, Koto T, Satofuka S, Ozawa Y, Yamashiro K, Inoue M, Tsubota K, Umezawa K, Ishida S. Suppression of diabetes-induced retinal inflammation by blocking the angiotensin II type 1 receptor or its downstream nuclear factor-kappaB pathway. Invest Ophthalmol Vis Sci. 2007;48:4342–50.
17. Nagai N, Noda K, Urano T, Kubota Y, Shinoda H, Koto T, Shinoda K, Inoue M, Shiomi T, Ikeda E, et al. Selective suppression of pathologic, but not physiologic, retinal neovascularization by blocking the angiotensin II type 1 receptor. Invest Ophthalmol Vis Sci. 2005;46:1078–84.
18. Nagai N, Oike Y, Izumi-Nagai K, Urano T, Kubota Y, Noda K, Ozawa Y, Inoue M, Tsubota K, Suda T, Ishida S. Angiotensin II type 1 receptor-mediated inflammation is required for choroidal neovascularization. Arterioscler Thromb Vasc Biol. 2006;26:2252–9.
19. Satofuka S, Ichihara A, Nagai N, Koto T, Shinoda H, Noda K, Ozawa Y, Inoue M, Tsubota K, Itoh H, et al. Role of nonproteolytically activated prorenin in pathologic, but not physiologic, retinal neovascularization. Invest Ophthalmol Vis Sci. 2007;48:422–9.
20. Satofuka S, Ichihara A, Nagai N, Noda K, Ozawa Y, Fukamizu A, Tsubota K, Itoh H, Oike Y, Ishida S. (Pro)renin receptor promotes choroidal neovascularization by activating its signal transduction and tissue renin-angiotensin system. Am J Pathol. 2008;173:1911–8.
21. Satofuka S, Ichihara A, Nagai N, Noda K, Ozawa Y, Fukamizu A, Tsubota K, Itoh H, Oike Y, Ishida S. (Pro)renin receptor-mediated signal transduction and tissue renin-angiotensin system contribute to diabetes-induced retinal inflammation. Diabetes. 2009;58:1625–33.
22. Satofuka S, Ichihara A, Nagai N, Yamashiro K, Koto T, Shinoda H, Noda K, Ozawa Y, Inoue M, Tsubota K, et al. Suppression of ocular inflammation in endotoxin-induced uveitis by inhibiting nonproteolytic activation of prorenin. Invest Ophthalmol Vis Sci. 2006;47:2686–92.
23. Nabi AH, Kageshima A, Uddin MN, Nakagawa T, Park EY, Suzuki F. Binding properties of rat prorenin and renin to the recombinant rat renin/prorenin receptor prepared by a baculovirus expression system. Int J Mol Med. 2006;18:483–8.
24. Satofuka S, Kanda A, Ishida S. Receptor-associated prorenin system in the pathogenesis of retinal diseases. Front Biosci. 2012;4:1449–60.
25. Biswas KB, Nabi AN, Arai Y, Nakagawa T, Ebihara A, Ichihara A, Inagami T, Suzuki F. Qualitative and quantitative analyses of (pro)renin receptor in the medium of cultured human umbilical vein endothelial cells. Hypertens Res. 2010;34:735–9.
26. Kanda A, Noda K, Saito W, Ishida S. (Pro)renin receptor is associated with angiogenic activity in proliferative diabetic retinopathy. Diabetologia. 2012;55:3104–13.
27. Kanda A, Noda K, Saito W, Ishida S. Vitreous renin activity correlates with vascular endothelial growth factor in proliferative diabetic retinopathy. Br J Ophthalmol. 2013;97:666–8.
28. Ishizuka ET, Kanda A, Kase S, Noda K, Ishida S. Involvement of the receptor-associated prorenin system in the pathogenesis of human conjunctival lymphoma. Invest Ophthalmol Vis Sci. 2015;56:74–80.
29. Kanda A, Noda K, Ishida S. ATP6AP2/(pro)renin receptor contributes to glucose metabolism via stabilizing the pyruvate dehydrogenase E1 beta subunit. J Biol Chem. 2015;290:9690–700.
30. Kanda A, Noda K, Yuki K, Ozawa Y, Furukawa T, Ichihara A, Ishida S. Atp6ap2/(pro)renin receptor interacts with Par3 as a cell polarity determinant required for laminar formation during retinal development in mice. J Neurosci. 2013;33:19341–51.
31. Danser AH, van den Dorpel MA, Deinum J, Derkx FH, Franken AA, Peperkamp E, de Jong PT, Schalekamp MA. Renin, prorenin, and immunoreactive renin in vitreous fluid from eyes with and without diabetic retinopathy. J Clin Endocrinol Metab. 1989;68:160–7.
32. Funatsu H, Yamashita H, Nakanishi Y, Hori S. Angiotensin II and vascular endothelial growth factor in the vitreous fluid of patients with proliferative diabetic retinopathy. Br J Ophthalmol. 2002;86:311–5.
33. Gao BB, Chen X, Timothy N, Aiello LP, Feener EP. Characterization of the vitreous proteome in diabetes without diabetic retinopathy and diabetes with proliferative diabetic retinopathy. J Proteome Res. 2008;7:2516–25.
34. Gao BB, Clermont A, Rook S, Fonda SJ, Srinivasan VJ, Wojtkowski M, Fujimoto JG, Avery RL, Arrigg PG, Bursell SE, et al. Extracellular carbonic anhydrase mediates hemorrhagic retinal and cerebral vascular permeability through prekallikrein activation. Nat Med. 2007;13:181–8.
35. Cousin C, Bracquart D, Contrepas A, Corvol P, Muller L, Nguyen G. Soluble form of the (pro)renin receptor generated by intracellular cleavage by furin is secreted in plasma. Hypertension. 2009;53:1077–82.
36. Yoshikawa A, Aizaki Y, Kusano K, Kishi F, Susumu T, Iida S, Ishiura S, Nishimura S, Shichiri M, Senbonmatsu T. The (pro)renin receptor is cleaved by ADAM19 in the Golgi leading to its secretion into extracellular space. Hypertens Res. 2011;34:599–605.

11

Therapeutic intervention of inflammatory/immune diseases by inhibition of the fractalkine (CX3CL1)-CX3CR1 pathway

Toshio Imai* and Nobuyuki Yasuda

Abstract

Inflammatory and immune responses are generated locally by the selective invasion and accumulation of the immune cells into the lesion site. The infiltration process of the immune cells into the tissue from the blood through the vascular endothelial cells is closely regulated by a number of chemotactic factors and cell adhesion molecules.

Fractalkine (FKN)/CX3CL1 is a membrane-bound chemokine possessing a chemokine/mucin hybrid structure and a transmembrane domain and has a dual function as an adhesion molecule and a chemoattractant. FKN is mainly expressed on activated endothelial cells, activated fibroblasts, and osteoblasts. Its receptor, CX3CR1, is expressed on cytotoxic effector lymphocytes, monocytes/macrophages, and osteoclasts. To date, a lot of key functional aspects of the FKN-CX3CR1 axis has been identified: (1) the rapid capture and firm adhesion of immune cells to vascular endothelial cells, (2) chemotaxis, (3) the enhancement of the transmigration to other chemokines, (4) the crawling behavior of the monocytes that patrol on vascular endothelial cells, (5) the retention of monocytes as the accessory cells of the inflamed endothelium to recruit inflammatory cells, and (6) the survival of the macrophage.

In this review, we will focus on the pathological role of FKN in rheumatoid arthritis (RA) and the physiological role of FKN on osteoclast differentiation. Furthermore, we will discuss the therapeutic potential of anti-FKN mAb for RA patients and its distinct mode of action from other cytokine inhibitors.

Keywords: Fractalkine/CX3CL1, CX3CR1, Osteoclast, Rheumatoid arthritis, E6011

Background

Rheumatoid arthritis (RA) is a long-lasting autoimmune disorder that primarily affects joints characterized by synovial hyperplasia and bone erosion associated with neovascularization, infiltration of proinflammatory cells, and increased cytokine production. Chemokines and their receptors control immune cell trafficking and are crucial for the inflammatory process. Fractalkine (FKN) is a unique membrane-bound chemokine possessing multiple biological functions. The FKN-CX3CR1 axis participates in the patrol for tissue damages and the quick mobilization and accumulation of immune cells to the sites of danger. The FKN-CX3CR1 axis is also involved in the pathogenesis in both bone-resorbing and inflammatory diseases. Taken together, FKN-CX3CR1 is expected to be a novel therapeutic target for RA by simultaneous direct inhibition of inflammation and bone resorption.

Introduction

Rheumatoid arthritis (RA) is a chronic inflammatory disease characterized by the synovial hyperplasia, joint destruction, and massive infiltration of lymphocytes and macrophages into the synovium. Fibroblast-like synoviocytes (FLSs) also play a major role in the pathogenesis of RA by producing a variety of cytokines, chemokines, and matrix-degrading enzymes that mediate the interaction with neighboring inflammatory and endothelial cells. Chronic inflammatory environments are responsible for the progressive inflammation in the joints and the destruction of the articular cartilage and bone [1].

* Correspondence: t-imai@kan.eisai.co.jp
KAN Research Institute, Inc., 6-8-2 Minatojima-minamimachi Chuo-ku, Kobe, Hyogo 650-0047, Japan

Chemokines are a family of small (8–10 kDa) proteins that play an important role in the recruitment and activation of immune cells. They are subdivided into four subfamilies, C, CC, CXC, and CX3C chemokines, based on the number and spacing of the amino-terminal, conserved cysteine residues. The biological effects of chemokines are mediated by their binding to the cognate receptors, seven-transmembrane G protein-coupled receptors (GPCRs). Over 50 chemokines and 19 receptors have been identified, for which complex ligand-receptor relationships are revealed with high redundancy [2].

Chemokines are originally identified as potent attractants for leukocytes such as neutrophils and monocytes and therefore are generally considered as mediators of acute inflammation (inflammatory chemokines). In addition, several chemokines have been found to be constitutively expressed in lymphoid and other tissues with individually characteristic patterns. Lymphocytes also express chemokine receptors with a cell-specific manner. Accumulating evidence indicates that chemokines are important not only in inflammation but also in the development, homeostasis, and functions of the immune system that should be shaped in a proper balance (immune or homeostatic chemokines).

In this review, we will discuss the roles of FKN, the only member of the CX3C chemokine family, on inflammatory/immune diseases and its potential as a new therapeutic target for RA.

Functions of the FKN-CX3CR1 axis

FKN is a membrane-bound chemokine possessing a chemokine/mucin hybrid structure followed by a transmembrane domain [3]. This interesting structure allows FKN to work as an adhesion molecule in the membrane-bound form or as a chemoattractant in the soluble form shed by metalloproteases, a disintegrin and metalloproteinase domain-containing protein (ADAM) 10 or 17. Soluble FKN acts as a chemoattractant for monocytes, natural killer (NK) cells, and T cells. The membrane-bound FKN on endothelial cells mediates the rapid capture, integrin-independent firm adhesion, and activation of circulating leukocytes under flow by its direct binding to CX3CR1 [4, 5].

FKN is expressed on vascular endothelial cells and is strongly enhanced by the stimulation with pro-inflammatory cytokines, such as tumor necrosis factor-α (TNF-α), interleukin-1 (IL-1), and interferon-γ (IFN-γ). CX3CR1 is expressed on monocytes/macrophages and perforin+/granzyme B+ cytotoxic lymphocytes including NK cells and terminally differentiated cytotoxic T cells [6]. Soluble FKN preferentially induced the migration of cytotoxic effector lymphocytes, and the membrane-bound FKN promoted their subsequent migration to the secondary chemokines, such as the macrophage inflammatory protein-1β/CCL4 or IL-8/

CXCL8. Thus, FKN expressed on the inflamed endothelium functions as a vascular regulator for cytotoxic effector lymphocytes. Interestingly, it is revealed that a subset of monocytes patrols healthy tissues through long-range crawling on the resting endothelium by the intravital imaging of blood monocytes [7]. This unique behavior depends on the physical interaction-mediated integrin LFA-1 and CX3CR1 and is required for rapid accumulation of the monocytes to the site of danger to initiate early immune response. Nr4a1-dependent Ly6C^{low} CX3CR1^{high} monocytes scan capillaries and scavenge micrometric particles from their luminal side in a steady state in the kidney cortex. Importantly, a local TLR7-dependent danger signal increases the retention time of Ly6C^{low} CX3CR1^{high} monocytes on the endothelium. These tethered monocytes are then activated and function as "accessory cells" of the endothelium by orchestrating the focal necrosis of endothelial cells by recruiting neutrophils and the in situ phagocytosis of cellular debris by monocytes [8]. The FKN-CX3CR1 axis also has been reported to increase the survival of microglia and smooth muscle cells by Akt activation in a PI3K-dependent manner [9]. Lionakis et al. demonstrated that CX3CR1 promotes resident macrophage survival by inhibiting caspase-dependent apoptosis in the kidney in a mouse model of systemic candidiasis [10].

These results indicate that the FKN-CX3CR1 axis participates in the patrol for tissue damages in normal conditions and the quick mobilization and accumulation of effector cells to the sites of danger (Fig. 1).

Role of the FKN-CX3CR1 axis in the pathogenesis of RA

FKN is expressed on fibroblast-like synoviocyte (FLS) cells and endothelial cells in the RA synovium and contributes to the accumulation of T cells and macrophages, which express CX3CR1. The interaction between FKN and CX3CR1 is involved in the adhesion of the inflammatory cells to endothelial cells, their migration into the synovium, and cytokine production [1]. Nanki et al. showed that the peripheral blood CX3CR1-expressing CD4+ and CD8+ T cells preferentially produce IFN-γ, TNF-α, granzyme A, and perforin and that these cells are increased in patients with RA [11]. Furthermore, FKN expression is up-regulated in endothelial cells and FLSs in the synovium of RA patients, but not in the osteoarthritis synovium. Thus, the FKN/CX3CR1 axis is likely to play an important role in the preferential infiltration of Th1 and Tc1 cells into the RA synovium, which contributes to the pathogenesis of RA.

Macrophages are the primary source of pro-inflammatory cytokines. A high percentage of macrophages within the rheumatoid synovium express the CX3CR1 receptor. Circulating CD16+ monocytes express higher levels

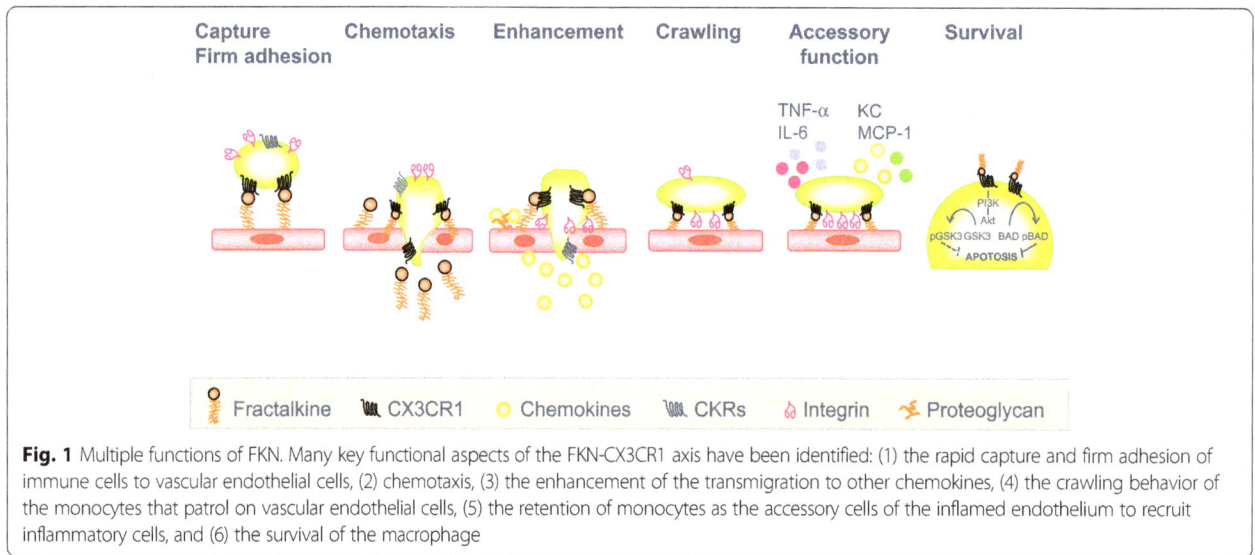

Fig. 1 Multiple functions of FKN. Many key functional aspects of the FKN-CX3CR1 axis have been identified: (1) the rapid capture and firm adhesion of immune cells to vascular endothelial cells, (2) chemotaxis, (3) the enhancement of the transmigration to other chemokines, (4) the crawling behavior of the monocytes that patrol on vascular endothelial cells, (5) the retention of monocytes as the accessory cells of the inflamed endothelium to recruit inflammatory cells, and (6) the survival of the macrophage

of CX3CR1 than CD16− monocytes in both RA patients and healthy subjects. High levels of CX3CR1 expression are also seen in CD16+ monocytes localized to the lining layer in RA synovial tissue, and soluble FKN efficiently induced the chemotaxis of these cell populations [12, 13]. Yano et al. postulated that the recruitment of CD16+ monocytes may be the result of the chemoattractant properties of FKN. Soluble FKN also induces IL-1 and IL-6 secretion from activated monocytes suggesting a crucial pro-inflammatory effect of FKN on monocyte function [12].

FLSs, which are resident cells in the sublining region and markedly expanded in the RA synovium, have been linked with a number of deleterious effects in RA. FLSs produce pro-inflammatory cytokines, exhibit a capacity for antigen presentation, and induce T cell expansion [14]. FKN is also expressed on cultured synovial fibroblasts and hyperplastic synoviocytes in RA. The senescent CD4+CD28− T cells that accumulate in the RA synovium aberrantly express CX3CR1. FKN, which is induced on FLSs by stimulation with pro-inflammatory cytokines, strongly induces the adhesion of CD4+CD28−CX3CR1+ T cells, provides survival signals and amplified proliferation, and stimulates the production of pro-inflammatory cytokines as well as the expulsion of cytoplasmic granules [15]. Thus, membrane-bound FKN may act as a co-stimulatory signal for CD4+CX3CR1 + T cells in the RA synovium.

In the collagen-induced arthritis (CIA) model in mice, the prophylactic treatment of anti-FKN monoclonal antibody (mAb) significantly improves the clinical arthritis score and reduces the infiltration of inflammatory cells, and bone erosion in the synovium, suggesting that anti-FKN mAb ameliorates arthritis by inhibiting the infiltration of inflammatory cells into the synovium [16].

In addition, our recent studies have shown that the therapeutic treatment of anti-FKN mAb also meliorates arthritis symptoms and radiological score in the CIA model (manuscript in preparation).

Role of the FKN-CX3CR1 axis in bone destruction

Osteoclast precursors selectively express CX3CR1, whereas FKN is expressed on osteoblasts. FKN on the osteoblasts is involved in the osteoblast-induced osteoclast differentiation [17]. Soluble FKN induces the migration of bone marrow cells containing osteoclast precursors, whereas immobilized FKN mediates the firm adhesion of osteoclast precursors. Furthermore, the blockade of FKN efficiently inhibits osteoclast differentiation from mouse bone marrow cells when co-cultured with osteoblasts. Consistently, an in vivo experiment in neonatal mice shows that anti-FKN mAb significantly suppresses bone resorption by reducing the number of bone-resorbing mature osteoclasts.

In the analysis of the femoral bone tissues of heterozygous CX3CR1−EGFP knock-in mice, CX3CR1−EGFP+ cells are shown to differentiate into tartrate-resistant acid phosphatase (TRAP)+ mature osteoclasts. CX3CR1−EGFP + but not CX3CR1−EGFP− cells sorted from bone marrow cells efficiently differentiate into TRAP+ mature osteoclast-like cells in vitro in the presence of RANKL, indicating that CX3CR1+ cells in the bone marrow are osteoclast precursors [18, 19].

The role of the FKN-CX3CR1 axis in osteoclast recruitment and osteoclastogenesis is evaluated by an irradiated murine model. FKN is dramatically up-regulated in the skeletal vascular endothelium after ionizing radiation (IR). The induced FKN promotes the recruitment of circulating CX3CR1+ osteoclast precursors toward the bone remodeling surface in the irradiated bones and enhances subsequent bone resorption. In vivo experiments also show that the blockade of the FKN-CX3CR1 axis ameliorates osteoclastogenesis and prevented bone loss after IR [20].

Collectively, FKN plays an important role in osteoclast recruitment and differentiation, possibly through its dual functions as a chemotactic factor and an adhesion molecule for CX3CR1+ osteoclast precursors. The FKN-CX3CR1 axis may be a novel target for the therapeutic intervention of bone-resorbing diseases such as RA and osteoporosis.

Development of the first humanized anti-FKN mAb, KANAb001 (E6011)

KANAb001 (E6011) is the first humanized anti-FKN mAb, generated by KAN Research Institute, Inc. Currently, phase 1/2 clinical studies of E6011 are ongoing in both RA and

Crohn's disease in Japan by Eisai Co., Ltd. Recently, we have reported that E6011 is safe and well tolerated and has a promising efficacy in active RA patients with MTX or TNF inhibitor-inadequate response (MTX-IR or TNFi-IR) at the American College of Rheumatology 2015. While further clinical studies are required, the results obtained to date indicate that a novel biological DMARD targeting the FKN-CX3CR1 axis will be clinically beneficial for active RA patients.

Most of current marketed mAbs inhibit specific cytokines and cytokine receptors, and JAK inhibitors block the effect of multiple cytokines by targeting cytokine signaling. On the other hand, E6011 targets the cell trafficking of immune cells, which produce multiple pro-inflammatory cytokines in the local inflamed sites. Previous studies have demonstrated that anti-FKN mAb inhibit the migration of both CX3CR1+ macrophages producing pro-inflammatory cytokines (TNF-α,

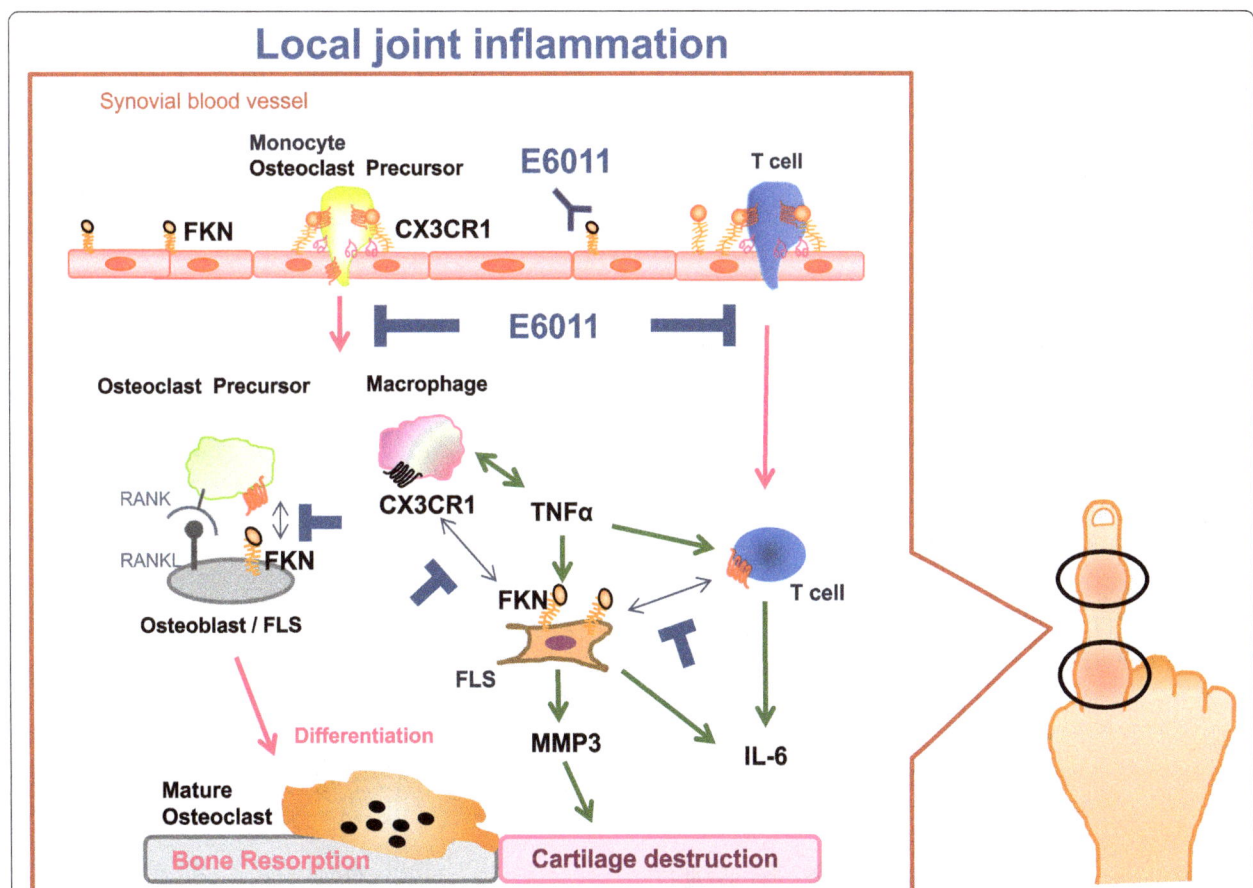

Fig. 2 E6011 targets CX3CR1+ cells in the inflammatory sites in RA. The interaction of the osteoclast precursor with osteoblasts via FKN-CX3CR1 promotes the osteoclast differentiation. The macrophage may be recruited by FLS-induced chemokine production through FKN-CX3CR1. In turn, the macrophage helps to activate the synovial sublining fibroblasts through the production of inflammatory cytokines such as TNF-α. CX3CR1 expressed on the cytotoxic effector CD4+ T cell binds to FKN on the fibroblast. And then, T cell-FLS communication activates the TNF-α production. TNF-α up-regulates FKN production as a growth factor of synovial fibroblasts, and TNF-α also induces the MMP3 expression, matrix metalloproteinase. Taken together, the interaction of FLS with the macrophage and T cells through FKN-CX3CR1 may contribute to the enhancement of inflammation and joint destruction

GM-CSF, and IL-6) and CX3CR1+ cytotoxic effector T cells containing cytotoxic molecules (granzyme B and perforin). These results indicate that anti-FKN mAb has a potential to block the most upstream step of the inflammation cascade in the local inflamed region. In addition, anti-FKN mAb suppresses the bone resorption by inhibiting osteoclast differentiation. Taken together, E6011 is expected to have strong preventive effects on joint destruction with a unique dual mode of action based on the inhibition of the immune cell trafficking and the direct suppression of osteoclastogenesis in local environments (Fig. 2).

Conclusions

FKN is a unique chemokine possessing a dual function as a chemoattractant and an adhesion molecule for CX3CR1-expressing monocytes, cytotoxic effector lymphocytes, and osteoclast precursors. Increasing evidence indicates that FKN is involved in the pathological roles of inflammatory disease such as RA. Now, clinical trials of E6011, the first humanized anti-FKN mAb, are ongoing in Japan. It is expected that E6011 will open up the possibility of a new therapeutic strategy for the treatment of RA with a novel mode of action distinct from other cytokine/cytokine receptor inhibitors (infliximab, tocilizumab, etc.) and modulator of T cell co-stimulation (abatacept).

Abbreviations
ADAM: metalloproteinase domain-containing protein; FKN: fractalkine (FKN); FLSs: fibroblast-like synoviocytes; IFN-γ: interferon-γ; IL-1: interleukin-1; IR: ionizing radiation; mAb: monoclonal antibody; MTX: methotrexate; NK cells: natural killer cells; RA: rheumatoid arthritis; TNF-α: tumor necrosis factor-α; TRAP: tartrate-resistant acid phosphatase.

Acknowledgements
We thank Prof. Yoshie of Kinki University; Dr. Nanki of Toho University; Dr. Umehara of Kyoto University; Dr. Koizumi of Toyama University; Prof. Takeuchi, Prof. Matsuo, and Dr. Kuroda of Keio University; and Prof. Tanaka of the University of Occupational and Environmental Health, Japan. We also thank all members of KAN Research Institute, Inc., and Eisai Co., Ltd., for the helpful discussion and advice.

Funding
We have received no specific grants.

Authors' contributions
The authors equally contributed to the preparation of this review. All authors read and approved the final manuscript.

Competing interests
The authors declare that they have no competing interests.

References
1. Murphy G, Caplice N, Molloy M. Fractalkine in rheumatoid arthritis: a review to date. Rheumatology (Oxford). 2008;47(10):1446–51.
2. Imai T, Nishimura M, Nanki T, Umehara H. Fractalkine and inflammatory diseases. Nihon Rinsho Meneki Gakkai Kaishi. 2005;28(3):131–9.
3. Bazan JF, Bcon KB, Hardiman G, Wang W, Soo K, Rossi D, et al. A new class of membrane-bound chemokine with a CX3C motif. Nature. 1997;385:640–4.
4. Imai T, Hieshima K, Haskell C, Baba M, Nagira M, Nishimura M, et al. Identification and molecular characterization of fractalkine receptor CX3CR1, which mediates both leukocyte migration and adhesion. Cell. 1997;91(4):521–30.
5. Fong AM, Robinson LA, Steeber DA, Tedder TF, Yoshie O, Imai T, et al. Fractalkine and CX3CR1 mediate a novel mechanism of leukocyte capture, firm adhesion, and activation under physiologic flow. J Exp Med. 1998; 188(8):1413–9.
6. Nishimura M, Umehara H, Nakayama T, Yoneda O, Hieshima K, Kakizaki M, et al. Dual functions of fractalkine/CX3C ligand 1 in trafficking of perforin +/granzyme B+ cytotoxic effector lymphocytes that are defined by CX3CR1 expression. J Immunol. 2002;168(12):6173–80.
7. Auffray C, Fogg D, Garfa M, Elain G, Join-Lambert O, Kayal S, et al. Monitoring of blood vessels and tissues by a population of monocytes with patrolling behavior. Science. 2007;317(5838):666–70.
8. Carlin LM, Stamatiades EG, Auffray C, Hanna RN, Glover L, Vizcay-Barrena G, et al. Nr4a1-dependent Ly6Clow monocytes monitor endothelial cells and orchestrate their disposal. Cell. 2013;153(2):362–75.
9. White GE, Greaves DR. Fractalkine: a survivor's guide: chemokines as antiapoptotic mediators. Arterioscler Thromb Vasc Biol. 2012;32(3):589–94.
10. Lionakis MS, Swamydas M, Fischer BG, Plantinga TS, Johnson MD, Jaeger M, et al. CX3CR1-dependent renal macrophage survival promotes Candida control and host survival. J Clin Invest. 2013;123(12):5035–51.
11. Nanki T, Imai T, Nagasaka K, Urasaki Y, Nonomura Y, Taniguchi K, et al. Migration of CX3CR1-positive T cells producing type 1 cytokines and cytotoxic molecules into the synovium of patients with rheumatoid arthritis. Arthritis Rheum. 2002;46(11):2878–83.
12. Yano R, Yamamura M, Sunahori K, Takasugi K, Yamana J, Kawashima M, et al. Recruitment of CD16+ monocytes into synovial tissues is mediated by fractalkine and CX3CR1 in rheumatoid arthritis patients. Acta Med Okayama. 2007;61(2):89–98.
13. McInnes IB, Leung BP, Liew FY. Cell-cell interactions in synovitis. Interactions between T lymphocytes and synovial cells. Arthritis Res. 2000;2:374–8.
14. Ruth JH, Volin MV, Haines 3rd GK, Woodruff DC, Katschke Jr KJ, Woods JM, et al. Fractalkine, a novel chemokine in rheumatoid arthritis and in rat adjuvant-induced arthritis. Arthritis Rheum. 2001;44(7):1568–81.
15. Sawai H, Park Y, Roberson J, Imai T, Goronzy J, Weyand C. T cell costimulation by fractalkine-expressing synoviocytes in rheumatoid arthritis. Arthritis Rheum. 2005;52:1392–401.
16. Nanki T, Urasaki Y, Imai T, Nishimura M, Muramoto K, Kubota T, et al. Inhibition of fractalkine ameliorates murine collagen-induced arthritis. J Immunol. 2004;173(11):7010–6.
17. Koizumi K, Saitoh Y, Minami T, Takeno N, Tsuneyama K, Miyahara T, et al. Role of CX3CL1/fractalkine in osteoclast differentiation and bone resorption. J Immunol. 2009;183(12):7825–31.
18. Ishii M, Egen JG, Klauschen F, Meier-Schellersheim M, Saeki Y, Vacher J, et al. Sphingosine-1-phosphate mobilizes osteoclast precursors and regulates bone homeostasis. Nature. 2009;458(26):524–9.
19. Ishii M, Kikuta J, Shimazu Y, Meier-Schellersheim M, Germain RN. Chemorepulsion by blood S1P regulates osteoclast precursor mobilization and bone remodeling in vivo. J Exp Med. 2010;207(13):2793–8.
20. Han KH, Ryu JW, Lim KE, Lee SH, Kim Y, Hwang CS, et al. Vascular expression of the chemokine CX3CL1 promotes osteoclast recruitment and exacerbates bone resorption in an irradiated murine model. Bone. 2014;61:91–101.

12

The crystal-induced activation of NLRP3 inflammasomes in atherosclerosis

Tadayoshi Karasawa* and Masafumi Takahashi

Abstract

Atherosclerosis is an inflammatory disease, which is accompanied by the deposition of cholesterol-rich lipids and the infiltration of macrophages. Other well-known features of atherosclerotic lesions include the deposition of cholesterol crystals and calcium phosphate crystals; however, their pathophysiological role remains unclear. Recent studies suggest that cholesterol crystals play a pivotal role in activation of NLRP3 inflammasomes, which regulate caspase-1 activation and the subsequent processing of IL-1β, in atherosclerotic lesions. NLRP3 inflammasomes are essential for the initiation of vascular inflammation during the progression of atherosclerosis. Therefore, the regulatory mechanisms of NLRP3 inflammasomes are regarded as potential targets for atherosclerosis treatment. Here, we review the current knowledge regarding the role of NLRP3 inflammasomes in the progression of atherosclerosis and the prospects for therapeutic approaches targeting NLRP3 inflammasomes.

Keywords: Cholesterol, Cytokines, Inflammation, Interleukin-1, Macrophages

Background

Atherosclerosis is an inflammatory disease characterized by the deposition of cholesterol-rich lipids and the macrophage infiltration of the vascular walls [1]. Infiltrated macrophages uptake cholesterol and cause inflammatory responses by producing various cytokines and chemokines. The mechanism of cholesterol accumulation in atherosclerotic lesions has been well described. For example, infiltrated macrophages incorporate modified low-density lipoprotein (LDL) via scavenger receptors and accumulate in the atherosclerotic lesions as lipid-loaded foam cells [2]. However, the molecular mechanisms by which lipids induce inflammatory responses are not been fully understood. In particular, the deposition of cholesterol crystals is a well-known feature of atherosclerosis [3], although the precise role of cholesterol crystals in the pathophysiology of atherosclerosis remains unclear. Recently, the molecular complexes called nucleotide-binding oligomerization domain-like receptor (NLR) family, pyrin domain containing 3 (NLRP3) inflammasomes have emerged as a key player for the crystal-induced inflammation in atherosclerosis [4, 5].

NLRP3 is a pattern recognition receptor (PRR), which participates in innate immune responses by recognizing danger signals, including pathogen-associated molecular patterns (PAMPs) and damage/danger-associated molecular patterns (DAMPs) [6]. The PRRs are evolutionarily conserved and expressed in the cells involved in the innate immune system such as macrophages, neutrophils, and dendritic cells [7]. The PRRs are classified into several groups according to their conserved structure and function. For instance, toll-like receptors (TLR) and C-type lectin receptors (CLRs) are expressed on the membrane surface, while NLRs and retinoic acid-inducible gene-I-like receptors (RLRs) exhibit intracellular localization. Recently, the involvement of several PRRs in the progression of atherosclerosis has been unveiled. Among PRRs, TLR2 and TLR4 are activated by inflammatory lipids, such as oxidized LDL and saturated fatty acids [1, 2]. Furthermore, NLRP3 is involved in the cholesterol crystal-mediated inflammatory response through the assembly of molecular complexes called inflammasomes. NLRP3 inflammasomes regulate inflammatory responses via processing of interleukin (IL)-1β, which is a potent inflammatory cytokine. Indeed, previous reports suggest that the development of atherosclerosis development was attenuated in the absence of NLRP3 inflammasomes [4, 8–10]. In this review, we describe the molecular mechanisms of

* Correspondence: tdys.karasawa@jichi.ac.jp
Division of Inflammation Research, Center for Molecular Medicine, Jichi Medical University, 3311-1 Yakushiji, Shimotsuke, Tochigi 329-0498, Japan

crystal-mediated NLRP3 inflammasome activation and the regulatory mechanisms of NLRP3 inflammasomes in the atherosclerotic lesions.

What is the inflammasome?

Inflammasomes are multiple cytoplasmic protein complexes, which are typically composed of NLRs, apoptosis-associated speck-like protein containing a caspase recruitment domain (CARD) (ASC), and caspase-1 (Fig. 1). In response to DAMPs or PAMPs, components of inflammasomes assemble through the interaction of pyrin domain (PYD) and caspase recruitment domain (CARD) [11]. Assembled inflammasomes form large molecular complexes and serve as a molecular platform for caspase-1 activation. Caspase-1 is a cysteine protease, which was originally identified as an interleukin-1 converting enzyme [12]. Therefore, inflammasome-mediated activation of caspase-1 converts inactive pro-IL-1β to its mature form. Among NLRs, at least NLRP1, NLRP3, NLRC4, NLRP6, and NLRP12 participate in inflammasomes as core components of the complexes [11]. Besides NLRs, PYHIN (pyrin and HIN domain-containing protein) family proteins, including absence in melanoma 2 (AIM2) and IFN-g-inducible protein 16 (IFI16), are also known as core components of inflammasomes. The adaptor protein ASC is necessary for several core components, such as NLRP3 and AIM2, for inflammasome assembly, while NLRC4 can assemble without ASC. Inflammasomes are named according to their core components. For example, the complexes composed of NLRP3, ASC, and caspase-1 are called NLRP3 inflammasomes. The core components of inflammasomes are activated by different danger signals. NLRC4 inflammasomes are activated by flagellin, a protein derived from flagellum of bacteria [13], while NLRP1 also recognizes, a lethal toxin derived from bacteria [14]. AIM2 functions as a sensor molecule for viral infection by recognizing cytosolic double-strand DNA [15]. NLRP3 is distinct from other core components because NLRP3 is activated by both DAMPs and PAMPs, while other core components are mainly activated by PAMPs and are involved in infection [6].

NLRP3 inflammasomes

NLRP3 inflammasomes are activated by DAMPs as well as PAMPs and thus involved in both sterile inflammation and host defense [6]. DAMPs, including extracellular adenosine triphosphate (ATP) and monosodium urate (MSU) crystals, induce the assembly of NLRP3 inflammasomes to activate caspase-1 (Fig. 1). The interaction among components of NLRP3 inflammasomes is mediated by conserved domains, which exhibit homophilic interaction. NLRP3 contains three domains: C-terminal leucine-rich repeats (LRRs), a central nucleotide domain termed the NACHT domain, and an N-terminal PYD. ASC can function as an adaptor molecule because it is composed of an N-terminal PYD and a C-terminal CARD. Caspase-1 also has a CARD and catalytic domains (p10 and p20). When cells are exposed to danger signals, NLRP3 assembles homotypically by the NACHT domain and offers scaffold for filamentous assembly of ASC by their interaction of PYD [16]. Subsequently, the assembled ASC promotes recruitment of caspase-1 via CARD–CARD interaction and subsequent auto-activation of caspase-1.

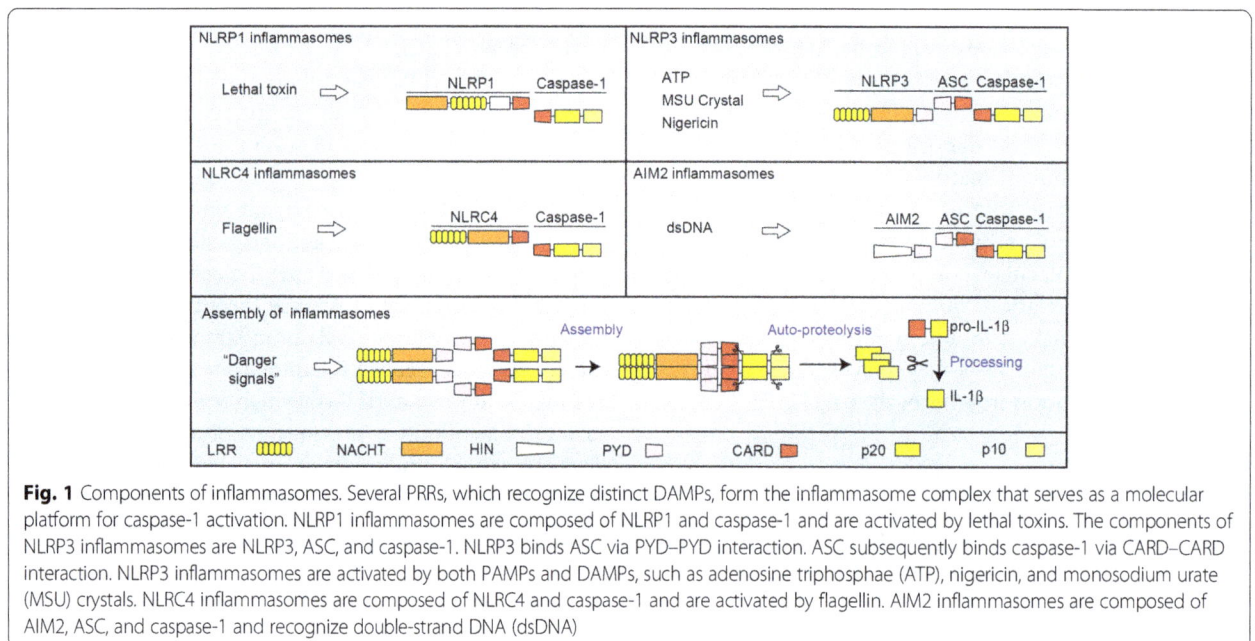

Fig. 1 Components of inflammasomes. Several PRRs, which recognize distinct DAMPs, form the inflammasome complex that serves as a molecular platform for caspase-1 activation. NLRP1 inflammasomes are composed of NLRP1 and caspase-1 and are activated by lethal toxins. The components of NLRP3 inflammasomes are NLRP3, ASC, and caspase-1. NLRP3 binds ASC via PYD–PYD interaction. ASC subsequently binds caspase-1 via CARD–CARD interaction. NLRP3 inflammasomes are activated by both PAMPs and DAMPs, such as adenosine triphosphae (ATP), nigericin, and monosodium urate (MSU) crystals. NLRC4 inflammasomes are composed of NLRC4 and caspase-1 and are activated by flagellin. AIM2 inflammasomes are composed of AIM2, ASC, and caspase-1 and recognize double-strand DNA (dsDNA)

The activated caspase-1 exerts proinflammatory effects by its proteolytic activity. Besides IL-1β, caspase-1 converts pro-IL-18 to its bioactive mature form. Furthermore, caspase-1 also cleaves gasdermin D (GSDMD) to induce pyroptosis, an inflammatory programed cell death accompanied by an increased permeability of the plasma membrane [17, 18]. Because IL-1β has no signal sequence for exocytosis, pyroptosis-mediated membrane permeabilization seems to be necessary for IL-1β release [19, 20].

The release of IL-1β is induced by a two-step regulation: transcriptional regulation called the priming step and processing by inflammasomes (Fig. 2). The transcriptional regulation of *Il1b* (signal 1) is mediated by PRRs or cytokine receptors including TLRs and IL-1 receptors (IL-1R). Besides NF-κB-mediated mRNA induction of *Il1b* and *Nlrp3*, activation of these receptors primes NLRP3 by posttranscriptional regulation, such as ubiquitination and deubiquitination [21, 22]. Then, accumulated cytosolic pro-IL-1β in cytosol is rapidly processed by caspase-1, which is activated by NLRP3 inflammasomes (signal 2). Since IL-1β exhibits potent proinflammatory effects, this two-step regulation is thought to be necessary for maintenance of immuno-homeostasis.

Although various endogenous or exogenous danger signals such as ATP, MSU crystals, and silica are known to activate NLRP3 inflammasomes, the precise mechanism by which NLRP3 recognizes the danger signals remains unclear [23, 24]. Unlike other PRRs, the direct ligands of NLRP3 are almost unknown and still controversial. Only a few reports suggest that mitochondrial DNA or mitochondria-derived cardiolipin functions as a direct ligand of NLRP3. Conversely, upstream molecular machineries of NLRP3 inflammasomes have been elucidated. Several common pathways including potassium (K⁺) efflux, generation of mitochondrial reactive oxygen species (ROS), and lysosomal destabilization are necessary for the activation of the NLRP3 inflammasome [6]. In particular, lysosomal destabilization and subsequent cathepsin B release is a common pathway for NLRP3 inflammasome activation by crystals and particulate matter. Thus, the regulatory mechanisms of NLRP3 inflammasomes have not been completely elucidated.

NLRP3 inflammasomes in the pathogenesis of diseases

Originally, NLRP3 was identified as a responsible gene for cryopyrin-associated periodic syndrome (CAPS), which includes three syndromes with differing severity [25]. Familial cold autoinflammatory syndrome (FCAS) is the mildest condition and is characterized by cold-induced fever and inflammation. Muckle–Wells syndrome (MWS) is a moderate condition and is characterized by episodic attacks with fever and urticaria-like rash. MWS patients also exhibit arthralgia and progressive hearing loss. Chronic infantile neurological cutaneous and articular

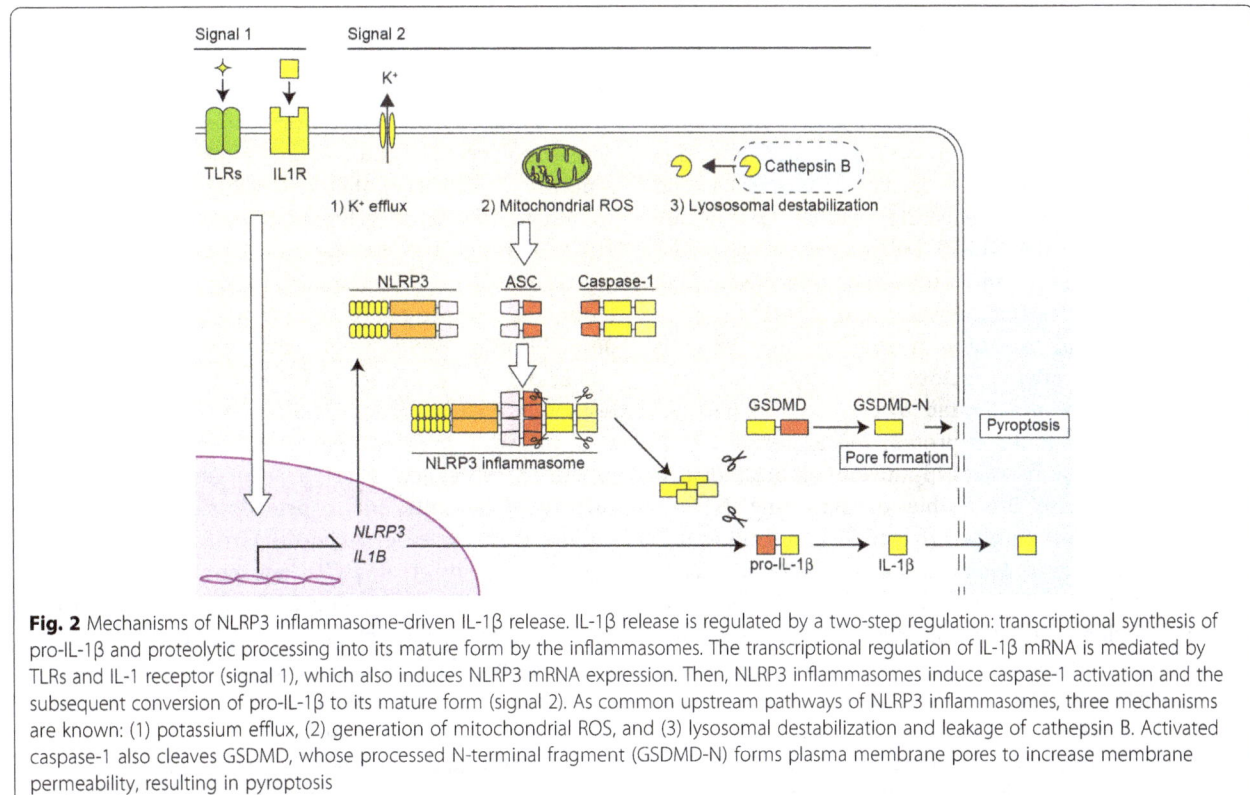

Fig. 2 Mechanisms of NLRP3 inflammasome-driven IL-1β release. IL-1β release is regulated by a two-step regulation: transcriptional synthesis of pro-IL-1β and proteolytic processing into its mature form by the inflammasomes. The transcriptional regulation of IL-1β mRNA is mediated by TLRs and IL-1 receptor (signal 1), which also induces NLRP3 mRNA expression. Then, NLRP3 inflammasomes induce caspase-1 activation and the subsequent conversion of pro-IL-1β to its mature form (signal 2). As common upstream pathways of NLRP3 inflammasomes, three mechanisms are known: (1) potassium efflux, (2) generation of mitochondrial ROS, and (3) lysosomal destabilization and leakage of cathepsin B. Activated caspase-1 also cleaves GSDMD, whose processed N-terminal fragment (GSDMD-N) forms plasma membrane pores to increase membrane permeability, resulting in pyroptosis

syndrome (CINCA) is the most severe condition with continuous inflammation, which results in neurological impairment. Since CAPS is a rare genetic disease, few investigations of NLRP3 inflammasomes had been performed until the link between NLRP3 inflammasomes and sterile inflammation was uncovered. However, the discovery that the NLRP3 inflammasome is activated by MSU crystals and associated with gout highlights the role of NLRP3 inflammasomes in sterile inflammatory diseases [23]. Indeed, we and others have revealed a pivotal role of NLRP3 inflammasomes in the development of cardiovascular and renal diseases including atherosclerosis [4, 8, 26–29]. Furthermore, in the last decade, numerous studies revealed that NLRP3 inflammasomes are activated by a broad variety of danger signals and are involved in various inflammatory diseases [6].

Crystal-induced NLRP3 inflammasome activation

Among danger signals that activate NLRP3 inflammasomes, crystals and particulate matter share similar molecular mechanisms to activate NLRP3 inflammasomes. Innate immune cells, including macrophages and neutrophils, engulf these particles to remove foreign substances. However, excess loads of particles in lysosome cause an indigestion called "frustrated lysosome," which in turn induces lysosome destabilization. As described above, the leakage of cathepsin B into the cytosol triggers NLRP3 inflammasome activation. Although downstream mechanisms of cathepsin B release are still unclear, K$^+$ efflux is regarded as essential for the activation of NLRP3 inflammasomes induced by lysosomal destabilization [30, 31].

NLRP3 inflammasome activation induced by crystals and particles is associated with various inflammatory diseases (Fig. 3). As endogenous crystals, MSU crystals and calcium pyrophosphate dehydrate (CPPD) crystals are known to activate the NLRP3 inflammasome and cause inflammation in gout and pseudo-gout, respectively [23]. Exogenous particles such as silica and asbestos are associated with inflammation in silicosis and asbestos lung [32, 33]. However, factors that induce lysosomal destabilization are not limited to crystals and particulate matter. Some kinds of protein aggregates also activate NLRP3 inflammasomes. β-amyloid associated with Alzheimer's disease is capable of activating NLRP3 inflammasomes [34]. Furthermore, NLRP3 inflammasome complex in the extracellular space can function as a danger signal of NLRP3 inflammasomes itself. The assembly of NLRP3 inflammasome components causes the formation of aggregates called speck, which are released to the extracellular space after NLRP3 inflammasome activation [35, 36]. The released NLRP3 inflammasomes are incorporated into neighbor cells in which they activate NLRP3 inflammasomes in part by lysosomal destabilization. Thus,

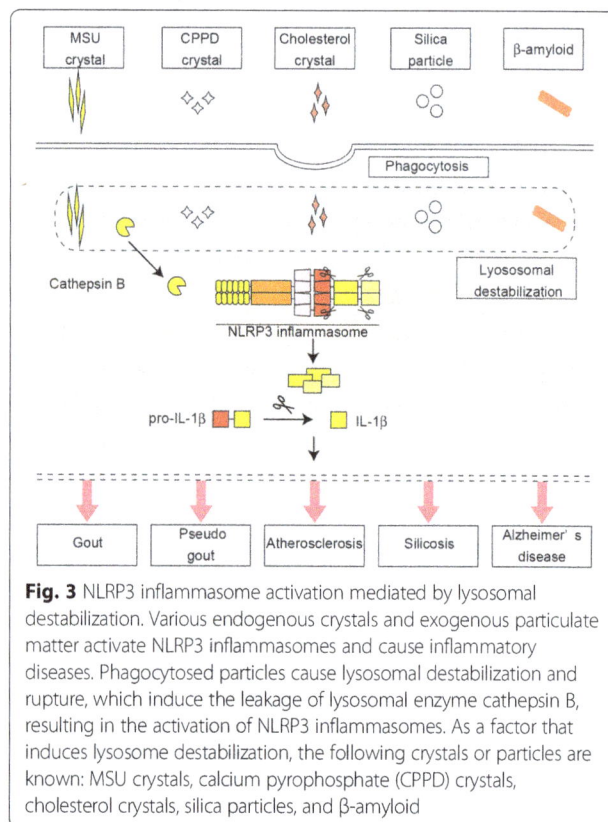

Fig. 3 NLRP3 inflammasome activation mediated by lysosomal destabilization. Various endogenous crystals and exogenous particulate matter activate NLRP3 inflammasomes and cause inflammatory diseases. Phagocytosed particles cause lysosomal destabilization and rupture, which induce the leakage of lysosomal enzyme cathepsin B, resulting in the activation of NLRP3 inflammasomes. As a factor that induces lysosome destabilization, the following crystals or particles are known: MSU crystals, calcium pyrophosphate (CPPD) crystals, cholesterol crystals, silica particles, and β-amyloid

various kinds of particles including crystals activate NLRP3 inflammasomes and initiate inflammatory responses.

NLRP3 inflammasomes in atherosclerosis

In the advanced atherosclerotic lesion, the deposition of cholesterol crystals and calcium phosphate crystals are reported [3]. However, their pathophysiological relevance to atherosclerosis development remained unclear. In 2010, Douwell et al. [4] revealed that cholesterol crystals are deposited even in the early stage of atherosclerotic lesion and activate NLRP3 inflammasomes via lysosomal destabilization. Interestingly, they further showed that oxidized LDL, a major lipid species in atherosclerotic lesions, not only induces cholesterol crystallization but also provides priming signals to induce NLRP3 and pro-IL-1β expression. Thus, it is suggested that oxidized LDL could be sufficient to provide signals 1 and 2 to induce IL-1β release. According to a subsequent report by Sheedy et al. [37], incorporation of oxidized LDL via scavenger receptor CD36 provokes intracellular crystallization of cholesterol. On the other hand, calcium phosphate is also particulate matter, which is accumulated in atherosclerotic lesions and associated with vascular calcification. In this regard, we and other investigators showed that calcium phosphate crystals, including hydroxyl apatite and tricalcium phosphate, activate NLRP3 inflammasomes through lysosomal rupture and subsequent cathepsin B release [8].

Since several studies have shown that IL-1β contributes to the progression of atherosclerosis [38, 39], it is expected that the deficiency of NLRP3 inflammasomes prevents atherosclerosis. Indeed, recent studies reported that the deficiency of NLRP3 inflammasome components prevents the atherosclerosis progression [4, 8–10]. However, Menu et al. [40] reported that deficiency of NLRP3 inflammasomes failed to prevent the development of atherosclerosis in ApoE$^{-/-}$ mice. The reason for this discrepancy is unclear, but the highly atherogenic diet used in the study by Menu et al., in comparison with other studies, may have influenced the immune status and inflammatory responses.

The regulatory mechanisms of NLRP3 inflammasomes

The regulatory mechanisms of NLRP3 inflammasomes may be a potential target for multiple inflammatory diseases including atherosclerosis. The possible mechanisms are the following: (1) modification of the inflammasome components including phosphorylation and ubiquitination, (2) modulation of the NLRP3 inflammasome assembly, (3) the upstream pathways of NLRP3 inflammasome activation, and (4) the destruction of NLRP3 inflammasome complexes. Among NLRP3 inflammasome components, the modification of NLRP3 is critical for inflammasome assembly. The priming signal provided by TLR or IL-1R promotes deubiquitination of NLRP3, which licenses the assembly of NLRP3 inflammasomes [41]. To date, BRCC3 has emerged as the only enzyme that can deubuiquitinate NLRP3 [22], while several E3 ubiquitine ligases such as FBXL12, MARCH7, and TRIM31 are reported to ubiquitinate NLRP3 [42–44]. Further reports suggest that protein kinase A directly inhibits NLRP3 via phosphorylation at Ser 291 and promotes the subsequent ubiquitination [45].

Since oligomerization of NLRP3 inflammasome components is a critical step for inflammasome activation, proteins which interact with the components can modify the assembly of NLRP3 inflammasomes. As a positive regulator of NLRP3 inflammasomes, NEK7 was found to participate in NLRP3 inflammasome complexes [46–48]. Additionally, negative regulatory proteins that prevent assembly of the NLRP3 inflammasomes by direct interaction with components are also reported. For example, CARD-only proteins (COPs) and PYD-only proteins (POPs) are typical molecules that modify NLRP3 inflammasome assembly [49]. These proteins are homologues of caspase-1 and ASC and consist of only CARD or PYD. Among these proteins, POP1 inhibits NLRP3 inflammasome activation by the prevention of ASC oligomerization [50]. Although all the COPs and POPs

were first reported as negative regulators of caspase-1 activation [51–53], the roles of COPs and POPs in NLRP3 inflammasome activation remain controversial. In this regard, we previously found that CARD16 induces caspase-1 activation by promoting filamentous assembly of caspase-1 [54]. Furthermore, β-arrestin-2, which functions as a downstream scaffold protein of G protein-coupled receptor 120 (GPR120), is suggested to be a potential negative regulator of NLRP3 inflammasome assembly. Yan et al. reported that the activation of GPR120 by polyunsaturated fatty acids inhibits NLRP3 inflammasomes via the direct interaction between β-arrestin-2 and NLRP3 [55].

The upstream pathways for NLRP3 inflammasome activation are also potential targets. Since mitochondria-derived ROS plays essential roles in the activation of NLRP3 inflammasomes, clearance of damaged mitochondria by autophagy (mitophagy) can inhibit the activation of NLRP3 inflammasomes [56]. Indeed, accelerated atherosclerotic lesion with enhanced NLRP3 inflammasome activation was observed in autophagy-defective Atg5-deficient mice [57]. Furthermore, lysosome biogenesis may protect against crystal-induced NLRP3 inflammasome activation. Activation of lysosome biogenesis by overexpression of TFEB, which regulates lysosome and autophagy-related genes, inhibits NLRP3 inflammasome activation induced by cholesterol crystals and attenuates the progression of atherosclerosis [58]. However, the regulatory mechanism for the destruction of NLRP3 inflammasomes is largely unknown. Although it is suggested that autophagy promotes destruction of the NLRP3 inflammasome complex in a ubiquitin-dependent manner [59], the regulatory mechanism to ubiquitinate the inflammasome complex is undetermined. Thus, the regulatory mechanisms of the NLRP3 inflammasomes are not fully elucidated. Further studies are necessary for the NLRP3 inflammasomes to be therapeutic targets in inflammatory diseases.

Conclusion

Accumulating evidence suggests that NLRP3 inflammasomes play an essential role in the progression of inflammatory diseases. Lysosome-destabilizing particles, including crystals and particulate matter, are common molecules that trigger activation of the NLRP3 inflammasomes in various diseases. In the progression of atherosclerosis, cholesterol crystals or calcium phosphate crystals are involved in NLRP3 inflammasome-mediated inflammatory responses. Further study clarifying the molecular mechanisms of NLRP3 inflammasome activation would serve to develop a novel therapeutic approach to atherosclerosis and other inflammatory diseases, which are caused by crystals and particulate matter.

Abbreviation

AIM2: Absence in melanoma 2; ASC: Apoptosis-associated speck-like protein containing a caspase recruitment domain; CAPS: Cryopyrin-associated periodic syndrome; CARD: Caspase recruitment domain; CINCA: Chronic infantile neurological cutaneous and articular syndrome; CLR: C-type lectin receptors; COPs: CARD-only proteins; CPPD: Calcium pyrophosphate dehydrate; DAMPs: Damage/danger-associated molecular patterns; FCAS: Familial cold autoinflammatory syndrome; GPR: G protein-coupled receptor; GSDMD: Gasdermin D; IFI16: IFN-g-inducible protein 16; IL: Interleukin; LDL: Low-density lipoprotein; LRR: Leucine-rich repeats; MSU: Monosodium urate; MWS: Muckle–Wells syndrome; NLR: Nucleotide-binding oligomerization domain-like receptor; NLRP3: NLR family, pyrin domain containing 3; PAMPs: Pathogen-associated molecular patterns; POPs: PYD-only proteins; PRR: Pattern recognition receptor; PYD: Pyrin domain; RLR: Retinoic acid-inducible gene-I-like receptors; ROS: Reactive oxygen species; TLR: Toll-like receptors

Acknowledgements

We are grateful to our colleagues, laboratory member, and collaborators for their helpful suggestions and experimental assistance.

Funding

TK is supported by "Grant-in-Aid for Young Scientists (B)" from Japan Society for the Promotion of Science, Japan Heart Foundation & Astellas Grant for Research on Atherosclerosis Update, and SENSIN Medical Research Foundation.

Authors' contributions

TK wrote the manuscript. MT critically revised the manuscript. Both authors read and approved the final manuscript.

Competing interests

The authors declare that they have no competing interests.

Reference

1. Tall AR, Yvan-Charvet L. Cholesterol, inflammation and innate immunity. Nat Rev Immunol. 2015;15:104–16.
2. Moore KJ, Tabas I. Macrophages in the pathogenesis of atherosclerosis. Cell. 2011;145:341–55.
3. Small D. M. George Lyman Duff memorial lecture. Progression and regression of atherosclerotic lesions. Insights from lipid physical biochemistry. Arteriosclerosis. 1988;8:103–29.
4. Duewell P, Kono H, Rayner KJ, Sirois CM, Vladimer G, Bauernfeind FG, Abela GS, Franchi L, Nunez G, Schnurr M, Espevik T, Lien E, Fitzgerald KA, Rock KL, Moore KJ, Wright SD, Hornung V, Latz E. NLRP3 inflammasomes are required for atherogenesis and activated by cholesterol crystals. Nature. 2010;464:1357–61.
5. Rajamaki K, Lappalainen J, Oorni K, Valimaki E, Matikainen S, Kovanen PT, Eklund KK. Cholesterol crystals activate the NLRP3 inflammasome in human macrophages: a novel link between cholesterol metabolism and inflammation. PLoS One. 2010;5:e11765.
6. Guo H, Callaway JB, Ting JP. Inflammasomes: mechanism of action, role in disease, and therapeutics. Nat Med. 2015;21:677–87.
7. Takeuchi O, Akira S. Pattern recognition receptors and inflammation. Cell. 2010;140:805–20.
8. Usui F, Shirasuna K, Kimura H, Tatsumi K, Kawashima A, Karasawa T, Hida S, Sagara J, Taniguchi S, Takahashi M. Critical role of caspase-1 in vascular inflammation and development of atherosclerosis in Western diet-fed apolipoprotein E-deficient mice. Biochem Biophys Res Commun. 2012;425:162–8.
9. Gage J, Hasu M, Thabet M, Whitman SC. Caspase-1 deficiency decreases atherosclerosis in apolipoprotein E-null mice. Can J Cardiol. 2012;28:222–9.
10. Hendrikx T, Jeurissen ML, van Gorp PJ, Gijbels MJ, Walenbergh SM, Houben T, van Gorp R, Pottgens CC, Stienstra R, Netea MG, Hofker MH, Donners MM, Shiri-Sverdlov R. Bone marrow-specific caspase-1/11 deficiency inhibits atherosclerosis development in Ldlr$^{-/-}$ mice. FEBS J. 2015;282:2327–38.
11. Lamkanfi M, Dixit VM. Mechanisms and functions of inflammasomes. Cell. 2014;157:1013–22.
12. Black RA, Kronheim SR, Merriam JE, March CJ, Hopp TP. A pre-aspartate-specific protease from human leukocytes that cleaves pro-interleukin-1β. J Biol Chem. 1989;264:5323–6.
13. Franchi L, Amer A, Body-Malapel M, Kanneganti TD, Ozoren N, Jagirdar R, Inohara N, Vandenabeele P, Bertin J, Coyle A, Grant EP, Nunez G. Cytosolic flagellin requires Ipaf for activation of caspase-1 and interleukin 1β in salmonella-infected macrophages. Nat Immunol. 2006;7:576–82.
14. Levin TC, Wickliffe KE, Leppla SH, Moayeri M. Heat shock inhibits caspase-1 activity while also preventing its inflammasome-mediated activation by anthrax lethal toxin. Cell Microbiol. 2008;10:2434–46.
15. Fernandes-Alnemri T, Yu JW, Datta P, Wu J, Alnemri ES. AIM2 activates the inflammasome and cell death in response to cytoplasmic DNA. Nature. 2009;458:509–13.
16. Lu A, Magupalli VG, Ruan J, Yin Q, Atianand MK, Vos MR, Schroder GF, Fitzgerald KA, Wu H, Egelman EH. Unified polymerization mechanism for the assembly of ASC-dependent inflammasomes. Cell. 2014;156:1193–206.
17. Kayagaki N, Stowe IB, Lee BL, O'Rourke K, Anderson K, Warming S, Cuellar T, Haley B, Roose-Girma M, Phung QT, Liu PS, Lill JR, Li H, Wu J, Kummerfeld S, Zhang J, Lee WP, Snipas SJ, Salvesen GS, Morris LX, Fitzgerald L, Zhang Y, Bertram EM, Goodnow CC, Dixit VM. Caspase-11 cleaves gasdermin D for non-canonical inflammasome signalling. Nature. 2015;526:666–71.
18. Shi J, Zhao Y, Wang K, Shi X, Wang Y, Huang H, Zhuang Y, Cai T, Wang F, Shao F. Cleavage of GSDMD by inflammatory caspases determines pyroptotic cell death. Nature. 2015;526:660–5.
19. He WT, Wan H, Hu L, Chen P, Wang X, Huang Z, Yang ZH, Zhong CQ, Han J. Gasdermin D is an executor of pyroptosis and required for interleukin-1β secretion. Cell Res. 2015;25:1285–98.
20. Martin-Sanchez F, Diamond C, Zeitler M, Gomez AI, Baroja-Mazo A, Bagnall J, Spiller D, White M, Daniels MJ, Mortellaro A, Penalver M, Paszek P, Steringer JP, Nickel W, Brough D, Pelegrin P. Inflammasome-dependent IL-1β release depends upon membrane permeabilisation. Cell Death Differ. 2016;23:1219–31.
21. Juliana C, Fernandes-Alnemri T, Kang S, Farias A, Qin F, Alnemri ES. Non-transcriptional priming and deubiquitination regulate NLRP3 inflammasome activation. J Biol Chem. 2012;287:36617–22.
22. Py BF, Kim MS, Vakifahmetoglu-Norberg H, Yuan J. Deubiquitination of NLRP3 by BRCC3 critically regulates inflammasome activity. Mol Cell. 2013; 49:331–8.
23. Martinon F, Petrilli V, Mayor A, Tardivel A, Tschopp J. Gout-associated uric acid crystals activate the NALP3 inflammasome. Nature. 2006;440:237–41.
24. Mariathasan S, Weiss DS, Newton K, McBride J, O'Rourke K, Roose-Girma M, Lee WP, Weinrauch Y, Monack DM, Dixit VM. Cryopyrin activates the inflammasome in response to toxins and ATP. Nature. 2006;440:228–32.
25. Agostini L, Martinon F, Burns K, McDermott MF, Hawkins PN, Tschopp J. NALP3 forms an IL-1β-processing inflammasome with increased activity in Muckle-Wells autoinflammatory disorder. Immunity. 2004;20:319–25.
26. Yajima N, Takahashi M, Morimoto H, Shiba Y, Takahashi Y, Masumoto J, Ise H, Sagara J, Nakayama J, Taniguchi S, Ikeda U. Critical role of bone marrow apoptosis-associated speck-like protein, an inflammasome adaptor molecule, in neointimal formation after vascular injury in mice. Circulation. 2008;117:3079–87.
27. Kawaguchi M, Takahashi M, Hata T, Kashima Y, Usui F, Morimoto H, Izawa A, Takahashi Y, Masumoto J, Koyama J, Hongo M, Noda T, Nakayama J, Sagara J, Taniguchi S, Ikeda U. Inflammasome activation of cardiac fibroblasts is essential for myocardial ischemia/reperfusion injury. Circulation. 2011;123: 594–604.
28. Komada T, Usui F, Shirasuna K, Kawashima A, Kimura H, Karasawa T, Nishimura S, Sagara J, Noda T, Taniguchi S, Muto S, Nagata D, Kusano E, Takahashi M. ASC in renal collecting duct epithelial cells contributes to inflammation and injury after unilateral ureteral obstruction. Am J Pathol. 2014;184:1287–98.
29. Komada T, Usui F, Kawashima A, Kimura H, Karasawa T, Inoue Y, Kobayashi M, Mizushina Y, Kasahara T, Taniguchi S, Muto S, Nagata D, Takahashi M. Role of NLRP3 inflammasomes for rhabdomyolysis-induced acute kidney injury. Sci Rep. 2015;5:10901.

30. Munoz-Planillo R, Kuffa P, Martinez-Colon G, Smith BL, Rajendiran TM, Nunez G. K+ efflux is the common trigger of NLRP3 inflammasome activation by bacterial toxins and particulate matter. Immunity. 2013;38:1142–53.

31. He Y, Hara H, Nunez G. Mechanism and regulation of NLRP3 inflammasome activation. Trends Biochem Sci. 2016;41:1012–21.

32. Hornung V, Bauernfeind F, Halle A, Samstad EO, Kono H, Rock KL, Fitzgerald KA, Latz E. Silica crystals and aluminum salts activate the NALP3 inflammasome through phagosomal destabilization. Nat Immunol. 2008;9:847–56.

33. Dostert C, Petrilli V, Van Bruggen R, Steele C, Mossman BT, Tschopp J. Innate immune activation through Nalp3 inflammasome sensing of asbestos and silica. Science. 2008;320:674–7.

34. Halle A, Hornung V, Petzold GC, Stewart CR, Monks BG, Reinheckel T, Fitzgerald KA, Latz E, Moore KJ, Golenbock DT. The NALP3 inflammasome is involved in the innate immune response to amyloid-β. Nat Immunol. 2008;9:857–65.

35. Franklin BS, Bossaller L, De Nardo D, Ratter JM, Stutz A, Engels G, Brenker C, Nordhoff M, Mirandola SR, Al-Amoudi A, Mangan MS, Zimmer S, Monks BG, Fricke M, Schmidt RE, Espevik T, Jones B, Jarnicki AG, Hansbro PM, Busto P, Marshak-Rothstein A, Hornemann S, Aguzzi A, Kastenmuller W, Latz E. The adaptor ASC has extracellular and 'prionoid' activities that propagate inflammation. Nat Immunol. 2014;15:727–37.

36. Baroja-Mazo A, Martin-Sanchez F, Gomez AI, Martinez CM, Amores-Iniesta J, Compan V, Barbera-Cremades M, Yague J, Ruiz-Ortiz E, Anton J, Bujan S, Couillin I, Brough D, Arostegui JI, Pelegrin P. The NLRP3 inflammasome is released as a particulate danger signal that amplifies the inflammatory response. Nat Immunol. 2014;15:738–48.

37. Sheedy FJ, Grebe A, Rayner KJ, Kalantari P, Ramkhelawon B, Carpenter SB, Becker CE, Ediriweera HN, Mullick AE, Golenbock DT, Stuart LM, Latz E, Fitzgerald KA, Moore KJ. CD36 coordinates NLRP3 inflammasome activation by facilitating intracellular nucleation of soluble ligands into particulate ligands in sterile inflammation. Nat Immunol. 2013;14:812–20.

38. Kirii H, Niwa T, Yamada Y, Wada H, Saito K, Iwakura Y, Asano M, Moriwaki H, Seishima M. Lack of interleukin-1β decreases the severity of atherosclerosis in ApoE-deficient mice. Arterioscler Thromb Vasc Biol. 2003;23:656–60.

39. Chi H, Messas E, Levine RA, Graves DT, Amar S. Interleukin-1 receptor signaling mediates atherosclerosis associated with bacterial exposure and/or a high-fat diet in a murine apolipoprotein E heterozygote model: pharmacotherapeutic implications. Circulation. 2004;110:1678–85.

40. Menu P, Pellegrin M, Aubert JF, Bouzourene K, Tardivel A, Mazzolai L, Tschopp J. Atherosclerosis in ApoE-deficient mice progresses independently of the NLRP3 inflammasome. Cell Death Dis. 2011;2:e137.

41. Pradeu T, Cooper EL. The danger theory: 20 years later. Front Immunol. 2012;3:287.

42. Han S, Lear TB, Jerome JA, Rajbhandari S, Snavely CA, Gulick DL, Gibson KF, Zou C, Chen BB, Mallampalli RK. Lipopolysaccharide primes the NALP3 inflammasome by inhibiting its ubiquitination and degradation mediated by the SCFFBXL2 E3 ligase. J Biol Chem. 2015;290:18124–33.

43. Yan Y, Jiang W, Liu L, Wang X, Ding C, Tian Z, Zhou R. Dopamine controls systemic inflammation through inhibition of NLRP3 inflammasome. Cell. 2015;160:62–73.

44. Song H, Liu B, Huai W, Yu Z, Wang W, Zhao J, Han L, Jiang G, Zhang L, Gao C, Zhao W. The E3 ubiquitin ligase TRIM31 attenuates NLRP3 inflammasome activation by promoting proteasomal degradation of NLRP3. Nat Commun. 2016;7:13727.

45. Guo C, Xie S, Chi Z, Zhang J, Liu Y, Zhang L, Zheng M, Zhang X, Xia D, Ke Y, Lu L, Wang D. Bile acids control inflammation and metabolic disorder through inhibition of NLRP3 inflammasome. Immunity. 2016;45:802–16.

46. He Y, Zeng MY, Yang D, Motro B, Nunez G. NEK7 is an essential mediator of NLRP3 activation downstream of potassium efflux. Nature. 2016;530:354–7.

47. Schmid-Burgk JL, Chauhan D, Schmidt T, Ebert TS, Reinhardt J, Endl E, Hornung V. A genome-wide CRISPR (Clustered Regularly Interspaced Short Palindromic Repeats) screen identifies NEK7 as an essential component of NLRP3 inflammasome activation. J Biol Chem. 2016;291:103–9.

48. Shi H, Wang Y, Li X, Zhan X, Tang M, Fina M, Su L, Pratt D, Bu CH, Hildebrand S, Lyon S, Scott L, Quan J, Sun Q, Russell J, Arnett S, Jurek P, Chen D, Kravchenko VV, Mathison JC, Moresco EM, Monson NL, Ulevitch RJ, Beutler B. NLRP3 activation and mitosis are mutually exclusive events coordinated by NEK7, a new inflammasome component. Nat Immunol. 2016;17:250–8.

49. Stehlik C, Dorfleutner A. COPs and POPs: modulators of inflammasome activity. J Immunol. 2007;179:7993–8.

50. de Almeida L, Khare S, Misharin AV, Patel R, Ratsimandresy RA, Wallin MC, Perlman H, Greaves DR, Hoffman HM, Dorfleutner A, Stehlik C. The PYRIN domain-only protein POP1 inhibits inflammasome assembly and ameliorates inflammatory disease. Immunity. 2015;43:264–76.

51. Guiet C, Vito P. Caspase recruitment domain (CARD)-dependent cytoplasmic filaments mediate bcl10-induced NF-κB activation. J Cell Biol. 2000;148:1131–40.

52. Humke EW, Shriver SK, Starovasnik MA, Fairbrother WJ, Dixit VM. ICEBERG: a novel inhibitor of interleukin-1β generation. Cell. 2000;103:99–111.

53. Lamkanfi M, Denecker G, Kalai M, D'Hondt K, Meeus A, Declercq W, Saelens X, Vandenabeele P. INCA, a novel human caspase recruitment domain protein that inhibits interleukin-1β generation. J Biol Chem. 2004;279:51729–38.

54. Karasawa T, Kawashima A, Usui F, Kimura H, Shirasuna K, Inoue Y, Komada T, Kobayashi M, Mizushina Y, Sagara J, Takahashi M. Oligomerized CARD16 promotes caspase-1 assembly and IL-1β processing. FEBS Open Bio. 2015;5:348–56.

55. Yan Y, Jiang W, Spinetti T, Tardivel A, Castillo R, Bourquin C, Guarda G, Tian Z, Tschopp J, Zhou R. Omega-3 fatty acids prevent inflammation and metabolic disorder through inhibition of NLRP3 inflammasome activation. Immunity. 2013;38:1154–63.

56. Zhou R, Yazdi AS, Menu P, Tschopp J. A role for mitochondria in NLRP3 inflammasome activation. Nature. 2011;469:221–5.

57. Razani B, Feng C, Coleman T, Emanuel R, Wen H, Hwang S, Ting JP, Virgin HW, Kastan MB, Semenkovich CF. Autophagy links inflammasomes to atherosclerotic progression. Cell Metab. 2012;15:534–44.

58. Emanuel R, Sergin I, Bhattacharya S, Turner JN, Epelman S, Settembre C, Diwan A, Ballabio A, Razani B. Induction of lysosomal biogenesis in atherosclerotic macrophages can rescue lipid-induced lysosomal dysfunction and downstream sequelae. Arterioscler Thromb Vasc Biol. 2014;34:1942–52.

59. Shi CS, Shenderov K, Huang NN, Kabat J, Abu-Asab M, Fitzgerald KA, Sher A, Kehrl JH. Activation of autophagy by inflammatory signals limits IL-1β production by targeting ubiquitinated inflammasomes for destruction. Nat Immunol. 2012;13:255–63.

13

Heart regeneration for clinical application update 2016: from induced pluripotent stem cells to direct cardiac reprogramming

Hiroyuki Yamakawa[1,2] (iD)

Abstract

Cardiovascular disease remains a major cause of death for which current therapeutic regimens are limited. Following myocardial injury, endogenous cardiac fibroblasts, which account for more than half of the cells in the heart, proliferate and synthesize extracellular matrix, leading to fibrosis and heart failure. As terminally differentiated cardiomyocytes have little regenerative capacity following injury, the development of cardiac regenerative therapy is highly desired. Embryonic stem and induced pluripotent stem (iPS) cells are promising tools for regenerative medicine. However, these stem cells demonstrate variable cardiac differentiation efficiency and tumorigenicity, which must be resolved prior to clinical regenerative applications. Until the last decade, an established theory was that cardiomyocytes could only be produced from fibroblasts through iPS cell generation. In 2010, we first reported cardiac differentiation from fibroblasts by direct reprogramming, and we demonstrated that various cardiac reprogramming pathways exist.

This review summarizes the latest trends in stem cell and regenerative research regarding iPS cells, a partial reprogramming strategy, and direct cardiac reprogramming. We also examine the many recent advances in direct cardiac reprogramming and explore the suitable utilization of these methods for regenerative medicine in the cardiovascular field.

Keywords: Cardiomyocytes, Cardiac fibroblasts, Myocardial infarction, Transcription factors, microRNAs, Cardiac regeneration, Induced cardiomyocytes, Direct reprogramming, iPS cells

Background

According to "the top 10 causes of death" announced by the World Health Organization (WHO), heart disease is a leading cause of death in the world. Current therapeutic regimens for heart disease are limited. Heart disease, including heart failure and myocardial infarction, is usually treated with medical therapy, mechanical device implantation, and surgical intervention. When a patient exhibits extremely poor cardiac function, a heart transplant is typically required; however, donor shortage is a major problem for heart transplantation (both in Japan and throughout the world). Thus, cardiac regenerative medicine is an attractive alternative therapy to heart transplantation. For the last two decades, embryonic stem (ES) cells have been used in the field of regenerative medicine due to their self-replication competence and cardiac differentiation ability; however, human ES cells are accompanied by ethical and legal concerns, as well as the threat of immunologic rejection. To solve these problems, Yamanaka and colleagues developed induced pluripotent stem (iPS) cells, which were created by introducing four stem cell-specific transcription factors (Oct3/4, Sox2, c-Myc, and Klf4; collectively, OSKM) into human dermal fibroblasts [1]. However, if iPS cells are to be used in clinical regenerative medicine applications in the future, several issues must be resolved. For example, these cells may demonstrate variable and low cardiomyocyte differentiation efficiency, may require a long time for cardiac maturation, and may show tumorigenicity.

Correspondence: yamakawa@cpnet.med.keio.ac.jp
[1]Department of Clinical and Molecular Cardiovascular Research, Keio University School of Medicine, Shinjuku-ku, Tokyo, Japan
[2]Department of Cardiology, Keio University School of Medicine, 35 Shinanomachi, Shinjuku-ku, Tokyo 160-8582, Japan

The skeletal muscle master gene, MyoD, was discovered in 1987 and spurred the search for a cardiomyocyte master gene, which has yet to be identified. However, the establishment of iPS cells suggested that cardiac reprogramming could be achieved by concurrent introduction of several transcription factors, rather than a single master gene, into fibroblasts. In fact, we first reported that induced cardiomyocyte-like cells or induced cardiomyocytes (iCMs) could be formed by transducing fibroblasts with genes encoding the cardiac-specific transcription factors, Gata4, Mef2c, and Tbx5 (collectively, GMT) [2]. Prior to our work, an established theory was that the reprogramming and subsequent differentiation of fibroblasts into cardiomyocytes required an iPS cell intermediate; however, our research introduced a new concept in which a direct reprogramming pathway exists for the production of cardiomyocytes from fibroblasts—one that does not involve iPS cells.

Here, we summarize current knowledge about cardiac reprogramming in vitro and in vivo. Furthermore, we discuss future applications of cardiac reprogramming in regenerative medicine.

Three pathways to generate new cardiomyocytes
The current methods of generating cardiomyocytes from fibroblasts are categorized into three general pathways (see Fig. 1):

(1) Full reprogramming of fibroblasts into iPS cells and subsequent cardiac differentiation

(2) Partial reprogramming of fibroblasts to cardiac progenitor cells and subsequent differentiation
(3) Direct reprogramming of fibroblasts into cardiomyocytes

The cardiomyocytes generated from any of these three pathways can be transplanted into an infarcted or failing heart. The direct reprogramming approach is particularly attractive, as transcription factors involved in cardiac reprogramming can be introduced directly into a heart, bypassing the need for engrafting of iCMs. In this section, we review preclinical and clinical data on these cardiac regeneration strategies and summarize the advantages of each of these three strategies [3].

1) Full reprogramming of fibroblasts into iPS cells and subsequent cardiac differentiation:
   Currently, the major strategy to generate cardiomyocytes requires the full reprogramming of fibroblasts into iPS cells and their subsequent differentiation. This strategy requires complete conversion of fibroblasts to undifferentiated cells (e.g., iPS cells) and differentiation of iPS cells into cardiomyocytes [4].
   Mouse and human iPS cells were established by Takahashi and Yamanaka in 2006 and 2007, respectively [1, 4]. In both instances, iPS cells were derived from fibroblasts by using retroviruses to transduce the fibroblasts with genes encoding four transcription factors (OSKM). iPS cells have brought

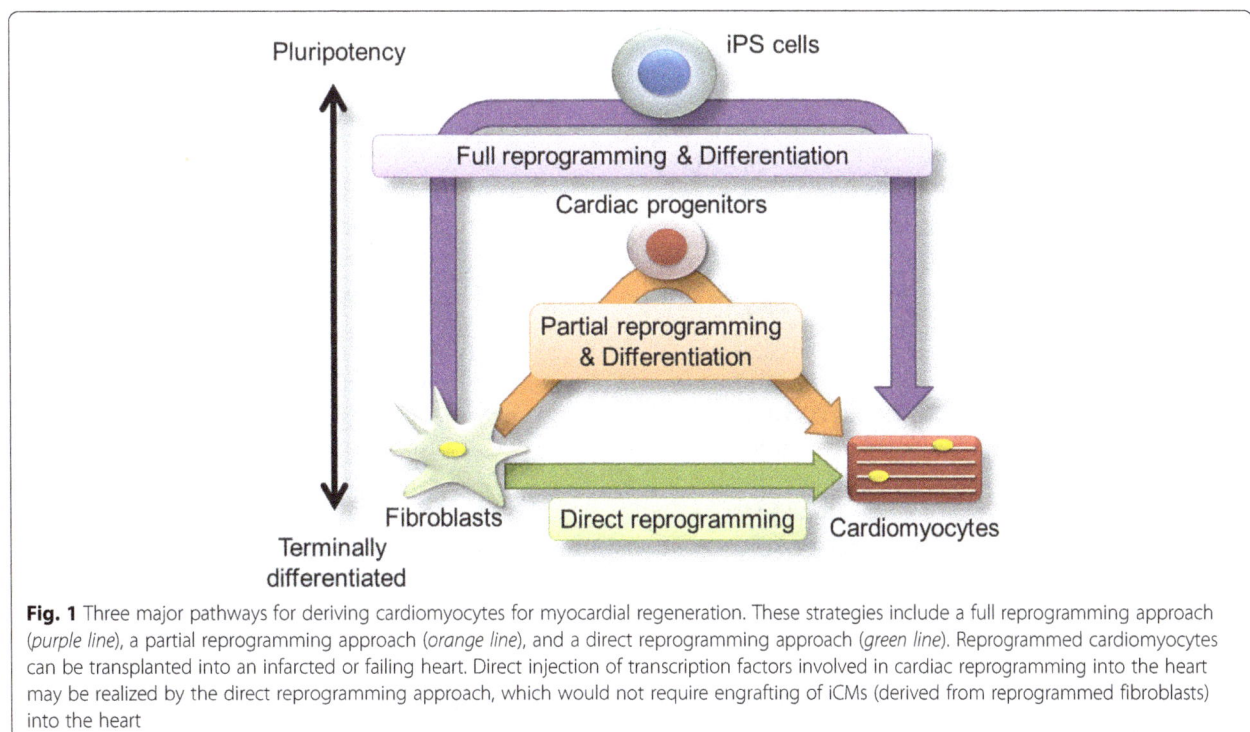

Fig. 1 Three major pathways for deriving cardiomyocytes for myocardial regeneration. These strategies include a full reprogramming approach (*purple line*), a partial reprogramming approach (*orange line*), and a direct reprogramming approach (*green line*). Reprogrammed cardiomyocytes can be transplanted into an infarcted or failing heart. Direct injection of transcription factors involved in cardiac reprogramming into the heart may be realized by the direct reprogramming approach, which would not require engrafting of iCMs (derived from reprogrammed fibroblasts) into the heart

about a major revolution in regenerative medicine [4]. Because they have a differentiation ability that is similar to ES cells, iPS cells can be exposed to cardiac differentiation protocols that were perfected in ES cells. Following the initial establishment of human iPS cells, functional analyses of iPS cell-derived cardiomyocytes showed that they are embryonic or immature cardiomyocytes rather than adult-type cardiomyocytes [5, 6]. Cardiomyocytes derived from human iPS cells have been used for disease modeling [7], and many laboratories have reported the analysis of models of various diseases using iPS cells from fibroblasts derived from patients or animals with those diseases.

2) Partial reprogramming of fibroblasts to cardiac progenitor cells and subsequent differentiation: The second strategy to generate cardiomyocytes requires the generation of partially reprogrammed cells, including cardiac progenitor cells. These cells can be generated during the process of iPS cell generation by exposing fibroblasts to OSKM and can be induced to differentiate into cardiomyocytes. Efe et al. reported an equivalent partial reprogramming method [8]. These researchers reported the successful induction of cardiomyocytes from fibroblast cultures transfected with OSKM, which were subsequently treated with cardiomyocyte-inducing factors.

If Efe's method induces partial reprogramming of fibroblasts into cardiac progenitor cells, several cardiomyocytes could be derived from a single fibroblast during this procedure. However, whether this strategy is applicable to human cells remains to be determined.

Wang et al. demonstrated that Oct4 alone, together with a small-molecule cocktail consisting of SB431542 (transforming growth factor beta (TGFβ) inhibitor), CHIR99021 (glycogen synthase kinase 3 (GSK3) inhibitor), Parnate (lysine-specific demethylase 1 (LSD1)/KDM1 (lysine(K)-specific demethylase1A) inhibitor), and Forskolin (adenylyl cyclase activator) (collectively, SCPF), is sufficient to "erase" the original cell identity, thereby enabling cell conversion with lineage-specific soluble signals [9]. In this case, bone morphogenetic protein (BMP) 4 was added beginning on day 6 after transduction to induce a cardiomyocyte phenotype. By using this strategy, they observed contracting clusters beginning on day 20 and generated 99 ± 17 beating clusters on day 30 after 10,000 mouse embryonic fibroblasts (MEFs) were initially plated [9]. Very recently, Lalit et al. [10] and Zhang et al. [11] reported two different strategies for reprogramming adult mouse fibroblasts into highly expandable cardiovascular progenitor cells [12]. They induced mouse fibroblasts with combinations of transcription

factors and small molecules and succeeded in expanding the cell populations they obtained in chemically defined conditions.

Lalit et al. [10] found that mouse fibroblasts can be infected with lentivirus harboring a doxycycline-inducible transgene encoding five reprogramming factors (Mesp1, Tbx5, Gata4, Nkx2.5, and Baf60c: collectively, MTGNB), and that self-expanding cardiac progenitor cells can be found with 6-bromoindirubin-30-oxime (BIO; canonical Wnt activator) and leukemia inhibitory factor (LIF; a JAK (Janus kinase) /STAT (signal transducer and activator of transcription) activator). These cells were called induced cardiac progenitor cells and can be expanded over 10^{15}-fold and differentiate into cardiomyocytes, endothelial cells, and smooth muscle cells. Transplantation of induced cardiac progenitor cells results in generation of all three of these lineages in vivo and improves survival of mouse after myocardial infarction [10].

Zhang et al. [11] utilized secondary MEFs, which transiently overexpress the four Yamanaka factors (OSKM) and showed that Yamanaka factor expression plus the JAK inhibitor JI1 and BACS (BMP4, activin A (the member of the transforming growth factor beta (TGF-β)), CHIR99021, and SU5402 (fibroblast growth factor receptor (FGFR)-specific tyrosine kinase inhibitor)) reprograms mouse fibroblasts into cardiac progenitor cells with a high capacity for expansion. These cells were named induced expandable cardiac progenitor cells, and they differentiate into cardiomyocytes, endothelial cells, and smooth muscle cells in vitro and after transplantation into myocardial infarcted hearts [11].

3) Direct reprogramming of fibroblasts into cardiomyocytes: Recently, a third strategy was developed as a new method to directly convert fibroblasts into another cell type by introducing single or multiple transcription factors. In 2010, Vierbuchen et al. succeeded in generating neuronal-like or induced neuronal cells by introducing three genes encoding transcription factors (Ascl1, Brn2, and Mytl1) necessary for neuronal differentiation into mouse fibroblasts [13]. This was the first successful report of direct reprogramming of fibroblasts into a specific cell type (without an iPS cell step) using organ-specific transcription factors.

Following the work of Vierbuchen and colleagues, we reported that neonatal mouse cardiac fibroblasts could be converted into cardiomyocyte-like cells or iCMs following introduction of genes encoding cardiac-specific transcription factors (Gata4, Mef2c, Tbx5: GMT) [2]. More recently, Sekiya et al.

reported the direct reprogramming of hepatocyte-like cells or induced hepatocytes from mouse fibroblasts [14]. Direct reprogramming technology converts terminally differentiated fibroblasts into another organ cell type and does not require the formation of iPS cells. In time, this strategy may provide a safe and novel alternative to heart transplants. We summarize the three strategies used to derive cardiomyocytes from fibroblasts in Table 1.

Direct cardiac reprogramming in vitro
Generation of mouse iCMs
Five years ago, we discovered that neonatal cardiac fibroblasts could be reprogrammed directly to form iCMs, without going through an intermediate iPS cell phase (see Table 2). Since then, multiple laboratories have reported the generation of iCMs using various methods. As cell sources for the generation of iCMs, we and others used cardiac fibroblasts, tail-tip fibroblasts, or MEFs derived from reporter mice that express a fluorescent protein when a cardiac-specific promoter, α-myosin heavy chain or cardiac troponin T (cTnT), is activated. To overexpress reprogramming factors in fibroblasts, researchers have used one of two techniques: (1) genes encoding cardiac-specific transcription factors (Gata4, Mef2c, Tbx5, Hand2, Myocd, etc.) were introduced into cells with viral vectors (retroviruses, lentiviruses, adenoviruses, etc.); or (2) the lipofection method was used to transfect cells with cardiac-specific microRNAs (miRs). The reprogramming efficiency can be quantified by counting the number of cells that express the cardiac reporter or protein (by flow cytometry or fluorescence-activated cell sorting) 1–3 weeks after introduction of reprogramming factors into fibroblasts. As part of the functional analysis, these cells were further evaluated for spontaneous beating, calcium homeostasis, and action potentials. Based on our epoch-making study, Song et al. were able to produce functional iCMs (identified as cTnT(+) cells) from adult cardiac fibroblasts and tail-tip fibroblasts by adding a gene encoding a fourth transcription factor—Hand2—to GMT (collectively GHMT) [15]. However, Chen et al. showed the difficulty in generating functional cardiomyocytes through induction with GMT and emphasized the need to examine the reprogramming mechanisms and epigenetic changes induced with this transcription factor cocktail [16].

Protze et al. introduced 120 combinations of factors into MEFs using a pool of 10 transcription factors in an attempt to induce cardiac differentiation and confirmed cardiomyocyte properties in treated cells through gene expression analyses. They showed that the 3F-Myocd combination (Mef2c, Tbx5, and Myocd, in which Myocd was substituted for Gata4) may result in cardiomyocytes that are more differentiated than with other combinations [17].

In addition, Jayawardena et al. introduced only the microRNAs, miR-1, miR-133, miR-208, and miR-499, into neonatal cardiac fibroblasts and succeeded in generating iCMs, distinguishing this report from other research. As microRNAs are not incorporated into host chromosomes during transient expression, microRNA-mediated induction may be safer for human applications [18]. This research also suggested that culture conditions are vital to cardiomyocyte induction, as expression of α-myosin heavy chain-cyan fluorescence protein (CFP) in transgenic mice increased nearly tenfold when a JAK inhibitor was added to the culture medium.

Table 1 Three strategies to generate cardiomyocytes from fibroblasts. The properties of the cells, advantages, and disadvantages of the strategies are shown

Strategy	Full reprogramming via iPS cells	Partial reprogramming via cardiac progenitor cells (CPCs)	Direct cardiac reprogramming
Cell state	iPS cells (pluripotent)	Cardiac progenitor cells (multipotent)	Differentiated cardiomyocytes (unipotent)
Properties	1. Pluripotent cells 2. Bypass ethical and legal problems (compared to ES cells) 3. Not accompanied by the problem of immunologic refusal	Multipotent CPCs can generate vascular and cardiac cells	Transdifferentiation without an undifferentiated (intermediate) state (i.e., iPS cells, CPCs)
Advantages	Engraftment of ES cell-derived cardiomyocytes is possible in large animal models, accompanied by improved heart function	A short culture period (weeks) required to produce cardiomyocytes, compared with iPSC-mediated cardiomyocytes	1. In vivo reprogramming 2. Takes 4 weeks to generate functional cardiomyocytes 3. Lack of tumor formation 4. Generating only cardiomyocytes
Disadvantages	1. Risk of teratoma formation 2. A long culture period (months) is required to generate cardiomyocytes 3. Immaturity of stem cell-derived cardiomyocytes	1. Uncertain mechanism of OSKM-mediated CPC induction 2. Risk of tumor formation	1. Immaturity of iCMs 2. Low efficiency of full reprogramming into functional cardiomyocytes 3. iCMs are not proliferative

Table 2 Direct/partial reprogramming of mouse/rat fibroblasts to cardiomyocytes in vitro

Reprogramming factors	Supplement agents	Species	Starting cell source	Efficiency	Comments	References
Gata4, Mef2c, Tbx5 (GMT)		Mouse	Adult cardiac fibroblasts (CFs) and tail-tip fibroblasts (TTFs)	20~30 % cTnT+ cells after 1 week	Beating after 4 weeks (CFs). Using retrovirus and lentivirus	[2]
Oct4, Sox2, Klf4 (, c-Myc)	JAK inhibitor I, BMP4	Mouse	Mouse embryonic fibroblasts (MEFs)	40 % cTnT(+) after 18 days	Partial reprogramming. Beating after 18 days in cluster. Using secondary MEFs harboring doxycycline-inducible transgenes encoding reprogramming factors.	[8]
Oct4	ALK4/5/7 inhibitor, GSK3 inhibitor, LSD/KDM1 inhibitor, BMP4	Mouse	MEFs, TTFs	Make clusters	Partial reprogramming. Beating after 20 days. Without any evidence of entrance into the pluripotent state. Using doxycycline inducible-expression lentivirus-based gene delivery system	[9]
Mesp1, Tbx5, Gata4, Nkx2-5, Baf60c (MTGNB)	BIO, LIF	Mouse	MEFs, CFs	Passage over 20 times, expand more than 10^{15}-fold	Partial reprogramming. Using a doxycycline-inducible lentivirus vector	[10]
Oct4, Sox2, Klf4, c-Myc (OSKM)	JAK inhibitor (JI1), BACS (BMP4, Activin A,CHIR99021, and SU5402)	Mouse	MEFs, TTFs	Expanded more than 10^{10}-fold	Partial reprogramming. Using secondary MEFs harboring doxycycline-inducible transgenes encoding reprogramming factors	[11]
Gata4, Mef2c, Tbx5 (GMT)		Mouse	CFs and TTFs	35 % cTnT+ cells	Beating after 4~5 weeks. Using retrovirus	[15]
Gata4, Mef2c, Tbx5 (GMT)		Mouse	CFs and TTFs	35 % cTnT+ cells	Beating after 4~5 weeks. Using lentivirus	[16]
Myocd, Mef2, Tbx5 (3F-Myocd)		Mouse	MEFs and neonatal CFs	2.5 % αMHC+ cells	Analysis of ion-channel. Using lentivirus	[17]
miR-1, miR-133, miR-208, miR-499	JAK inhibitor 1	Mouse	CFs	13~28 % αMHC+ cells	Added JAK inhibitor. Only micro RNAs	[18]
GMT, Hand2, Nkx2-5 (HNGMT)		Mouse	MEFs, CFs	Almost 5 % the calcium indicator GCaMP(+) cells	Using the induction of calcium oscillation for screening. Utilizing an inducible-expression lentivirus-based gene delivery system (lentivirus)	[19]
GMT, Mesp1, Myocd, Smarcd3 (Baf60c), SRF		Mouse	MEFs	2.4 % αMHC+ cells	Using lentivirus	[20]
GMT, miR-133		Mouse	MEFs, CFs	40~50 % αMHC+ cells (MEFs)	Beating after 10 days. Using retrovirus	[21]
Gata4, Mef2c-MyoD fusion, Tbx5, Hand2		Mouse	MEFs, TTFs	10~20 % cTnT(+) cells	Beating after 7 days. Using retrovirus	[22]
Mef2c-P2A-Gata4-T2A-Tbx5		Mouse	Adult CFs	Tenfold increase in beating iCMs	Using polycistronic vectors (retrovirus)	[23]
Gata4, Mef2c, Tbx5, Hand2, Nkx2-5 (HNGMT)	TGFβ inhibitor	Mouse	MEFs, CFs	17 % the calcium indicator GCaMP(+) cells	Beating approximately fivefold compared to 16). Using a doxycycline-inducible lentivirus vector	[24]

Table 2 Direct/partial reprogramming of mouse/rat fibroblasts to cardiomyocytes in vitro *(Continued)*

Gata4, Mef2c, Tbx5, Hand2 (GHMT)	Akt1	Mouse	MEFs, CFs, TTFs	50 % of reprogrammed MEFs beating	Beating after 3 weeks Using retrovirus	[25]
(−)	CHIR99021, RepSox, Forskolin, VPA, Parnate, TTNPB, DZnep	Mouse	MEFs, TTFs		Chemical reprogramming Beating after 20–24 days	[26]
Gata4, Mef2c, Tbx5, Hand2 (GHMT), miR-1, miR-133	A83-01 (inhibitor of TGF-β1), Y-27632 (inhibitor of ROCK)	Mouse	MEFs, CFs	60 % cTnT(+) cells after	Beating 2 weeks Using retrovirus	[27]
Gata4, Mef2c, Tbx5 (Hand2)	FGF2, FGF10, VEGF, IWR-1	Mouse	MEFs, CFs, TTFs	10–20 % αMHC(+) cells after 1 week	1 % Beating after 4 weeks (GMT) 5~9 % Beating after 4 weeks (GHMT) Using retrovirus	[28]
Mef2c, Tbx5	FGF2, FGF10, VEGF	Mouse	MEFs	3 % αMHC(+) cells after 1 week	Beating after 4 weeks Using retrovirus	[28]

Addis et al. reported the benefits of adding Nkx2-5 and Hand2 to GMT if both factors were added to GMT. Using a transgenic calcium fluorescent reporter driven by a cardiomyocyte-specific gene promoter, they demonstrated that infection with GMT, Hand2, and Nkx2-5 (collectively HNGMT) results in the most efficient generation of functional cardiomyocytes [19]. Christoforou et al. determined that overexpression of Myocd and Srf (serum response factor) transcription factors, alone or in conjunction with Mesp1 and Smardcd3 (Baf60c), enhances the basal cardiac-inducing effects of GMT. Through global gene expression analysis, they demonstrated the significantly greater cardiac-inducing effects of Myocd and Srf compared to GMT alone [20].

In 2014, we demonstrated that miR-133 overexpression paired with GMT generates sevenfold more beating iCMs from MEFs compared to GMT treatment alone; this treatment also shortened the duration required to induce beating iCMs (from 30 to 10 days). Furthermore, we found that miR-133-mediated Snail repression is critical for cardiac reprogramming in adult mouse (and human cardiac) fibroblasts, and that silencing fibroblast signatures via miR-133/Snail is a key molecular roadblock during cardiac reprogramming [21]. Importantly, this was the first study to demonstrate a molecular mechanism underlying cardiac reprogramming by defined factors.

Hirai et al. fused a transactivation domain from MyoD to individual factors in the GHMT cocktail and found that fusion of the Mef2c C-terminus with the MyoD transactivation domain plus wild-type Gata4, Hand2, and Tbx5 accelerates cardiac reprogramming and generates larger beating clusters from MEFs with a 15-fold greater efficiency than GHMT without the fusion [22]. This result is consistent with the observation that reprogramming requires high levels of gene expression and activity to overcome the high barrier of cellular stability that is inherently present in adult somatic cells.

Wang et al. generated six polycistronic constructs to include all ordered combinations of Gata4, Mef2c, and Tbx5 with identical self-cleaving 2A sequences and showed distinct protein levels of the three transcription factors based on the splicing order [23]. They further demonstrated that relatively higher protein levels of Mef2c with modest levels of Gata4 and Tbx5 lead to more efficient cardiac reprogramming, and an optimized MGT combination with puromycin selection results in an over tenfold increase in beating iCMs. This report convincingly showed that the protein ratio of cardiac reprogramming factors could greatly influence the efficiency and quality of iCMs.

Small molecules promote the reprogramming of mouse iCMs
Recently, multiple groups have shown that modification of reprogramming factors can promote cardiac reprogramming. In particular, by stimulating or inhibiting the signaling pathways involved in generation of cardiomyocytes, they could improve cardiac reprogramming efficiency. Cardiac reprogramming can also be affected by cell culture conditions. These recent findings provide new insights into the molecular mechanisms underlying cardiac conversion of fibroblasts and will enhance efforts to generate cardiomyocytes for clinical applications (see Table 2).

Ifkovits et al. visualized the induction of calcium oscillations in reprogrammed cells with a transgenic calcium reporter, GCaMP5 (Ca^{2+} probe composed of a single GFP 5), driven by a cardiac-specific gene promoter. They found that a combination of five cardiac transcription factors, GMT, Hand2, and Nkx2.5 (GMTHN), more efficiently reprograms MEFs. They also found that GCaMP5 helps track the location of rare beating iCMs that represent fully reprogrammed cells. With the same method, they found that a small molecule inhibitor of TGF-β, SB431542, increases reprogramming efficiency via GMTHN up to nearly fivefold and generates more beating iCMs from MEFs [24].

Zhou et al. discovered that Akt/protein kinase B dramatically improves the efficiency of reprogramming fibroblasts to iCMs by the cardiac transcription factors GHMT. Approximately 50 % of reprogrammed MEFs displayed spontaneous beating after 3 weeks of induction by Akt plus GHMT. Insulin-like growth factor 1 and phosphoinositol 3-kinase act upstream of Akt, whereas the mitochondrial target of rapamycin complex 1 and forkhead box O3 act downstream of Akt to influence fibroblast-to-cardiomyocyte reprogramming [25].

Fu et al. reported generation of automatically beating cardiomyocyte-like cells from mouse fibroblasts using only chemical cocktails (CHIR99021, RepSox (inhibitor of the TGFβ receptor-1/ALK5), Forskolin, VPA (valproic acid; histone deacetylase inhibitor), Parnate, TTNPB (Arotinoid acid; a synthetic stilbene analog of retinoic acid (RA)), DZnep (3-Deazaneplanocin A hydrochloride; histone methyltransferase EZH2 (enhancer of zeste homolog 2) inhibitor)) [26]. These chemically induced cardiomyocyte-like cells express cardiomyocyte-specific markers and possess typical cardiac calcium transients and electrophysiological features [26].

Zhao et al. reported that inhibition of the TGF-β1 or Rho-associated kinase (ROCK) pathways converts embryonic fibroblasts into functional cardiomyocyte-like cells by forced expression of GMT or GHMT, with an efficiency of up to 60 %. Furthermore, inhibition of TGF-β1 or ROCK signaling dramatically enhances full reprogramming, with spontaneously beating cardiomyocytes emerging in less than 2 weeks with GHMT alone [27].

In 2015, we demonstrated that a combination of fibroblast growth factor (FGF) 2, FGF10, and vascular endothelial growth factor (VEGF) promotes cardiac reprogramming in defined serum-free conditions, increasing spontaneously beating iCMs by 100-fold compared with other conventional serum-based conditions. Mechanistically, FGF2, FGF10, and VEGF activate multiple cardiac transcriptional regulators and convert partially reprogrammed cells into functional iCMs through the p38 mitogen-activated protein kinase and phosphoinositol 3-kinase/AKT pathways. Moreover, our cocktail enables cardiac reprogramming with only Mef2c and Tbx5 [28].

Generation of human iCMs

Three studies including ours applied the concept of direct reprogramming to neonatal and adult human fibroblasts in 2013 [29–31] (see Table 3). Nam et al. reported that a combination of genes encoding four transcription factors (Gata4, Hand2, Tbx5, and Myocd) and two muscle-specific microRNAs (miR-1 and miR-133) can reprogram up to 20 % of human fibroblasts into cTnT(+) cells (presumptive cardiomyocytes). Furthermore, a subset of iCMs derived from human cardiac fibroblasts demonstrated spontaneous beating after 11 weeks in culture [29]. Similarly, Fu et al. reported that a mixture of genes encoding seven transcription factors (Gata4, Mef2c, Tbx5, Mesp1, Myocd, Zfpm2, Esrrg) can induce human cardiomyocyte gene expression in treated fibroblasts [30]. This work also demonstrated that this mixture of reprogramming factors generates epigenetically stable human iCMs, and that TGF-β signaling improves the efficiency of human iCM reprogramming [30]. Finally, we found that a combination of genes encoding five transcription factors (Gata4, Mef2c, Tbx5, Mesp1, and Myocd) can reprogram human fibroblasts into beating, cardiomyocyte-like cells with action potentials when co-cultured with rat cardiomyocytes [31]. Islas et al. used two transcription factors (Mesp1 and Ets-2) in activin A- and BMP2-treated cells to reprogram human dermal fibroblasts into cardiac progenitor-like cells, which could then differentiate into cardiomyocyte-like cells [32]. Despite these promising results, direct cardiac reprogramming is less efficient in human cells compared to mouse fibroblasts.

Muraoka et al. induced 2–8 % of α-actin(+)/cTnT(+) cells with lentiviral transduction of Gata4, Mef2c, Tbx5, Mesp1, and Myocd into human cardiac fibroblasts (HCFs). Interestingly, by adding miR-133 to the reprogramming cocktail, they increased the efficiency of iCM generation to 23–27 % [21].

In 2015, Li et al. reported that the combination of QQ-reagent-modified Gata4, Hand2, Mef2c, and Tbx5 and sevral cytokines (BMP4, activin A, FGF2, IWR1 (Wnt pathway inhibitor)) reprogrammed human dermal fibroblasts (HDFs) into CPCs [33]. Like what Yamamakawa et al. pointed out [28], the protein-transduction method can directrely program with high efficiency. And finally, Cao

et al. demonstrated that cardiomyocyte-like cells can be generated by treating human fibroblasts with a combination of nine compounds (CHIR99021, A83-01 (Inhibitor of TGF-beta type I receptor), BIX01294 (a histone methyltransferase (HMTase) inhibitor), SC1 (ERK 1 inhibitor), Y27632 (ROCK inhibitor), OAC2 (Oct4-activating compound 2), SU16F (inhibitor of platelet-derived growth factor receptor-beta (PDGFR beta), and JNJ10198409 (inhibitor of platelet-derived growth factor receptor tyrosine kinase (PDGF-RTK))). The chemically induced cardiomyocyte-like cells uniformly contracted and resembled human cardiomyocytes in their transcriptome, epigenetic, and electrophysiological properties [34].

These protein reprogramming strategies have the promising approaches for future regenerative medicine both in vitro and in vivo. But the conversion of fibroblasts into human iCMs is not easy, compared with mouse iCMs. Therefore, further research is essential to identify optimal reprogramming factors (transcription factors, microRNAs, etc.) as well as culture conditions (small molecules, cytokines, etc.) for improving reprogramming efficiency and use in clinical applications [33, 34].

Direct cardiac reprogramming in vivo

The most exciting potential for cardiac transcription factor-based reprogramming is the possibility of using this technology in vivo. Injection of reprogramming factors directly into the damaged heart may convert endogenous cardiac fibroblasts, which represent >50 % of all cardiac cells, into new functional cardiomyocytes. This in vivo reprogramming approach may have several advantages over cell transplantation-based therapy. First, the process is simple. Second, avoiding the induction of pluripotent cells before cardiac differentiation would greatly lower the risk of tumor formation. Third, direct injection of defined factors obviates the need for cell transplantation, for which long-term cell survival remains challenging [35–37] (see Table 4).

For example, cardiac fibroblasts in an infarcted area of a heart could be targeted for cardiogenic reprogramming, resulting in the formation of new cardiomyocytes in situ. In 2012, multiple groups including us demonstrated the transdifferentiation of fibroblasts into cardiomyocytes in vivo. Olson's and Srivastava's groups used the Cre recombinase driven by fibroblast-specific promoters to trace the cell fate of cardiac fibroblasts and subsequent cardiomyocyte transdifferentiation.

Qian et al. used the periostin and fibroblast-specific protein 1 (FSP-1) promoter Cre transgenic mice and found that fibroblasts in infarcted hearts are converted into cardiomyocyte-like cells by GMT retroviral gene transfer; global function also restored in treated hearts [38]. Following direct injection of GMT retroviruses into infarcted mouse hearts, this work demonstrated

Table 3 Direct reprogramming of human fibroblasts to cardiomyocytes in vitro

Reprogramming factors	Supplement agents	Species	Starting cell type	Efficiency	Comments	References
Gata4, Hand2, Myocd, Tbx5, miR-1, miR-133,		Human	Human neonatal foreskin fibroblasts (HFF), adult human cardiac fibroblasts (AHCFs) and and adult human dermal fibroblasts (AHDFs)	~20 % cTnT(+) cells (HFF) 13 % cTnT(+) cells (AHCFs) 9.5 % cTnT(+) cells (AHDFs)	Bating after 11 weeks (AHCFs) Using retrovirus	[29]
Gata4, Mef2c, Tbx5, Mesp1, Myocd, Zfp42/Rex1, ESRRG		Human	Human cardiac fibroblasts (HCF)	35 % cTnT(+) cells	Using retrovirus and lentivirus	[30]
Gata4, Mef2c, Tbx5, Mesp1, Myocd		Human	Adult cardiac human fibroblasts (AHCFs) and adult dermal fibroblasts (AHDFs)	5 % αactinin(+) and cTnT(+) cells	Beating co-cultured with mouse cardiomyocytes Using retrovirus	[31]
Ets2, Mesp1		Human	Adult dermal human fibroblasts (AHDFs)	2.3 % αMHC(+) cells	Cells expressing the cardiac mesoderm marker KDR(+) using lentivirus	[32]
Gata4, Mef2c, Tbx5, Mesp1, Myocd, miR-133		Human	Human cardiac fibroblasts (HCFs)	23~27 % cTNT(+) cells	Using retrovirus	[21]
Gata4, Mef2c, Tbx5, Hand2	Add supplement agents (BMP4, activin A, FgF2, IWR1)	Human	Adult human dermal human fibroblasts (AHDFs)		Cardiac progenitor cells (?) Using retrovirus	[33]
(–)	9 compounds (9C; CHIR99021, A83-01, BIX01294, SC1, Y27632, OAC2, SU16F, and JNJ10198409)	Human	Human foreskin fibroblast (HFF) Human fetal lung fibroblasts (HLFs)	6.6 ± 0.4 % of cTNT(+) cells	Chemical reprogramming	[34]

Table 4 Direct reprogramming of fibroblasts to cardiomyocytes in vivo

Reprogramming factors	Gene transduction	Species	Disease model	Comments	References
Gata4, Mef2c, Tbx5 (GMT)	Retrovirus	Mouse	Myocardial infarction (MI)	Injected reprogrammed cells	[2]
Mesp1, Tbx5, Gata4, Nkx2.5, Baf60c (MTGNB)	Using a doxycycline-inducible lentivirus vector	Mouse	MI	Improved survival after myocardial infarction (MI) Differentiate into cardiomyocytes, smooth muscle cells, and endothelial cells	[10]
Oct4, Sox2, Klf4, c-Myc (OSKM)	(–) Using secondary MEFs harboring doxycycline-inducible transgenes encoding reprogramming factors	Mouse	MI	Improves heart function after MI Reduce infarct area Differentiate into cardiomyocytes, smooth muscle cells, and endothelial cells	[11]
Gata4, Hand2, Mef2c, Tbx5 (GHMT)	Retrovirus	Mouse	MI	Injected virus 2.4~6.5 % (border zone) reduction of 50 % in scar zone	[15]
Gata4, Mef2c, Tbx5 (GMT)	Lentivirus	Mouse	MI	Injected reprogrammed cells	[16]
Gata4, Mef2c, Tbx5 (GMT)	Retrovirus	Mouse	MI	Injected virus Almost 35 % of iCMs in the border/infarct area Improvement 10 % in ejection fraction	[38]
Gata4, Mef2c, Tbx5 (GMT) 3F-2A system	Polycistronic vectors (retrovirus)	Mouse	MI	Injected virus 1~3 % (border zone)	[31]
miR-1, miR-133, miR-208, miR-499	microRNA	Mouse	MI	Added JAK inhibitor ~1 % (border zone)	[18]
GMT and Vegf (GMT/VEGF)	Lentivirus	Rat	MI	Injected virus Improvement in ejection fraction fourfold greater in GMT/VEGF vs GMT only	[40]

that almost 35 % of cardiomyocytes in the infarcted area or its border were newly generated iCMs derived from resident cardiac fibroblasts. Furthermore, half of these iCMs showed well-organized sarcomeric structures and exhibited functional characteristics of adult ventricular cardiomyocytes, including cellular contraction, electrophysiological properties, and functional coupling to other cardiac cells. These observations suggested that in vivo reprogramming generates functional iCMs more efficiently than in vitro reprogramming [38]. In contrast to the work of Qian et al., Song et al. added Hand2 to the GMT cocktail (creating a GHMT cocktail) and utilized FSP-1 promoter Cre transgenic and Tcf21-iCre knock-in mice for fibroblast lineage tracing. They reported that GHMT retroviral injection into mouse infarcted hearts converts endogenous cardiac fibroblasts into functional cardiomyocyte-like cells in vivo [15]. These researchers also demonstrated that approximately 6 % of cardiomyocytes in the infarcted area or its border were newly generated cardiomyocyte-like cells with clear striations and functional properties similar to those of endogenous ventricular cardiomyocytes. Twelve weeks after myocardial infarction, Song et al. also demonstrated that the scar zone of infarcted hearts was reduced by 50 %, and the ejection fraction was increased twofold in GHMT-treated mice compared to controls [15].

We generated a polycistronic retrovirus expressing GMT. This polycistronic retrovirus, which expresses GMT at near equimolar levels from the same promoter, was generated using self-cleaving 2A peptides [39]. We co-injected polycistronic GMT (3F2A) and reporter genes (e.g., GFP) to determine cardiac induction from non-myocytes. We found that gene transfer of this polycistronic GMT retrovirus induces more mature cardiomyocyte-like cells (as evidenced by sarcomeric structures) than those generated by the injection of three separate vectors.

Mathison et al. injected a mixture of GMT retroviruses and VEGF into infarcted myocardium areas in rats. Infarcted areas were reduced in rats treated with VEGF compared to those only treated with GMT. This reduction in the scar in the infarcted area may be due to VEGF-mediated neovascularization or some other unknown mechanisms [40].

Direct injection of lentiviruses containing four microRNAs (miR-1, miR-133, miR-208, and miR-499) into mouse infarcted hearts converts resident cardiac fibroblasts into cardiomyocyte-like cells in vivo. After injection of these microRNAs, Jayawardena et al. reported that approximately 1 % of the infarcted area contained new iCMs; however, this work did not report on whether ejection fraction improved after microRNA injection [18].

For clinical applications, the development of a non-viral delivery method, including chemically synthesized molecules and microRNAs, may be a very attractive therapeutic approach, because non-viral factors do not integrate into the host chromosomes. Of note, these results suggest that the abundant pool of endogenous cardiac fibroblasts could be a cell source for new cardiomyocytes via direct reprogramming and that this new technology may improve cardiac function and reduce scar size after myocardial infarction. These studies clearly demonstrate that iCMs reprogrammed in vivo are more mature than those reprogrammed in vitro, suggesting that the effects of the in vivo environment, such as mechanical stretch, local signals, and the extracellular matrix, enhance the quality of iCMs in the native heart.

Conclusions

We reviewed the three different reprogramming strategies that are being developed in the field of cardiac regenerative medicine. Although all strategies (iPS cell approach, partial reprogramming, and direct reprogramming) have been utilized by many researchers, these strategies each have several problems that must be overcome prior to clinical application [41, 42].

The heart is composed of various groups of cells, including blood vessel endothelial cells, smooth muscle cells, nerve cells, and cardiac fibroblasts. Judging from the absolute number of cells comprising the heart, cardiomyocytes only account for approximately 30 % of heart cells, whereas cardiac fibroblasts constitute approximately 50 % of this organ. When a large number of cardiomyocytes die due to necrosis caused by myocardial infarction, the number of cardiac fibroblasts increases in the infarcted area. Heart rupture can be prevented by replacing an infarcted area with fibrous tissue; however, fibroblasts can result in low cardiac function and a potentially fatal arrhythmic focus. Direct reprogramming technology may provide an ideal treatment that could bypass the formation of cardiac fibroblasts in an infarcted region, instead resulting in new cardiomyocyte formation if certain genes are efficiently introduced into cardiac tissue [43].

Today, almost all reports of successful direct cardiac reprogramming have been generated with retroviruses or lentiviruses (Tables 2, 3, and 4). These reports involve integration in the host cell genome with an identified risk for insertional mutagenesis. To circumvent such risks which are deemed incompatible with therapeutic prospects, significant progress has been made with transgene-free reprogramming methods based on other kinds of virus, microRNA [15], or the cocktail of small molecules [26, 34] to achieve conversion into cardiomyocytes.

In the future, many scientists will examine the feasibility of a novel reprogramming process based on transgene-free methods using adenovirus, microRNAs, non-viral episomal expression vectors, and protein transduction.

However, for direct reprogramming to be used in clinical applications, the cardiac reprogramming efficiency induced by this method must be optimized. The generation of sufficient numbers of fully reprogrammed cells in vitro will also be valuable for drug toxicity studies and drug screening. Currently, the reprogramming efficiency of fibroblasts into mature cardiomyocytes is variable and low. Although several reports have described direct reprogramming of human cardiac fibroblasts into cardiomyocytes, further study is required for optimization.

On the other hand, current iCM technology is quite efficient for in vivo reprogramming, and the iCM in vivo reprogramming approach has several advantages over cell-based transplantation therapy. Because reprogramming factors are directly injected into the heart, no issues arise concerning the homing, survival, or migration of transplanted cells.

Future identification of small molecules or secreted proteins that could replace each transcription factor, as has been performed for iPS cell reprogramming, may allow an alternative to gene therapy. We hope to utilize regenerative medicine-based therapies to treat patients with severe heart failure, potentially employing cardiac muscle cells derived from iPS cells and iCMs.

Abbreviations

A83-01: Inhibitor of TGF-β type I receptor, ALK5 kinase; ADHF: Adult human dermal fibroblasts; AHCF: Adult human cardiac fibroblasts; ALK: Activin receptor-like kinase; AS8351: 2-Hydroxy-1-naphthylaldehyde isonicotinoyl hydrazine, histone demethylase inhibitor; BIO: 6-Bromoindirubin-30-oxime, canonical Wnt activator; BIX01294: (2-(Hexahydro-4-methyl-1H-1,4-diazepin-1-yl)-6,7-dimethoxy-N-[1-(phenylmethyl)-4-piperidinyl]-4-quinazolinamine trihydrochloride), a histone methyltransferase (HMTase) inhibitor; BMP: Bone morphogenetic protein; CF: Cardiac fibroblast; CFP: Cyan fluorescence protein; CHIR99021: 6-{2-[4-(2,4-Dichloro-phenyl)-5-(5-methyl-1H-imidazol-2-yl)-pyrimidin-2-ylamino]-ethylamino}-nicotinonitrile), GSK3 inhibitor; cTnT: Cardiac troponin T; DZnep: 3-Deazaneplanocin A hydrochloride; histone methyltransferase (EZH2 inhibitor); ERK: Extracellular signal-regulated kinase; ES cells: Embryonic stem cells; EZH2: Enhancer of zeste homolog 2; FGF: Fibroblast growth factor; FGFR: Fibroblast growth factor receptor; FSP-1: Periostin and fibroblast-specific protein 1; GCaMP: Ca2+ probe composed of a single GFP; GMT: Gata4, Mef2c, and Tbx5; GSK3: Glycogen synthase kinase 3; HCF: Human cardiac fibroblasts; HFF: Human neonatal foreskin fibroblasts; HLF: Human fetal lung fibroblasts; HMTase: Methyltransferase inhibitor; iCMs: Induced cardiomyocytes; iPS cells: Induced pluripotent stem cells; IWR1: 4-[(3aR,4S,7R,7aS)-1,3,3a,4,7,7a-hexahydro-1,3-dioxo-4,7-methano-2H-isoindol-2-yl]-N-8-quinolinyl-benzamide, Wnt pathway inhibitor; JAK: Janus kinase; JI1: JAK inhibitor 1; JNJ10198409: N-(3-Fluorophenyl)-2,4-dihydro-6,7-dimethoxyindeno[1,2-c]pyrazol-3-amine, inhibitor of platelet-derived growth factor receptor tyrosine kinase (PDGF-RTK); KDM1: Lysine(K)-specific demethylase1A; LIF: Leukemia inhibitory factor, a JAK/STAT activator; LSD1: Lysine-specific demethylase 1; MEF: Mouse embryonic fibroblast; miR: microRNA; OAC2: N-1H-indol-5-yl-benzamide, Oct4-activating compound 2; OKSM: Oct3/4, Sox2, c-Myc, and Klf4; Parnate: Tranylcypromine, LSD1/KDM1 inhibitor); RepSox: E-616452, 2-(3-(6-Methylpyridine-2-yl)-1H-pyrazol-4-yl)-1,5-naphthyridine; ROCK: Rho-associated kinase; SB431542: 4-[4-(1,3-Benzodioxol-5-yl)-5-(pyridin-2-yl)-1H-imidazol-2-yl]benzamide, TGFβ inhibotor; SB431542: 4-[4-(1,3-Benzodioxol-5-yl)-5-(2-pyridinyl)-1H-imidazol-2-yl]-benzamide, ALK4/5/7 inhibitor; SC1: N-(3-(7-(1,3-dimethyl-1H-pyrazol-5-ylamino)-1-methyl-2-oxo-1,2-dihydropyrimido[4,5-d]pyrimidin-3(4H)-yl)-4-methylphenyl)-3-(trifluoromethyl)benzamide, Pluripotin, ERK 1 inhibitor; Srf: Serum response factor; STAT: Signal transducer and activator of transcription; SU16F: 5-[1,2-Dihydro-2-oxo-6-phenyl-3H-indol-3-ylidene)methyl]-2,4-dimethyl-1H-pyrrole-3-propanoic acid, inhibitor of platelet-derived growth factor receptor-beta (PDGFRβ); SU5402: 3-[3-(2-Carboxyethyl)-4-methylpyrrol-2-methylidenyl]-2-indolinone, fibroblast growth factor receptor (FGFR)-specific tyrosine kinase inhibitor; TGF-β: Transforming growth factor beta; TTF: tail tip fibroblast; TTNPB: 4-[(E)-2-(5,6,7,8-Tetrahydro-5,5,8,8-tetramethyl-2-naphthalenyl)-1-propenyl]benzoic acid (Arotinoid acid; a synthetic stilbene analog of retinoic acid (RA)); VEGF: Vascular endothelial growth factor; VPA: Valproic acid; WHO: the World Health Organization; Y-27632: (trans-4-[(1R)-1-Aminoethyl]-N-4-pyridinylcyclohexanecarboxamide), inhibitor of ROCK

Acknowledgements

I thank all the members of the Department of Clinical and Molecular Cardiovascular Research and Department of Cardiology, Keio University School of Medicine, especially Ieda M. and Fukuda K.

Funding

H.Y. was supported by research grants from Japan Society for the Promotion of Science (JSPS) KAKENHI Grant Number 15K09147 (Grant-in-aid for Scientific Research (C)).

Competing interests

The author declares that they he has no competing interests.

References

1. Takahashi K, Tanabe K, Ohnuki M, et al. Induction of pluripotent stem cells from adult human fibroblasts by defined factors. Cell. 2007;131:861–72.

2. Ieda M, Fu JD, Delgado-Olguin P, et al. Direct reprogramming of fibroblasts into functional cardiomyocytes by defined factors. Cell. 2010;142:375–86.

3. David R, Franz WM. From pluripotency to distinct cardiomyocytes subtypes. Physiology. 2011;27:119–29.

4. Takahashi K, Yamanaka S. Induction of pluripotent stem cells from mouse embryonic and adult fibroblast cultures by defined factors. Cell. 2006;126:663–76.

5. Narazaki G, Uosaki H, Teranishi M, et al. Directed and systematic differentiation of cardiovascular cells from mouse induced pluripotent stem cells. Circulation. 2008;118:498–506.

6. Zhang J, Wilson GF, Soerens AG, et al. Functional cardiomyocytes derived from human induced pluripotent stem cells. Circ Res. 2009;104:e30–41.

7. Moretti A, Bellin M, Welling A, et al. Patient-specific induced pluripotent stem-cell models for long QT-syndrome. N Engl J Med. 2010;363:1397–409.

8. Efe JA, Hilcove S, Kim J, et al. Conversion of mouse fibroblasts into cardiomyocytes using a direct reprogramming strategy. Nat Cell Biol. 2011;13:215–22.

9. Wang H, Cao N, Spencer CI, et al. Small molecules enable cardiac reprogramming of mouse fibroblasts with a single factor, Oct4. Cell Rep. 2014;13:951–60.

10. Lalit PA, Salick MR, Nelson DO, et al. Lineage reprogramming of fibroblasts into proliferative induced cardiac progenitor cells by defined factors. Cell Stem Cell. 2016;18:354–67.

11. Zhang Y, Cao N, Huang Y, et al. Expandable cardiovascular progenitor cells reprogrammed from fibroblasts. Cell Stem Cell. 2016;18:368–81.

12. Yamashita JK. Expanding reprogramming to cardiovascular progenitors. Cell Stem Cell. 2016;18:299–301.

13. Vierbuchen T, Ostermeier A, Pang ZP, et al. Direct conversion of fibroblasts to functional neurons by defined factors. Nature. 2010;463:1035–41.

14. Sekiya S, Suzuki A. Direct conversion of mouse fibroblasts to hepatocyte-like cells by defined factors. Nature. 2011;475:390–3.

15. Song K, Nam YJ, Luo X, et al. Heart repair by reprogramming non-myocytes with cardiac transcription factors. Nature. 2012;485:599–604.

16. Chen JX, Krane M, Deutsch MA, et al. Inefficient reprogramming of fibroblasts into cardiomyocytes using Gata4, Mef2c, and Tbx5. Circ Res. 2012;111:50–5.

17. Protze S, Khattak S, Poulet C, et al. A new approach to transcription factor screening for reprogramming of fibroblasts to cardiomyocyte-like cells. J Mol Cell Cardiol. 2012;53:323–32.

18. Jayawardena TM, Egemnazarov B, Finch EA, et al. MicroRNA-mediated in vitro and in vivo direct reprogramming of cardiac fibroblasts to cardiomyocytes. Circ Res. 2012;110:1465–73.

19. Addis RC, Ifkovits JL, Pinto F, et al. Optimization of direct fibroblast reprogramming to cardiomyocytes using calcium activity as a functional measure of success. J Mol Cell Cardiol. 2013;60:97–106.

20. Christoforou N, Chellappan M, Adler AF, et al. Transcription factors MYOCD, SRF, Mesp1 and SMARCD3 enhance the cardio-inducing effect of GATA4, TBX5, and MEF2C during direct cellular reprogramming. PLoS One. 2013;8:e63577.

21. Muraoka N, Yamakawa H, Miyamoto K, et al. MiR-133 promotes cardiac reprogramming by directly repressing Snai1 and silencing fibroblast signatures. EMBO J. 2013;33:1565–81.

22. Hirai H, Katoku-Kikyo N, Keirstead SA, et al. Accelerated direct reprogramming of fibroblasts into cardiomyocyte-like cells with the MyoD transactivation domain. Cardiovasc Res. 2013;100:105–13.

23. Wang L, Liu Z, Yin C, et al. Stoichiometry of Gata4, Mef2c, and Tbx5 influences the efficiency and quality of induced cardiac myocyte reprogramming. Circ Res. 2015;116:237–44.

24. Ifkovits JL, Addis RC, Epstein JA, et al. Inhibition of TGFβ signaling increases direct conversion of fibroblasts to induced cardiomyocytes. PLoS ONE. 2014;9:e89678.

25. Zhou H, Dickson ME, Kim MS, et al. Akt1/protein kinase B enhances transcriptional reprogramming of fibroblasts to functional cardiomyocytes. Natl Acad Sci USA. 2015;112:11864–9.

26. Fu Y, Huang C, Xu X, et al. Direct reprogramming of mouse fibroblasts into cardiomyocytes with chemical cocktails. Cell Res. 2015;25:1013–24.

27. Zhao Y, Londono P, Cao Y, et al. High-efficiency reprogramming of fibroblasts into cardiomyocytes requires suppression of pro-fibrotic signalling. Nat Commun. 2015;10:8243.

28. Yamakawa H, Muraoka N, Miyamoto K, et al. Fibroblast growth factors and vascular endothelial growth factor promote cardiac reprogramming under defined conditions. Stem Cell Rep. 2015;5:1128–42.

29. Nam YJ, Song K, Luo X, et al. Reprogramming of human fibroblasts toward a cardiac fate. Proc Natl Acad Sci U S A. 2013;110(14):5588–93.

30. Fu JD, Stone NR, Liu L, et al. Direct reprogramming of human fibroblasts toward a cardiomyocyte-like state. Stem Cell Rep. 2013;1:235–47.

31. Wada R, Muraoka N, Inagawa K, et al. Induction of human cardiomyocyte-like cells from fibroblasts by defined factors. Proc Natl Acad Sci U S A. 2013;110:12667–72.

32. Islas JF, Liu Y, Weng KC, et al. Transcription factors ETS2 and MESP1 transdifferentiate human dermal fibroblasts into cardiac progenitors. Proc Natl Acad Sci U S A. 2012;109:13016–21.

33. Blum B, Benvenisty N. The tumorigenicity of human embryonic stem cells. Adv Cancer Res. 2008;100:133–58.

34. Tsuji O, Miura K, Okada Y, et al. Therapeutic potential of appropriately evaluated safe-induced pluripotent stem cells for spinal cord injury. Proc Natl Acad Sci U S A. 2010;107:12704–9.

35. Muraoka N, Ieda M. Direct reprogramming of fibroblasts into myocytes to reverse fibrosis. Annu Rev Physiol. 2014;76:21–37.

36. Qian L, Huang Y, Spencer CI, et al. In vivo reprogramming of murine cardiac fibroblasts into induced cardiomyocytes. Nature. 2012;485:593–8.

37. Inagawa K, Miyamoto K, Yamakawa H, et al. Induction of cardiomyocyte-like cells in infarct hearts by gene transfer of Gata4, Mef2c, and Tbx5. Circ Res. 2012;111:1147–56.

38. Mathison M, Gersch RP, Nasser A, et al. In vivo cardiac cellular reprogramming efficacy is enhanced by angiogenic preconditioning of the infarcted myocardium with vascular endothelial growth factor. J Am Heart Assoc. 2012;1:e005652.

39. Sadahiro T, Yamanaka S, Ieda M. Direct cardiac reprogramming: progress and challenges in basic biology and clinical applications. Circ Res. 2015;116:1378–91.

40. Doppler SA, Deutsch MA, Lange R, et al. Direct reprogramming—the future of cardiac regeneration? Int J Mol Sci. 2015;16:17368–93.

41. Yamakawa H, Ieda M. Strategies for heart regeneration: approaches ranging from induced pluripotent stem cells to direct cardiac reprogramming. Int Heart J. 2015;56:1–5.

42. Cao N, Huang Y, Zheng J, et al. Conversion of human fibroblasts into functional cardiomyocytes by small molecules. Science. 2016;352:1216–20.

43. Li XH, Li Q, Jiang L, et al. Generation of functional human cardiac progenitor cells by high-efficiency protein transduction. Stem Cells Transl Med. 2015;4:1415–24.

14

Inflammatory responses in the initiation of lung repair and regeneration: their role in stimulating lung resident stem cells

Mitsuhiro Yamada*, Naoya Fujino and Masakazu Ichinose

Abstract

The lungs are the primary organs for respiration, the process by which carbon dioxide and oxygen are exchanged. The alveolus, which is the site of gas exchange in the lungs, consists of multiple cell types including alveolar epithelial cells, lung capillary endothelial cells and fibroblasts. Because of their complexity, lung parenchymal cells including epithelial lineage have been thought to have a lower rate of cellular turnover in adult lung. However, accumulating observations suggest that the turnover of parenchymal cells in adult lungs is essential for maintaining homeostasis during the steady state as well as for the repair and regeneration after lung injury. After lung injury by harmful pathogens, inflammation occurs to protect the host. Although excessive inflammation damages lung tissue, inflammatory cells are essential for regeneration because they remove harmful pathogens as well as debris derived from apoptotic and necrotic cells. In addition, subsets of inflammatory cells, especially phagocytic monocytes, produce cytokines and growth factors to resolve inflammation and promote tissue regeneration by stimulating tissue-resident stem cells. Recent advances in the biology of lung-resident stem cells, especially those addressing epithelial lineage, have revealed that there are several cellular populations capable of self-renewal that can differentiate into airway and/or alveolar epithelial cells. A part of these populations does not exist in the steady state but emerges after lung injury, suggesting that signals induced by inflammation may play an important role in initiating the proliferation and differentiation of lung stem or progenitor cells. Understanding the interaction between inflammatory responses and tissue-resident stem cells would help elucidate the pathogenesis of inflammatory lung diseases and promote the discovery of new therapeutic targets.

Keywords: Inflammation, Tissue-resident stem cells, Progenitor cells, M2 macrophage

Background

The lungs are the primary organs for respiration, the process by which carbon dioxide and oxygen are exchanged. The air enters the trachea from the laryngopharynx and continues further into the right and left bronchi. These bronchi split into secondary and tertiary bronchi as the lobes of the lungs. These finally split into smaller bronchioles until they become the respiratory bronchioles. The respiratory bronchioles supply air through alveolar ducts into the alveoli, which are the main place for exchange of the gases. The alveolus is composed of mixed lineage cells including alveolar epithelial cells, lung capillary endothelial cells and fibroblasts. The alveolus is a functional organ unit that provides both efficient gas exchange and a barrier against the external environment. The total surface area of alveoli in human is approximately 60 m². Because of the complexity of the alveolus, lung parenchymal cells including epithelial cells lining the respiratory tract have a lower rate of cellular turnover in adult lung compared to high turnover organs such as the intestine. However, experiments using calorie restriction of adult rodents showed that starvation induced alveolar destruction [1–4] and refeeding induced alveolar regeneration [4, 5]. Starvation in adult humans also leads to alveolar destruction in the lung, suggesting this phenomenon is conserved in humans. These findings imply that the turnover of the parenchymal cells in adult lungs is also essential to maintain homeostasis during the steady state. Moreover, it has

* Correspondence: yamitsu@med.tohoku.ac.jp
Department of Respiratory Medicine, Graduate School of Medicine, Tohoku University, 1-1 Seiryo-machi, Aoba-ku, Sendai 980-8574, Japan

been shown that the lung has tissue-resident stem or progenitor cells for regeneration after lung injury. Disruption of the regenerative capacity supported by these resident stem or progenitor cells can cause lung diseases such as emphysema and lung fibrosis [6, 7]. Therefore, to understand the mechanism of regeneration in the lung after lung injury mainly induced by inflammation is likely to be important for understanding the pathogenesis of lung diseases and finding new therapeutic targets. In this review, we focus on the mechanism by which inflammation is resolved and on the initiation of lung tissue regeneration. We then provide an overview of the behaviours of lung stem or progenitor cells, especially focusing on cells of the lung alveolar epithelial lineage, during inflammation after lung injury.

Resolution of inflammation and initiation of regeneration: roles of inflammatory cells in lung tissue repair

Inflammation is a nonspecific biological response of tissues to harmful stimuli including pathogens. Inflammation promotes protective responses involving the immune system. Although inflammation is a beneficial and indispensable response to protect an individual organism against both external and internal harmful stimuli, inflammation induces significant injury to cells, tissues and organs. Excess or prolonged inflammatory responses cause a wide variety of acute and chronic diseases in various organs including the lungs. Therefore, the resolution of inflammation is important for the repair and regeneration of the lungs after injury.

During acute lung injury induced by harmful stimuli such as pathogenic bacteria, the acute inflammatory response is characterized initially by the generation of mediators (cytokines, chemokines, etc.) that induce the accumulation of neutrophils in alveoli. The emigration of neutrophils from alveolar capillaries to the airspace impairs the alveolar function by damaging alveolar epithelial cells. Therefore, neutrophil accumulation actually worsens the lung injury during the acute phase [8]. However, the neutrophil accumulation also has a role in the repair and regeneration of the lung epithelium. This reparative function of the neutrophil accumulation is partially due to the clearance of cellular debris from the damaged cells in order to create a new matrix sheet for regeneration of the epithelium [9]. It has been also reported that neutrophils directly activate the response for repair of the epithelium. β-catenin signalling is activated in lung epithelial cells during neutrophil transmigration, via the elastase-mediated cleavage of E-cadherin. This activation of β-catenin signalling promotes epithelial repair [10].

During the acute phase of inflammation in the lungs, the alveoli are filled with debris derived from apoptotic or necrotic cells, apoptotic bodies, harmful foreign materials including pathogens, and microvesicles from inflammatory cells and parenchymal cells. These materials must be removed if the alveoli are to be repaired. The cells important for clearing the debris and apoptotic cells are mononuclear-linage phagocytes including alveolar macrophages and monocytes. In alveoli, alveolar macrophages are the tissue-resident phagocytes that defend against harmful exogenous materials including pathogenic microbes. They have various kinds of receptors to sense harmful agents including pathogens [11, 12]. Alveolar macrophages first initiate a proinflammatory reaction to remove harmful agents and propagate the innate immune response. As well as neutrophils, macrophages are also important inflammatory cells that clear pathogens by releasing toxic mediators including reactive oxygen species and phagocytize pathogens or other inflammatory debris. Proinflammatory macrophages (M1 macrophages) can induce tissue damage through the release of toxic species and enzymes including matrix metalloproteinases. M1 macrophages also enhance lung tissue injury through augmenting neutrophil recruitment by releasing chemokines [13, 14].

On the other hand, macrophages have the ability to change their phenotype to anti-inflammatory and tissue-repairing phenotypes [11, 15], and both resident and recruited macrophages play a significant role in repair and regeneration after lung injury. The engulfment of apoptotic cells, called efferocytosis, is one of the important processes by which macrophages change toward M2 macrophages, which are anti-inflammatory macrophages [16]. Efferocytosis induces a decrease in the release of proinflammatory cytokines and chemokines and augments the production of anti-inflammatory cytokines and growth factors that promote the proliferation of lung parenchymal cells (such as TGF-β, IL-10, VEGF and HGF) [17, 18]. Efferocytosis also reduces the release of nitric oxide by inhibiting its synthesis [18]. M2-derived cytokines, including IL-4 and IL-10, increase the expression of mannose receptor, which augments efferocytosis [19].

The recognition of phosphatidylserine (PS) structures by mononuclear phagocytes is an important step in the initiation of efferocytosis (Fig. 1a). PS normally exists in the inner cell membrane but rapidly emerges on the cell surface during apoptosis. Several membranous proteins have been identified as receptors that recognize PS. Tim4 is a type I membrane protein that is expressed on phagocytic monocytes including macrophages [20]. It has been shown that Tim4 can bind PS strongly and specifically [20]. A study using Tim4-deficient mice showed that Tim4-deficient macrophages lack the ability to phagocytize apoptotic cells. Other membrane proteins, including CD300 [21–23], phosphatidylserine receptor

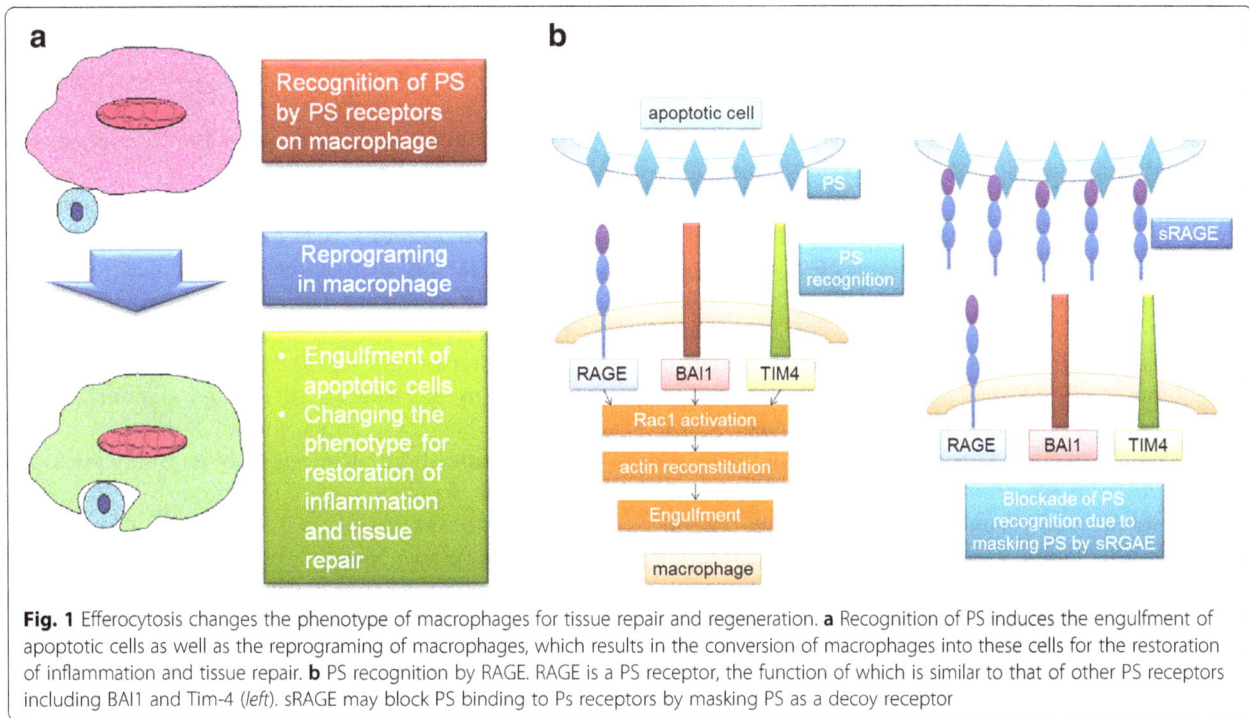

Fig. 1 Efferocytosis changes the phenotype of macrophages for tissue repair and regeneration. **a** Recognition of PS induces the engulfment of apoptotic cells as well as the reprograming of macrophages, which results in the conversion of macrophages into these cells for the restoration of inflammation and tissue repair. **b** PS recognition by RAGE. RAGE is a PS receptor, the function of which is similar to that of other PS receptors including BAI1 and Tim-4 (*left*). sRAGE may block PS binding to Ps receptors by masking PS as a decoy receptor

(PSR) [24], TAM receptor tyrosine kinase Axl [25] and brain-specific angiogenesis inhibitor 1 (BAI1) [26], have been shown to be PS receptors or receptors that promote apoptotic cell engulfment.

We have also identified that the receptor for advanced glycation end products (RAGE) functions as a receptor for PS [27]. RAGE is a membranous protein of the immunoglobulin superfamily [28]. RAGE is expressed on various parenchymal cells, including endothelial cells, and mononuclear phagocytes, including macrophages [29]. It has been reported that RAGE recognizes various ligands including HMGB1, and the binding of RAGE to such ligands is involved in the pathogenesis of various diseases including diabetic vascular disorders, malignancy and inflammation [30]. RAGE is expressed in both a membrane-bound (mRAGE) and soluble form (sRAGE) lacking the transmembrane domain. sRAGE is produced by either the proteolysis of mRAGE or mRNA alternative splicing [31]. sRAGE can work as an inhibitor of RAGE like a decoy receptor for RAGE ligands [32]. We used fluorochrome-labelled sRAGE and found that sRAGE bound to apoptotic thymocytes, indicating that RAGE recognizes and binds to a material expressed on the surface of apoptotic cells. We hypothesized that RAGE could recognize PS and performed a protein–lipid overlay assay, which showed that sRAGE specifically binds to phosphatidylserine. We then performed a surface plasmon resonance analysis to examine the binding affinity of sRAGE to PS and found that the binding response was concentration-dependent with a KD of

0.563 μM. We further performed both FRET analysis and confocal image analysis and found that PS expressed on apoptotic thymocytes binds to full-length mRAGE located in macrophages. Our findings suggest that RAGE can bind specifically to phosphatidylserine.

Using RAGE-deficient mice, we found that alveolar macrophages from RAGE-deficient mice impaired the phagocytic capacity for apoptotic cells, indicating that alveolar macrophages can recognize and phagocytize apoptotic cells through RAGE. We then examined whether sRAGE administration influenced macrophage phagocytosis because sRAGE functions as an endogenous competitive inhibitor of ligand engagement by cell-surface RAGE. sRAGE administration attenuated the phagocytosis of apoptotic cells by wild-type alveolar macrophages, also confirming that RAGE plays a role in the phagocytosis of apoptotic cells. sRAGE also decreased the phagocytic activity of RAGE-deficient alveolar macrophages, possibly suggesting that sRAGE also blocks other types of PS receptor-mediated phagocytosis. We also investigated the intracellular signalling and revealed that Rac1 is activated due to PS recognition through RAGE in alveolar macrophages. These results suggest that RAGE is one of the PS receptors that recognize apoptotic cells. We also examined whether RAGE works for the clearance of apoptotic cells in vivo. We administrated lipopolysaccharide (LPS) into mouse airway, which induced neutrophil migration into the airspace. Once neutrophils migrate, they undergo programmed cell death [33] and are then removed from the airspace through phagocytosis by alveolar macrophages [34]. This resolution process starts in the first few hours after inflammation begins [35]. We observed that more apoptotic neutrophils existed in RAGE-deficient mice during LPS-induced lung injury. RAGE-deficient mice showed a significant increase in the accumulation of inflammatory cells, demonstrating that the deletion of RAGE in macrophages impairs the clearance of apoptotic cells. In summary, the results of our study suggest that RAGE may be one of the PS receptors that recognize apoptotic cells and initiate the clearance of those cells (Fig. 1b). Moreover, sRAGE might inhibit the recognition of PS by cell-surface RAGE and other PS receptors during phagocytosis (Fig. 1b). The balance between sRAGE and mRAGE could modify the phagocytotic activity of macrophages, which might be important in the resolution of inflammation and in tissue regeneration after lung injury. Therefore, RAGE is a PS receptor that may play a role in the resolution of inflammation and in promoting tissue repair and regeneration after lung injury, suggesting that RAGE could be a potential new target for the treatment of human diseases.

Epithelial cells with the capacities of stem cells and their behaviours in lung injury and inflammation

Although inflammatory cells including mononuclear phagocytes contribute to repair and regeneration by clearing debris and producing growth factors, tissue-resident stem cells are critical for tissue repair and regeneration because apoptotic or necrotic parenchymal cells must be replaced by new cells derived from tissue-resident stem cells (Fig. 2a). Recent advances including the analysis of cell fate by in vivo lineage tracing and the identification of new stem cell markers revealed the presence of potential stem cells in the lung, especially in the epithelial cell linage (Table 1).

The airways of human lungs are covered by a pseudostratified epithelium made of basal cells, secretory cells including CC10+ club cells and goblet cells, ciliated cells and neuroendocrine cells. Basal cells are characterized by the expression of P63, nerve growth factor receptor (NGFR) and cytokeratin5 (KRT5) [36, 37]. These cells are capable of self-renewal and can differentiate into ciliated and secretory cells [37, 38]. Some of the basal cells that express KRT14 in the steady state have been shown to be a self-renewing population that maintains the KRT5+ basal cell population. A naphthalene-induced injury mouse model showed that this KRT14+ KRT5+ double-positive cell population is significantly increased [39, 40]. These double-positive cells can directly differentiate into ciliated and secretory cells [41]. Recently, two distinct populations of basal cells were then identified in the adult lung. One is basal stem cells (BSCs) and

the other population is referred to as basal luminal precursor cells (BLPCs). Both cell populations express both KRT5 and P63 but do not express KRT14, indicating that KRT14 is not a general marker for identifying stem cell populations [42]. In the steady state, BSCs divide via asymmetric division to produce one new BSC and one BLPC. The BLPCs can further differentiate into neuroendocrine and secretory cells but have a low ability for self-renewal [42]. BLPCs can become distinct from BSCs through KRT8 expression [42]. KRT8 and KRT5 double-positive cells were also identified in mice as progenitor cells during repair and regeneration after injury induced by reactive oxygen species (ROS) and sulphur dioxide (SO_2) [43]. This SO_2 injury model showed that P63+ basal cell populations divide into other subpopulations prior to the formation of KRT8 and KRT5 double-positive progenitor cells. One of the populations is active Notch2 intracellular domain positive cells, which can differentiate into secretory cells. The other is c-myb positive cells which can differentiate into ciliated cells [44]. This division was not observed in the steady state, suggesting that post-injury mechanisms including inflammatory responses possibly induce different cellular populations of progenitor cells [44]. Tadokoro et al. focused on the potential role of inflammatory cytokine signalling between stem/progenitor cells of a pseudostratified epithelium and their niche [45]. First, they sorted NGFR+ basal cells from mouse trachea and performed a clonal 3D organoid assay. They found that IL-6 promoted the differentiation of mouse basal progenitors into ciliated cells, whereas STAT3 inhibitors inhibited the differentiation. The following in vitro experiments also suggested that IL-6/STAT3 signalling promotes the differentiation into ciliated cells by an increase in multicilin and FOXJ1 expression and inhibition of the Notch signalling pathway. To confirm their in vitro findings, they used an SO_2 injury model and found the activation of STAT3 in basal cells as well as an increase in IL-6 in stromal mesenchymal cells. Using conditional-deficient mice, they found that conditional deletion in basal cells of SOCS3, which is a negative regulator of the STAT3 pathway, resulted in an increase in multiciliated cells after SO_2 injury, whereas IL-6-deficient mice regenerated fewer ciliated cells after injury. These findings suggest that inflammatory responses possibly function to stimulate stem/progenitor cells for the repair and regeneration of lung tissue.

In the distal lung including the alveolar region, there are candidate stem cells that can differentiate into alveolar epithelial cells. Broncho-alveolar stem cells (BASCs) expressing both CC10 and pro-surfactant protein C (pro-SPC) were identified as cells that can differentiate into both bronchiolar and alveolar epithelial cells in vitro. These cells are located at the broncho-alveolar

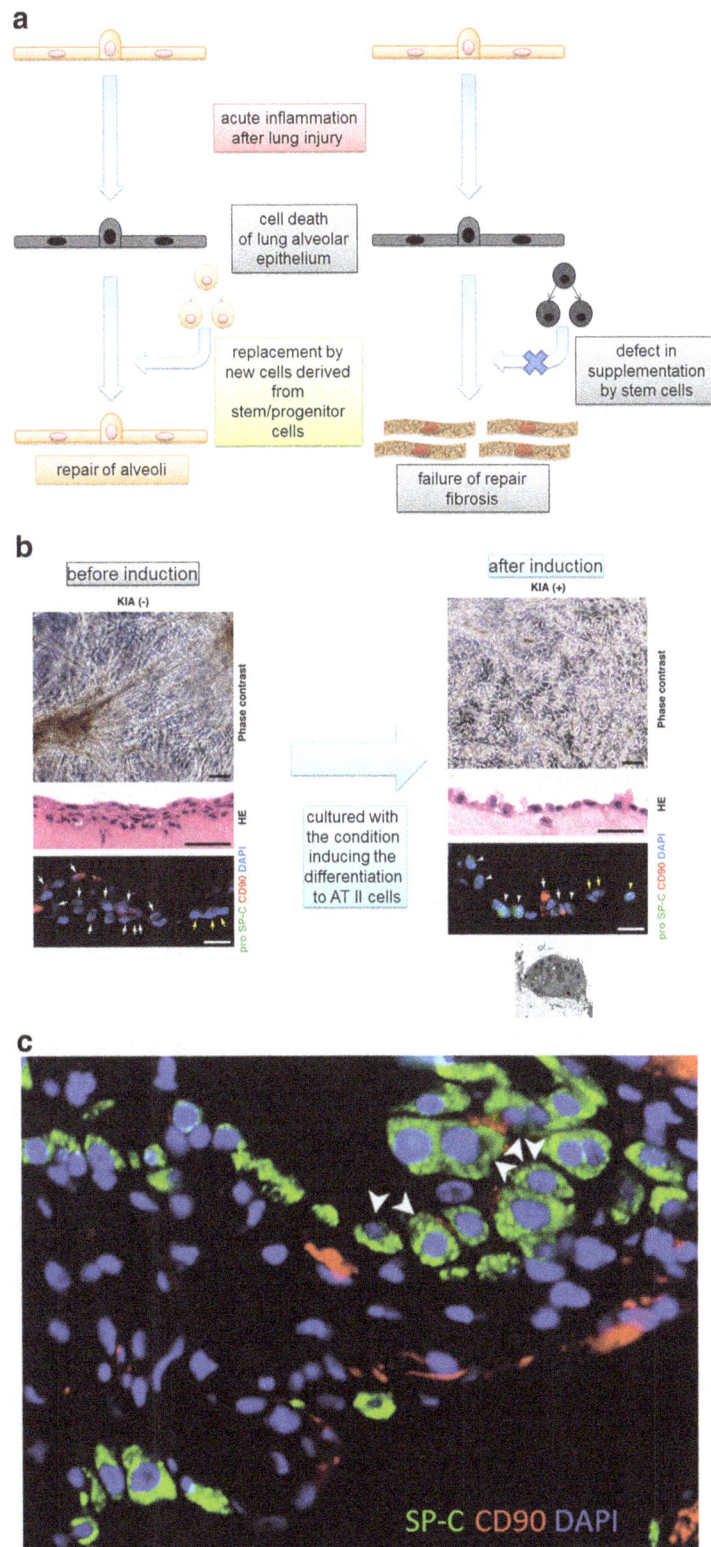

Fig. 2 Tissue-resident stem cells for repair and regeneration after lung injury and acute inflammation. **a** Schematic image of the roles of epithelial stem/progenitor cells during lung injury. **b** AEPCs can differentiate to AT II cells in vitro culture. **c** Alveolar epithelial progenitor cells (AEPCs; *arrowheads*) express both CD90 (mesenchymal marker) and pro-SPC (AT II marker) and are localized in the regions of hyperplasia of AT II cells in the lungs of IPF patients

Table 1 Candidate populations as lung epithelial stem cells

Populations	Markers	Cell types into which they can differentiate
Basal stem cells (BSCs)	P63$^+$, KRT5$^+$, KRT14$^{+\ or\ -}$	BLPCs
Basal luminal precursor cells (BLPCs)	P63+, KRT5$^+$, KRT8$^+$	ciliated cells, club cells, neuroendocrine cells
Broncho-alveolar stem cells	CC10$^+$, pro-SPC$^+$	AT II cells, ciliated cells, club cells
ITGα6$^+$, ITGβ4$^+$ alveolar progenitor cells	CC10$^-$, pro-SPC$^-$, ITGα6$^+$, ITGβ4$^+$	AT II cells, club cells
Alveolar type 2 cells (AT II cells)	pro-SPC$^+$	AT I cells
Distal alveolar stem cells (DASCs)	P63$^+$, KRT5$^+$	AT II cells, club cells
Alveolar Epithelial Progenitor cells (AEPCs)	CD90$^+$, pro-SPC$^+$	AT II cells

duct junction (BADJ) [46]. Alveolar type II cells (AT II cells) expressing surfactant protein C were shown to have the ability for self-renewal. Some alveolar type II cells can differentiate into alveolar type I cells (AT I cells) for homeostasis and after injury [47, 48]. In addition to AT II cells, another progenitor subpopulation for alveolar epithelial cells has been identified. These cells are located in both the alveoli and the BADJ and express both α6 and β4 integrin but do not express either CC10 or pro-SPC. During lung injury, these cells proliferate and differentiate into alveolar type II cells and club cells. Distal alveolar stem cells (DASCs) expressing both P63 and Krt5 cells are present in the distal airways during lung injury induced by influenza virus infection. These cells have the ability to differentiate into alveolar epithelial cells [49–51]. KRT5 lineage tracing studies revealed that these cells were not present in the steady state and emerged after injury.

We also isolated colony-forming cells, called alveolar epithelial progenitor cells (AEPCs), which have the ability for self-renewal and the potential to generate alveolar type II cells in vitro (Fig. 2b) [52]. These progenitor cells expressed surface markers of mesenchymal stem cells and surfactant proteins associated with alveolar type II cells, such as CD90 and pro-SPC, respectively (Fig. 2c). Comprehensive expression analyses by microarray revealed that transcripts associated with lung development were enriched in AEPCs compared with bone marrow-mesenchymal stem cells. Histological evaluation indicated that AEPCs were present within alveolar walls in normal lungs. However, these cells significantly increased in the region of AT II cell hyperplasia, suggesting that these cells contribute to alveolar epithelial repair in damaged lungs.

As mentioned above, several cellular populations have been identified as lung epithelial stem/progenitor cells that differentiate into airway and/or alveolar epithelial cells. A part of these populations only emerge during lung injury, suggesting that unidentified inflammatory stimuli induce the emergence or proliferation of lung epithelial stem/progenitor cells. So far, it is still unknown whether these different stem/progenitor cells are really different cells or cells derived from the same origin but

phenotypically changed according to circumstances. Further studies including a comprehensive RNA expression assay in a single cell will be necessary to elucidate these issues.

Conclusions

After lung injury by various harmful stimuli including pathogenic microbes, inflammation occurs for the host defence. Although excessive inflammatory responses are harmful to lung tissue, inflammatory cells are essential for repair and regeneration because these cells are important cleaners that remove harmful pathogens as well as debris derived from apoptotic and necrotic cells. Moreover, inflammatory cells, especially phagocytic monocytes including alveolar macrophages, produce cytokines and growth factors to resolve inflammation and promote tissue repair and regeneration by inducing tissue-resident stem cells. Recent advances in the biology of lung-resident stem cells, especially those of the epithelial lineage, revealed that there are several populations that can self-renew and differentiate into airway and/or alveolar epithelial cells. Interestingly, some of these populations do not exist in the steady state but emerge during inflammation after lung injury, suggesting that signals induced by inflammation may play an important role in initiating the proliferation and differentiation of lung stem/progenitor cells. Further investigation will be needed to understand the interactions between inflammatory responses and tissue-resident stem cells that contribute to lung tissue regeneration in the pathogenesis of inflammatory lung diseases.

Abbreviations
AEPCs, alveolar epithelial progenitor cells; AT I cells, alveolar type I cells; AT II cells, alveolar type II cells; BADJ, broncho-alveolar duct junction; BASC, broncho-alveolar stem cell; BLPC, basal luminal precursor cells; BSC, basal stem cell; CC10, the club cell 10-kDa protein; FOXJ1, forkhead box protein J1; HGF, hepatocyte growth factor; HMGB1, high-mobility group protein-1; IL-10, interleukin-10; ITG, integrin; KRT14, cytokeratin; KRT5, cytokeratin5; LPS, lipopolysaccharide; mRAGE; membrane-bound receptor for advanced glycation end products; NGFR, nerve growth factor receptor; P63, transformation-related protein 63; Pro-SPC, pro-surfactant protein C; SOCS, suppressor of cytokine signalling; sRAGE, soluble RAGE; STAT, signal transducers and activator of transcription; TGF-β, transforming

growth factor-β; Tim4, T cell immunoglobulin and mucin domain-containing molecule 4; VEGF, vascular endothelial growth factor

Acknowledgements
We thank Mr. Brent K Bell for critical reading of the manuscript.

Funding
This work was supported by Grants-in-Aid for Scientific Research (24591148 and 15K09206 to M Yamada) from the Japan Society for the Promotion of Science (JSPS).

Authors' contributions
All authors contributed to writing the manuscript. All authors read and approved the final version of the manuscript.

Competing interests
The authors declare that they have no competing interests.

References

1. Harkema JR, Mauderly JL, Gregory RE, Pickrell JA. A comparison of starvation and elastase models of emphysema in the rat. Am Rev Respir Dis. 1984;129:584–91.
2. Karlinsky JB, Goldstein RH, Ojserkis B, Snider GL. Lung mechanics and connective tissue levels in starvation-induced emphysema in hamsters. Am J Physiol. 1986;251:R282–288.
3. Kerr JS, Riley DJ, Lanza-Jacoby S, Berg RA, Spilker HC, Yu SY, et al. Nutritional emphysema in the rat. Influence of protein depletion and impaired lung growth. Am Rev Respir Dis. 1985;131:644–50.
4. Sahebjami H, Wirman JA. Emphysema-like changes in the lungs of starved rats. Am Rev Respir Dis. 1981;124:619–24.
5. Massaro GD, Radaeva S, Clerch LB, Massaro D. Lung alveoli: endogenous programmed destruction and regeneration. Am J Physiol Lung Cell Mol Physiol. 2002;283:L305–309.
6. Sisson TH, Mendez M, Choi K, Subbotina N, Courey A, Cunningham A, et al. Targeted injury of type II alveolar epithelial cells induces pulmonary fibrosis. Am J Respir Crit Care Med. 2010;181:254–63.
7. Kasahara Y, Tuder RM, Taraseviciene-Stewart L, Le Cras TD, Abman S, Hirth PK, et al. Inhibition of VEGF receptors causes lung cell apoptosis and emphysema. J Clin Invest. 2000;106:1311–9.
8. Grommes J, Soehnlein O. Contribution of neutrophils to acute lung injury. Mol Med. 2011;17:293–307.
9. Hyde DM, Miller LA, McDonald RJ, Stovall MY, Wong V, Pinkerton KE, et al. Neutrophils enhance clearance of necrotic epithelial cells in ozone-induced lung injury in rhesus monkeys. Am J Physiol. 1999;277:L1190–1198.
10. Zemans RL, Briones N, Campbell M, McClendon J, Young SK, Suzuki T, et al. Neutrophil transmigration triggers repair of the lung epithelium via beta-catenin signaling. Proc Natl Acad Sci U S A. 2011;108:15990–5.
11. Henson PM, Bratton DL. Antiinflammatory effects of apoptotic cells. J Clin Invest. 2013;123:2773–4.
12. Aggarwal NR, King LS, D'Alessio FR. Diverse macrophage populations mediate acute lung inflammation and resolution. Am J Physiol Lung Cell Mol Physiol. 2014;306:L709–725.
13. Robbe P, Draijer C, Borg TR, Luinge M, Timens W, Wouters IM, et al. Distinct macrophage phenotypes in allergic and nonallergic lung inflammation. Am J Physiol Lung Cell Mol Physiol. 2015;308:L358–367.
14. Zhang S, Hwaiz R, Rahman M, Herwald H, Thorlacius H. Ras regulates alveolar macrophage formation of CXC chemokines and neutrophil activation in streptococcal M1 protein-induced lung injury. Eur J Pharmacol. 2014;733:45–53.
15. Johnston LK, Rims CR, Gill SE, McGuire JK, Manicone AM. Pulmonary macrophage subpopulations in the induction and resolution of acute lung injury. Am J Respir Cell Mol Biol. 2012;47:417–26.
16. McCubbrey AL, Curtis JL. Efferocytosis and lung disease. Chest. 2013;143:1750–7.
17. Huynh ML, Fadok VA, Henson PM. Phosphatidylserine-dependent ingestion of apoptotic cells promotes TGF-beta1 secretion and the resolution of inflammation. J Clin Invest. 2002;109:41–50.
18. Freire-de-Lima CG, Xiao YQ, Gardai SJ, Bratton DL, Schiemann WP, Henson PM. Apoptotic cells, through transforming growth factor-beta, coordinately induce anti-inflammatory and suppress pro-inflammatory eicosanoid and NO synthesis in murine macrophages. J Biol Chem. 2006;281:38376–84.
19. Linehan SA, Coulson PS, Wilson RA, Mountford AP, Brombacher F, Martinez-Pomares L, et al. IL-4 receptor signaling is required for mannose receptor expression by macrophages recruited to granulomata but not resident cells in mice infected with Schistosoma mansoni. Lab Invest. 2003;83:1223–31.
20. Miyanishi M, Tada K, Koike M, Uchiyama Y, Kitamura T, Nagata S. Identification of Tim4 as a phosphatidylserine receptor. Nature. 2007;450:435–9.
21. Murakami Y, Tian L, Voss OH, Margulies DH, Krzewski K, Coligan JE. CD300b regulates the phagocytosis of apoptotic cells via phosphatidylserine recognition. Cell Death Differ. 2014;21:1746–57.
22. Simhadri VR, Andersen JF, Calvo E, Choi SC, Coligan JE, Borrego F. Human CD300a binds to phosphatidylethanolamine and phosphatidylserine, and modulates the phagocytosis of dead cells. Blood. 2012;119:2799–809.
23. Choi SC, Simhadri VR, Tian L, Gil-Krzewska A, Krzewski K, Borrego F, et al. Cutting edge: mouse CD300f (CMRF-35-like molecule-1) recognizes outer membrane-exposed phosphatidylserine and can promote phagocytosis. J Immunol. 2011;187:3483–7.
24. Li MO, Sarkisian MR, Mehal WZ, Rakic P, Flavell RA. Phosphatidylserine receptor is required for clearance of apoptotic cells. Science. 2003;302:1560–3.
25. Fujimori T, Grabiec AM, Kaur M, Bell TJ, Fujino N, Cook PC, et al. The Axl receptor tyrosine kinase is a discriminator of macrophage function in the inflamed lung. Mucosal Immunol. 2015;8:1021–30.
26. Park D, Tosello-Trampont AC, Elliott MR, Lu M, Haney LB, Ma Z, et al. BAI1 is an engulfment receptor for apoptotic cells upstream of the ELMO/Dock180/Rac module. Nature. 2007;450:430–4.
27. He M, Kubo H, Morimoto K, Fujino N, Suzuki T, Takahasi T, et al. Receptor for advanced glycation end products binds to phosphatidylserine and assists in the clearance of apoptotic cells. EMBO Rep. 2011;12:358–64.
28. Neeper M, Schmidt AM, Brett J, Yan SD, Wang F, Pan YC, et al. Cloning and expression of a cell surface receptor for advanced glycosylation end products of proteins. J Biol Chem. 1992;267:14998–5004.
29. Brett J, Schmidt AM, Yan SD, Zou YS, Weidman E, Pinsky D, et al. Survey of the distribution of a newly characterized receptor for advanced glycation end products in tissues. Am J Pathol. 1993;143:1699–712.
30. Ramasamy R, Yan SF, Schmidt AM. RAGE: therapeutic target and biomarker of the inflammatory response—the evidence mounts. J Leukoc Biol. 2009;86:505–12.
31. Raucci A, Cugusi S, Antonelli A, Barabino SM, Monti L, Bierhaus A, et al. A soluble form of the receptor for advanced glycation endproducts (RAGE) is produced by proteolytic cleavage of the membrane-bound form by the sheddase a disintegrin and metalloprotease 10 (ADAM10). FASEB J. 2008;22:3716–27.
32. Santilli F, Vazzana N, Bucciarelli LG, Davi G. Soluble forms of RAGE in human diseases: clinical and therapeutical implications. Curr Med Chem. 2009;16:940–52.
33. Watson RW, Redmond HP, Wang JH, Condron C, Bouchier-Hayes D. Neutrophils undergo apoptosis following ingestion of Escherichia coli. J Immunol. 1996;156:3986–92.
34. Cox G, Crossley J, Xing Z. Macrophage engulfment of apoptotic neutrophils contributes to the resolution of acute pulmonary inflammation in vivo. Am J Respir Cell Mol Biol. 1995;12:232–7.
35. Serhan CN, Savill J. Resolution of inflammation: the beginning programs the end. Nat Immunol. 2005;6:1191–7.
36. Daniely Y, Liao G, Dixon D, Linnoila RI, Lori A, Randell SH, et al. Critical role of p63 in the development of a normal esophageal and tracheobronchial epithelium. Am J Physiol Cell Physiol. 2004;287:C171–181.
37. Rock JR, Onaitis MW, Rawlins EL, Lu Y, Clark CP, Xue Y, et al. Basal cells as stem cells of the mouse trachea and human airway epithelium. Proc Natl Acad Sci U S A. 2009;106:12771–5.
38. Rock JR, Gao X, Xue Y, Randell SH, Kong YY, Hogan BL. Notch-dependent differentiation of adult airway basal stem cells. Cell Stem Cell. 2011;8:639–48.
39. Prytherch Z, Job C, Marshall H, Oreffo V, Foster M, BeruBe K. Tissue-specific stem cell differentiation in an in vitro airway model. Macromol Biosci. 2011;11:1467–77.

40. Ghosh M, Helm KM, Smith RW, Giordanengo MS, Li B, Shen H, et al. A single cell functions as a tissue-specific stem cell and the in vitro niche-forming cell. Am J Respir Cell Mol Biol. 2011;45:459–69.

41. Tsao PN, Vasconcelos M, Izvolsky KI, Qian J, Lu J, Cardoso WV. Notch signaling controls the balance of ciliated and secretory cell fates in developing airways. Development. 2009;136:2297–307.

42. Watson JK, Rulands S, Wilkinson AC, Wuidart A, Ousset M, Van Keymeulen A, et al. Clonal dynamics reveal two distinct populations of basal cells in slow-turnover airway epithelium. Cell Rep. 2015;12:90–101.

43. Paul MK, Bisht B, Darmawan DO, Chiou R, Ha VL, Wallace WD, et al. Dynamic changes in intracellular ROS levels regulate airway basal stem cell homeostasis through Nrf2-dependent Notch signaling. Cell Stem Cell. 2014;15:199–214.

44. Pardo-Saganta A, Law BM, Tata PR, Villoria J, Saez B, Mou H, et al. Injury induces direct lineage segregation of functionally distinct airway basal stem/progenitor cell subpopulations. Cell Stem Cell. 2015;16:184–97.

45. Tadokoro T, Wang Y, Barak LS, Bai Y, Randell SH, Hogan BL. IL-6/STAT3 promotes regeneration of airway ciliated cells from basal stem cells. Proc Natl Acad Sci U S A. 2014;111:E3641–3649.

46. Kim CF, Jackson EL, Woolfenden AE, Lawrence S, Babar I, Vogel S, et al. Identification of bronchioalveolar stem cells in normal lung and lung cancer. Cell. 2005;121:823–35.

47. Yee M, Gelein R, Mariani TJ, Lawrence BP, O'Reilly MA. The oxygen environment at birth specifies the population of alveolar epithelial stem cells in the adult lung. Stem Cells. 2016;34:1396–406.

48. Barkauskas CE, Cronce MJ, Rackley CR, Bowie EJ, Keene DR, Stripp BR, et al. Type 2 alveolar cells are stem cells in adult lung. J Clin Invest. 2013;123:3025–36.

49. Deuse T, Schrepfer S. Distal airway stem cells are essential for lung regeneration. Transplantation. 2015;99:1540–1.

50. Zuo W, Zhang T, Wu DZ, Guan SP, Liew AA, Yamamoto Y, et al. p63(+)Krt5(+) distal airway stem cells are essential for lung regeneration. Nature. 2015;517:616–20.

51. Kumar PA, Hu Y, Yamamoto Y, Hoe NB, Wei TS, Mu D, et al. Distal airway stem cells yield alveoli in vitro and during lung regeneration following H1N1 influenza infection. Cell. 2011;147:525–38.

52. Fujino N, Kubo H, Suzuki T, Ota C, Hegab AE, He M, et al. Isolation of alveolar epithelial type II progenitor cells from adult human lungs. Lab Invest. 2011;91:363–78.

15

Role of fibroblast growth factors in bone regeneration

Pornkawee Charoenlarp, Arun Kumar Rajendran and Sachiko Iseki[*]

Abstract

Bone is a metabolically active organ that undergoes continuous remodeling throughout life. However, many complex skeletal defects such as large traumatic bone defects or extensive bone loss after tumor resection may cause failure of bone healing. Effective therapies for these conditions typically employ combinations of cells, scaffolds, and bioactive factors. In this review, we pay attention to one of the three factors required for regeneration of bone, bioactive factors, especially the fibroblast growth factor (FGF) family. This family is composed of 22 members and associated with various biological functions including skeletal formation. Based on the phenotypes of genetically modified mice and spatio-temporal expression levels during bone fracture healing, FGF2, FGF9, and FGF18 are regarded as possible candidates useful for bone regeneration. The role of these candidate FGFs in bone regeneration is also discussed in this review.

Keywords: Bone regeneration, FGFs, FGF2, FGF9, FGF18, Osteogenesis, Tissue engineering

Background

Tissue engineering is an interdisciplinary field of research and clinical applications, which focuses on restoration of impaired function and morphology of tissues and organs by repair, replacement, or regeneration. It uses a combination of several technological approaches beyond traditional transplantation and replacement therapies. The key components of these approaches are using of cells, scaffolds, and bioactive factors.

Bone is a specialized connective tissue that is being continuously remodeled throughout life. However, many complex clinical conditions such as large traumatic bone defects, osteomyelitis, tumor resection, or skeletal abnormalities can impair normal bone healing. Bone tissue engineering is required for regenerating tissue from these conditions. Studies on the mechanisms of physiological, pathological skeletal development and fracture healing have provided a wealth of information towards potential methods for regulating osteoblast proliferation and differentiation to regenerate bone.

Here, we focus on one of the main components of tissue engineering, bioactive factors, especially fibroblast growth factors (FGFs) and their roles in bone regeneration.

FGF signaling in skeletal formation has been demonstrated by identification of gain-of-function mutations in human FGF receptor (FGFR) genes in craniosynostosis and dwarfism patients and skeletal phenotypes in genetically modified mice for FGFs and FGFRs [1]. FGFRs are transmembrane tyrosine kinase receptors that belong to the immunoglobulin (Ig) superfamily consisting of extracellular, transmembrane, and intracellular tyrosine kinase domains. Binding of FGFs to FGFRs activates intracellular downstream signaling pathways such as RAS-MAP and PI3K-AKT [2]. The FGFR family consists of four members, FGFR1 to FGFR4. Among the four FGFRs, skeletal mutations have been found in FGFRs1–3 expressed in the osteoblast cell lineage. Most of the mutations are point mutations, and distinct mutation sites result in different syndromes [1]. Some of the mutations have been introduced into mice and confirmed to affect skeletal development.

FGFs and bone regeneration

The mammalian FGF family contains 22 members. Some of them are intracellular FGFs (iFGFs), FGFs 11–14, which are expected to function without binding to FGFRs. FGF19 (FGF15 for mice), FGF21, and FGF23 are hormone-like FGFs which act in an endocrine manner

* Correspondence: s.iseki.emb@tmd.ac.jp
Section of Molecular Craniofacial Embryology, Tokyo Medical and Dental University Graduate School of Medical and Dental Sciences, 1-5-45 Yushima, Bunkyo-ku, Tokyo 113-8549, Japan

in postnatal life. All other FGFs have high affinity to heparin and act in a paracrine manner by binding to the four receptors with different levels of affinities [3–5]. The roles of various FGFs are compiled in Table 1. Skeletal phenotypes after deletion of FGFs in mice are found in FGFs 2, 8, 9, 10, 18, and 23 [6], which confirm the indispensable function of FGF/FGFR signaling in the process of osteogenesis. It is of note that FGF/FGFR signaling does not directly induce osteoblast differentiation but is known to modulate osteoblast differentiation. However, the exact mechanism of FGF/FGFR signaling in bone healing or regeneration has not been elucidated. Schmid et al. [7] reported expression levels of different FGFs by reverse transcriptase polymerase chain reaction (RT-PCR) during normal healing of tibial fracture in mice. Throughout the healing process, FGFs 2, 5, and 6 were upregulated with different levels. FGF9 was highly expressed at the early stage of healing. FGFs 16 and 18 were transcribed at the late stage. Upregulation of FGFs 1 and 17 was delayed after callus formation. This study also identified concordance between the expression of the particular FGFs and their known receptors during different stages of fracture repair. Among three FGFRs

expressed in the osteoblast cell lineage, FGFR3 showed the greatest change in expression levels. This study provided the idea of how FGFs work at the different stages of healing, which could be applied to bone regenerative therapy.

Considering clinical applications, studies involving modification of FGF signaling by ligands are more practical compared to those involving modulating FGFRs. Animal studies revealed that the expression of FGFs 8 and 10 is required for the early stage of limb development, which suggests that they are not directly involved in osteogenesis. Among FGFs which change their expression levels during bone fracture healing, FGF1 protects the osteoblast cell lineage from cell death [8]. FGF5 is associated with the hair follicle cycle. FGF6 is involved in muscle regeneration and those events that occur during the healing process. Therefore, in this review, we chose FGFs 2, 9, and 18 to discuss about their properties and applications for bone regeneration.

FGF2

FGF2 is the most common FGF ligand that is being used in the regenerative medicine field including bone regeneration.

Table 1 List of FGFs and their various functions

Subfamily	FGFs	Manner of action	Prime functions	References
FGF1/2	FGF1	Paracrine	Patterning of optical vesicle	[36]
	FGF2	Paracrine	Neuronal, skeletal, vascular tone; heart repair	[37–39]
FGF4/5/6	FGF4	Paracrine	Proliferation of inner cell mass	[40]
	FGF5	Paracrine	Hair growth cycle regulator	[41]
	FGF6	Paracrine	Regulation of muscle regeneration	[42]
FGF3/7/10/22	FGF3	Paracrine	Inner ear formation, regulation of tooth morphogenesis	[43, 44]
	FGF7	Paracrine	Modulation of hair growth, kidney development	[45, 46]
	FGF10	Paracrine	Regulator of development of many organs such as brain, limb, lung, pancreas	[47, 48]
	FGF22	Paracrine	Presynaptic organization in brain development, hair development	[49, 50]
FGF9/16/20	FGF9	Paracrine	Lung development, maintenance of stemness in nephrons, bone repair, mammalian sex determination	[51–53]
	FGF16	Paracrine	Heart development	[54]
	FGF20	Paracrine	Inner ear development, maintenance of stemness in nephrons	[52, 55]
FGF8/17/18	FGF8	Paracrine	Development of brain, limbs, cardiovascular system, craniofacial region	[56–59]
	FGF17	Paracrine	Brain development	[60]
	FGF18	Paracrine	Bone and cartilage development, lung development	[22, 61]
FGF11/12/13/14	FGF11	Intracrine	Signalling functions during tooth development	[62]
	FGF12	Intracrine	Unclear	
	FGF13	Intracrine	Signaling functions during tooth development	[62]
	FGF14	Intracrine	Regulation of neurotransmission of motor functions	[63]
FGF15/19/21/23	FGF15/19	Endocrine	Regulates hepatic glucose metabolism	[64]
	FGF21	Endocrine	Lipid metabolism regulator	[65]
	FGF23	Endocrine	Phosphate and vitamin D metabolism	[66]

The table shows the subfamilies of various FGFs, FGFs under each subfamily, the manner of action of each FGF, and their prime functions

It has been well known that FGF2 is a critical component of maintenance of many kinds of stem cell cultures [9]. Stabilization of FGF2 levels in a culture medium using polyesters of glycolic and lactic acid (PLGA) microspheres as a FGF2 release controller successfully improved the expression of stem cell markers, increased stem cell numbers, and decreased spontaneous differentiation [10].

FGF2-deleted mice showed a significant decrease in bone mass and bone formation without gross abnormalities. Bone marrow stromal cells (BMSCs) from the $FGF2^{-/-}$ mice demonstrated decreased osteoblast differentiation, which can be partially rescued by addition of exogenous FGF2 in vitro [11]. Furthermore, $FGF2^{-/-}$ BMSC-derived osteoblasts displayed a marked reduction in inactive phosphorylated glycogen synthase kinase-3 (GSK-3) as well as a significant decrease in Dkk2 mRNA, which plays important roles in osteoblast differentiation. These results suggested that FGF2 is an endogenous, positive regulator of bone mass [12]. In contrast, non-specific overexpression of FGF2 (Tg-*FGF2*) in mice exhibits a dwarf phenotype with impaired bone mineralization and osteopenia [13]. Addition of FGF2 into a culture medium of a mouse osteoblast-like cell line, MC3T3-E1, activated cell proliferation and suppressed mineralization [14]. In this study, treatment of the cells with FGF10 as an experimental control did not show any effects. These observations suggested that FGF2 could work in both directions for osteogenesis promotion and inhibition. It is important to elucidate conditions for positive and negative osteogeneses.

FGF9

$FGF9^{-/-}$ mice showed disproportionate shortening of the proximal skeletal elements (rhizomelia), which suggests that FGF9 promotes chondrocyte hypertrophy and vascularization of the cartilage anlagen [15]. A missense mutation of *FGF9* in mice resulted in decreased heparin binding, which caused elbow-knee synostosis [16]. A similar mutation was also found in humans [17]. $FGF9^{+/-}$ mice did not seem to have a particular phenotype. However, bone healing of a 1-mm unicortical defect was impaired with decreased levels of neovascularization and osteoclast recruitment. This condition was rescued by exogenous addition of FGF9 (2 µg) with collagen sponge but not by exogenous FGF2 application [18]. These reports elucidated the specific functions of FGF9 in bone healing.

Bone healing of a 1-mm unicortical defect in diabetic model mice (*db/db*) was significantly delayed with decreased levels of osteogenesis marker expressions. Treatment of FGF9 with collagen sponge to the defect in the *db/db* mice induced better bone healing [19]. Treatment with FGF9-soaked collagen sponge to mouse circular calvarial bone defects of a diameter of 2 mm showed sufficient bone regeneration in postnatal day 7 (P7) mice

but not in postnatal day 60 (P60) mice [20]. Addition of FGF9 with various concentrations into dexamethasone-containing media for inducing osteogenesis of BMSCs and dental pulp stem cells resulted in stimulation of proliferation but not differentiation [21].

FGF18

Deletion of FGF18 in mice resulted in delayed suture formation, reduced osteoblast lineage cell proliferation, delayed osteoblast differentiation, and perinatal death. The long bones of $FGF18^{-/-}$ mice showed reduced osteoblast differentiation but increased chondrocyte proliferation and differentiation. These results suggested that FGF18 demonstrated a positive effect on osteogenesis by enhancing cell proliferation and differentiation but a negative effect on chondrogenesis [22, 23]. However, it was also proposed that FGF18 transduced the signal through FGFR3 to enhance cartilage formation [24].

In vitro analysis on mesenchymal stem cells (MSCs) derived from the bone marrow suggested that FGF18 enhanced osteoblast differentiation by activation of FGFR1 or FGFR2 signaling [25]. They also showed that overexpression of FGF18 by lentiviral infection or direct addition of FGF18 into the culture medium could induce the expression of osteoblast marker genes in C3H10T1/2 fibroblastic cells. Treatment of FGF18 on rat-derived MSCs under a differentiation-inducing condition showed elevated expression of osteoblast differentiation markers and mineralization [26]. Low-dose FGF18 treatment with bone morphogenetic protein 2 (BMP2)-dependent osteogenic induction of MC3T3-E1 cells enhanced mineralization whereas high-dose treatment inhibited the process (unpublished observation of Sachiko Iseki). FGF18-soaked heparin-coated acrylic beads accelerated osteoblast differentiation in mouse fetuses by upregulating the expression of BMP2 in osteoblast cell lineage cells [27]. In accordance with the above reports, FGF18 application with BMP2 in cholesteryl group- and acryloyl group-bearing pullulan (CHPOA) nanogels stabilized BMP2-dependent bone regeneration of critical-sized bone defects on mouse calvarium [28].

Application of FGFs in bone regeneration

The above discussions suggest that although FGFs do not have osteoinductive property, they function as an accelerator of osteogenesis under the appropriate conditions. It is possible that FGF2 and FGF9 work on proliferation of osteoblast cell lineage as well as induction of angiogenesis, and FGF18 functions in promotion of osteoblast differentiation. Tables 2 and 3 show some of the in vivo experiments in which FGFs were applied to non-critical- and critical-sized bone defects for bone healing, respectively. Further applications of FGFs have been elaborated by Du et al. and Gothard et al. [29, 30].

Table 2 Application of different FGFs in non-critical-sized bone defect in vivo models

Growth factor	Dose	In vivo model	Carrier	Investigations	Effect	References
FGF2	200 µg	Monkey ulna fracture	Injectable gelatin hydrogel	Bone mineral content and mechanical properties	Accelerates fracture healing and prevents nonunion	[67]
FGF2	2.5 µg	Rat periodontal defect (2 × 2 × 1.7 mm)	Injectable calcium phosphate cement	Histology and histomorphometry of bone	Increased periodontal regeneration	[68]
FGF2	50 µg	Rat calvarial defect (4-mm diameter)	PLGA/β-TCP	Histomorphometry of bone	Enhanced bone regeneration	[69]
FGF2	50 µg/ml	Rat calvarial defect (5-mm diameter)	Collagen and nano-bioactive glass hybrid membrane	Histomorphometry of bone	Accelerated bone regeneration	[70]
FGF2	45 µg	Rabbit femoral condyle (4-mm diameter and 6 mm long)	Hydrogel polymer	Bone mass and microarchitecture	Enhanced bone regeneration	[32]
FGF2 Melatonin	10 µg 100 mg/kg i.p.	Rat tibia (2-mm diameter, 4 mm long)	Titanium implant	Bone histomorphometry	Synergistically enhanced new bone formation	[71]
FGF2	200, 400, or 800 µg	Human tibia (high tibial osteotomy)	Gelatin hydrogel	Radiographic assessment of bone	Dose dependently accelerated bone union	[72]
FGF2	100 µg	Rabbit femoral condyle (10 mm^2 × 5 mm depth)	Interconnected porous calcium hydroxyapatite ceramic	Bone histomorphometry	Decreases lamellar bone formation, increases vascularization and osseointegration	[73]
FGF2 BMP2	0, 25, or 250 ng 0.1 mg/ml	Rat calvarial defect (3.5-mm diameter)	PLGA/gelatin	Radiological, histological, and biochemical examination	Low-dose administration enhanced the degree of calcification and ALP activity	[74]
FGF9	2 µg	Mouse tibia (1-mm defect)	Collagen sponge	Bone histomorphometry	Enhances angiogenesis and bone regeneration	[19]

The table shows the various growth factors and their combinations used for regeneration of non-critical-sized defects, their dose, the site of application, the carrier used for the application, and the investigations through which the effects of bone healing have been studied
i.p. intraperitoneal injection

Systemic or subcutaneous injections of FGF2 could enhance osteogenesis. However, it was shown that systemic injections of FGF2 caused adverse extraskeletal effects [31]. Therefore, local administration has been chosen as a more preferable method for applying bioactive factors.

FGF2 has been used for inducing angiogenesis and enhancing osteogenesis in non-critical-sized bone defects by activating proliferation of osteoblast cell lineages. FGF9 is also suggested to be involved in angiogenesis by controlling VEGFa expression [18]. As long as osteogenesis is

Table 3 Application of different FGFs in critical-sized bone defect in vivo models

Growth factor	Dose	In vivo model	Carrier	Investigations	Effect	References
FGF2 BMP2	5 ng 2 µg	Mouse calvarial defect (3.5-mm diameter)	Col-HA/PEG hydrogel	Micro CT and histology of bone	Enhanced bone regeneration	[34]
FGF2	10 ng, 100 µg, and 1 µg	Rat mandibular defect (5-mm diameter)	Collagen sponge	Radiological and histological examination	Promotes osteogenesis	[75]
FGF2	200 µg	Beagle dog periodontal defect (6 × 5 mm: vertical × horizontal)	β-TCP	Bone histomorphometry	Enhances formation of new bone and cementum	[76]
FGF18 BMP2	0.5 µg 0.5 µg	Mouse calvaria (3-mm diameter)	CHPOA/hydrogel	Micro CT assessment of bone	Synergistically enhanced new bone formation	[28]
FGF2 or FGF9 or FGF18	250 ng (P7 mice) or 2.5 µg (P60 mice)	Mouse calvaria defect (2-mm diameter)	Collagen sponge	Micro CT assessment of bone	All FGF ligands promote healing rate in P7 mice. Only FGF18 promotes healing rate in P60 mice	[20]

The table shows the various growth factors and their combinations used for regeneration of critical-sized defects, their dose, the site of application, the carrier used for the application, and the investigations through which the effects of bone healing have been studied taking place to recover the bone defect, FGF2 can support or even enhance the healing. Recent studies suggest that high-dose FGF2 inhibits progression of osteoblast differentiation [20, 32, 33] (also unpublished observation of Sachiko Iseki) and low concentration of FGF2 enhanced osteogenesis [33, 34]. In contrast, it is likely that high-dose FGF18 can promote osteoblast differentiation in vivo [20, 28], while FGF18 treatment in vitro inhibits mineralization [14].

Kang et al. developed a sequential delivery system with fiber scaffolds in which FGF2 was released first and then FGF18 [35]. Applying this scaffold to rat calvarial critical-sized bone defects resulted in better bone volume and density, although the amount of FGFs applied to the defect was not clear. This study suggested that it is critical to control the amount or release speed of soluble factors for the bone regeneration process.

Conclusions

FGFs play an important role in the development and regeneration of various tissues. In this article, we have summarized the prime functions of all FGFs, and further, we have discussed elaborately about FGFs 2, 9 and 18, which play a major role in bone regeneration. We have also discussed about different carrier systems for FGF delivery in different animal models for bone regeneration. With the ongoing advancements in the field of cellular and molecular biology, we could expect that more detailed functioning of FGF/FGFR will be elucidated. Further, with the advent of novel carriers and protein delivery systems, it could be possible that the spatio-temporal release of FGFs can be controlled precisely as needed. This would improve our understanding and help us to clinically translate the use of FGFs to achieve effective bone regeneration.

Abbreviations

BMP2: Bone morphogenetic protein 2; BMSC: Bone marrow stromal cells; CHPOA: Cholesteryl group- and acryloyl group-bearing pullulan; Col-HA/PEG: Collagen-hydroxyapatite/polyethylene glycol; Dkk2: Dickkopf-related protein 2; FGF: Fibroblast growth factor; FGFR: Fibroblast growth factor receptor; GSK-3: Glycogen synthase kinase-3; iFGF: Intracellular fibroblast growth factor; Ig: Immunoglobulin; MSC: Mesenchymal stem cells; PLGA: Polyesters of glycolic and lactic acid; RT-PCR: Reverse transcriptase polymerase chain reaction; Tg-FGF2: Transgenic fibroblast growth factor 2; VEGFa: Vascular endothelial growth factor A; β-TCP: Beta tricalcium phosphate

Acknowledgements

We would like to express our sincere gratitude to all the researchers, collaborators, technical assistants, and secretaries for contributing to the research cited in the present manuscript.

Funding

Not applicable.

Authors' contributions

All authors contributed equally to drafting the manuscript. All authors read, revised, and approved the final manuscript.

Competing interests

The authors declare that they have no competing interests.

References

1. Wilkie AO. Bad bones, absent smell, selfish testes: the pleiotropic consequences of human FGF receptor mutations. Cytokine Growth Factor Rev. 2005;16:187–203.
2. Goetz R, Mohammadi M. Exploring mechanisms of FGF signalling through the lens of structural biology. Nat Rev Mol Cell Biol. 2013;14:166–80.
3. Itoh N, Ornitz DM. Functional evolutionary history of the mouse Fgf gene family. Dev Dyn. 2008;237:18–27.
4. Ornitz DM, Xu J, Colvin JS, McEwen DG, MacArthur CA, Coulier F, et al. Receptor specificity of the fibroblast growth factor family. J Biol Chem. 1996;271:15292–7.
5. Zhang X, Ibrahimi OA, Olsen SK, Umemori H, Mohammadi M, Ornitz DM. Receptor specificity of the fibroblast growth factor family. The complete mammalian FGF family. J Biol Chem. 2006;281:15694–700.
6. Itoh N. The Fgf families in humans, mice, and zebrafish: their evolutional processes and roles in development, metabolism, and disease. Biol Pharm Bull. 2007;30:1819–25.
7. Schmid GJ, Kobayashi C, Sandell LJ, Ornitz DM. Fibroblast growth factor expression during skeletal fracture healing in mice. Dev Dyn. 2009;238:766–74.
8. Kelpke S, Reiff D, Prince C, Thompson J. Acidic fibroblast growth factor signaling inhibits peroxynitrite-induced death of osteoblasts and osteoblast precursors. J Bone Miner Res. 2001;16:1917–25.
9. Levenstein ME, Ludwig TE, Xu RH, Llanas RA, VanDenHeuvel-Kramer K, Manning D, et al. Basic fibroblast growth factor support of human embryonic stem cell self-renewal. Stem Cells. 2006;24:568–74.
10. Lotz S, Goderie S, Tokas N, Hirsch SE, Ahmad F, Corneo B, et al. Sustained levels of FGF2 maintain undifferentiated stem cell cultures with biweekly feeding. PLoS One. 2013;8:e56289.
11. Montero A, Okada Y, Tomita M, Ito M, Tsurukami H, Nakamura T, et al. Disruption of the fibroblast growth factor-2 gene results in decreased bone mass and bone formation. J Clin Invest. 2000;105:1085–93.
12. Fei Y, Xiao L, Doetschman T, Coffin DJ, Hurley MM. Fibroblast growth factor 2 stimulation of osteoblast differentiation and bone formation is mediated by modulation of the Wnt signaling pathway. J Biol Chem. 2011;286:40575–83.
13. Coffin J, Florkiewicz R, Neumann J, Mort-Hopkins T, Gn D, Lightfoot P, et al. Abnormal bone growth and selective translational regulation in basic fibroblast growth factor (FGF-2) transgenic mice. Mol Biol Cell. 1995;6:1861–73.
14. Shimoaka T, Ogasawara T, Yonamine A, Chikazu D, Kawano H, Nakamura K, et al. Regulation of osteoblast, chondrocyte, and osteoclast functions by fibroblast growth factor (FGF)-18 in comparison with FGF-2 and FGF-10. J Biol Chem. 2002;277:7493–500.
15. Hung IH, Yu K, Lavine KJ, Ornitz DM. FGF9 regulates early hypertrophic chondrocyte differentiation and skeletal vascularization in the developing stylopod. Dev Biol. 2007;307:300–13.
16. Harada M, Murakami H, Okawa A, Okimoto N, Hiraoka S, Nakahara T, et al. FGF9 monomer–dimer equilibrium regulates extracellular matrix affinity and tissue diffusion. Nat Genet. 2009;41:289–98.
17. Wu X-l, Gu M-m, Huang L, Liu X-s, Zhang H-x, Ding X-y, et al. Multiple synostoses syndrome is due to a missense mutation in exon 2 of FGF9 gene. Am J Hum Genet. 2009;85:53–63.
18. Behr B, Leucht P, Longaker MT, Quarto N. Fgf9 is required for angiogenesis and osteogenesis in long bone repair. Proc Natl Acad Sci U S A. 2010;107: 11853–8.
19. Wallner C, Schira J, Wagner JM, Schulte M, Fischer S, Hirsch T, et al. Application of VEGFA and FGF9 enhances angiogenesis, osteogenesis and bone remodeling in type 2 diabetic long bone regeneration. PLoS One. 2015;10:e0118823.
20. Behr B, Panetta NJ, Longaker MT, Quarto N. Different endogenous threshold levels of fibroblast growth factor-ligands determine the healing potential of frontal and parietal bones. Bone. 2010;47:281–94.

21. Lu J, Dai J, Wang X, Zhang M, Zhang P, Sun H, et al. Effect of fibroblast growth factor 9 on the osteogenic differentiation of bone marrow stromal stem cells and dental pulp stem cells. Mol Med Rep. 2015;11:1661–8.

22. Ohbayashi N, Shibayama M, Kurotaki Y, Imanishi M, Fujimori T, Itoh N, et al. FGF18 is required for normal cell proliferation and differentiation during osteogenesis and chondrogenesis. Genes Dev. 2002;16:870–9.

23. Liu Z, Xu J, Colvin JS, Ornitz DM. Coordination of chondrogenesis and osteogenesis by fibroblast growth factor 18. Genes Dev. 2002;16:859–69.

24. Davidson D, Blanc A, Filion D, Wang H, Plut P, Pfeffer G, et al. Fibroblast growth factor (FGF) 18 signals through FGF receptor 3 to promote chondrogenesis. J BiolChem. 2005;280:20509–15.

25. Hamidouche Z, Fromigué O, Nuber U, Vaudin P, Ebert R, Jakob F, et al. Autocrine fibroblast growth factor 18 mediates dexamethasone-induced osteogenic differentiation of murine mesenchymal stem cells. J Cell Physiol. 2010;224:509–15.

26. Jeon E, Yun Y-R, Kang W, Lee S, Koh Y-H, Kim H-W, et al. Investigating the role of FGF18 in the cultivation and osteogenic differentiation of mesenchymal stem cells. PLoS One. 2012;7:e43982.

27. Nagayama T, Okuhara S, Ota MS, Tachikawa N, Kasugai S, Iseki S. FGF18 accelerates osteoblast differentiation by upregulating Bmp2 expression. Congenit Anom. 2013;53:83–8.

28. Fujioka-Kobayashi M, Ota MS, Shimoda A, Nakahama K-I, Akiyoshi K, Miyamoto S, et al. Cholesteryl group- and acryloyl group-bearing pullulan nanogel to deliver BMP2 and FGF18 for bone tissue engineering. Biomaterials. 2012;33:7613–20.

29. Du X, Xie Y, Xian CJ, Chen L. Role of FGFs/FGFRs in skeletal development and bone regeneration. J Cell Physiol. 2012;227:3731–43.

30. Gothard D, Smith E, Kanczler J, Rashidi H, Qutachi O, Henstock J, et al. Tissue engineered bone using select growth factors: a comprehensive review of animal studies and clinical translation studies in man. Eur Cell Mater. 2014;28:166–208.

31. Wamsley HL, Iwaniec UT, Wronski TJ. Selected extraskeletal effects of systemic treatment with basic fibroblast growth factor in ovariectomized rats. Toxicol Pathol. 2005;33:577–83.

32. Mabilleau G, Aguado E, Stancu IC, Cincu C, Baslé MF, Chappard D. Effects of FGF-2 release from a hydrogel polymer on bone mass and microarchitecture. Biomaterials. 2008;29:1593–600.

33. Nakamura Y, Tensho K, Nakaya H, Nawata M, Okabe T, Wakitani S. Low dose fibroblast growth factor-2 (FGF-2) enhances bone morphogenetic protein-2 (BMP-2)-induced ectopic bone formation in mice. Bone. 2005; 36:399–407.

34. Charles LF, Woodman JL, Ueno D, Gronowicz G, Hurley MM, Kuhn LT. Effects of low dose FGF-2 and BMP-2 on healing of calvarial defects in old mice. Exp Geront. 2015;64:62–9.

35. Kang MS, Kim J-H, Singh RK, Jang J-H, Kim H-W. Therapeutic-designed electrospun bone scaffolds: mesoporous bioactive nanocarriers in hollow fiber composites to sequentially deliver dual growth factors. Acta Biomater. 2015;16:103–16.

36. Hyer J, Mima T, Mikawa T. FGF1 patterns the optic vesicle by directing the placement of the neural retina domain. Development. 1998;125: 869–77.

37. Dono R, Texido G, Dussel R, Ehmke H, Zeller R. Impaired cerebral cortex development and blood pressure regulation in FGF-2-deficient mice. EMBO J. 1998;17:4213–25.

38. Zhou M, Sutliff RL, Paul RJ, Lorenz JN, Hoying JB, Haudenschild CC, et al. Fibroblast growth factor 2 control of vascular tone. Nat Med. 1998;4:201.

39. Van Gastel N, Stegen S, Van Looveren R, Stockmans I, Schrooten J, Graf D, et al. FGF2 primes periosteal cells for endochondral ossification via maintenance of skeletal precursors and modulation of BMP signaling. 35th Annual Meeting of the American Society for Bone and Mineral Research (ASBMR); Baltimore, Maryland, USA 2013.

40. Feldman B, Poueymirou W, Papaioannou VE, DeChiara TM, Goldfarb M. Requirement of FGF-4 for postimplantation mouse development. Science. 1995;267:246.

41. Hébert JM, Rosenquist T, Götz J, Martin GR. FGF5 as a regulator of the hair growth cycle: evidence from targeted and spontaneous mutations. Cell. 1994;78:1017–25.

42. Armand A-S, Laziz I, Chanoine C. FGF6 in myogenesis. BBA Mol Cell Res. 2006;1763:773–8.

43. Maroon H, Walshe J, Mahmood R, Kiefer P, Dickson C, Mason I. Fgf3 and Fgf8 are required together for formation of the otic placode and vesicle. Development. 2002;129:2099–108.

44. Kettunen P, Laurikkala J, Itäranta P, Vainio S, Itoh N, Thesleff I. Associations of FGF-3 and FGF-10 with signaling networks regulating tooth morphogenesis. Dev Dyn. 2000;219:322–32.

45. Guo L, Degenstein L, Fuchs E. Keratinocyte growth factor is required for hair development but not for wound healing. Gene Dev. 1996;10:165–75.

46. Qiao J, Uzzo R, Obara-Ishihara T, Degenstein L, Fuchs E, Herzlinger D. FGF-7 modulates ureteric bud growth and nephron number in the developing kidney. Development. 1999;126:547–54.

47. Sekine K, Ohuchi H, Fujiwara M, Yamasaki M, Yoshizawa T, Sato T, et al. Fgf10 is essential for limb and lung formation. Nat Genet. 1999;21:138–41.

48. Bhushan A, Itoh N, Kato S, Thiery JP, Czernichow P, Bellusci S, et al. Fgf10 is essential for maintaining the proliferative capacity of epithelial progenitor cells during early pancreatic organogenesis. Development. 2001;128:5109–17.

49. Umemori H, Linhoff MW, Ornitz DM, Sanes JR. FGF22 and its close relatives are presynaptic organizing molecules in the mammalian brain. Cell. 2004; 118:257–70.

50. Nakatake Y, Hoshikawa M, Asaki T, Kassai Y, Itoh N. Identification of a novel fibroblast growth factor, FGF-22, preferentially expressed in the inner root sheath of the hair follicle. BBA Gene Struct Expr. 2001;1517:460–3.

51. Colvin JS, White AC, Pratt SJ, Ornitz DM. Lung hypoplasia and neonatal death in Fgf9-null mice identify this gene as an essential regulator of lung mesenchyme. Development. 2001;128:2095–106.

52. Barak H, Huh S-H, Chen S, Jeanpierre C, Martinovic J, Parisot M, et al. FGF9 and FGF20 maintain the stemness of nephron progenitors in mice and man. Dev Cell. 2012;22:1191–207.

53. Kim Y, Kobayashi A, Sekido R, DiNapoli L, Brennan J, Chaboissier M-C, et al. Fgf9 and Wnt4 act as antagonistic signals to regulate mammalian sex determination. PLoS Biol. 2006;4:e187.

54. Lu SY, Sheikh F, Sheppard PC, Fresnoza A, Duckworth ML, Detillieux KA, et al. FGF-16 is required for embryonic heart development. Biochem Biophys Res Commun. 2008;373:270–4.

55. Hayashi T, Ray CA, Bermingham-McDonogh O. Fgf20 is required for sensory epithelial specification in the developing cochlea. J Neurosci. 2008;28:5991–9.

56. Reifers F, Bohli H, Walsh EC, Crossley PH, Stainier D, Brand M. Fgf8 is mutated in zebrafish acerebellar (ace) mutants and is required for maintenance of midbrain-hindbrain boundary development and somitogenesis. Development. 1998;125:2381–95.

57. Crossley PH, Minowada G, MacArthur CA, Martin GR. Roles for FGF8 in the induction, initiation, and maintenance of chick limb development. Cell. 1996;84:127–36.

58. Abu-Issa R, Smyth G, Smoak I, Yamamura K-i, Meyers EN. Fgf8 is required for pharyngeal arch and cardiovascular development in the mouse. Development. 2002;129:4613–25.

59. Albertson RC, Yelick PC. Roles for fgf8 signaling in left–right patterning of the visceral organs and craniofacial skeleton. Dev Biol. 2005;283:310–21.

60. Cholfin JA, Rubenstein JL. Patterning of frontal cortex subdivisions by Fgf17. Proc Natl Acad Sci U S A. 2007;104:7652–7.

61. Usui H, Shibayama M, Ohbayashi N, Konishi M, Takada S, Itoh N. Fgf18 is required for embryonic lung alveolar development. Biochem Biophys Res Commun. 2004;322:887–92.

62. Kettunen P, Furmanek T, Chaulagain R, Hals Kvinnsland I, Luukko K. Developmentally regulated expression of intracellular Fgf11-13, hormone-like Fgf15 and canonical Fgf16, -17 and -20 mRNAs in the developing mouse molar tooth. Acta Odontol Scand. 2011;69:360–6.

63. Zhang X, Bao L, Yang L, Wu Q, Li S. Roles of intracellular fibroblast growth factors in neural development and functions. Sci China Life Sci. 2012;55: 1038–44.

64. Potthoff MJ, Boney-Montoya J, Choi M, He T, Sunny NE, Satapati S, et al. FGF15/19 regulates hepatic glucose metabolism by inhibiting the CREB-PGC-1α pathway. Cell Metab. 2011;13:729–38.

65. Chui PC, Antonellis PJ, Bina HA, Kharitonenkov A, Flier JS, Maratos-Flier E. Obesity is a fibroblast growth factor 21 (FGF21)-resistant state. Diabetes. 2010;59:2781–9.

66. Shimada T, Kakitani M, Yamazaki Y, Hasegawa H, Takeuchi Y, Fujita T, et al. Targeted ablation of Fgf23 demonstrates an essential physiological role of FGF23 in phosphate and vitamin D metabolism. J Clin Invest. 2004;113:561–8.

67. Kawaguchi H, Nakamura K, Tabata Y, Ikada Y, Aoyama I, Anzai J, et al. Acceleration of fracture healing in nonhuman primates by fibroblast growth factor-2. J Clin Endocrinol Metab. 2001;86:875–80.

68. Oortgiesen DA, Walboomers XF, Bronckers AL, Meijer GJ, Jansen JA. Periodontal regeneration using an injectable bone cement combined with BMP-2 or FGF-2. J Tissue Eng Regen Med. 2014;8:202–9.

69. Yoshida T, Miyaji H, Otani K, Inoue K, Nakane K, Nishimura H, et al. Bone augmentation using a highly porous PLGA/β-TCP scaffold containing fibroblast growth factor-2. J Periodont Res. 2015;50:265–73.

70. Hong KS, Kim EC, Bang SH, Chung CH, Lee YI, Hyun JK, et al. Bone regeneration by bioactive hybrid membrane containing FGF2 within rat calvarium. J Biomed Mater Res A. 2010;94:1187–94.

71. Takechi M, Tatehara S, Satomura K, Fujisawa K, Nagayama M. Effect of FGF-2 and melatonin on implant bone healing: a histomorphometric study. J Mater Sci Mater Med. 2008;19:2949–52.

72. Kawaguchi H, Jingushi S, Izumi T, Fukunaga M, Matsushita T, Nakamura T, et al. Local application of recombinant human fibroblast growth factor-2 on bone repair: a dose-escalation prospective trial on patients with osteotomy. J Orthop Res. 2007;25:480–7.

73. Nakasa T, Ishida O, Sunagawa T, Nakamae A, Yokota K, Adachi N, et al. Feasibility of prefabricated vascularized bone graft using the combination of FGF-2 and vascular bundle implantation within hydroxyapatite for osteointegration. J Biomed Mater Res A. 2008;85:1090–5.

74. Tanaka E, Ishino Y, Sasaki A, Hasegawa T, Watanabe M, Dalla-Bona DA, et al. Fibroblast growth factor-2 augments recombinant human bone morphogenetic protein-2-induced osteoinductive activity. Ann Biomed Eng. 2006;34:717–25.

75. Zellin G, Linde A. Effects of recombinant human fibroblast growth factor-2 on osteogenic cell populations during orthopic osteogenesis in vivo. Bone. 2000;26:161–8.

76. Ishii Y, Fujita T, Okubo N, Ota M, Yamada S, Saito A. Effect of basic fibroblast growth factor (FGF-2) in combination with beta tricalcium phosphate on root coverage in dog. Acta Odontol Scand. 2013;71:325–32.

16

The pathological role of vascular aging in cardio-metabolic disorder

Goro Katsuumi[1†], Ippei Shimizu[1,2*†], Yohko Yoshida[1,2] and Tohru Minamino[1*]

Abstract

Chronological aging is linked to cellular senescence, and there is accumulating evidence for a pathological role of cellular senescence in age-related disorders such as obesity, diabetes, and heart failure. The protein p53 has a central role in cellular senescence, and p53 expression in cardiomyocytes, vascular endothelial cells, adipocytes, and immune cells leads to the development of heart failure and diabetes. It is widely accepted that formation of capillary networks is critical for morphogenesis of organs and maintenance of homeostasis. Capillary rarefaction and hypoxia promote pathological changes in the myocardium of the failing heart, causing systolic dysfunction. Capillary rarefaction and hypoxia also cause dysfunction of brown adipose tissue (BAT), leading to systemic metabolic disorders with promotion of diabetes. Vascular endothelial cell senescence develops in heart failure and diabetes and is responsible for progression of these age-related disorders. In a murine model of left ventricular pressure overload, increased expression of p53 in vascular endothelial cells and bone marrow cells promotes inflammatory cell infiltration into the heart, contributing to cardiac remodeling and systolic dysfunction. Metabolic stress up-regulates p53 expression in endothelial cells, while reducing the phosphorylation of endothelial nitric oxide synthase (eNOS) and glucose transporter (GLUT)1 expression in these cells. These changes lead to suppression of mitochondrial biogenesis and glucose uptake in the skeletal muscle and promote the development of systemic metabolic dysfunction. Suppression of vascular aging and vascular dysfunction is critically important for maintenance of organ homeostasis and is essential for prevention or treatment of heart failure, obesity, and diabetes.

Keywords: p53, Cellular senescence, Endothelial cell, Heart failure, Diabetes

Background

Chronological aging increases the risk of age-related disorders such as obesity, diabetes, and heart failure. Aging also occurs at the cellular level. Shortening of telomeres associated with cell division triggers the DNA damage response and cellular senescence, which is known as replicative senescence and is mainly mediated via a p53 signaling pathway [10, 12]. In addition, stress due to factors such as cytokines and reactive oxygen species also leads to p53-mediated cellular senescence that is termed premature senescence [27]. Senescent cells are characterized by growth arrest associated with various alterations of gene expression [10, 24, 32, 37].

Obesity and its associated disorders are among the top health problems in many societies. Obesity promotes pathological processes that contribute to atherosclerotic disease, heart failure, and diabetes, and there is evidence for a causal role of cellular senescence in these diseases. Metabolic stress leads to p53-induced cellular senescence in adipocytes, resulting in adipose tissue inflammation and systemic metabolic dysfunction [16]. Obesity has also been linked to elevated p53 expression in vascular endothelial cells, which reduces the activation of endothelial nitric oxide synthase (eNOS) and glucose transporter (GLUT)1 in these cells and contributes to suppression of mitochondrial biogenesis and glucose uptake in the skeletal muscle, leading to systemic metabolic dysfunction [41]. In addition, capillary rarefaction and hypoxia cause dysfunction of brown adipose tissue (BAT) and promote systemic metabolic abnormalities [28]. Recently, vascular senescence was shown to have a

* Correspondence: ippeishimizu@yahoo.co.jp; t_minamino@yahoo.co.jp
†Equal contributors
[1]Department of Cardiovascular Biology and Medicine, Niigata University Graduate School of Medical and Dental Sciences, 1-757 Asahimachidori, Chuo-ku, Niigata 951-8510, Japan
Full list of author information is available at the end of the article

pathological role in the progression of heart failure. In a murine model of left ventricular pressure overload, increased adrenergic signaling associated with heart failure was found to up-regulate p53 expression in both endothelial cells and bone marrow cells, contributing to cardiac inflammation and remodeling [42]. Heart failure also promotes p53-induced adipocyte senescence and visceral fat inflammation, leading to the development of systemic insulin resistance and hyperinsulinemia. In turn, hyperinsulinemia contributes to cardiac hypertrophy via the Akt signaling pathway, possibly because cardiac tissue is slow to develop insulin resistance, and activation of this pathway has a detrimental effect on cardiac homeostasis by promoting pathological cardiomyocyte hypertrophy, cardiomyocyte/capillary mismatch, and hypoxia [29].

It is widely accepted that formation of vascular networks is critically important for organ morphogenesis and for maintenance of homeostasis, while cellular senescence has a pathological role in promoting vascular dysfunction that leads to organ dysfunction and systemic metabolic disorders [6, 28, 41, 42]. In this review, we discuss the role of vascular aging in cardio-metabolic disorders.

Pathological role of vascular aging/dysfunction in heart failure

The prognosis of severe heart failure is still very poor, and it is urgent to find new therapeutic targets for this disorder [2]. Hypertensive heart disease is among the chief causes of heart failure. When cardiac tissue is exposed to pressure overload, cardiac hypertrophy occurs in step with angiogenesis as an adaptive response to maintain systolic function. Sustained pressure overload promotes the transition to decompensated heart failure, which features excessive cardiomyocyte hypertrophy uncoordinated with the angiogenic response [33]. The resulting capillary rarefaction and hypoxia contribute to cardiac remodeling and systolic dysfunction. It was reported that increased cardiac expression of p53, which induces cellular senescence, promotes cardiac dysfunction in a murine model of pressure overload. In addition, p53 suppresses cardiac angiogenesis via inhibition of hypoxia-inducible factor 1α (Hif-1α) and vascular endothelial growth factor (VEGF), thus promoting cardiac hypoxia and remodeling [25]. It is well accepted that sterile inflammation contributes to the progression of cardiac remodeling associated with heart failure, but the mechanistic link between p53 and inflammation in the failing heart has been unclear [7]. Recently, activation of p53 signaling in vascular endothelial cells and bone marrow cells was reported to be the underlying cause of cardiac inflammation in a murine model of left ventricular (LV) pressure overload [42]. In this model, p53 expression was significantly increased in cardiac microvascular

endothelial cells and bone marrow cells, leading to up-regulation of intercellular adhesion molecule (ICAM)-1 expression by endothelial cells and an increase of integrin alpha-L in macrophages. Genetic deletion of p53 in endothelial cells or bone marrow cells reduced the expression of these adhesion molecules, suppressed inflammatory cell infiltration into cardiac tissue, inhibited production of pro-inflammatory cytokines, and ameliorated cardiac dysfunction due to LV pressure overload. Conversely, forced expression of p53 in bone marrow cells led to exacerbation of cardiac inflammation and systolic dysfunction. It is well known that activation of the sympathetic nervous system (SNS) occurs in heart failure patients and is associated with a poor prognosis [3]. In the LV pressure overload model, norepinephrine markedly increased the level of reactive oxygen species (ROS) and p53 expression in macrophages and endothelial cells, while inhibition of adrenergic signaling through suppression of beta-2 adrenergic receptor expression in endothelial cells or bone marrow cells decreased ROS and p53 levels, and also ameliorated cardiac inflammation and systolic dysfunction due to pressure overload. These results suggest that activation of SNS/ROS/p53 signaling promotes interaction between endothelial cells and bone marrow-derived inflammatory cells via up-regulation of ICAM-1 and integrin expression, resulting in exacerbation of cardiac dysfunction [42] (Fig. 1). It was also reported that increased p53 signaling in endothelial cells led to capillary rarefaction in cardiac tissue in a murine model of LV pressure overload, while depletion of endothelial cell p53 ameliorated capillary rarefaction, improved cardiac function, and suppressed cardiac fibrosis/remodeling [8]. Cardiac expression of p53 is up-regulated by LV pressure overload, but this change is significantly suppressed by endothelial cell p53 depletion. These results indicate that infiltration of inflammatory cells into cardiac tissue (promoted by endothelial cell senescence) is the initial step in the process of cardiac remodeling due to LV pressure overload, and this process is accelerated by capillary rarefaction and hypoxia [8, 25, 42]. It is well accepted that the non-selective β-blocker, carvedilol, has a cardioprotective effect contributing for the better clinical outcomes in severe heart failure patients with reduced ejection fraction. Carvedilol is known to bind preferentially to beta-2 adrenergic receptor, and it may exert its biological effects via the suppression of SNS/ROS/p53 signaling mediated via beta-2 adrenergic receptor in endothelial cells. Accordingly, suppression of endothelial cell senescence could be a new therapeutic target for heart failure associated with reduced cardiac systolic function.

It is well known that approximately half of the heart failure is classified as heart failure with preserved ejection fraction (HFpEF). HFpEF is known to be predominant

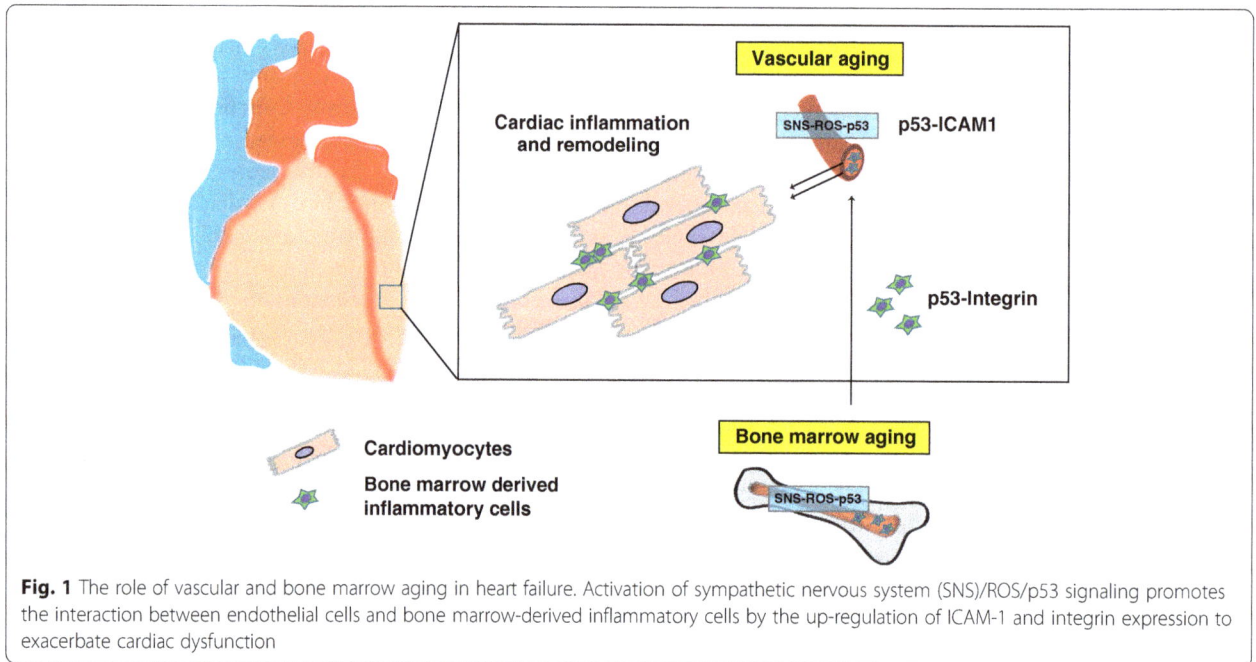

Fig. 1 The role of vascular and bone marrow aging in heart failure. Activation of sympathetic nervous system (SNS)/ROS/p53 signaling promotes the interaction between endothelial cells and bone marrow-derived inflammatory cells by the up-regulation of ICAM-1 and integrin expression to exacerbate cardiac dysfunction

among elderly individuals. Overweight/obesity, hypertension, and diabetes mellitus are also known to become the risk factors for promoting this pathological condition. Cardiomyocyte hypertrophy and interstitial fibrosis, associated with incomplete relaxation of myocardial strips and cardiomyocyte stiffness, develop in HFpEF [13, 26, 38]. Recently, coronary microvascular inflammation is thought crucial for the development of HFpEF [22]. Considering that cellular senescence has a central role in inducing vascular dysfunction, it is highly possible that this would promote pathologies in HFpEF. Further studies are needed to analyze the role of vascular aging in this critical disorder.

Pathological role of vascular aging/dysfunction in obesity

Skeletal muscle

The skeletal muscle makes a major contribution to glucose disposal, so maintenance of skeletal muscle homeostasis is crucial for metabolic health. Metabolic stress induces accumulation of lipids and causes inflammation that promotes insulin resistance in the skeletal muscle, contributing to the development of systemic insulin resistance [15, 23]. Capillaries have an important role in the regulation of skeletal muscle metabolism. An increase of p53 in the vascular endothelium was reported in a murine model of dietary obesity [41]. In this model, genetic depletion of endothelial p53 reduced the accumulation of visceral and subcutaneous fat and led to improvement of systemic insulin resistance. eNOS up-regulates peroxisome proliferator-activated receptor-γ coactivator-1α (PGC1-α) in the skeletal muscle, while p53 suppresses the activation of eNOS. It was found that the

depletion of endothelial cell p53 promoted glucose uptake by the skeletal muscle via up-regulation of GLUT1 expression in endothelial cells. These findings suggest that suppression of vascular aging contributes to better metabolic health by promoting mitochondrial biogenesis in the skeletal muscle [41] (Fig. 2).

Brown adipose tissue

Several types of fat exist in the body, including white, brown, and beige adipose tissue. BAT was initially characterized as a thermogenic organ that is abundantly expressed in newborn infants and small rodents, but subsequent studies have shown that adult humans also have BAT [4]. In addition to its role in thermogenesis, BAT is now known to make a large contribution to the regulation of systemic metabolism [1, 18, 34]. In adults, BAT activity was found to decline with obesity and aging, but the detailed mechanisms involved were uncertain. BAT is highly vascular, and metabolic stress was recently shown to suppress angiogenesis by reducing the expression of vascular endothelial growth factor-A (VEGF-A), a major pro-angiogenic molecule, in brown adipocytes due to accumulation of fatty acids. This leads to capillary rarefaction and hypoxia, which affect BAT much more prominently than white adipose tissue (WAT), leading to "whitening" of BAT that is associated with diminished β-adrenergic signaling, accumulation of large lipid droplets, and mitochondrial dysfunction or loss. These changes of the BAT microenvironment impair thermogenesis and promote systemic metabolic dysfunction. Whitening of BAT has also been observed after ablation of *Vegfa* in the adipose tissue of non-obese

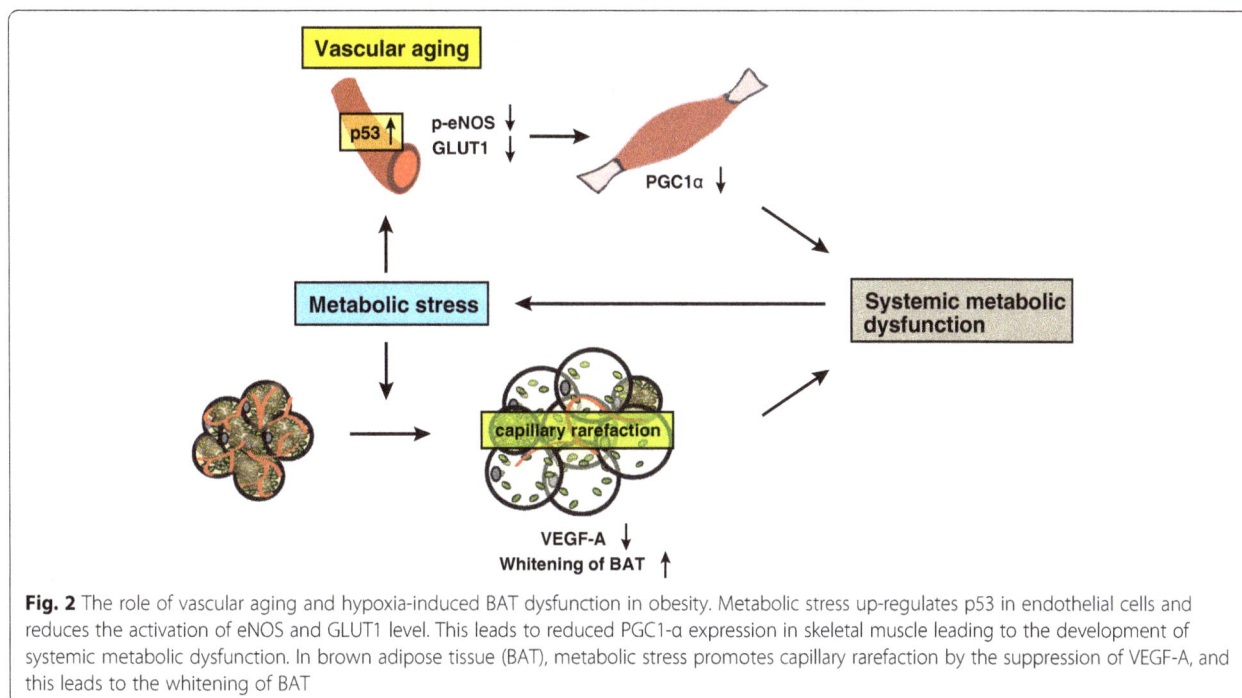

Fig. 2 The role of vascular aging and hypoxia-induced BAT dysfunction in obesity. Metabolic stress up-regulates p53 in endothelial cells and reduces the activation of eNOS and GLUT1 level. This leads to reduced PGC1-α expression in skeletal muscle leading to the development of systemic metabolic dysfunction. In brown adipose tissue (BAT), metabolic stress promotes capillary rarefaction by the suppression of VEGF-A, and this leads to the whitening of BAT

mice, which demonstrated impairment of systemic glucose metabolism and reduction of thermogenesis. Importantly, specific introduction of *Vegfa* into the BAT of mice with dietary obesity restored its vascularity and ameliorated brown adipocyte dysfunction, and this re-browning of BAT was associated with improvement of insulin sensitivity. These data indicate that overnutrition promotes hypoxia in BAT, causing it to whiten through mitochondrial dysfunction and loss, and subsequently contributing to impaired systemic glucose metabolism [28] (Fig. 2). Recently, the expression of an anti-angiogenic VEGF-A splice isoform (VEGF-A165b) was shown to increase upon metabolic stress and inhibit vascularization in ischemic hind limbs [14]. The role of VEGF-A165b in the maintenance of BAT homeostasis remains an open question.

White adipose tissue

WAT was initially thought to be mainly involved in energy storage, but it is now well known to be an active endocrine organ secreting humoral mediators called "adipokines" [20]. Metabolic stress induces the influx of fatty acids into white adipocytes, leading to increased production of inflammatory cytokines and promoting systemic metabolic dysfunction. Angiogenic factors have been reported to have a critical role in the maintenance of homeostasis in WAT [5, 35, 36]. In obese patients and obese mice, WAT displays capillary rarefaction and hypoxia associated with the infiltration of macrophages and increased production of pro-inflammatory cytokines. In obesity, the VEGF-A level has variously been reported to be increased [11, 40], decreased [9, 17, 21], or unchanged [39], but there is a consensus that inadequate angiogenesis occurs during WAT expansion associated with metabolic stress. Disruption of VEGF expression in the fat cells of mice leads to capillary rarefaction and hypoxia in visceral WAT along with increased *Tnf* expression, and the mice develop systemic metabolic dysfunction when fed a high-calorie diet. In contrast, forced VEGF expression in fat cells increases the vascularity of adipose tissue and ameliorates systemic metabolic dysfunction in mice with dietary obesity. These findings indicate that capillary network formation has a crucial role in WAT homeostasis and metabolic health [5, 35, 36].

Recently, impaired angiogenesis in visceral adipose tissue was reported to associate with high VEGF-A165b expression in the fat, suggesting that the inhibition of VEGF-A165b would have a therapeutic potential to maintain homeostasis in visceral fat, contributing to the suppression of systemic metabolic dysfunction [19].

In both white and brown adipose tissue, molecules or mechanisms contributing to the up-regulation of angiogenic VEGF are yet to be defined. Studies indicate that hypoxia-inducible factor 1α (HIF1α) in the visceral fat is increased in response to obesity. In cardiac tissue and other organs, HIF1α is well accepted as a critical regulator for angiogenesis [25]. Interestingly, in both fats, HIF1α does not induce angiogenesis; instead, it activates fibrotic response or autophagy and disturbs homeostasis in these organs [9, 28]. Further studies are needed to explore mechanisms that would promote angiogenesis in white and brown adipose tissue.

Conclusions

Capillaries are critically involved in maintenance of homeostasis in the heart, BAT and WAT, and skeletal muscle [5, 25, 28, 35, 36, 41, 42]. Studies have shown that endothelial cell senescence leads to cardiac inflammation, capillary rarefaction, and hypoxia, thereby promoting pathologic cardiac remodeling in response to LV pressure overload [25, 42]. In a murine model of LV pressure overload, the downregulation of endothelial cell expression of p53 (a critical regulator of cellular senescence) has been shown to inhibit cardiac inflammation, promote angiogenesis, and protect cardiac function [42]. Studies performed in murine models of obesity have shown that capillary rarefaction also develops in BAT as a response to metabolic stress. Accumulation of lipids leads to the suppression of VEGF-A, a critical regulator of angiogenesis, and induces capillary rarefaction and hypoxia, promoting the whitening of brown fat and systemic metabolic dysfunction. Conversely, up-regulation of *Vegfa* expression promotes the re-browning of whitened BAT and improves systemic metabolic health [28]. Endothelial cell senescence is linked with metabolic dysfunction in skeletal muscle via suppression of mitochondrial biogenesis and contributes to systemic metabolic dysfunction [41]. These results provide evidence that maintenance of vascular homeostasis through regulation of endothelial cell senescence is critically important for suppressing pathologic changes associated with heart failure, obesity, and diabetes. It has been reported that systemic insulin resistance develops during heart failure in humans and mice. Excessive lipolysis in visceral fat promotes adipose tissue inflammation during LV pressure overload and leads to systemic insulin resistance with hyperinsulinemia [30], while excessive insulin signaling has been reported to induce pathological cardiac hypertrophy associated with capillary rarefaction and hypoxia [29]. Studies have shown that p53-induced senescence of adipocytes causes the development of adipose tissue inflammation and systemic insulin resistance in animal models of obesity or heart failure, contributing to the progression of these age-related disorders [16, 30, 31]. Recent studies have also indicated that endothelial cell senescence has a pathological role in systemic insulin resistance through impairment of skeletal muscle metabolism [41]. Thus, maintenance of vascular homeostasis is essential in the management of obesity, diabetes, and heart failure.

Acknowledgements

This work was supported by a Grant-in-Aid for Scientific Research, a Grant-in-Aid for Scientific Research on Innovative Areas (Stem Cell Aging and Disease), and a Grant-in-Aid for Exploratory Research from the Ministry of Education, Culture, Sports, Science and Technology (MEXT) of Japan and grants from the Ono Medical Research Foundation, the Japan Diabetes Foundation, the Takeda Science Foundation, and the Takeda Medical Research Foundation (to TM) as well as by a Grants-in-Aid for Young Scientists (Start-up) (JSPS

KAKENHI Grant Number 26893080), and grants from the Uehara Memorial Foundation, Takeda Science Foundation, Kowa Life Science Foundation, Manpei Suzuki Diabetes Foundation, Kanae Foundation, Japan Heart Foundation Research Grant, Senri Life Science Foundation, SENSHIN Medical Research Foundation, ONO Medical Research Foundation, Tsukada Grant for Niigata University Medical Research, The Nakajima Foundation, Suzuken Memorial Foundation, HOKUTO Corporation, Inamori Foundation, Mochida Memorial Foundation for Medical & Pharmaceutical Research, Banyu Foundation Research Grant, and Grant for Basic Science Research Projects from The Sumitomo Foundation (to IS) and by a Grant-in-Aid for Young Scientists from MEXT, a Japan Heart Foundation Dr. Hiroshi Irisawa & Dr. Aya Irisawa Memorial Research Grant, Senshin Medical Research Foundation grant, Suzuken memorial foundation, Takeda Science Foundation, ONO Medical Research Foundation, Uehara Memorial Foundation, and Research Foundation for Community Medicine (to YY) and by a grant from Bourbon (to TM, IS, and YY).

Authors' contributions

GK, IS, YY, and TM wrote the paper. IS and TM supervised the manuscript preparation. All authors read and approved the final manuscript.

Competing interests

The authors declare that they have no competing interests.

Author details

[1]Department of Cardiovascular Biology and Medicine, Niigata University Graduate School of Medical and Dental Sciences, 1-757 Asahimachidori, Chuo-ku, Niigata 951-8510, Japan. [2]Division of Molecular Aging and Cell Biology, Niigata University Graduate School of Medical and Dental Sciences, 1-757 Asahimachidori, Chuo-ku, Niigata 951-8510, Japan.

References

1. Bartelt A, Bruns OT, Reimer R, Hohenberg H, Ittrich H, Peldschus K, Kaul M.G, Tromsdorf, UI, Weller, H, Waurisch, C et al. Brown adipose tissue activity controls triglyceride clearance. Nat Med. 2010;17:200–5.
2. Braunwald E. The war against heart failure: the Lancet lecture. Lancet. 2015; 385:812–24.
3. Cohn JN, Levine TB, Olivari MT, Garberg V, Lura D, Francis GS, Simon AB, Rector T. Plasma norepinephrine as a guide to prognosis in patients with chronic congestive heart failure. N Engl J Med. 1984;311:819–23.
4. Cypess AM, Lehman S, Williams G, Tal I, Rodman D, Goldfine AB, Kuo, FC, Palmer, E.L, Tseng, YH, Doria, A et al. Identification and importance of brown adipose tissue in adult humans. N Engl J Med. 2009;360:1509–17.
5. Elias I, Franckhauser S, Ferre T, Vila L, Tafuro S, Munoz S, Roca C, Ramos D, Pujol A, Riu E et al. Adipose tissue overexpression of vascular endothelial growth factor protects against diet-induced obesity and insulin resistance. Diabetes. 2012;61:1801–13.
6. Ferrara N. Vascular endothelial growth factor: basic science and clinical progress. Endocr Rev. 2004;25:581–611.
7. Frieler RA, Mortensen RM. Immune cell and other noncardiomyocyte regulation of cardiac hypertrophy and remodeling. Circulation. 2015;131: 1019–30.
8. Gogiraju R, Xu X, Bochenek ML, Steinbrecher JH, Lehnart SE, Wenzel P, Kessel M, Zeisberg E.M, Dobbelstein, M, Schafer K. Endothelial p53 deletion improves angiogenesis and prevents cardiac fibrosis and heart failure induced by pressure overload in mice. J Am Heart Assoc. 2015;4:e001770.
9. Halberg N, Khan T, Trujillo ME, Wernstedt-Asterholm I, Attie AD, Sherwani S, Wang ZV, Landskroner-Eiger S, Dineen S, Magalang UJ et al. Hypoxia-inducible factor 1alpha induces fibrosis and insulin resistance in white adipose tissue. Mol Cell Biol. 2009;29:4467–83.
10. Hayflick L, Moorhead PS. The serial cultivation of human diploid cell strains. Exp Cell Res. 1961;25:585–621.
11. He Q, Gao Z, Yin J, Zhang J, Yun Z, Ye J. Regulation of HIF-1{alpha} activity in adipose tissue by obesity-associated factors: adipogenesis, insulin, and hypoxia. Am J Physiol Endocrinol Metab. 2011;300:E877–885.
12. Jaskelioff M, Muller FL, Paik JH, Thomas E, Jiang S, Adams AC, Sahin E, Kost-Alimova M, Protopopov A, Cadinanos J et al. Telomerase reactivation reverses tissue degeneration in aged telomerase-deficient mice. Nature. 2011;469:102–6.

13. Kasner M, Westermann D, Lopez B, Gaub R, Escher F, Kuhl U, Schultheiss HP, Tschope C. Diastolic tissue Doppler indexes correlate with the degree of collagen expression and cross-linking in heart failure and normal ejection fraction. J Am Coll Cardiol. 2011;57:977–85.

14. Kikuchi R, Nakamura K, MacLauchlan S, Ngo DT, Shimizu I, Fuster JJ, Katanasaka Y, Yoshida S, Qiu Y, Yamaguchi TP et al. An antiangiogenic isoform of VEGF-A contributes to impaired vascularization in peripheral artery disease. Nat Med. 2014;20:1464–71.

15. Lumeng CN, Saltiel AR. Inflammatory links between obesity and metabolic disease. J Clin Invest. 2011;121:2111–7.

16. Minamino T, Orimo M, Shimizu I, Kunieda T, Yokoyama M, Ito T, Nojima A, Nabetani A, Oike Y, Matsubara H et al. A crucial role for adipose tissue p53 in the regulation of insulin resistance. Nat Med. 2009;15:1082–7.

17. Miranda M, Escote X, Ceperuelo-Mallafre V, Megia A, Caubet E, Naf S, Gomez JM, Gonzalez-Clemente JM, Vicente V, Vendrell J. Relation between human LPIN1, hypoxia and endoplasmic reticulum stress genes in subcutaneous and visceral adipose tissue. Int J Obes (Lond). 2010;34:679–86.

18. Nedergaard J, Cannon B. The changed metabolic world with human brown adipose tissue: therapeutic visions. Cell Metab. 2010;11:268–72.

19. Ngo DT, Farb MG, Kikuchi R, Karki S, Tiwari S, Bigornia SJ, Bates DO, LaValley MP, Hamburg NM, Vita JA et al. Antiangiogenic actions of vascular endothelial growth factor-A165b, an inhibitory isoform of vascular endothelial growth factor-A, in human obesity. Circulation. 2014;130:1072–80.

20. Ouchi N, Parker JL, Lugus JJ, Walsh K. Adipokines in inflammation and metabolic disease. Nat Rev Immunol. 2011;11:85–97.

21. Pasarica M, Sereda OR, Redman LM, Albarado DC, Hymel DT, Roan LE, Rood JC, Burk DH, Smith SR. Reduced adipose tissue oxygenation in human obesity: evidence for rarefaction, macrophage chemotaxis, and inflammation without an angiogenic response. Diabetes. 2009;58:718–25.

22. Paulus WJ, Tschope C. A novel paradigm for heart failure with preserved ejection fraction: comorbidities drive myocardial dysfunction and remodeling through coronary microvascular endothelial inflammation. J Am Coll Cardiol. 2013;62:263–71.

23. Pillon NJ, Bilan PJ, Fink LN, Klip A. Cross-talk between skeletal muscle and immune cells: muscle-derived mediators and metabolic implications. Am J Physiol Endocrinol Metab. 2013;304:E453–465.

24. Rodier F, Coppe JP, Patil CK, Hoeijmakers WA, Munoz DP, Raza SR, Freund A, Campeau E, Davalos AR, Campisi J. Persistent DNA damage signalling triggers senescence-associated inflammatory cytokine secretion. Nat Cell Biol. 2009;11:973–9.

25. Sano M, Minamino T, Toko H, Miyauchi H, Orimo M, Qin Y, Akazawa H, Tateno K, Kayama Y, Harada M et al. p53-induced inhibition of Hif-1 causes cardiac dysfunction during pressure overload. Nature. 2007;446:444–8.

26. Selby DE, Palmer BM, LeWinter MM, Meyer M. Tachycardia-induced diastolic dysfunction and resting tone in myocardium from patients with a normal ejection fraction. J Am Coll Cardiol. 2011;58:147–54.

27. Serrano M, Lin AW, McCurrach ME, Beach D, Lowe SW. Oncogenic ras provokes premature cell senescence associated with accumulation of p53 and p16INK4a. Cell. 1997;88:593–602.

28. Shimizu, I., Aprahamian, T., Kikuchi, R., Shimizu, A., Papanicolaou, K.N., MacLauchlan, S., Maruyama, S., and Walsh, K. (2014a). Vascular rarefaction mediates whitening of brown fat in obesity. J Clin Invest 124, 2099-2112.

29. Shimizu I, Minamino T, Toko H, Okada S, Ikeda H, Yasuda N, Tateno K, Moriya J, Yokoyama M, Nojima A et al. Excessive cardiac insulin signaling exacerbates systolic dysfunction induced by pressure overload in rodents. J Clin Invest. 2010;120:1506–14.

30. Shimizu I, Yoshida Y, Katsuno T, Tateno K, Okada S, Moriya J, Yokoyama M, Nojima A, Ito T, Zechner R et al. p53-induced adipose tissue inflammation is critically involved in the development of insulin resistance in heart failure. Cell Metab. 2012;15:51–64.

31. Shimizu I, Yoshida Y, Moriya J, Nojima A, Uemura A, Kobayashi Y, Minamino T. Semaphorin3E-induced inflammation contributes to insulin resistance in dietary obesity. Cell Metab. 2013;18:491–504.

32. Shimizu, I., Yoshida, Y., Suda, M., and Minamino, T. (2014b). DNA damage response and metabolic disease. Cell Metab 20, 967-977.

33. Shiojima I, Sato K, Izumiya Y, Schiekofer S, Ito M, Liao R, Colucci WS, Walsh K. Disruption of coordinated cardiac hypertrophy and angiogenesis contributes to the transition to heart failure. J Clin Invest. 2005;115:2108–18.

34. Stanford KI, Middelbeek RJ, Townsend KL, An D, Nygaard EB, Hitchcox KM, Markan KR, Nakano K, Hirshman MF, Tseng YH et al. Brown adipose tissue regulates glucose homeostasis and insulin sensitivity. J Clin Invest. 2013;123:215–23.

35. Sun K, Wernstedt Asterholm I, Kusminski CM, Bueno AC, Wang ZV, Pollard JW, Brekken RA, Scherer PE. Dichotomous effects of VEGF-A on adipose tissue dysfunction. Proc Natl Acad Sci U S A. 2012;109:5874–9.

36. Sung HK, Doh KO, Son JE, Park JG, Bae Y, Choi S, Nelson, SM, Cowling R, Nagy K, Michael IP et al. Adipose vascular endothelial growth factor regulates metabolic homeostasis through angiogenesis. Cell Metab. 2013;17:61–72.

37. Tchkonia T, Zhu Y, van Deursen J, Campisi J, Kirkland JL. Cellular senescence and the senescent secretory phenotype: therapeutic opportunities. J Clin Invest. 2013;123:966–72.

38. van Heerebeek L, Borbely A, Niessen HW, Bronzwaer JG, van der Velden J, Stienen GJ, Linke WA, Laarman GJ, Paulus WJ. Myocardial structure and function differ in systolic and diastolic heart failure. Circulation. 2006;113: 1966–73.

39. Voros G, Maquoi E, Demeulemeester D, Clerx N, Collen D, Lijnen HR. Modulation of angiogenesis during adipose tissue development in murine models of obesity. Endocrinology. 2005;146:4545–54.

40. Ye J, Gao Z, Yin J, He Q. Hypoxia is a potential risk factor for chronic inflammation and adiponectin reduction in adipose tissue of ob/ob and dietary obese mice. Am J Physiol Endocrinol Metab. 2007;293:E1118–1128.

41. Yokoyama M, Okada S, Nakagomi A, Moriya J, Shimizu I, Nojima A, Yoshida Y, Ichimiya H, Kamimura N, Kobayashi Y et al. Inhibition of endothelial p53 improves metabolic abnormalities related to dietary obesity. Cell Rep. 2014; 7(5):1691–703.

42. Yoshida Y, Shimizu I, Katsuumi G, Jiao S, Suda M, Hayashi Y, Minamino T. p53-induced inflammation exacerbates cardiac dysfunction during pressure overload. J Mol Cell Cardiol. 2015;85:183–98.

17

Roles of nitric oxide and ethyl pyruvate after peripheral nerve injury

Sandesh Panthi[1][*] and Kripa Gautam[2]

Abstract

Short-lived reactive nitrogen species and reactive oxygen species have acquired significant attention in the field of biomedical science. Nitric oxide (NO), which was thought to be an unstable gas and pollutant, is now regarded as a gas transmitter like H_2S and CO. NO is synthesized inside the mammalian body by L-arginine via three different isoforms of NO synthase whereas pyruvate is a glycolysis product and substrate for TCA cycle. Due to poor solubility and stability, therapeutic potential of pyruvate is limited. Ethyl pyruvate (EP) is now considered as a suitable replacement of pyruvate. In this paper, we will try to focus the effect of NO and EP in Schwann cell dedifferentiation, proliferation, nerve degeneration, and regeneration during Wallerian degeneration (WD) of peripheral nerve injury along with their neuroprotective effects, cardiovascular functioning, support in hepatic complication, etc.

Keywords: Nitric oxide, Ethyl pyruvate, Peripheral nerve injury, Gasotransmitter, Wallerian degeneration

Background

Nitric oxide is a unique biological messenger which was thought to be an unstable gas and noxious pollutant for all these years, but recently, it is regarded as a fascinating gasotransmitter [1, 2]. The finding of neuromodulators like CO, NO, and H_2S has entirely changed the prospect of synaptic transmission, and discovery of NO as a neurotransmitter has uncovered the leads for CO [3]. NO was first discovered to be a substance formed by macrophages, and they had the ability to kill tumor cells and fungi and was found to be an endothelium-derived relaxing factor [4]. All these melodramatic properties led researchers to an impression that NO is formed in the brain and finally all observations came true [5–7].

The beneficial roles of nitric oxide are changing periodically based on the research and successful discovery via several animal experiments. It was first linked with noradrenergic non-cholinergic neurotransmission in the end of the nineteenth century [8], and now it is seen as a major chemical messenger [9] and mediator of synaptic transmission and plasticity with its most appealing role in peripheral nerve injury [10, 11]. Various studies are also performed to find the role of NO in cardiovascular

reflexes and vaso-neuronal coupling in CNS [12, 13]. Claimed as the molecule of the year in 1992 by Journal Science [14], the discovery of pathways and roles of NO was acknowledged by scientists with the noble prize in physiology and medicine after 6 years [15].

In addition to the physiological role of NO, this study will be mainly focused on the role of nitric oxide during Wallerian degeneration in peripheral nerves, including its role in peripheral nerve degeneration and regeneration where we will try to find its therapeutic potential in peripheral demyelination disorder.

Synthesis and regulation of NO in nervous system

NO is biologically synthesized/produced from the amino acid L-arginine molecular oxygen as substrate via the members of NO synthase (NOS) [16]. There are three isoforms of nitric oxide synthase which are genetically different and required for NO production [17]. Three isoforms include:

1. Inducible nitric oxide synthase
2. Endothelial nitric oxide synthase
3. Neuronal nitric oxide synthase

Within the brain, NOS has been found in gamma-aminobutyric acid interneurons, aminergic, and peptidergic

* Correspondence: sanpan276@gmail.com
[1]Otago School of Biomedical Sciences, University of Otago, Otago, New Zealand
Full list of author information is available at the end of the article

neurons and in neurons that use excitatory amino acid glutamate transmitter [15].

NO from nNOS and eNOS are produced in low concentration, and they act as a messenger for signal transduction while NO liberated from iNOS are in high concentration provide immunological support [18]. Under normal physiological condition, it was found that the concentration of NO fluctuates in the range of low values [19]. In the brain, during ischemia or other injuries, the level of NO rises due to production via nNOS which is triggered and modulated via glutamate [20]. On other conditions like inflammation, the level of NO, produced by iNOS, is high but temporary. So, it is often termed as a double-edged sword [21]. nNOS and eNOS are regulated via a calcium-dependent manner but iNOS via gene transcription [22]. Tissue distribution of nNOS includes CNS, PNS, skeletal muscle, and lung epithelia whereas iNOS is primarily found in macrophages, glial cells, and hepatocytes [23]. eNOS is found in endothelial cells, smooth muscle cells, and hippocampus [24].

Nitric oxide and peripheral nerve injury

Peripheral nerve injury is a complex histopathological event often termed as Wallerian degeneration (WD) [25]. This type of injury results in hyperalgesia and allodynia which are a part of neuropathic pain. It is a well-established fact that unlike the central nervous system, peripheral nerve axons can regenerate [26]. However, due to poor axonal growth, there is a loss of sensation and muscle weakness. Some components of inflammation are helpful or sometimes harmful for nerve regeneration after peripheral nerve injury [27].

After peripheral nerve injury, a broad range of mechanisms are initiated in the proximal and distal stump of a neuron [28]. For successful growth and reinnervation of the target organ and subsequently for a successful regeneration, the following series of events occur and it is compulsory, i.e.,

1. WD including myelin breakdown and clearance of distal stump.
2. Dedifferentiation of previously myelinating Schwann cell to regeneration.

The cellular events in WD can be further reclassified into neuronal reaction, response of Schwann cell, infiltration of hematogenes cell, and their relationship with other cell of distal nerve stump [29].

And, it was found that iNOS and nNOS are both important during peripheral nerve injury, and NO released by them participates in successful WD and peripheral nerve regeneration [30, 31].

To date, few animal experiments demonstrated the effect of iNOS and nNOS in peripheral nerve degeneration

and regeneration and are summarized as the critical factors in the repair of injured nerve tissues. Levy et al. used iNOS-knockout mice to observe how peripheral nerve responds in chronic constriction partial nerve injury (neuropathic pain), crush of nerve trunk, and complete nerve transection. For chronic constriction injury, they evaluated iNOS mRNA and protein expression, whereas for nerve crush and nerve transection, they used myelinated fiber morphometry and electrophysiological recording. They were able to conclude that mice lacking iNOS (iNOS-KO) has delay in the breakdown of myelinated fiber and myelinated fiber regeneration and also failed to upregulate iNOS mRNA and protein reaction. Delay in the fiber breakdown distal to injury site also delayed the whole procedure of WD of myelinated fiber. Chronic constriction model was also associated with slowed breakdown of myelinated fiber with normal initiation but dally the expression of behavioral characteristics of neuropathic pain [32, 33].

The presence of superoxide in the injury site forms peroxynitrite with NO, which is a powerful antioxidant that helps in the initiation of lipid peroxidation [34]. Lipid peroxidation assists the dissolution of myelin sheath or phagocytic effect of myelin by macrophages [35, 36]. Besides this, peripheral nerve injury is also correlated with supervision of iNOS in macrophages and Schwann cells [37]. iNOS is believed to be a contributing enzyme, and production of NO via iNOS has a role in wound healing [38], traumatic brain injury [39], MPTP-induced dopaminergic neurodegeneration [40], and cerebral ischemia [41, 42]. The level of NO is also found to be increased in the patient with Alzheimer's disease and HIV infection [16, 32]. Another finding suggests that local non-direct inflammation of peripheral nerve after injury blocks the nerve regeneration and over production of NO via iNOS-pathway can block the repair [37]. This study used sciatic nerve transection of male SD rats as an experimental model. Using adult male wistar rats, Campuzano et al. [43] found that there are age-dependent changes in the macrophage response to injury and iNOS expression is reduced which also can affect the neurodegeneration process and injury outcome in aged individuals. Some researchers tried to find out the outcomes by disrupting the mouse iNOS gene. They carried out by deleting the promoter region of axons and disrupting some important binding domains of iNOS. In their conclusion, they stated the role of NO in septic shock and mortality [38].

Sciatic nerve model of mice is an ideal way for the study of effect of production of NO by three different isoforms of NOS. One study also suggests the similar type of result, where by blocking endogenous supply of NO in peripheral nerve via knocking out iNOS leads to the delay in WD which impedes the regenerative outcome [32, 43, 44]. Acetylcholinesterase histochemistry was used to examine WD. The hindered nerve regeneration in iNOS-KO mice foreground the significance of iNOS expression and liberation of NO after injury underpin the notion that effective regeneration in PNS depend on the exact timeframe of cellular and molecular degeneration procedure [18, 45, 46]. NO is also found to be connected with the removal of misdirected axons, and absence of NO or knocking out NOS also causes the disturbance in the pruning mechanism [47]. Neuroprotective and neurodegenerative roles of NO based on iNOS, eNOS, and nNOS are explained in Fig. 1.

Ethyl pyruvate and its roles

Reactive oxygen species (ROS) scavenging property of pyruvate is well explained via various in vivo and in vitro experiments. It is found to be neuroprotective against H_2O_2 [48], hemorrhagic shock [49, 50], cerebral ischemic

injury, zinc toxicity, pressure-induced retinal damage, and acute renal failure. It is also found to provide neuroprotective action against β-amyloid and zinc [51, 52].

A recent investigation also demonstrated the role of ethyl pyruvate in long-term neurological improvement after traumatic injury. Use of sensorimotor and cognitive neurobehavioral tests in this study suggested that ethyl pyruvate may cease the outrageous cycle of blood brain barrier disruption and damage leading to the long-term neuroprotective role. Lots of pre-clinical studies already had concluded the role of ethyl pyruvate from amelioration of hepatic neurons to acute lung injury and preservation of renal function to T-cell functions.

Recently, the effect of ethyl pyruvate in peripheral nerve injury is also identified, and it became one of the novel findings in the field of neuroscience. Park et al. [53] used 5-week-old mice to study the dedifferentiation and proliferation pattern of a Schwann cell using ethyl pyruvate during a process of WD in peripheral nerve injury. Results in this study were achieved by using antibodies against p75NGFR (p75 nerve growth factor receptor), LAMP1 (lysosomal associated membrane protein1), phosphor-p44/43MPK, and Ki67. From immunostaining and Western blot analysis, it was detected that ethyl pyruvate inhibits p-ERK1/2 expression, lysosomal activation, p75NGFR, and Ki67 expression. Sciatic explants of mice were treated with ethyl pyruvate and proved its role to inhibit Schwann cell dedifferentiation by inhibiting p-ERK1/2 and p75NGFR expression in denervated Schwann cells. It is also a well-established fact that during WD, lysosomal proteosomal protein are activated in dedifferentiated Schwann cells to remove myelin sheath debris. They remarkably observed reduced LAMP1 expression in explants treated with ethyl pyruvate. A similar type of result was discovered using cell proliferation marker Ki67 which led them to a conclusion that ethyl pyruvate also inhibits Schwann cell proliferation during WD stage of peripheral nerve injury. Effect of EP in paclitaxel-induced neuropathic pain was also investigated by researchers, but they were not able to relate mechanical allodynia of this type of neuropathic pain with EP [54].

Conclusions

Regeneration is possible in peripheral nervous system even after nerve damage which is not possible in CNS. Peripheral nerve regeneration involves a series of events where WD is the major phenomenon. Study of these processes and effects is crucial for the treatment of demyelinating and peripheral degenerative disorders. This study tried to brief the discussion of recent findings on the importance of nitric oxide and ethyl pyruvate on peripheral nerve regeneration. Disruption of binding domains of iNOS or use of iNOS-KO mice gave the impression of delayed WD. Additionally, neurodegeneration and regeneration process is also affected

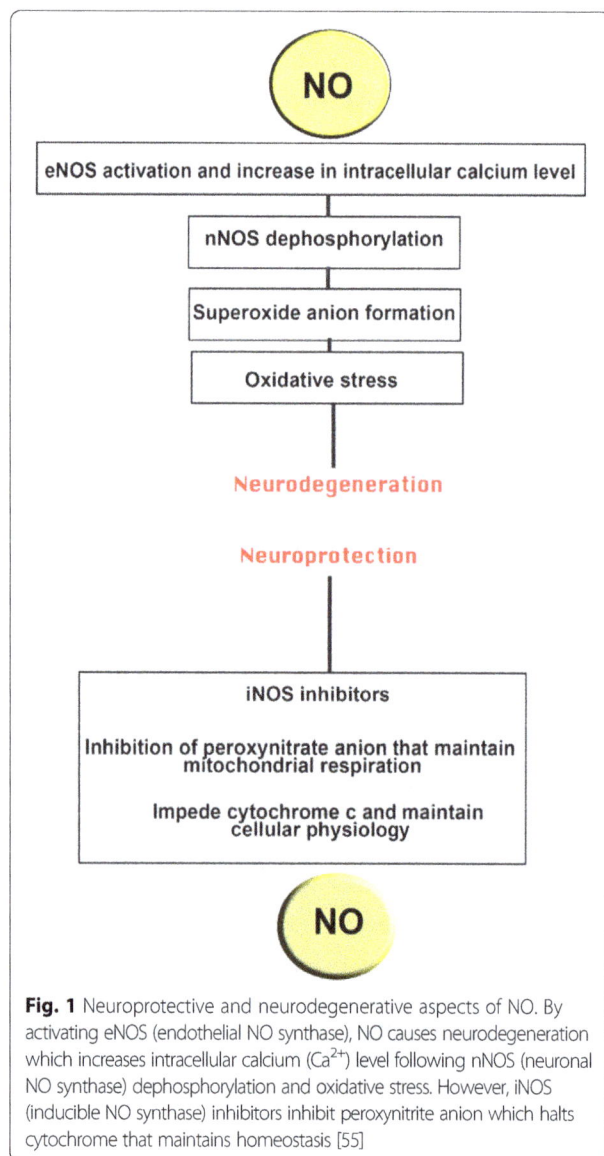

Fig. 1 Neuroprotective and neurodegenerative aspects of NO. By activating eNOS (endothelial NO synthase), NO causes neurodegeneration which increases intracellular calcium (Ca^{2+}) level following nNOS (neuronal NO synthase) dephosphorylation and oxidative stress. However, iNOS (inducible NO synthase) inhibitors inhibit peroxynitrite anion which halts cytochrome that maintains homeostasis [55]

by the age of an individual. The role of NO is also found in removal of misdirected axons and enhance the pruning mechanism of axons. Importance and role of ethyl pyruvate in and after peripheral nerve injury are still in the infant stage of finding. However, recently, few researchers claimed that ethyl pyruvate inhibits Schwann cell dedifferentiation and proliferation. It is also believed that reduction of oxidative stress is the result of this inhibition. Thus, for the treatment of disorders related to peripheral nerve injury, new strategy and finding will be helpful.

Abbreviations
CNS: Central nervous system; CO: Carbon-monoxide; eNOS: Endothelial nitric oxide synthase; EP: Ethyl pyruvate; H_2O_2: Hydrogen peroxide; H_2S: Hydrogen sulfide; HIV: Human immuno virus; iNOS: Inducible nitric oxide synthase; LAMP1: Lysosomal-associated membrane protein; MPK: Mitogen-activated protein kinase; mRNA: Messenger ribonucleic acid; nNOS: Neuronal nitric oxide synthase; NO: Nitric oxide; NOS: Nitric oxide synthase; p75NGFR: p75 nerve growth factor receptor; p-ERK1/2: p-extracellular regulated kinase 1/2; PNS: Peripheral nervous system; ROS: Reactive oxygen species; TCA: Tricarboxylic acid; WD: Wallerian degeneration

Acknowledgements
Not any

Funding
Not any

Authors' contributions
SP and KP designed and planned about the review topic. SP wrote the manuscript. KG provided intellectual input to the manuscript. Both authors read and approved the final manuscript.

Competing interests
The authors declare that they have no competing interests.

Author details
[1]Otago School of Biomedical Sciences, University of Otago, Otago, New Zealand. [2]China Medical University, Shenyang, People's Republic of China.

References
1. Toledo JC, Augusto O. Connecting the chemical and biological properties of nitric oxide. Chem Res Toxicol. 2012;25:975–89.
2. Basudhar D, Ridnour LA, Cheng R, Kesarwala AH, Heinecke J, Wink DA. Biological signaling by small inorganic molecules. Coord Chem Rev. 2016; 306:708–23.
3. Panthi S, Chung H-J, Jung J, Jeong NY. Physiological importance of hydrogen sulfide: emerging potent neuroprotector and neuromodulator. In: Oxidative Medicine and Cellular Longevity 2016; 2016.
4. Loscalzo J. The identification of nitric oxide as endothelium-derived relaxing factor. Circ Res. 2013;113:100–3.
5. Faro MLL, Fox B, Whatmore JL, Winyard PG, Whiteman M. Hydrogen sulfide and nitric oxide interactions in inflammation. Nitric Oxide. 2014;41:38–47.
6. Ersoy A, Koc ER, Sahin S, Duzgun U, Acar B, Ilhan A. Possible effects of rosuvastatin on noise-induced oxidative stress in rat brain. Noise Health. 2014;16:18.
7. Garry P, Ezra M, Rowland M, Westbrook J, Pattinson K. The role of the nitric oxide pathway in brain injury and its treatment—from bench to bedside. Exp Neurol. 2015;263:235–43.
8. Rajfer J, Aronson WJ, Bush PA, Dorey FJ, Ignarro LJ. Nitric oxide as a mediator of relaxation of the corpus cavernosum in response to nonadrenergic, noncholinergic neurotransmission. N Engl J Med. 1992; 326:90–4.
9. Lamattina L, García-Mata C, Graziano M, Pagnussat G. Nitric oxide: the versatility of an extensive signal molecule. Annu Rev Plant Biol. 2003;54:109–36.
10. Zochodne D, Levy D. Nitric oxide in damage, disease and repair of the peripheral nervous system. Cell Mole Biol (Noisy-le-Grand, France). 2005;51: 255–67.
11. Tanabe M, Nagatani Y, Saitoh K, Takasu K, Ono H. Pharmacological assessments of nitric oxide synthase isoforms and downstream diversity of NO signaling in the maintenance of thermal and mechanical hypersensitivity after peripheral nerve injury in mice. Neuropharmacology. 2009;56:702–8.
12. Zanzinger J. Role of nitric oxide in the neural control of cardiovascular function. Cardiovasc Res. 1999;43:639–49.
13. Gkaliagkousi E, Ferro A. Nitric oxide signalling in the regulation of cardiovascular and platelet function. Front Biosci (Landmark edition). 2010; 16:1873–97.
14. Cech TR, Bennett D, Jasny B, Kelner KL, Miller LJ, Szuromi PD, Voss DF, Kiberstis PA, Parks S, Ray LB. The molecule of the year. Science. 1992; 258:1861.
15. Zhou L, Zhu D-Y. Neuronal nitric oxide synthase: structure, subcellular localization, regulation, and clinical implications. Nitric Oxide. 2009;20:223–30.
16. Calabrese V, Mancuso C, Calvani M, Rizzarelli E, Butterfield DA, Stella AMG. Nitric oxide in the central nervous system: neuroprotection versus neurotoxicity. Nat Rev Neurosci. 2007;8:766–75.
17. Boissel J-P, Schwarz PM, Förstermann U. Neuronal-type NO synthase: transcript diversity and expressional regulation. Nitric Oxide. 1998;2:337–49.
18. Prast H, Philippu A. Nitric oxide as modulator of neuronal function. Prog Neurobiol. 2001;64:51–68.
19. Tieu K, Ischiropoulos H, Przedborski S. Nitric oxide and reactive oxygen species in Parkinson's disease. IUBMB Life. 2003;55:329–35.
20. Keynes RG, Garthwaite J. Nitric oxide and its role in ischaemic brain injury. Curr Mol Med. 2004;4:179–91.
21. Mocellin S, Bronte V, Nitti D. Nitric oxide, a double edged sword in cancer biology: searching for therapeutic opportunities. Med Res Rev. 2007;27:317–52.
22. Kim Y, Moon JS, Lee KS, Park SY, Cheong J, Kang HS, Lee HY, Do Kim H. Ca 2+/calmodulin-dependent protein phosphatase calcineurin mediates the expression of iNOS through IKK and NF-κB activity in LPS-stimulated mouse peritoneal macrophages and RAW 264.7 cells. Biochem Biophys Res Commun. 2004;314:695–703.
23. Förstermann U, Sessa WC. Nitric oxide synthases: regulation and function. Eur Heart J. 2012;33:829–37.
24. Albrecht EW, Stegeman CA, Heeringa P, Henning RH, van Goor H. Protective role of endothelial nitric oxide synthase. J Pathol. 2003;199:8–17.
25. Dubový P. Wallerian degeneration and peripheral nerve conditions for both axonal regeneration and neuropathic pain induction. Ann Anat Anat Anz. 2011;193:267–75.
26. Gaudet AD, Popovich PG, Ramer MS. Wallerian degeneration: gaining perspective on inflammatory events after peripheral nerve injury. J Neuroinflammation. 2011;8:110.
27. Coleman MP, Freeman MR. Wallerian degeneration, wlds, and nmnat. Annu Rev Neurosci. 2010;33:245–67.
28. Burnett MG, Zager EL. Pathophysiology of peripheral nerve injury: a brief review. Neurosurg Focus. 2004;16:1–7.
29. Mcdonald D, Cheng C, Chen Y, Zochodne D. Early events of peripheral nerve regeneration. Neuron Glia Biol. 2006;2:139–47.
30. Martucci C, Trovato AE, Costa B, Borsani E, Franchi S, Magnaghi V, Panerai AE, Rodella LF, Valsecchi AE, Sacerdote P. The purinergic antagonist PPADS reduces pain related behaviours and interleukin-1β, interleukin-6, iNOS and nNOS overproduction in central and peripheral nervous system after peripheral neuropathy in mice. Pain. 2008;137:81–95.

31. Guan Y, Yaster M, Raja SN, Tao Y-X. Genetic knockout and pharmacologic inhibition of neuronal nitric oxide synthase attenuate nerve injury-induced mechanical hypersensitivity in mice. Mol Pain. 2007;3:29.

32. Levy D, Kubes P, Zochodne DW. Delayed peripheral nerve degeneration, regeneration, and pain in mice lacking inducible nitric oxide synthase. J Neuropathol Exp Neurol. 2001;60:411–21.

33. Levy D, Höke A, Zochodne DW. Local expression of inducible nitric oxide synthase in an animal model of neuropathic pain. Neurosci Lett. 1999;260:207–9.

34. Hogg N, Kalyanaraman B. Nitric oxide and lipid peroxidation. Biochim Biophys Acta Bioenerg. 1999;1411:378–84.

35. Rubbo H, Radi R, Trujillo M, Telleri R, Kalyanaraman B, Barnes S, Kirk M, Freeman BA. Nitric oxide regulation of superoxide and peroxynitrite-dependent lipid peroxidation. Formation of novel nitrogen-containing oxidized lipid derivatives. J Biol Chem. 1994;269:26066–75.

36. Radi R, Beckman JS, Bush KM, Freeman BA. Peroxynitrite-induced membrane lipid peroxidation: the cytotoxic potential of superoxide and nitric oxide. Arch Biochem Biophys. 1991;288:481–7.

37. McDonald DS, Cheng C, Martinez JA, Zochodne DW. Regenerative arrest of inflamed peripheral nerves: role of nitric oxide. Neuroreport. 2007;18:1635–40.

38. Yamasaki K, Edington HD, McClosky C, Tzeng E, Lizonova A, Kovesdi I, Steed DL, Billiar TR. Reversal of impaired wound repair in iNOS-deficient mice by topical adenoviral-mediated iNOS gene transfer. J Clin Investig. 1998;101:967.

39. Sinz EH, Kochanek PM, Dixon CE, Clark RS, Carcillo JA, Schiding JK, Chen M, Wisniewski SR, Carlos TM, Williams D. Inducible nitric oxide synthase is an endogenous neuroprotectant after traumatic brain injury in rats and mice. J Clin Invest. 1999;104:647–56.

40. Liberatore GT, Jackson-Lewis V, Vukosavic S, Mandir AS, Vila M, McAuliffe WG, Dawson VL, Dawson TM, Przedborski S. Inducible nitric oxide synthase stimulates dopaminergic neurodegeneration in the MPTP model of Parkinson disease. Nat Med. 1999;5:1403–9.

41. Nogawa S, Forster C, Zhang F, Nagayama M, Ross ME, Iadecola C. Interaction between inducible nitric oxide synthase and cyclooxygenase-2 after cerebral ischemia. Proc Natl Acad Sci. 1998;95:10966–71.

42. Iadecola C, Zhang F, Xu S, Casey R, Ross ME. Inducible nitric oxide synthase gene expression in brain following cerebral ischemia. J Cereb Blood Flow Metab. 1995;15:378–84.

43. Campuzano O, Castillo-Ruiz M, Acarin L, Castellano B, Gonzalez B. Distinct pattern of microglial response, cyclooxygenase-2, and inducible nitric oxide synthase expression in the aged rat brain after excitotoxic damage. J Neurosci Res. 2008;86:3170–83.

44. Keilhoff G, Fansa H, Wolf G. Differences in peripheral nerve degeneration/regeneration between wild type and neuronal nitric oxide synthase knockout mice. J Neurosci Res. 2002;68:432–41.

45. Turner JE, Glaze KA. The early stages of Wallerian degeneration in the severed optic nerve of the newt (Triturus viridescens). Anat Rec. 1977;187:291–309.

46. Yuan Q, Su H, Chiu K, Lin Z-X, Wu W. Assessment of the rate of spinal motor axon regeneration by choline acetyltransferase immunohistochemistry following sciatic nerve crush injury in mice: laboratory investigation. J Neurosurg. 2014;120:502–8.

47. Rabinovich D, Yaniv SP, Alyagor I, Schuldiner O. Nitric oxide as a switching mechanism between axon degeneration and regrowth during developmental remodeling. Cell. 2016;164:170–82.

48. Wang X, Perez E, Liu R, Yan L-J, Mallet RT, Yang S-H. Pyruvate protects mitochondria from oxidative stress in human neuroblastoma SK-N-SH cells. Brain Res. 2007;1132:1–9.

49. Mongan PD, Capacchione J, West S, Karaian J, Dubois D, Keneally R, Sharma P. Pyruvate improves redox status and decreases indicators of hepatic apoptosis during hemorrhagic shock in swine. Am J Phys Heart Circ Phys. 2002;283:H1634–44.

50. Mongan PD, Capacchione J, Fontana JL, West S, Bunger R. Pyruvate improves cerebral metabolism during hemorrhagic shock. Am J Phys Heart Circ Phys. 2001;50:H854.

51. Fink M. Ethyl pyruvate: a novel anti-inflammatory agent. J Intern Med. 2007;261:349–62.

52. Kawahara M, Kato-Negishi M, Kuroda Y. Rapid communication: pyruvate blocks zinc-induced neurotoxicity in immortalized hypothalamic neurons. Cell Mol Neurobiol. 2002;22:87–93.

53. Park BS, et al. A novel effect of ethyl pyruvate in Schwann cell de differentiation and proliferation during Wallerian degeneration. Anim Cells Syst. 2015;19(4):262–8.

54. Choi SS, et al. Effect of ethyl pyruvate on Paclitaxel-induced neuropathic pain in rats. Kor J Pain. 2013;26(2):135–41.

55. Shefa U, Geun Yeo S, Kim MS, et al. Role of gasotransmitters in oxidative stresses, neuroinflammation, and neuronal repair. Biomed Res Int. 2017;2017:15. Article ID 1689341

18

CTGF in kidney fibrosis and glomerulonephritis

Naohiro Toda[1], Masashi Mukoyama[2], Motoko Yanagita[1] and Hideki Yokoi[1*]

Abstract

Background: Glomerulonephritis, which causes inflammation in glomeruli, is a common cause of end-stage renal failure. Severe and prolonged inflammation can damage glomeruli and lead to kidney fibrosis. Connective tissue growth factor (CTGF) is a member of the CCN matricellular protein family, consisting of four domains, that regulates the signaling of other growth factors and promotes kidney fibrosis.

Main body of the abstract: CTGF can simultaneously interact with several factors with its four domains. The microenvironment differs depending on the types of cells and tissues and differentiation stages of these cells. The diverse biological actions of CTGF on various types of cells and tissues depend on this difference in microenvironment. In the kidney, CTGF is expressed at low levels in normal condition and its expression is upregulated by kidney fibrosis. CTGF expression is known to be upregulated in the extra-capillary and mesangial lesions of glomerulonephritis in human kidney biopsy samples. In addition to involvement in fibrosis, CTGF modulates the expression of inflammatory mediators, including cytokines and chemokines, through distinct signaling pathways, in various cell systems. In anti-glomerular basement membrane (GBM) glomerulonephritis, systemic CTGF knockout (Rosa-CTGF cKO) mice exhibit 50% reduction of proteinuria and decreased crescent formation and mesangial expansion compared with control mice. In addition to fibrotic markers, the glomerular mRNA expression of *Ccl2* is increased in the control mice with anti-GBM glomerulonephritis, and this increase is reduced in Rosa-CTGF cKO mice with nephritis. Accumulation of MAC2-positive cells in glomeruli is also reduced in Rosa-CTGF cKO mice. These results suggest that CTGF may be required for the upregulation of *Ccl2* expression not only in anti-GBM glomerulonephritis but also in other types of glomerulonephritis, such as IgA nephropathy; CTGF expression and accumulation of macrophages in the mesangial area have been documented in these glomerular diseases. CTGF induces the expression of inflammatory mediators and promotes cell adhesion.

Short conclusion: CTGF plays an important role in the development of glomerulonephritis by inducing the inflammatory process. CTGF is a potentiate target for the treatment of glomerulonephritis.

Keywords: CTGF, Glomerulonephritis, Inflammation, Macrophage, Chemokine

Background

Glomerulonephritis causes inflammation in glomeruli and occurs alone or as part of diseases such as vasculitis, systemic lupus erythematosus, cancer, and infections. Glomerulonephritis is a common cause of end-stage renal failure. Severe and prolonged inflammation can damage glomeruli and lead to kidney fibrosis. Kidney fibrosis is the unifying pathological feature of diverse renal disease. Emerging evidence suggests that connective tissue growth factor (CTGF) is a key player in the progression of kidney fibrosis. In addition, CTGF is known to participate in cell migration, proliferation, and inflammation. The efficacy of CTGF inhibition previously observed in a wide variety of animal models is now being evaluated in clinical trials. Therefore, CTGF appears to be a candidate therapeutic target for kidney disease. In this review, we present the current knowledge of the involvement of CTGF in kidney disease, especially glomerulonephritis.

Connective tissue growth factor

CTGF/CCN2 is a member of CCN family of matricellular proteins. CTGF was isolated with an antiserum

* Correspondence: yokoih@kuhp.kyoto-u.ac.jp
[1]Department of Nephrology, Graduate School of Medicine, Kyoto University, 54 Shogoin Kawahara-cho, Sakyo-ku, Kyoto 606-8507, Japan
Full list of author information is available at the end of the article

directed against the platelet growth factor from human endothelial cells in 1991. CTGF is a 36- to 38-kDa cysteine-rich secreted protein with 349 amino acids [1]. CCN family of human proteins contains six members. The name of CCN family is derived from the first letter of the first three identified members of the family CCN1-CCN3. The family members other than CTGF are cysteine-rich angiogenic inducer 61 (Cyr61/CCN1), nephroblastoma overexpressed genes (Nov/CCN3), and Wnt-inducible signaling pathway proteins 1–3 (WISP1-3/CCN4-6). CCN proteins are numbered in the order of their discovery, as proposed in 2003 [2]. Except for CCN5 which lacks domain 4, these proteins share a multimodular structure, with an N-terminal secretory signal peptide followed by four distinct conserved domains: the insulin-like growth factor-binding protein domain (domain 1; IGFBP), von Willebrand factor domain (domain 2; vWC), thrombospondin type 1 repeat (domain 3; TSP1), and a cystine knot (domain 4; CT). A hinge region susceptible to protease cleavage links domains 1 and 2, and domains 3 and 4 (Fig. 1). Human CTGF gene is located on chromosome 6q23.1 and has five exons that each encodes a signal peptide and domains 1 to 4 [3].

CTGF not only acts through their own putative receptors but also modifies various growth factors and cytokines. The specific receptor of CTGF has not been identified, and each domain of CTGF can bind to multiple ligands. These includes insulin-like growth factor-1 (IGF-1), fibronectin (domain 1: IGFBP), TGF-β1, bone morphogenetic factors, α5β3 integrin (domain 2: vWC), low-density lipoprotein receptor-related protein 1 (LRP-1), VEGF (domain 3: TSP1) and Wnt, integrins, heparan sulfate proteoglycan, LRPs, and epidermal growth factor receptor (EGFR; domain 4: CT). Thus, CTGF can

simultaneously interact with several factors with their four hands. As the microenvironment differs depending on the types of cells and tissues and differentiation stages of these cells, the diverse biological actions of CTGF on various types of cells and tissues would depend on this difference in microenvironment [4].

CTGF and development, and physiological functions

CTGF is expressed in various tissues in midgestation embryos, with the highest levels found in vascular tissues and maturing chondrocytes. Analysis of CTGF knockout mice reveals that CTGF deficiency leads to skeletal dysmorphisms due to impaired chondrocyte proliferation and extracellular matrix composition. CTGF is important for cell proliferation and matrix remodeling during chondrogenesis and is a key regulator coupling extracellular matrix remodeling to angiogenesis at the growth plate [5]. In kidney development, CTGF mRNA is presented in the immediate precursors of glomerular visceral and parietal epithelial cells in the comma- and S-shaped stages, but not in the earlier stages of nephron development. During the maturating glomerular stages, CTGF mRNA expression is maximal and present only in differentiating glomerular epithelial cells. CTGF protein is also present in the precursors of mesangial cells and glomerular endothelium [6]. The role of CTGF in kidney development cannot be excluded, but Falk et al. reported that 90% CTGF reduction does not lead to structural changes and albuminuria [7].

CTGF and kidney fibrosis

Kidney fibrosis is a common pathological feature in chronic kidney disease and characterized by glomerulosclerosis and

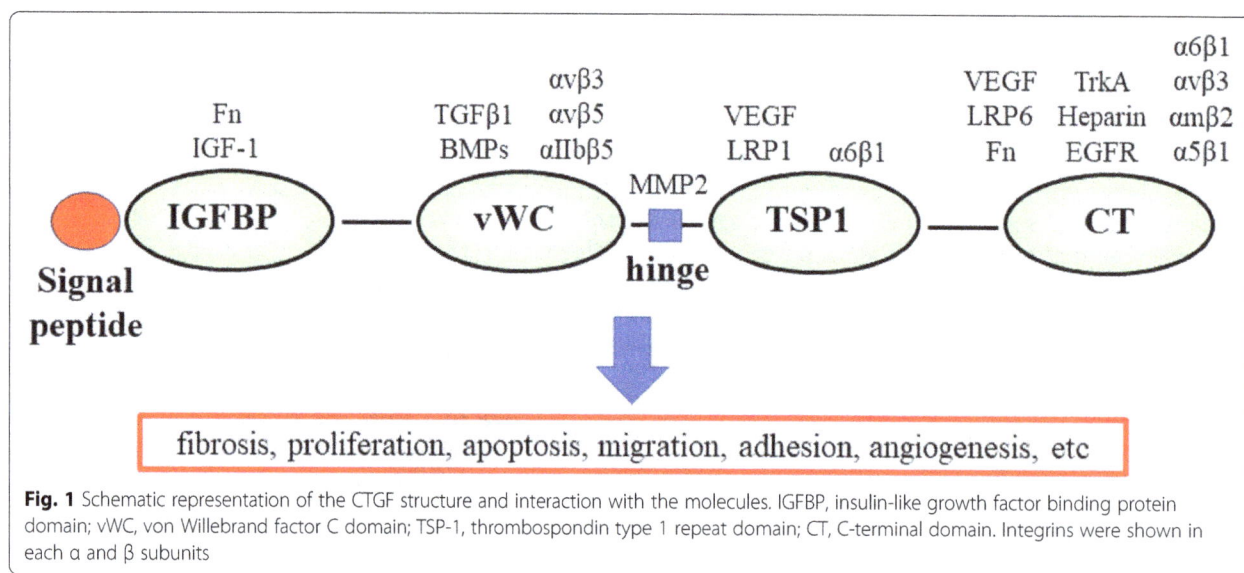

Fig. 1 Schematic representation of the CTGF structure and interaction with the molecules. IGFBP, insulin-like growth factor binding protein domain; vWC, von Willebrand factor C domain; TSP-1, thrombospondin type 1 repeat domain; CT, C-terminal domain. Integrins were shown in each α and β subunits

tubulointerstitial fibrosis. Various cytokines and growth factors are reportedly involved and associated with fibrogenic and inflammatory processes. Of these, TGF-β has been shown to play a central role in the development of renal fibrosis [8]. Igarashi et al. reported that CTGF is induced by TGF-β1 in wound healing and that there is a strong correlation between skin sclerosis and CTGF expression in the dermal fibroblasts of patients with systemic sclerosis [9, 10]. Mice overexpressing CTGF in fibroblast are susceptible to acceleration of tissue fibrosis that affects the skin, lung, kidney, and vascular system, most notably the small arteries [11]. In addition, CTGF-dependent activation of the tropomyosin-related kinase A receptor induces TIEG-1, a transcriptional receptor of Smad7, which represses Smad7, a natural receptor of TGF-β signaling. Thus, activation of CTGF increases phosph-Smad2/3, promoting transcription of Smad-responsive genes including CTGF itself. These results indicate that CTGF may be involved in fibrosis.

CTGF expression in fibrosis is also reported to occur in the kidney area. Exposure of mesangial cell to recombinant human CTGF significantly increased production of fibronectin and collagen type I. Induction of CTGF in rat mesangial cells due to high glucose levels is mediated by TGF-β [12]. The study of human kidney biopsy samples from various kidney diseases has revealed that CTGF expression level is increased in glomerulosclerosis and tubulointerstitial fibrosis [13]. Thereafter, many animal and in vitro experiments have demonstrated the pivotal role of CTGF in kidney fibrosis.

Relationship of CTGF expression levels in plasma or urine with kidney function has been reported [14, 15]. In patients with CKD, an independent association is observed between plasma CTGF level and estimated glomerular filtration rate (eGFR). In addition, plasma CTGF level correlates with residual kidney function in patients with end-stage kidney disease [14].

An interventional study of an animal model is first reported by Yokoi et al. Treatment of CTGF antisense oligonucleotide markedly attenuates the induction of fibronectin and collagen expressions in the rat unilateral ureteral obstruction (UUO) model [15]. Another study also showed the efficacy of CTGF inhibition by CTGF antisense oligonucleotide in subtotal nephrectomy of TGF-β transgenic mice [16].

In diabetes, the role of CTGF in disease development has been reported. Increased CTGF expression has been documented both in glomeruli and in tubulointerstitium [13]. Urinary CTGF is elevated as a result of both increased local production and reduced reabsorption due to tubular dysfunction and correlates with albuminuria and GFR. Thus, urinary CTGF might be as a suitable marker of diabetic nephropathy [17]. Overexpression of CTGF in the podocytes of a streptozotocin (STZ)-induced diabetes model is sufficient to exacerbate

proteinuria and mesangial expansion through functional impairment and loss of podocytes [18]. In a 16-week STZ-induced diabetic nephropathy model, CTGF heterozygous mice (CTGF +/−) with 50% lower CTGF expression develop less albuminuria, mesangial expansion, and glomerular basement thickness [19]. In cultured embryonic fibroblasts from wild-type mice, glucose increases the expressions of pro-collagens 1 and 4, fibronectin, and TSP1. By contrast, activation of these genes by high glucose is attenuated in CTGF+/− embryonic fibroblasts from wild-type mice [20]. On the other hand, Falk et al. reported that a heterozygous deletion of CTGF does not prevent severe kidney fibrosis. They examined the effect of CTGF on the progression of renal scarring in long-term STZ-induced diabetic nephropathy, in the advanced stage of obstructive nephropathy following UUO and in aristolochic acid (AA)-induced tubulotoxic nephritis by using heterozygous CTGF knockout mice. Unlike in mild and relatively early STZ-induced diabetic nephropathy, scarring of severely and chronically damaged kidneys induced by STZ, UUO, and AA is not attenuated by a 50% reduction in CTGF levels relative to normal levels [21].

Possible efficacy of anti-CTGF therapy has been explored by a genetic deletion and neutralizing antibody. Of these, FG-3019, a human monoclonal antibody to CTGF, has been used in some animal models, including pulmonary fibrosis, peritoneal fibrosis, and systemic sclerosis. These studies showed successful treatment for fibrosis by inhibition of CTGF [22]. In addition, FG-3019 has also humper tumor growth in mouse models of pancreatic cancer, ovarian cancer, and melanoma [23, 24]. Moreover, FG-3019 has been used in clinical trials for pulmonary fibrosis and pancreatic cancer and no serious adverse effects have been observed [25]. Although treatment for diabetic kidney disease with microalbuminuria using FG-3019 is well tolerated and associated with decreased albuminuria, there are no active trials in renal field [26].

CTGF and glomerulonephritis

Acute and chronic inflammation usually precedes the development of organ fibrosis. Activated inflammatory cells release many factors, including profibrotic cytokines such as TGF-β, and chronic inflammation leads to the development of fibrosis. CTGF is well known to participate in this fibrotic process. Apart from this fibrotic effect, several reports have showed the upregulation of CTGF expression in glomerulonephritis. Glomerulonephritis often develops from intra-glomerular activation via the classical or alternative complement pathway. Immune complexes can form different compartment of the glomerulus, which determines the resulting histopathological lesion, as different glomerular cell types are primarily activated. The result of histological lesions determined the classification of glomerulonephritis. Immune complex deposition in mesangial cell activates mesangial cells lead to mesangioproliferative glomerulonephritis, such as IgA nephropathy. Subendothelial immune complex deposition activates endothelial cells, as seen in lupus nephritis classes III and IV. Subepithelial immune complex deposition activate podocytes, as seen in membranous nephropathy usually cause massive proteinuria. Immune complex deposition in glomerular basement membrane (GBM) induces anti-GBM disease. Anti-neutrophil cytoplasmic antibody (ANCA)-associated glomerulonephritis develops the absence of immune complex deposits, as it is driven by both ANCA and cellular immunity [27]. Ito et al. showed that CTGF is strongly upregulated in the extra-capillary and severe mesangial proliferative lesions of IgA nephritis, crescentic glomerulonephritis, and focal segmental sclerosis in various human kidney biopsy samples [6, 13]. Another study reported that CTGF is strongly expressed in cellular and fibrocellular crescents and proposed that it is involved in extracellular matrix production by parietal epithelial cells [28]. The mRNA expression of CTGF in kidney biopsy samples from chronic glomerulonephritis is higher than that in control samples [29].

Animal models of glomerulonephritis also reported increased expression of CTGF. In anti-Thy-1.1 nephritis, CTGF mRNA expression is strongly increased in mesangial proliferative and extra-capillary lesions. Glomerular CTGF expression is maximal on day 7, in association with increased TGF-β1 mRNA and protein expression levels. The kinetics of CTGF expression strongly suggests a role in glomerular repair, possibly downstream of TGF-β, in this model of transient renal injury [30]. In the acute phase of rat crescentic glomerulonephritis, a major component of crescents was macrophages, which do not express CTGF mRNA. However, in the advanced phase, crescentic cells strongly express CTGF mRNA and epithelial marker but do not express the macrophage marker ED1, which suggests that parietal epithelial cells synthesize CTGF. Blockade of endogenous CTGF using antisense oligonucleotide significantly attenuates TGF-β1 and PDGF-BB-induced extracellular matrix accumulation in parietal epithelial glomerular cells [28].

The relationship of plasma and urine CTGF levels with kidney function in glomerulonephritis was previously reported. CTGF mRNA is expressed at the site of chronic tubulointerstitial damage and correlated with the degree of damage [13]. In patients with anti-neutrophil cytoplasmic antibodies-associated glomerulonephritis, plasma CTGF levels are associated with cellular crescents but are not correlated with renal function. The plasma CTGF level at baseline predicted renal

survival more accurately than the acute glomerular nephritis classification [31]. In lupus nephritis, renal CTGF mRNA expression correlates inversely with baseline GFR and was also higher in patients with subsequent decline in GFR [32]. These results indicate the relationship of CTGF with glomerulonephritis.

Anti-GBM nephritis is an animal model commonly used to study a type of immune complex-mediated glomerulonephritis [33]. Anti-GBM nephritis is caused by autoantibodies specific for α3 chain of type IV collagen. Neutrophil recruitment to the kidney starts several hours after the induction of anti-GBM nephritis and its mediated by interleukin-17A (IL-17)-producing γδT cell. The adaptive immune response is initiated by mature dendritic cells that depend on CC-chemokine receptor 2 (CCR2). In earlier stage, immune responses that are mediated by Th17 cells which recruit neutrophils and macrophages cause sustained kidney inflammation [27]. Usually, CTGF is known to be a downstream mediator of TGF-β. Blockade of TGF-β in the early stage of anti-GBM nephritis in rat ameliorates renal function and histological changes such as crescentic formation and interstitial fibrosis [34]. The gene expression profile of anti-GBM glomerulonephritis revealed that CTGF is expressed as early as on the first day of disease induction preceding TGF-β1 expression [35]. Rodrigues-Diez et al. showed that the C-terminal domain 4 of CTGF induced renal Th17 inflammatory response. In vitro, stimulation of human CD4+ T lymphocytes with CTGF domain 4 results in differentiation of the Th17 phenotype [36]. These results mean that CTGF might be involved in inflammatory responses and is a candidate for therapeutic target for glomerulonephritis.

Complete deletion of CTGF is a desired in an experimental approach for evaluating the contribution of CTGF to the development of renal disease. However, CTGF knockout mice die shortly after birth. To investigate the role of CTGF in the glomerulonephritis model and the contribution of endogenous CTGF expression, we generated a full length of CTGF floxed mice and established tamoxifen-inducible systemic CTGF knockout (Rosa-CTGF cKO) mice by crossing Rosa-CreER^{T2} mice [37]. The gene expression of CTGF in the kidneys of Rosa-CTGF cKO mice is decreased by 80%. After induction of anti-GBM nephritis, Rosa-CTGF cKO mice exhibit 50% reduction of proteinuria and decreased crescent formation and mesangial expansion as compared with the control mice. In addition to the increases in the expression levels of fibrotic makers such as *Tgfβ1*, *Acta2*, and *Fn1*, the glomerular mRNA expression of MCP-1 (*Ccl2*) and F4/80 (*Adgre1*) is increased in the control mice with anti-GBM nephritis, and this increase is reduced in the Rosa-CTGF cKO mice with nephritis. Accumulation of MAC2-positive cells in glomeruli is also reduced in Rosa-CTGF cKO mice. It is interesting that this amelioration of anti-GBM nephritis is not observed in podocyte-specific CTGF deletion. Furthermore, mesangial cell CTGF cKO mice with nephritis show similar phenotype to Rosa-CTGF cKO mice [38]. In addition, Rosa-CTGF cKO mice with peritoneal fibrosis also exhibit almost 50% reduction in MAC-2 (macrophage marker)-positive cell infiltration and *Cd68* mRNA expression in the peritoneum (Fig. 2) [39]. These results suggest that CTGF from mesangial cell, not podocytes, may be required for the upregulation of MCP-1expression not only in anti-GBM nephritis but also in other types of glomerulonephritis, such as IgA nephropathy, because CTGF expression and accumulation of macrophages in the mesangial area are documented in these glomerular diseases [38].

Role of CTGF in adhesion and migration

During development of inflammation, transmigration of leukocytes to the inflammatory site is a major step. Inflammatory stimuli activate endothelial cells to express adhesion molecules and chemokines which recruit leukocytes. An increasing number of studies have shown the function of CTGF in adhesion and migration.

CTGF modulates the expression of inflammatory mediators, including cytokines and chemokines through distinct signaling pathways in various cell systems [40]. Direct application of CTGF osteoarthritis synovial fibroblast increases the MCP-1 expression in a time- and dose-dependent manner. CTGF-mediated MCP-1 production is attenuated by $\alpha_V\beta 1$ integrin-neutralized

antibody. Pretreatment with focal adhesion kinase (FAK) , MEK, AP-1, and NF-κB inhibitor also inhibits the potentiating action of CTGF. CTGF-mediated increase in NF-κB and AP-1 luciferase activities are inhibited by FAK, MEK, and ERK inhibitors [41]. In vivo, Sanchez-Lopes reported that systemic administration of CTGF in mice for 24 h induces marked infiltration of T lymphocytes and macrophages in the renal interstitium and leads to elevated renal NF-κB activity. Administration of CTGF increases the renal expression of chemokines (MCP-1 and RANTES) and cytokines (INF-Υ and IL-6) that recruit immune cells and promote inflammation [42]. In rat mesangial cells, CTGF expression induces production of fractalkine, MCP-1, and RANTES in a time- and dose-dependent manner via the p42/44 MAPK-, PI3-K/AKT-, and NF-κB-dependent signal pathways [43]. MCP-1 expression is reduced by CTGF inhibition in TGF-β1-treated mesangial cells. Treatment with recombinant CTGF can overcome this effect of endogenous CTGF inhibition. In tubule-epithelial cells, CTGF increases MCP-1 gene expression through activation of NF-κB and mitogen-activated protein kinase [42]. Thus, CTGF is thought to regulate proinflammatory cytokines and chemokines and induces leukocyte migration in kidney inflammation.

Previous reports have demonstrated that CTGF enhances adhesion through interactions with integrins and fibronectin in various cell types. These results showed that the absence of CTGF prevents cell adhesion and treatment of CTGF increases cell adhesion. This CTGF-mediated adhesion occurs through integrin and

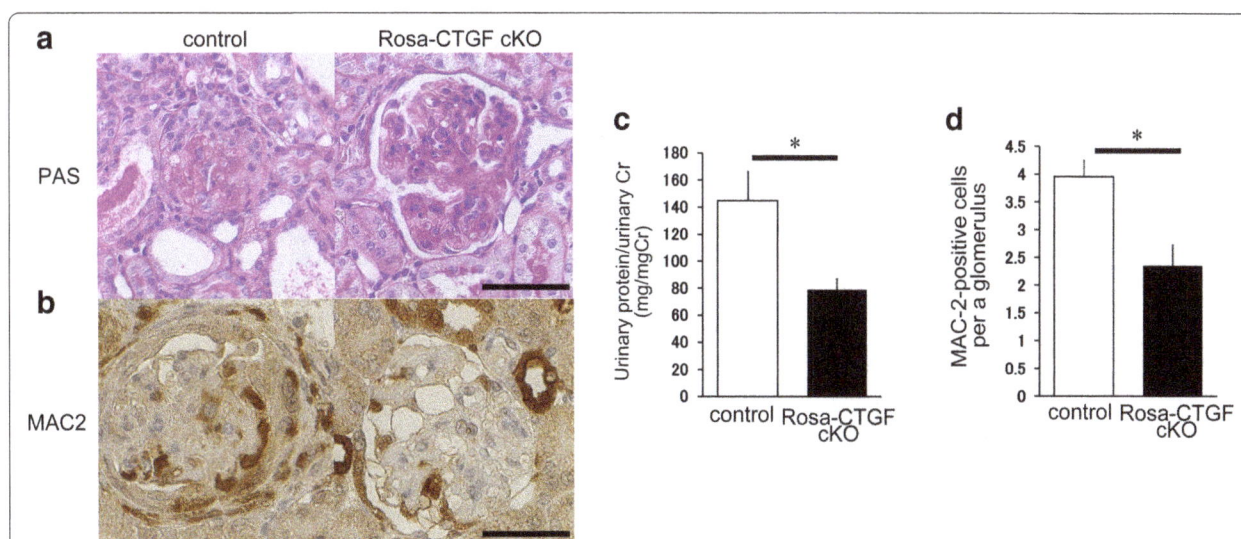

Fig. 2 Macrophage recruitment in Rosa-CTGF cKO mice with anti-GBM nephritis at the earlier stage. **a** Representative photomicrographs of the kidneys at 1 week after induction of anti-GBM nephritis (PAS staining). Left upper panel, control mice with anti-GBM nephritis; right upper panel show, Rosa-CTGF cKO mice with anti-GBM nephritis. Bar represents 50 μm. **b** Immunohistochemical studies for MAC-2 at 1 week after induction of anti-GBM nephritis. Bar represents 50 μm. **c** Changes in proteinuria at 1 week after induction of anti-GBM nephritis. **d** The number of MAC-2-positive cells at 1 week after induction of anti-GBM nephritis. Values are expressed as means ± s.e. *$P < 0.05$, **$P < 0.01$ vs. control GBM

fibronectin expressions [44]. As regards macrophage or monocyte adhesion, Schober et al. reported that activated monocytes adhere to Cyr61 (CCN1) and CTGF through $\alpha_M\beta2$ integrin and cell surface heparan sulfate proteoglycans [45]. Another report showed that CTGF induces peripheral blood mononuclear cell (PBMC) migration in a dose-dependent manner. In the presence of heparin, which binds to CTGF, the chemotactic response to CTGF is reduced. Cell surface heparin sulfate is required for CTGF-mediated PBMC migration [46]. Osteoarthritis synovial fluid and supernatants from CTGF-treated osteoarthritis synovial fibroblasts increase migration of monocytes. In addition, CTGF-mediated migration is inhibited by MEK and ERK inhibitors [41]. Mesangial cell adhesion and CTGF are also reported. CTGF significantly increases cell surface $\alpha5\beta1$ integrin levels relative to the basal levels in human mesangial cells (HMC). CTGF and TGF-β increased cell adhesion to fibronectin, the main $\alpha5\beta1$ substrate. Antisense CTGF reduces the number of adherent cells with TGF-β stimulation. CTGF controls $\alpha5\beta1$ expression by HMC in vitro [47]. We investigated the effects of CTGF on the adhesion of macrophages to activated mesangial cells. Fluorescein-dye-labeled RAW264.7 cells are co-cultured with recombinant TNF-α-stimulated mesangial cells on culture plates. The increase in macrophage adhesion by TNF-α stimulation is significantly inhibited by CTGF knockdown in mesangial cells, and this reduction is negated by exogenous CTGF administration. These results suggest that CTGF induces macrophage accumulation in

glomerulonephritis by enhancing both chemotaxis and adhesion and that reduction of CTGF expression, particularly in mesangial cells, ameliorates nephritis via inhibition of macrophage infiltration (Fig. 3) [38].

CTGF and inflammatory mediator

The regulation of CTGF expression by an inflammatory mediator has been reported. It was found that the effect of TNF-α on CTGF expression is dependent on cell systems or exposure time. The sequences between -244 and -166 of the CTGF promoter were necessary for TNF-α to modulate CTGF expression [48]. TGF-$\beta1$ induces CTGF gene expression via Smad-binding element (SBE) and a unique TGF-$\beta1$ response element which is located between -162 and -128 of the CTGF promoter [49]. Short-term treatment of mesangial cells with TNF-α, like with TGF-β, significantly increases secreted CTGF per cell. TNF-α combined with TGF-β further increases CTGF secretion and mRNA levels and reduces proliferation. However, long-term treatment with TNF-α or TGF-β alone does not increase CTGF protein levels [50]. In synovial cells, TNF-α can also induce CTGF production [51]. By contrast, TNF-α downregulated CTGF in human lung endothelial cells and in normal and scleroderma fibroblasts in a dose- and time-dependent manner [52, 53].

Several reports indicated that CTGF modulates the expression of inflammatory mediators. Stimulation with CTGF induces TNF-α expression in macrophage [38]. Osteoarthritis synovial fibroblast stimulation with CTGF

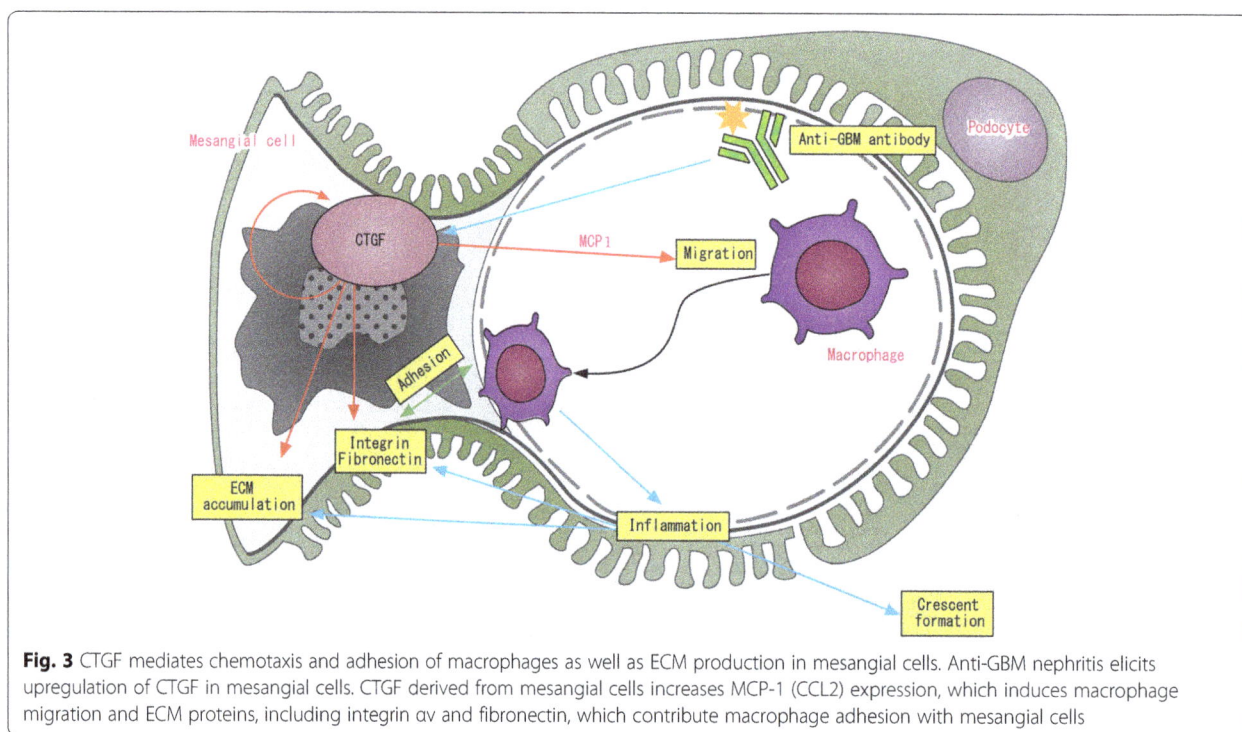

Fig. 3 CTGF mediates chemotaxis and adhesion of macrophages as well as ECM production in mesangial cells. Anti-GBM nephritis elicits upregulation of CTGF in mesangial cells. CTGF derived from mesangial cells increases MCP-1 (CCL2) expression, which induces macrophage migration and ECM proteins, including integrin αv and fibronectin, which contribute macrophage adhesion with mesangial cells

induces concentration-dependent increases in IL-6 expression level. CTGF-mediated IL-6 production is attenuated by $\alpha v \beta 5$ integrin-neutralized antibody [54]. In tubule-epithelial cells, CTGF increases the IL-6 gene expression through activation of NF-κB and mitogen-activated protein kinase [42]. In clinical, the serum level of CTGF in rheumatoid arthritis (RA) was higher than in normal controls and active RA patients showed higher serum CTGF level than inactive RA patients. Furthermore, CTGF level was decreased by infliximab, anti-TNF-α antibody [55]. These results suggest that CTGF induces inflammatory mediators.

Conclusions

CTGF is a downstream mediator of the profibrotic properties of TGF-β. In addition to fibrosis, CTGF has multiple functions, including cell adhesion and migration. CTGF expression is upregulated in glomerulonephritis. Deletion of CTGF can ameliorate anti-GBM glomerulonephritis by reducing macrophage accumulation in mice. Further studies are required to investigate the use of CTGF as a potential target for the treatment of glomerulonephritis.

Abbreviations
CTGF: Connective tissue growth factor; GBM: Glomerular basement membrane; GFR: Glomerular filtration rate; IFN-γ: Interferon-gamma; IL-6: Interleukin-6; MCP-1: Monocyte chemoattractant protein-1; RANTES: Regulation and activation, normal T cell expressed and secreted; STZ: Streptozotocin; TGF-β1: Transforming growth factor beta1; TNF-α: Tumor necrosis factor alpha; VEGF: Vascular endothelial growth factor

Acknowledgements
The authors would like to express science appreciation to Prof. Hideyuki Okano for giving us the opportunity to write this review article and to all lab members and collaborators.

Funding
This work was supported in part by research grants from JSPS KAKENHI (Grant Numbers 17K16080 to N.T. and 25461246, 26461225, 17K09697 to H.Y.)

Authors' contributions
NT and HY wrote the paper. MH and MM revised it. All authors read and approved the final manuscript.

Competing interests
The authors declare that they have no competing interests.

Author details
[1]Department of Nephrology, Graduate School of Medicine, Kyoto University, 54 Shogoin Kawahara-cho, Sakyo-ku, Kyoto 606-8507, Japan. [2]Department of Nephrology, Kumamoto University Graduate School of Medical Sciences, Kumamoto, Japan.

References
1. Bradham DM, Igarashi A, Potter RL, Grotendorst GR. Connective tissue growth factor: a cysteine-rich mitogen secreted by human vascular endothelial cells is related to the SRC-induced immediate early gene product CEF-10. J Cell Biol. 1991;114(6):1285–94.
2. Brigstock DR, Goldschmeding R, Katsube KI, Lam SC, Lau LF, Lyons K, et al. Proposal for a unified CCN nomenclature. Mol Pathol. 2003;56(2):127–8.
3. Perbal B. CCN proteins: multifunctional signalling regulators. Lancet. 2004; 363(9402):62–4.
4. Takigawa M. The CCN protein: an overview. Methods Mol Biol. 2017;1489:1–8.
5. Ivkovic S, Yoon SB, Popoff NS, Safadi FF, Libuda ED, Stephenson CR, et al. Connective tissue growth factor coordinates chondrogenesis and angiogenesis during skeletal development. Development. 2003;130(12): 2779–91.
6. Ito Y, Goldschmeding R, Kasuga H, Claessen N, Nakayama M, Yuzawa Y, et al. Expression patterns of connective tissue growth factor and of TGF-β isoforms during glomerular injury recapitulate glomerulogenesis. Am J Physiol Renal Physiol. 2010;299(3):F545–58.
7. Falke LL, Goldschmeding R, Nguyen TQ. A perspective on anti-CCN2 therapy for chronic kidney disease. Nephrol Dial Transplant. 2014;29(supple 1):30–7.
8. Yokoi H, Mukoyama M. Analysis of pathological activities of CCN proteins in fibrotic disease: kidney fibrosis. Methods Mol Biol. 2017;1489:431–43.
9. Igarashi A, Okochi H, Bradham DM, Grotendorst GR. Regulation of connective tissue growth factor gene expression in human skin fibroblasts and during wound repair. Mol Biol Cell. 1993;4(6):637–45.
10. Igarashi A, Nashiro K, Kikuchi K, Sato S, Ihn H, Grotendorst GR, et al. Significant correlation between connective tissue growth factor gene expression and skin sclerosis in tissue sections from patients with systemic sclerosis. J Invest Dermatol. 1995;105(2):280–4.
11. Sonnylal S, Shi-wen X, Leoni P, Naff K, van Pelt CS, Nakamura H, et al. Selective expression of connective tissue growth factor in fibroblast in vivo promotes systemic tissue fibrosis. Arthritis Rheum. 2010;62(5):1523–32.
12. Riser BL, Denichilo M, Cortes P, Baker C, Grondin JM, Yee J, et al. Regulation of connective tissue growth factor activity in cultured rat mesangial cells and its expression in experimental diabetic glomerulosclerosis. J Am Soc Nephrol. 2000;11(1):25–38.
13. Ito Y, Aten J, Bende JR, Oemar SB, Rabelink JT, Weening JJ, Goldschmeding R. Expression of connective tissue growth factor in human renal fibrosis. Kidney Int. 1998;53(4):853–61.
14. Gerristen KG, Abrahams AC, Peters HP, Nguyen TQ, Koeners MP, den Hoedt CH, et al. Effect of GFR on plasma N-terminal connective tissue growth factor (CTGF) concentrations. Am J Kidney Dis. 2012;59(5):619–27.
15. Yokoi H, Mukoyama M, Nagae T, Mori K, Suganami T, Sawai K, et al. Reduction in connective tissue growth factor by antisense treatment ameliorates renal tubulointerstitial fibrosis. J Am Soc Nephrol. 2004;15(6): 1430–40.
16. Okada H, Kikuta T, Kobayashi T, Inoue T, Kanno Y, Takigawa M, et al. Connective tissue growth factor expressed in tubular epithelium plays a pivotal role in renal fibrogenesis. J Am Soc Nephrol. 2005;16(1):133–43.
17. Gerritsen KG, Leeuwis JW, Koeners MP, Bakker SJ, van Oeveren W, Aten J, et al. Elevated urinary connective tissue growth factor in diabetic nephropathy is caused by local production and tubular dysfunction. J Diabetes Res. 2015;2015:539787.
18. Yokoi H, Mukoyama M, Mori K, Kasahara M, Suganami T, Sawai K, et al. Overexpression of connective tissue growth factor in podocytes worsens diabetic nephropathy in mice. Kidney Int. 2008;73(4):446–55.
19. Nguyen QT, Roestenberg P, Nieuwenhoven vAF, Bovenschen N, Li Z, Xu L, et al. CTGF inhibits BMP-7 signaling in diabetic nephropathy. J Am Soc Nephrol 2008; 19(11): 2098–2107.
20. James LR, Le C, Doherty H, Kim HS, Maeda N. Connective tissue growth factor expression modulates response to high glucose. PLoS One. 2013;8(8):e70441.
21. Falke LL, Dendooven A, Leeuwis JW, Geest R, Giezen DM, Broekhuizen R, et al. Hemizygous deletion of CTGF/CCN2 dose not suffice to prevent fibrosis of severely injured kidney. Matrix Biol. 2012;31(7–8):421–31.
22. Sakai N, Nakamura M, Lipson KE, Miyake T, Kamikawa Y, Sagara A, et al. Inhibition of CTGF ameliorates peritoneal fibrosis through suppression of fibroblast and myofibroblast accumulation and angiogenesis. Sci Rep. 2017;7(1):5392.

23. Dornhofer N, Spong S, Bennewith K, Salim A, Klaus S, Kambham N, et al. Connective tissue growth factor-specific monoclonal antibody therapy inhibits pancreatic tumor growth and metastasis. Cancer Res. 2006;66(11):5816–27.

24. Moran-Jones K, Gloss BS, Murail R, Chang DK, Colvin EK, et al. Connective tissue growth factor as a novel therapeutic target in high grade serous ovarian cancer. Int J Exp Path. 2015;6(42):44551–62.

25. Raghu G, Scholand MB, Andrade J, Lancaster L, Mageto Y, Goldin J, et al. FG3019 anti-connective tissue growth factor antibody: results of an open-label clinical trial in idiopathic pulmonary fibrosis. Eur Respir J. 2016;47(5):1481–91.

26. Adler SG, Schwartz S, Williams ME, Arauz-Pacheco C, Bolton WK, Lee T, et al. Phase 1 study of anti-CTGF monoclonal antibody in patients with diabetes and microalbuminuria. Clin J Am Soc Nephrol. 2010;19(8):1420–8.

27. Kurts C, Panzer U, Anders HJ, Rees AJ. The immune system and kidney disease: basic concepts and clinical implications. Nat Rev Immunol. 2013;13(10):738–53.

28. Kanemoto K, Usui J, Tomari S, Yokoi H, Mukoyama M, Aten J, et al. Connective tissue growth factor participates in scar formation of crescentic glomerulonephritis. Lab Investig. 2003;83(11):1615–25.

29. Donderski R, Szczepanek J, Domagalski K, Tretyn A, Korenkiewicz MA, et al. Analysis of relative expression level of VEGF, HIF-1α and CTGF genes in chronic glomerulonephritis patients. Kidney Blood Press Res. 2013;38(1):83–91.

30. Ito Y, Goldschmeding R, Bende R, Claessen N, Chand M, Kieij L, et al. Kinetics of connective tissue growth factor expression during experimental proliferative glomerulonephritis. J Am Soc Nephrol. 2001;12(3):472–84.

31. Hilhorst M, Kok HM, Broekhuizen R, van Passen P, Vriesman PB, et al. Connective tissue growth factor and the cicatrization of cellular crescents in ANCA-associated glomerulonephritis. Nephrol Dial Transplant. 2015;30(8):1291–9.

32. Tachaudomdach C, Kantachuvesiri S, Changsirikulchai S, Wimolluck S, Pinpradap K, Kitiyakara C. Connective tissue growth factor gene expression and decline in renal function in lupus nephritis. Exp Ther Med. 2012;3(4):713–8.

33. Artinger K, Kirsch AH, Aringer I, Moschovaki-Filippidou F, Eller P, Rosenkranz AR, et al. Innate and adaptive immunity in experimental glomerulonephritis: a pathfinder tale. Pediatr Nephrol. 2017;32(6):943–7.

34. Zhou A, Ueno H, Shimomura M, Tanaka R, Shirakawa T, Nakamura H, et al. Blockade of TGF-β action ameliorates renal dysfunction and histologic progression in anti-GBM nephritis. Kidney Int. 2003;64(1):92–101.

35. Kim JH, Ha IS, Hwang CI, Lee YJ, Kim J, Yang SH, et al. Gene expression profiling of anti-GBM glomerulonephritis model: the role of NF-κB in immune complex kidney disease. Kidney Int. 2004;66(5):1826–37.

36. Rodrigues-Diez R, Rodrigues-Diez RR, Rayego-Mateos S, Suarez-Alvarez B, Lavoz C, Aroeira SL, et al. The C-terminal module IV of connective tissue growth factor is a novel immune modulator of the Th17 response. Lab Investig. 2013;93(7):812–24.

37. Toda N, Yokoi H, Mukoyama M. Production and analysis of conditional KO mice of CCN2 in kidney. Methods Mol Biol. 2017;1489:377–90.

38. Toda N, Mori K, Kasahara M, Ishii A, Koga K, Ohno S, et al. Crucial role of mesangial cell-derived connective tissue growth factor in a mouse model of anti-glomerular basement membrane glomerulonephritis. Sci Rep. 2017;7:42114.

39. Toda N, Mori K, Kasahara M, Koga K, Ishii A, Mori PK, et al. Deletion of connective tissue growth factor ameliorates peritoneal fibrosis by inhibiting angiogenesis and inflammation. Nephrol Dial Transplant. 2017;17 in press

40. Kular L, Pakradouni J, Kitabgi P, Laurent M, Martinerie C. The CCN family: a new class of inflammation modulators? Biochimie. 2011;93(3):377–88.

41. Liu SC, Hsu CJ, Fong YC, Chuang SM, Tang CH. CTGF induces monocyte chmoattractant protein-1 expression to enhance monocyte migration in human synovial fibroblasts. Biochim Biophys Acta. 2013;1833(5):1114–24.

42. Sanchez-Lopez E, Rayego S, Rodrigues-Diez R, Rodriguez SJ, Rodrigues-Diez R, Rodriguez-Vita J, et al. CTGF promotes inflammatory cell infiltration of the renal interstitium by activating NF-κB. J Am Soc Nephrol. 2009;20(7):1513–26.

43. Wu HS, Wu HX, Lu C, Dong L, Zhou PG, Chen QZ. Lipoxin A4 inhibits connective tissue growth factor-induced production of chemokines in rat mesangial cells. Kidney Int. 2006;69(2):248–56.

44. Aguiar DP, de Farias GC, de Sousa EB, de Mattos C-AJ, Lobo JC, et al. New strategy to control cell migration and metastasis regulated by CCN2/CTGF. Cancer Cell Int. 2014;14:61.

45. Schober MJ, Chen N, Grzeszkiewicz MT, Jovanovic I, Emeson EE, Ugarova PT, et al. Identification of integrin $\alpha_M\beta_2$ as an adhesion receptor on peripheral blood monocytes for Cyr61 (CCN1) and connective tissue growth factor (CCN2): immediate-early gene products expressed in atherosclerotic lesions. Blood. 2002;99(12):4457–65.

46. Iwano C, Yilmaz A, Klein M, Raithel D, Brigstock DR, Daniel WG, et al. Connective tissue growth factor is overexpressed in complicated atherosclerotic plaques and induces mononuclear cell chemotaxis in vitro. Arterioscler Thromb Vasc Biol. 2005;25(5):1008–13.

47. Weston BS, Wahab NA, Mason RM. CTGF mediates TGF-β-induced fibronectin matrix deposition by upregulating active α5β1 integrin in human mesangial cells. J Am Soc Nephrol. 2003;14(3):601–10.

48. Abraham DJ, Shiwen X, Black CM, Sa S, Xu Y, Leask A, et al. Tumor necrosis factor alpha suppresses the induction of connective tissue growth factor by transforming growth factor-beta in normal and scleroderma fibroblasts. J Biol Chem. 2002;275(20):15220–5.

49. Grotendorst GR, Okochi H, Hayashi N. A novel transforming growth factor beta response element controls the expression of the connective tissue growth factor gene. Cell Growth Differ. 1996;7(4):469–80.

50. Cooker LA, Peterson D, Rambow J, Riser ML, Riser RE, Najmabadi F, et al. TNF-α, but not IFN-γ, regulates CCN2 (CTGF), collagen type I, and proliferation in mesangial cells: possible roles in the progression of renal fibrosis. Am J Physiol Renal Physiol. 2007;293(1):F157–65.

51. Miyashita T, Morimoto S, Fujishiro M, Hayakawa K, Suzuki S, Ikedda K, et al. Inhibition of each module of connective tissue growth factor as a potential therapeutic target for rheumatoid arthritis. Autoimmunity. 2016;49(2):109–14.

52. Laug R, Fehrholz M, Schutze N, Kramer BW, Krump-Konvalinkova V, Speer CP, et al. IFN-γ and TNF-α synergize to inhibit CTGF expression in human lung endothelial cells. PLoS One. 2012;7(9):e45430.

53. Abraham DJ, Shiwen X, Black CM, Sa S, Xu Y, Leask A. Tumor necrosis factor α suppresses the induction of connective tissue growth factor by transforming growth factor β in normal and scleroderma fibroblast. J Biol Chem. 2000;275(20):15220–5.

54. Liu SC, Hsu CJ, Chen HT, Tsou HK, Chuang SM, Tang CH. CTGF increases IL-6 expression in human synovial fibroblast through integrin-dependent signaling pathway. PLoS One. 2012;7(12):e51097.

55. Nozawa K, Fujishiro M, Kawasaki M, Kaneko H, Iwabuchi K, Yanagida M, et al. Connective tissue growth factor promotes articular damage by increased osteoclastogenesis in patients with rheumatoid arthritis. Arthritis Res Ther. 2009;11(6):R174.

19

Human LYPD8 protein inhibits motility of flagellated bacteria

Chiao-Ching Hsu[1,2,3], Ryu Okumura[1,2,3] and Kiyoshi Takeda[1,2,3*]

Abstract

Background: We previously reported that the mouse Ly6/Plaur domain containing 8 (mLypd8), a GPI-anchored protein highly and selectively expressed on colonic epithelia, contributes to segregation of intestinal microbiota and intestinal epithelia and is critical for prevention of intestinal inflammation. In addition, it was found that human LYPD8 (hLYPD8) is expressed in the colonic epithelia and expression of hLYPD8 is reduced in some ulcerative colitis patients. However, the molecular characteristics and functions of hLYPD8 remain unclear. In this study, we generated the hLYPD8 protein and characterized its functions.

Methods: To analyze the characteristics and functions of the hLYPD8 protein, recombinant FLAG-tagged hLYPD8 protein was generated by two kinds of protein expression systems: a mammalian cell expression system and a *Pichia pastoris* expression system. Recombinant hLYPD8 protein was analyzed by western blot analysis or deglycosylation assay. The effect of the protein on flagellated bacteria was examined by ELISA assay and motility assay using semi-agar plates.

Results: hLYPD8 was a highly *N*-glycosylated GPI-anchored protein, like mLypd8. Moreover, recombinant hLYPD8 protein generated by the *Pichia pastoris* expression system using the SuperMan$_5$ strain, which enabled production of a large number of proteins with human-like glycosylation, presented the high binding affinity and the motility inhibitory function to flagellated bacteria, such as *Proteus mirabilis*.

Conclusions: These results demonstrated that hLYPD8 inhibits the motile activity of flagellated bacteria, many of which are involved in intestinal inflammation. The supplementation of recombinant hLYPD8 protein might be a novel therapeutic approach for intestinal inflammation of inflammatory bowel diseases.

Keywords: LYPD8, Glycosylation, *Pichia Pastoris*, Flagellated bacteria, Intestinal inflammation

Background

Intestinal epithelial cells play important roles in the regulation of intestinal inflammation by generating several kinds of mucosal barriers, including mucus and antimicrobial peptides. These barriers contribute to the segregation of intestinal bacteria and the intestinal mucosa, which is indispensable for homeostatic maintenance of the gut where tremendous numbers of microorganisms live symbiotically [1–5]. Therefore, the dysfunction of mucosal barriers leads to the excessive immune response in the intestinal mucosa, which causes inflammatory bowel disease (IBD) represented by ulcerative colitis (UC) and Crohn's disease (CD) [6]. Indeed, it has been reported that increased intestinal permeability and penetration of intestinal bacteria into the mucus layer due to barrier dysfunction are found in the intestine of IBD patients [7, 8].

In the colon, where tremendous numbers of microorganisms exist, intestinal microbiota and intestinal epithelial cells are clearly segregated by the thick mucus layer to maintain the symbiotic relationship between commensal microorganisms and the host [2, 3]. We previously demonstrated that the Ly6/Plaur domain containing 8 (Lypd8) expressed in intestinal epithelial cells promotes the segregation of intestinal bacteria and epithelial cells in the colon [9]. This molecule is an *N*-glycosylated GPI-anchored protein, and it binds to

* Correspondence: ktakeda@ongene.med.osaka-u.ac.jp
[1]Department of Microbiology and Immunology, Graduate School of Medicine, Osaka University, Osaka 565-0871, Japan
[2]WPI Immunology Frontier Research Center, Osaka University, Osaka 565-0871, Japan
Full list of author information is available at the end of the article

flagella and suppresses the motility of flagellated bacteria to prevent bacterial invasion of colonic mucosa. Furthermore, it was found that human LYPD8 (hLYPD8) is also expressed in the colonic epithelia, and the expression of LYPD8 is reduced in the colon of some UC patients. However, the molecular characteristics and functions of hLYPD8 remain unclear. We therefore analyzed the molecular characteristics and function of recombinant hLYPD8 protein generated by both mammalian cellexpression system and *Pichia pastoris* expression system.

Methods

Generation of HEK293T cells stably expressing mLypd8 and hLYPD8

Mouse Lypd8 (mLypd8) and human LYPD8 (hLYPD8) genes were amplified by PCR from mouse and human colonic cDNA. A FLAG-tagged sequence was inserted into the total mLypd8 and hLYPD8 coding sequence immediately downstream of the predicted N-terminal signal sequence. HEK293T cells obtained from ATCC were transfected with linearized pcDNA3.1 (+) vector (Invitrogen) inserted the sequence for FLAG-tagged mLypd8 or hLYPD8 using Lipofectamine2000 (Invitrogen). These cells were cultured in G418-containing medium. The surviving cells were stained with anti-FLAG M2 monoclonal antibody (cat F3165: Sigma-Aldrich) and Alexa Fluor 488 goat anti-mouse IgG antibody (cat A11001: Molecular Probes), and cells expressing FLAG-tagged mLypd8 or hLYPD8 were sorted using FACSAria (BD Biosciences).

Purification of FLAG-tagged hLYPD8 proteins from HEK293T cells

Recombinant hLYPD8 protein was purified from HEK293T cells stably expressing FLAG-tagged hLYPD8 using FLAG M2 Purification Kit (Sigma-Aldrich). As a negative control, non-transfected cells were used.

Assay for GPI cleaving activity

HEK293T cells stably expressing hLYPD8 (1×10^6 cells) were rinsed twice with cold PBS and incubated with 0.5 ml of PBS containing 0.5 units of *Bacillus cereus* phosphatidylinositol-specific phospholipase C (PI-PLC, Molecular Probes) at 4 °C for 20 min. These cells were stained with anti-FLAG M2 mAb (Sigma-Aldrich) and Alexa Fluor 488 goat anti-mouse IgG (Invitrogen). The surface expression of hLYPD8 was analyzed using FACS-Canto II (BD Biosciences).

Deglycosylation assay

Recombinant hLYPD8 protein (1 μg) was incubated with PNGase F, sialidase A, and *O*-glycanase (Prozyme) at

37 °C for 3 h. Recombinant hLYPD8 protein treated with glycanase was separated with SDS-PAGE and transferred to polyvinylidene fluoride membranes (Millipore) that were incubated with horseradish peroxidase (HRP)-conjugated anti-FLAG M2 mAb (Sigma-Aldrich). Immunoreactivity was detected using Chemi-Lumi One (Nacalai Tesque).

ELISA assay of LYPD8 binding to bacteria

Bacterial strains including *Escherichia coli* JCM 1649[T], *Enterococcus gallinarum* JCM 8728[T], *Bacteroides sartrii* JCM 17136[T], and *Bifidobacterium breve* JCM 1192[T] were obtained from the Japan Collection of Microorganisms. *Proteus mirabilis* was isolated from the colonic tissue of *Lypd8*[−/−] mice as described previously [9]. These bacteria were cultured at 37 °C for 16 h in an anaerobic chamber, fixed by 4% PFA, and stained with DAPI. The cell numbers were quantified by a confocal microscope. Each bacterium was centrifuged at 5000×*g* for 5 min, and the pellet was resuspended in 0.05 M sodium carbonate. The bacteria (1×10^7 cells/ ml) were coated on 96-well plates (Corning) and incubated for 16 h at 4 °C. The plates were then washed with PBS and blocked with 1% BSA/PBS. After the plates were washed, the increasing concentrations of FLAG-tagged hLYPD8 protein diluted in PBS were added and incubated for 2 h at room temperature. Next, after the plates were washed, HRP-conjugated anti-FLAG M2 mAb (Sigma-Aldrich) in PBS was added and incubated for 1 h at room temperature. The plates were then washed, and 3,3′,5,5′-tetramethylbenzidine (TMB) substrate was added. Stop solution 1 M H_2SO_4 was then added, and the plates were read at 450 nm with a spectrometer.

Pull-down assay for LYPD8 binding to flagella

Bacterial suspension of *P. mirabilis* or *E. coli* JCM 1649[T] in PBS was shaken 300 times per min for 60 min to remove flagella from bacterial bodies. Bacterial bodies were pelleted by centrifuging at 4000×*g* for 20 min. The supernatants were ultracentrifuged at 80,000×*g* for 60 min to obtain flagella. Bacterial bodies or flagella were mixed with the solution of FLAG-tagged recombinant LYPD8 (10 ng/μl) and incubated for 3 h at 4 °C. After incubation, the bacterial bodies or flagella were pelleted down by centrifugation or ultracentrifugation, respectively. Then, the supernatant was collected and the pellet was resuspended in PBS. The supernatant and pellet suspension were separated with SDS-PAGE and transferred to polyvinylidene fluoride membranes (Millipore) that were incubated with HRP-conjugated anti-FLAG M2 mAb (Sigma-Aldrich). Immunoreactivity was detected using Chemi-Lumi One (Nacalai Tesque).

Generation of *Pichia pastoris* expressing glycosylated hLYPD8 protein

The host strain *Pichia pastoris* SuperMan$_5$ strain (*HIS*$^+$) and the expression vector pJAZ-aMF vector were purchased from Biogrammatics Inc. (Carlsbad, USA). The FLAG-tagged LYPD8 gene without C-terminal signal sequence was amplified by PCR and ligated into pJAZ-aMF vector.

P. pastoris SuperMan$_5$ competent cells were prepared by a high-efficiency transformation condition suggested by Wu et al. [10]. Adequate amounts of constructed plasmids were digested with *Pme* I or *Sac* I to linear form and purified, then added to *P. pastoris* competent cells and well mixed. The mixed sample was added into a 2-mm gap cuvette (Bio-Rad, USA) and placed on ice for 5 min. The linearized DNA fragment was transformed into *P. pastoris* competent cells by the electroporation condition of 1.5 kV, 25 µF, and 200 Ω. Then, 1 ml of 1 M sorbitol was added into the sample and incubated at 30 °C for 1 h. At last, the sample was poured evenly into YPDSZ (1% yeast extract, 2% peptone, 2% dextrose, 1 M sorbitol, 100 µg/mL zeocin) agar plates then cultured at 30 °C for 2–3 days. Fifty colonies were selected to the new YPDZ agar plates with different zeocin gradients (100, 300, and 500 µg/ml) for testing the zeocin resistance and cultured at 30 °C for 1–2 days. Few transformants with better zeocin resistance were selected for further analysis.

Purification of FLAG-tagged hLYPD8 proteins generated by a *Pichia pastoris* expression system

The selected transformants were inoculated in 4 ml of YPDZ for 24 h as a seed culture, then transferred into 500 ml BMGY (1% yeast extract, 2% peptone, pH 6.0 100 mM potassium phosphate, 1% glycerol, 1.34% yeast nitrogen base, and 4×10^{-5}% biotin) and cultured at 30 °C, 200 rpm for 24 h. The medium of each transformant was replaced with 100 ml of BMMY (1% yeast extract, 2% peptone, pH 6.0 100 mM potassium phosphate, 1.34% yeast nitrogen base, 2% methanol, and 4×10^{-5}% biotin). The transformants were then cultured for 48 h at 20 °C, 200 rpm. At the 24-h time point, 2% methanol (2 ml) was added to the culture. Soluble FLAG-tagged hLYPD8 protein was purified from 100 ml of the supernatant by column chromatography according to the FLAG M2 Purification Kit (Sigma-Aldrich).

Motility assay of *Proteus mirabilis* and *Escherichia coli* in semisolid agar

HEK293T cells (5×10^7 cells) with or without FLAG-tagged hLYPD8 were lysed with 1 ml of CelLytic M Cell Lysis Reagent (Sigma-Aldrich). After centrifuging at 13,000×g for 10 min, the supernatant was incubated with 150 µl of anti-FLAG M2 affinity gel (Sigma-Aldrich) for

3 h. The resin was centrifuged and washed with Tris-buffered saline three times. The resin containing FLAG-tagged hLYPD8 was mixed with 2 ml of lysogeny broth (LB) medium containing 0.3% agar. The final concentration of hLYPD8 protein in the LB agar was estimated by SDS-PAGE and was approximately 1.5 µg/ml. In the case of usage of soluble hLYPD8 protein generated by *P. pastoris*, 0.5 ml of recombinant soluble hLYPD8 protein was mixed with 1.5 ml of the LB medium containing 0.3% agar. The final concentration of hLYPD8 protein in the LB agar was estimated by SDS-PAGE and BCA assay, and it was approximately 50 µg/ml.

P. mirabilis or *E. coli* was cultured in the LB medium at 37 °C until OD$_{600}$ was 0.6. The semisolid LB agar (0.3%) containing hLYPD8 protein was centrally inoculated with 1 µl of bacterial culture and incubated at 37 °C. Motility was assessed by examining circular migration. The radius of circles formed by bacterial migration was measured at 4 h after the bacterial inoculation.

ELISA assay for LYPD8 binding to flagella

Several 96-well plates (Corning) were coated with 100 µg/ml flagella of *P. mirabilis* or 1% BSA/PBS for 16 h at 4 °C. The plates were then washed, and increasing concentrations of FLAG-tagged hLYPD8 protein diluted in 1% BSA/PBS were added and incubated for 2 h at room temperature. The plates were then washed, and HRP-conjugated anti-FLAG M2 mAb (Sigma-Aldrich) diluted in 1% BSA/PBS was added and incubated for 2 h at room temperature. The plates were then washed, and TMB substrate was added. The plates were then read at 450 nm with a spectrometer.

Statistical analysis

Data are presented as mean ± s.d., as indicated in the figure legends. Differences between control and experimental groups were evaluated using a two-tailed unpaired Student's *t* test. A *P* value of < 0.05 was considered significant. No statistical methods were used to predetermine sample size. No sample was excluded from the analysis.

Results

Molecular characteristics of the hLYPD8 protein

LYPD8 is broadly conserved in mammalian species, including human, mouse, and rat. We previously showed that mouse Lypd8 (mLypd8) is a highly *N*-glycosylated protein. The hLYPD8 protein also contains eight glycosylation sites predicted by the amino acid sequence (Fig. 1a). We first purified recombinant hLYPD8 protein from HEK293T cells stably expressing FLAG-tagged hLYPD8 and analyzed the protein by SDS-PAGE and western blot analysis. Although the expected molecular weight from amino acid length is about 20 kDa, a band

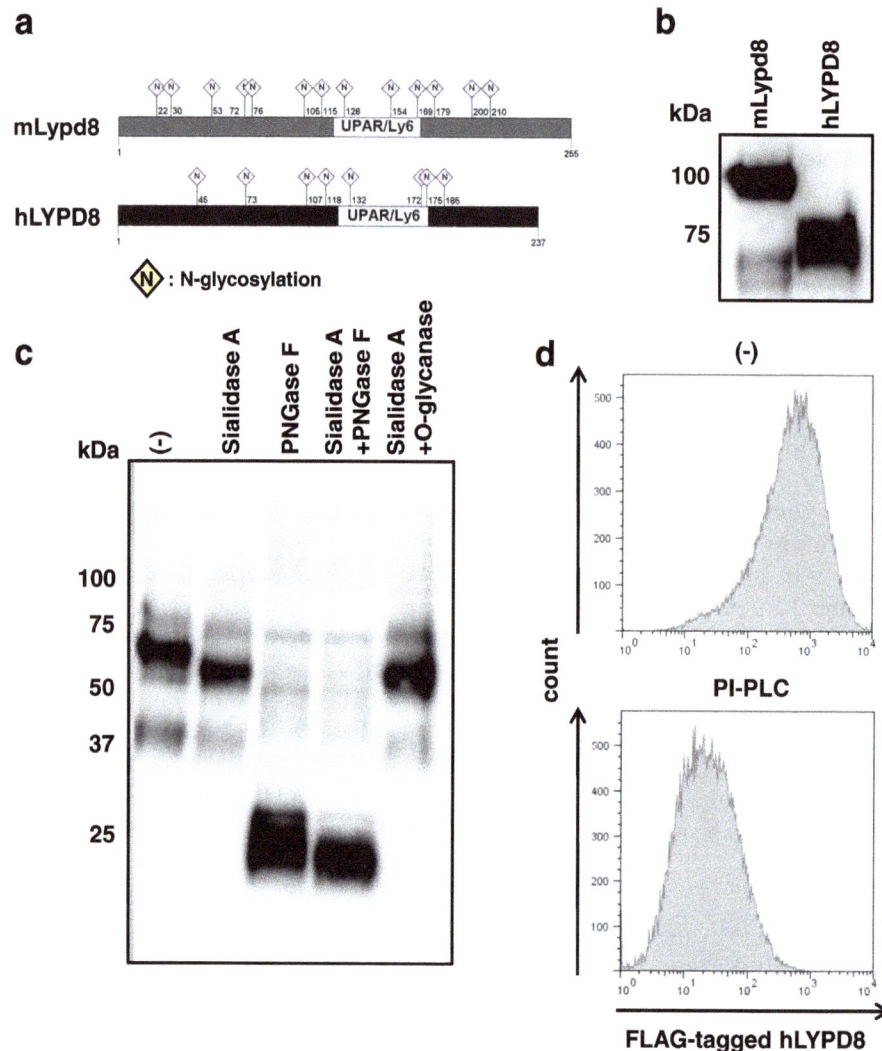

Fig. 1 Molecular characteristics of the hLYPD8 protein. **a** Predicted glycosylation sites of the mLypd8 and hLYPD8 proteins. Glycosylation sites were referred to the UniProt database, and the picture was drawn by a group-based predictive system (IBS 1.0.2). **b** Immunoblotting for whole cell lysates of HEK293T cells expressing mLypd8 and hLYPD8. **c** Immunoblotting for recombinant hLYPD8 protein untreated or treated with sialidase A, PNGase F, or O-glycanase. **d** Flow cytometric analysis of HEK239T cells expressing FLAG-tagged LYPD8 before (upper) and after (lower) treatment with PI-PLC

for recombinant hLYPD8 protein was observed at about the 75-kDa position (Fig. 1b). In addition, the treatment with peptide-N-glycosidase F (PNGase F), which cleaves N-oligosaccharide chains from glycoproteins, substantially reduced the molecular weight of the hLYPD8 protein. In contrast, treatment with sialidase A and O-glycanase did not markedly change the molecular weight of the hLYPD8 protein (Fig. 1c). These data indicate that hLYPD8 is a highly N-glycosylated protein, like mLypd8. We next treated HEK293T cells expressing FLAG-tagged hLYPD8 with phosphatidylinositol-phospholipase C (PI-PLC), which cleaves GPI-anchored proteins from the cell membrane, and analyzed hLYPD8 surface expression by flow cytometry. Treatment of PI-PLC

severely reduced hLYPD8 surface expression, indicating that hLYPD8 is a GPI-anchored protein, similar to mLypd8 (Fig. 1d).

Functions of the hLYPD8 protein generated by a mammalian cell expression system

The molecular characteristics of hLYPD8 are similar to those of mLypd8. Therefore, we next investigated the functions of recombinant hLYPD8 protein generated by a mammalian cell expression system. In the previous study, the mLypd8 protein was found to preferentially bind to flagellated bacteria, such as *E. coli* and *P. mirabilis*. Hence, we examined whether the hLYPD8 protein produced in mammalian cells bind to various kinds of intestinal bacteria including *P. mirabilis*, *E. coli*, *E. gallinarum*, *B. sartrii*, and *B. breve* by an ELISA assay (Fig. 2a). The hLYPD8 protein preferentially bound to *E. coli* and *P. mirabilis*, both of which are flagellated bacteria. Next, isolated flagella and bacterial bodies from cultured *P. mirabilis* were incubated with the hLYPD8 protein and then pelleted down by centrifuging. The hLYPD8 protein and the flagella were coprecipitated (Fig. 2b). After incubation with increasing flagella concentration, the amount of the hLYPD8 protein in the supernatants was decreased, whereas it was increased in the pellets (Fig. 2c). The incubation with bacterial bodies did not alter the amount of hLYPD8 in the supernatants (Fig. 2d). These data indicate that the hLYPD8 protein binds

to flagella of *P. mirabilis*. Therefore, we tested whether recombinant hLYPD8 protein inhibits the motile activity of *P. mirabilis* in a semi-agar plate. The swarm circle diameter was reduced in the semi-agar plate containing the hLYPD8 protein (Fig. 2e, f), indicating that the hLYPD8 protein inhibits the swarming motility of *P. mirabilis*, as does the mLypd8 protein.

Generation of the hLYPD8 protein by a *Pichia pastoris* expression system

To extensively explore the functions of hLYPD8, a high quantity and quality of recombinant hLYPD8 protein are required. Considering the limitation of the protein-expressing ability of mammalian cells, we established another recombinant protein expression system for

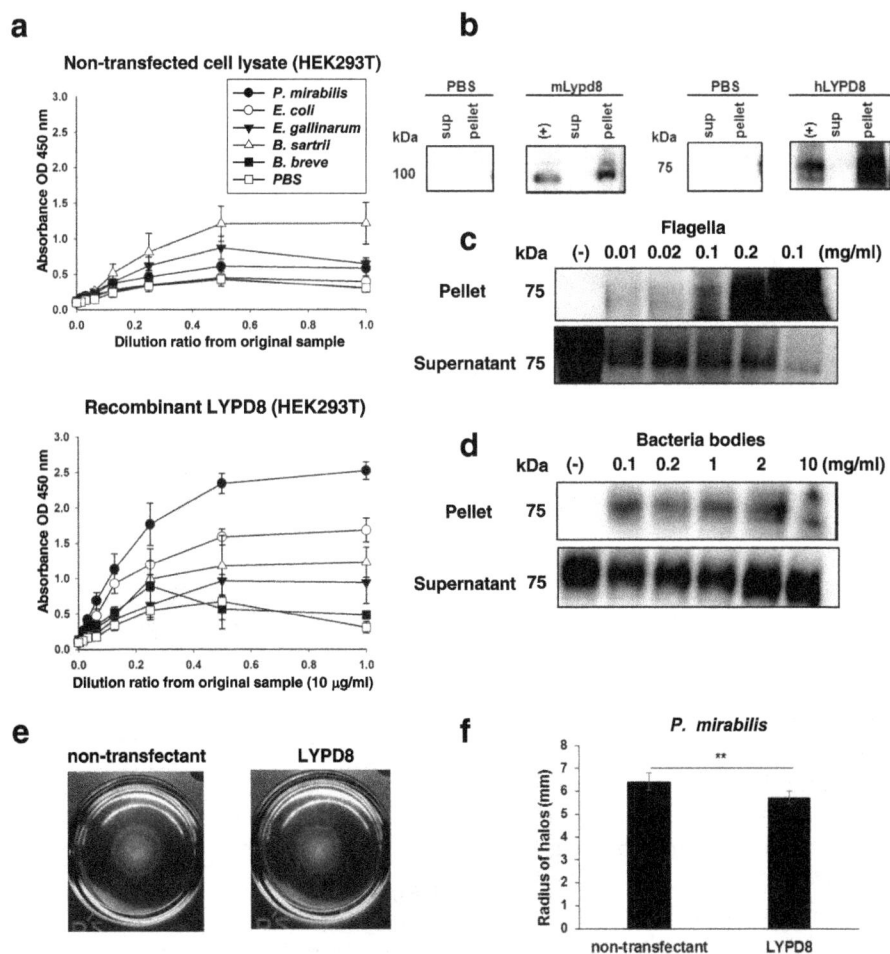

Fig. 2 Function of the hLYPD8 protein generated by a mammalian cell expression system. **a** ELISA assay for hLYPD8 binding to intestinal bacteria. The quantified bacteria were coated onto microtiter plates and incubated with a dilution series of purified FLAG-tagged hLYPD8 (lower) or control sample (purified sample of non-transfected HEK293T cell lysate) (upper). **b–d** Immunoblot analysis with the anti-FLAG antibody for the supernatant and pellet of the mixture of FLAG-tagged mLypd8 or hLYPD8 and flagella from *P. mirabilis* (**b**) and the mixture of hLYPD8 and a gradient dose of flagella (**c**) or bacterial bodies (**d**) from *P. mirabilis*. **e, f** Motility of *P. mirabilis* in semisolid agar with the hLYPD8 protein or a control sample (a purified sample of non-transfected HEK293T cell lysate). Representative photos were shown (**e**). The radii of motility halos were measured at 4 h (**f**). Data are mean ± s.d. (*n* = 6 per group). **p < 0.01

hLYPD8 by using the *Pichia* GlycoSwitch system [11]. This system uses the *Pichia pastoris* SuperMan$_5$ strain, a methylotrophic yeast, which has strong promoters to drive the expression of a foreign gene. Moreover, it is a genetically modified strain that enable the production of large amounts of human-like glycosylated proteins with an easier technique and lower cost than other eukaryotic systems. Our previous mouse study revealed that the soluble form of mLypd8, shed from intestinal epithelial surface, acts on intestinal bacteria. Therefore, we constructed a soluble hLYPD8 expression vector by inserting a FLAG-tagged hLYPD8 sequence without a C-terminal signal sequence to the original *Pichia* GlycoSwitch vector. Recombinant hLYPD8 protein purified from the culture supernatant of *P. pastoris* transformed with the hLYPD8 expression vector was analyzed by SDS-PAGE and western blot analysis (Fig. 3a, b). Two bands for soluble hLYPD8 protein were observed at around the 50 and 30-kDa positions. These analyses suggested that the purified soluble hLYPD8 protein solution included about 50 kDa molecular weight of completely glycosylated hLYPD8 protein and 30 kDa molecular weight of partially glycosylated hLYPD8 protein. We next tested whether soluble hLYPD8 protein generated from *P. pastoris* was *N*-glycosylated, like GPI-anchored hLYPD8 protein generated by the mammalian cell expression system. The treatment of PNGaseF reduced the molecular weight of soluble hLYPD8 protein, indicating that soluble hLYPD8 protein generated by the *Pichia* GlycoSwitch system is *N*-glycosylated (Fig. 3c).

Functions of the hLYPD8 protein generated by a *Pichia pastoris* expression system

We next examined the functions of soluble hLYPD8 protein generated by the *P. pastoris* expression system. We analyzed the binding of soluble hLYPD8 protein to several kinds of intestinal bacteria by an ELISA assay. We found that soluble hLYPD8 protein showed the stronger binding to *P. mirabilis* and *E. coli*, compared with the other non-flagellated bacteria (Fig. 4a). We then analyzed whether soluble hLYPD8 protein binds to flagella of *P. mirabilis* by the ELISA and pull-down assays (Fig. 4b–d). The results of both binding assays revealed that soluble hLYPD8 protein binds to flagella of *P. mirabilis* with high affinity. Subsequently, we analyzed the effect on the motile activity of bacteria. Soluble hLYDP8 protein remarkably inhibited the swarming ability of *P. mirabilis* in a dose-dependent manner (Fig. 4e–g). Moreover, soluble hLYPD8 protein also inhibited the motility of *E. coli* (Fig. 4h, i). These data clearly demonstrated that highly glycosylated soluble hLYPD8 protein generated by the *P. pastoris* expression

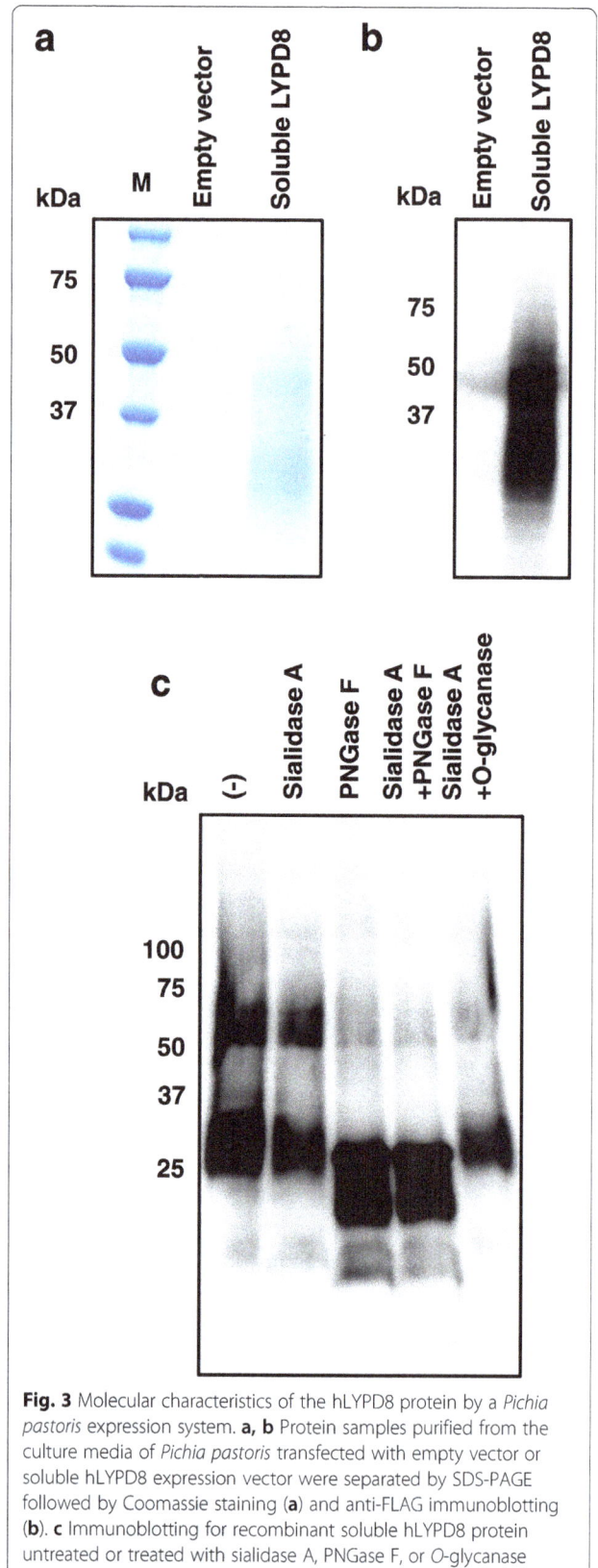

Fig. 3 Molecular characteristics of the hLYPD8 protein by a *Pichia pastoris* expression system. **a, b** Protein samples purified from the culture media of *Pichia pastoris* transfected with empty vector or soluble hLYPD8 expression vector were separated by SDS-PAGE followed by Coomassie staining (**a**) and anti-FLAG immunoblotting (**b**). **c** Immunoblotting for recombinant soluble hLYPD8 protein untreated or treated with sialidase A, PNGase F, or *O*-glycanase

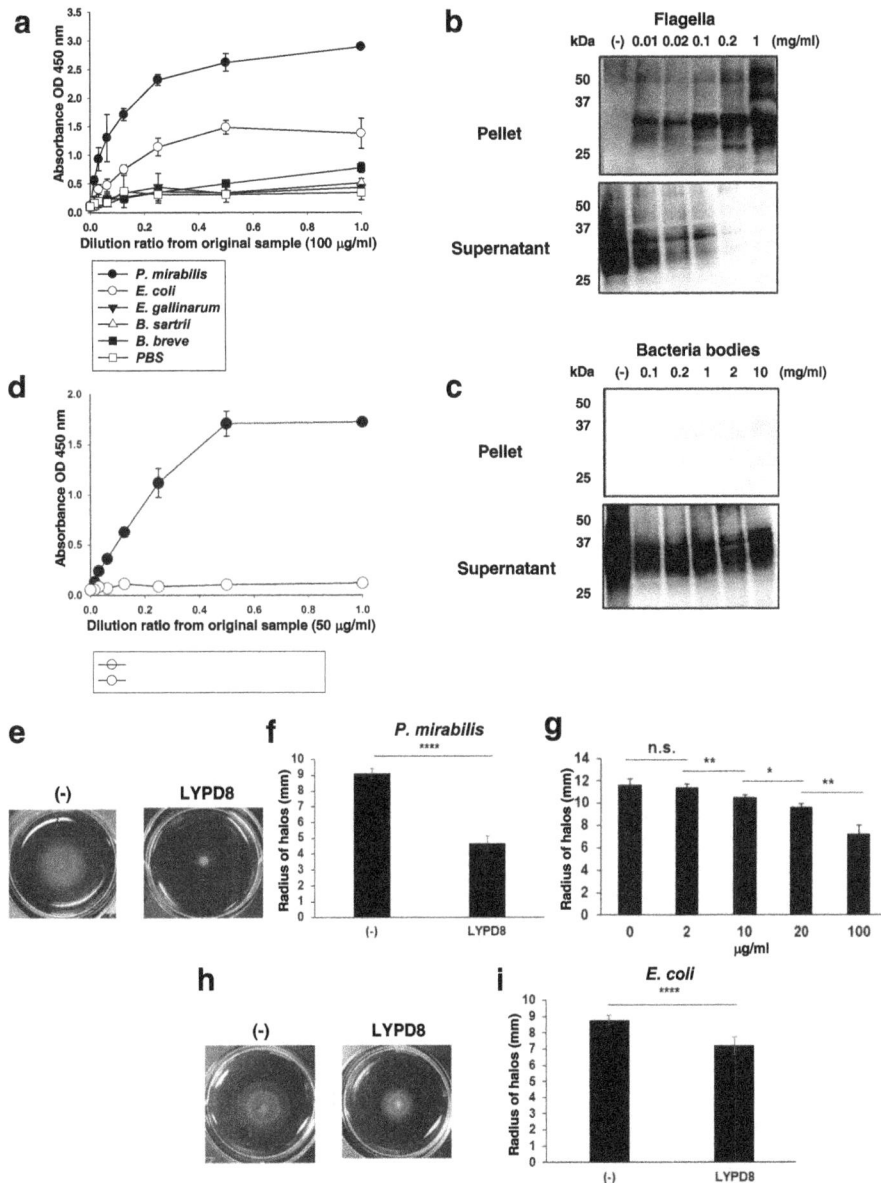

Fig. 4 Function of the hLYPD8 protein generated by a *Pichia pastoris* expression system. **a** ELISA assay for binding of soluble hLYPD8 protein from *P. pastoris* to the indicated species of intestinal bacteria. **b, c** Immunoblot analysis with anti-FLAG antibody for the supernatant and pellet of the mixture of soluble hLYPD8 protein and a gradient dose of flagella (**b**) or bacterial bodies (**c**) from *P. mirabilis*. **d** ELISA assay of LYPD8 binding to flagella of *P. mirabilis*. **e, f** Motility of *P. mirabilis* in semisolid agar with or without soluble hLYPD8 protein. Representative photos are shown (**e**). The radii of motility halos were measured at 4 h (**f**). Data are mean ± s.d. (*n* = 6 per group). **g** Motility of *P. mirabilis* in semisolid agar with a gradient concentration of soluble hLYPD8 protein. The radii of motility halos were measured at 4 h. Data are mean ± s.d. (*n* = 6 per group). **h, i** Motility of *E. coli* in semisolid agar with or without soluble hLYPD8 protein. Representative photos are shown (**h**). The radii of motility halos were measured at 4 h (**i**). Data are mean ± s.d. (*n* = 6 per group). *$p < 0.05$, **$p < 0.01$, ****$p < 0.001$. n.s. not significant

system suppresses the motility of flagellated bacteria by binding to the flagella.

Discussion

We previously demonstrated that mLypd8 contributes to the segregation of intestinal bacteria and intestinal epithelial cells through inhibiting bacterial invasion of colonic epithelia [9]. In this study, we characterized the

hLYPD8 protein. We found that the hLYPD8 protein generated by the mammalian cell expression system was a highly *N*-glycosylated GPI-anchored protein. In addition, the ELISA binding assay showed that the hLYPD8 protein preferentially bound to flagellated bacteria such as *P. mirabilis* and *E. coli*. The motility assay revealed that the hLYPD8 protein inhibited the motility of flagellated bacteria in a semi-agar plate.

These results indicate that hLYPD8 has the same characteristics and functions as mLypd8.

Glycans of secretory or membrane proteins such as mucins, produced by intestinal epithelial cells, are critical for the maintenance of mucosal barriers [12, 13]. In the case of mLypd8, PNGase F treatment reduced the inhibitory function of mLypd8 on intestinal epithelial cells, suggesting that N-glycans are important in the function of Lypd8 [9]. N-glycosylation varies across species and types of cells. The glycosylation in mammalian cells is the most suitable for mammalian glycosylated proteins to function appropriately. However, the ability of protein expression in mammalian cells is limited. Therefore, we generated soluble hLYPD8 protein by using a *Pichia* GlycoSwitch system, which makes it possible to generate large amounts of humanized-glycosylated protein at a relatively low cost. Both recombinant hLYPD8 proteins generated by mammalian cells and *P. pastoris* were highly N-glycosylated, which suggests that both recombinant proteins include similar glycans. However, the molecular weight of both proteins was different, indicating that there seems to exist some dissimilarity in the glycosylation pattern between both proteins. Although the *Pichia* strain we used for heterologous protein expression has been engineered to generate more human-like product by mutating the yeast *OCH1* gene which encodes α-1,6-mannosyltransferase resulting in high mannose-type of N-glycan and introducing heterologous enzyme activities [11], there remain many differences in glycosylation pathway between yeasts and mammalian cells [14]. Hence, the glycosylation pattern of *Pichia pastoris* generated protein is similar but not completely same as that of the protein produced by mammalian cells, and it is important to analyze the glycosylation pattern of both recombinant hLYPD8 proteins using mass spectrometry or lectin array analysis in the future. Despite the different glycosylation patterns, soluble hLYPD8 protein from *P. pastoris* showed a strong inhibitory effect for bacterial motility of flagellated bacteria. This result suggests that the difference in glycosylation between the mammalian cell expression system and the *Pichia* GlycoSwitch system does not affect the protein conformation influencing the protein activity. In addition, the purified soluble hLYPD8 protein solution included two forms of hLYPD8 proteins, fully or not fully glycosylated. Although soluble hLYPD8 protein contained a large amount of the immature form of the protein, it represented the inhibitory function against flagellated bacteria. Therefore, soluble hLYPD8 protein from *P. pastoris* can be used for further analyses of hLYPD8 protein function.

Conclusion

Collectively, we found that hLYPD8 has the same characteristics and functions as mLypd8, and we successfully generated the functional highly glycosylated hLYPD8 protein by using the *P. pastoris* expression system, which enables generation of large amounts of recombinant protein. However, it remains unclear how the LYPD8 protein inhibits the motility of flagellated bacteria. Therefore, it is crucial to analyze the mechanism by which the LYPD8 protein binds to the flagella and inhibits the flagellar motile activity. Nonetheless, there is no convincing therapeutic approach targeting the dysfunction of mucosal barriers in IBD patients. Thus, a challenge exists in examining whether the supplementation of the hLYPD8 protein can reduce the severity of intestinal inflammation by regulating the motile activity of flagellated bacteria, many of which are related to intestinal inflammation [15, 16].

Abbreviations
CD: Crohn's disease; HRP: Horseradish peroxidase; IBD: Inflammatory bowel diseases; Lypd8: Ly6/Plaur domain containing 8; PI-PLC: Phosphatidylinositol-specific phospholipase C; PNGase F: Peptide-N-Glycosidase; TMB: 3, 3',5,5'-Tetramethylbenzidine; UC: Ulcerative colitis

Acknowledgements
We thank T. Kondo and Y. Magota for their technical assistance and C. Hidaka for secretarial assistance.

Funding
This work was supported by grants from the Ministry of Education, Culture, Sports, Science and Technology of Japan, the Japan Agency for Medical Research and Development (to KT), Project MEET, Osaka University Graduate School of Medicine, Mitsubishi Tanabe Pharma Corporation, and Senri Life Science Foundation and Terumo Foundation for Life Science and Arts (to RO).

Authors' contributions
CH and RO designed and performed the experiments, analyzed the data, and wrote the manuscript. KT supervised the study and revised the manuscript. All authors read and approved the final manuscript.

Competing interests
The authors declare that they have no competing interests.

Author details
[1]Department of Microbiology and Immunology, Graduate School of Medicine, Osaka University, Osaka 565-0871, Japan. [2]WPI Immunology Frontier Research Center, Osaka University, Osaka 565-0871, Japan. [3]Core Research for Evolutional Science and Technology, Japan Agency for Medical Research and Development, Tokyo 100-0004, Japan.

References

1. Ayabe T, Satchell DP, Wilson CL, Parks WC, Selsted ME, Ouellette AJ. Secretion of microbicidal alpha-defensins by intestinal Paneth cells in response to bacteria. Nat Immunol. 2000;1(2):113–8.

2. Johansson ME, Phillipson M, Petersson J, Velcich A, Holm L, Hansson GC. The inner of the two Muc2 mucin-dependent mucus layers in colon is devoid of bacteria. Proc Natl Acad Sci U S A. 2008;105(39):15064–9.

3. Johansson ME, Larsson JM, Hansson GC. The two mucus layers of colon are organized by the MUC2 mucin, whereas the outer layer is a legislator of host-microbial interactions. Proc Natl Acad Sci U S A. 2011;108(Suppl 1): 4659–65.

4. Vaishnava S, Yamamoto M, Severson KM, Ruhn KA, Yu X, Koren O, Ley R, Wakeland EK, Hooper LV. The antibacterial lectin RegIIIgamma promotes the spatial segregation of microbiota and host in the intestine. Science (New York, NY). 2011;334(6053):255–8.

5. Maynard CL, Elson CO, Hatton RD, Weaver CT. Reciprocal interactions of the intestinal microbiota and immune system. Nature. 2012;489(7415):231–41.

6. Ahmad R, Sorrell MF, Batra SK, Dhawan P, Singh AB. Gut permeability and mucosal inflammation: bad, good or context dependent. Mucosal Immunol. 2017;10(2):307–17.

7. Chang J, Leong RW, Wasinger V, Ip M, Yang M, Phan TG. Impaired intestinal permeability contributes to ongoing bowel symptoms in patients with inflammatory bowel disease and mucosal healing. Gastroenterology. 2017; 153(3):723-31.

8. Johansson ME, Gustafsson JK, Holmen-Larsson J, Jabbar KS, Xia L, Xu H, Ghishan FK, Carvalho FA, Gewirtz AT, Sjovall H, et al. Bacteria penetrate the normally impenetrable inner colon mucus layer in both murine colitis models and patients with ulcerative colitis. Gut. 2014;63(2):281–91.

9. Okumura R, Kurakawa T, Nakano T, Kayama H, Kinoshita M, Motooka D, Gotoh K, Kimura T, Kamiyama N, Kusu T, et al. Lypd8 promotes the segregation of flagellated microbiota and colonic epithelia. Nature. 2016; 532(7597):117–21.

10. Wu S, Letchworth GJ. High efficiency transformation by electroporation of Pichia pastoris pretreated with lithium acetate and dithiothreitol. BioTechniques. 2004;36(1):152–4.

11. Jacobs PP, Geysens S, Vervecken W, Contreras R, Callewaert N. Engineering complex-type N-glycosylation in Pichia pastoris using GlycoSwitch technology. Nat Protoc. 2009;4(1):58–70.

12. Fu J, Wei B, Wen T, Johansson ME, Liu X, Bradford E, Thomsson KA, McGee S, Mansour L, Tong M, et al. Loss of intestinal core 1-derived O-glycans causes spontaneous colitis in mice. J Clin Invest. 2011;121(4): 1657–66.

13. Goto Y, Obata T, Kunisawa J, Sato S, Ivanov II, Lamichhane A, Takeyama N, Kamioka M, Sakamoto M, Matsuki T, et al. Innate lymphoid cells regulate intestinal epithelial cell glycosylation. Science (New York, NY). 2014; 345(6202):1254009.

14. Vervecken W, Kaigorodov V, Callewaert N, Geysens S, De Vusser K, Contreras R. In vivo synthesis of mammalian-like, hybrid-type N-glycans in Pichia pastoris. Appl Environ Microbiol. 2004;70(5):2639–46.

15. Garrett WS, Gallini CA, Yatsunenko T, Michaud M, DuBois A, Delaney ML, Punit S, Karlsson M, Bry L, Glickman JN, et al. Enterobacteriaceae act in concert with the gut microbiota to induce spontaneous and maternally transmitted colitis. Cell Host Microbe. 2010;8(3):292–300.

16. Rigottier-Gois L. Dysbiosis in inflammatory bowel diseases: the oxygen hypothesis. ISME J. 2013;7(7):1256–61.

20

Control of articular synovitis for bone and cartilage regeneration in rheumatoid arthritis

Hiromu Ito[1*], Furu Moritoshi[1], Motomu Hashimoto[2], Masao Tanaka[2] and Shuichi Matsuda[1]

Abstract

Background: Rheumatoid arthritis is an autoimmune inflammatory disease, the specific feature of which is progressive joint destruction induced by synovitis. The universal consensus is that alleviation of the synovitis is essential to prevent joint destruction and achieve clinical remission.

Main text: We have shown that not only achieving but also maintaining remission is crucial to prevent the progression of joint destruction. Although regeneration of the damaged joints is considered very rare, accumulating evidence shows that it actually occurs in routine clinical practice as a result of strong inhibition of synovitis using highly potent medications. Oral and intravenous medications affect the whole body, but to promote joint regeneration in a particular joint, two potent options are intra-articular steroid injection and synovectomy.

Conclusion: In situations where strong inhibition of synovitis combined with self-regeneration cannot repair severe joint destruction, regenerative medicine may in the future play a crucial role in the regeneration of damaged joints.

Keywords: Rheumatoid arthritis, Joint destruction, Synovitis, Articular cartilage, Regeneration

Background

RA pathology: joint destruction and synovitis

Rheumatoid arthritis (RA) is characterized by spontaneous progressive joint destruction that is predominantly caused by persistent, chronic synovitis in the joint [1]. Treatment with disease-modifying anti-rheumatic drugs (DMARDs) improves RA disease activities, but even with the best currently available treatment, residual disease activity can induce inflammatory joint damage such as erosion and joint-space narrowing that can be progressive and irreversible and that results in functional impairment [2–4].

The loss of the articular cartilage in RA is evident on X-ray as joint-space narrowing, but in most cases, erosion and joint-space narrowing progress coordinately. Therefore, most studies show combined data for erosion and joint-space narrowing as exemplified by one of the most widely used joint destruction scores, the modified total Sharp score [5–7]. Moreover, although they do not progress separately, it is considered that erosion and joint-space narrowing can affect one another. Because joint destruction is mostly irreversible and directly causes joint pain and functional disability, a key target of treatment is prevention of joint destruction, and it is a fundamental rule of treatment that results should be determined, at least partially, by how well the treatment can prevent joint destruction [8].

As indicated above, synovitis is a fundamental clinical and pathological feature of RA and is largely responsible for the disease-associated joint destruction. Therefore, the basic strategy of treatment is to inhibit or alleviate synovitis; numerous clinical and basic studies have shown that this can prevent joint destruction. Most studies, guidelines, and recommendations have suggested that prevention of joint destruction can be achieved by decreasing disease activity and maintaining this lower activity as remission [9, 10]. Moreover, to suppress the progression of joint destruction, alleviation of synovitis should be achieved as early as possible within the (therapeutic) *window of opportunity* [11, 12].

* Correspondence: hiromu@kuhp.kyoto-u.ac.jp
[1]The Department of Orthopaedic Surgery, Kyoto University Graduate School of Medicine, 54 Kawahara-cho, Shogoin, Sakyo, Kyoto 606-8507, Japan
Full list of author information is available at the end of the article

Clinical remission and joint destruction

The main goal of RA treatment is to suppress disease activity as early in the disease process as possible, thereby achieving clinical remission and preventing radiographic damage and disability. Several sets of criteria to define clinical remission in RA have been proposed and applied, starting with the 1981 American College of Rheumatology (ACR) definition of remission [13], followed by the definition of remission as a disease activity score of less than 1.6 based on 44 joints (DAS44) [14], later modified to a score of less than 2.6 involving 28 joints (DAS28) [15], a clinical disease activity index (CDAI) of less than 2.8 [16], and a simplified disease activity index (SDAI) of less than 3.3 [17]. More recently, the ACR and the European League Against Rheumatism (EULAR) collaborated to propose that remission in RA can be defined either according to the remission criteria of both the CDAI and the SDAI or the new Boolean-based set of criteria (ACR/EULAR remission criterion) [18].

Treat to target (T2T) is considered a key strategy in the induction of remission in individual RA patients [19]. DAS28 remission is a feasible goal in daily clinical practice with the application of a T2T strategy of early and intensive treatment of patients with early RA, which leads to high remission rates [20] and limited radiographic progression after 1 year of follow-up [21]. However, clinical trials have demonstrated that some patients with RA in remission defined by DAS28 showed residual joint swelling and radiographic progression compared with patients in remission defined by ACR/EULAR. However, the ACR/EULAR remission criteria are difficult to achieve in patients with established RA. It is unclear which criteria should be used and how often clinical remission can be achieved in daily clinical practice.

Sustained clinical remission contributes to functional remission and less radiological progression

On the basis of these considerations, we conducted a retrospective longitudinal study to investigate whether sustained clinical remission would reduce functional disability and radiological progression, to identify which remission criteria best reflected functional and radiological remission, and how often clinical remission should be achieved in daily clinical practice. The results of this study were partially described in an article in the official journal of the Japanese Orthopaedic Association [22].

Materials and methods

In 2012, we enrolled 384 patients from the Kyoto University Rheumatoid Arthritis Management Alliance (KURAMA) cohort [23], and complete datasets for 170 of these patients, with both more than 6 months of follow-up and with more than three visits during follow-up, were used in this study. The data collected included age, sex, disease duration, Steinbrocker class, Steinbrocker stage, swollen joint count based on assessment of 28 joints (SJC28), tender joint count based on assessment of 28 joints (TJC28), the presence of rheumatoid factor (RF) and/or anti-citrullinated protein antibodies, C-reactive protein level, erythrocyte sedimentation rate (ESR), score on the Health Assessment Questionnaire disability index (HAQ-DI) [24], the patient's assessment of pain measured using a 100-mm visual analogue scale (VAS), and global assessments of disease activity by evaluators (EGA) and patients (PGA). The radiographs were scored according to the van der Heijde-modified Sharp scoring method by two trained physicians blinded to the sequence of the radiographs [6]. The change in the Sharp/van der Heijde score (SHS) during follow-up was the main outcome of the study and was divided by the years of follow-up to calculate the annual rate of change. Patients with more than 1 unit change in SHS per year were classified as "progressors" [25]. Patients with 5 or more unit change in SHS per year were classified as showing rapid radiographic progression (RRP). Four different remission criteria were evaluated in this study: DAS28–ESR calculated including ESR (mm/h), TJC28, SJC28, and the PGA. Remission was defined as reported previously [16, 17]. The rate of remission maintenance was calculated by dividing the length of time for each remission by the number of patient visits throughout the follow-up period. "Complete sustained remission" was defined as a maintenance rate of 100%, "nearly sustained remission" was defined as a maintenance rate of 50% or more, "incomplete sustained remission" was defined as a maintenance rate of less than 50%, and "no remission" was defined as a maintenance rate of 0%.

Results

The demographic characteristics of the patients are shown in Table 1. Among the 170 patients, the mean (SD) maintenance rates of clinical remission were 38.4% (38.3%) using DAS28, 23.0% (31.5%) using CDAI, 25.0% (32.7%) using SDAI, and 15.0% (25.7%) using Boolean-based remission criteria (Table 2). To determine whether biological DMARDs (bDMARDs) maintained clinical remission better than conventional synthetic DMARDs (csDMARDs), we compared the maintenance rates for each remission definition between the 62 patients treated with bDMARDs and the 108 patients treated with csDMARDs. The maintenance rate of remission defined according to DAS28–ESR was higher with bDMARDs than with csDMARDs (bDMARDs: mean 48.9%, csDMARDs: mean 32.4%; $P < 0.01$). However, there were no significant differences between bDMARDs and csDMARDs in the maintenance rates of remission defined according to CDAI, SDAI, and Boolean-based criteria. Analysis of functional

Table 1 Characteristics of the patient population

	Mean ± SD or n (percent)	Median (range)
Age, years	62.7 ± 12.4	64.5 (31~85)
Disease duration, years	13.6 ± 11.5	11.25 (0.4~64.3)
Women	140 patients (82.4%)	
Steinbrocker's stage, I/II/III/IV	23 (13.5%)/53 (31.2%)/27 (15.9%)/67 (39.4%)	
Steinbrocker's class, 1/2/3/4	41 (24.1%)/103 (60.6%)/25 (14.7%)/1 (0.01%)	
Rheumatoid factor positive	133 (78.2%)	
Anti-citrullinated protein antibody positive	135 (79.4%)	
C-reactive protein, mg/dl	0.61 ± 1.13	0.1 (0~5.4)
Erythrocyte sedimentation rate, mm/h	25.4 ± 21.1	18.5 (0~117)
Tender joint count, 0 to 28joints	1.1 ± 2.0	0 (0~14)
Swollen joint count, 0 to 28joints	1.2 ± 1.7	0 (0~9)
Patient's global assessment, 0 to 100 mm	36.8 ± 26.3	32 (1~100)
Evaluator's global assessment, 0 to 100 mm	14.6 ± 15.1	10 (0~73)
Disease activity score in 28 joints at endpoint	3.05 ± 1.22	2.94 (0.00~5.90)
Simplified disease activity index at endpoint	7.99 ± 6.51	5.90 (0.20~30.40)
Clinical disease activity index at endpoint	7.37 ± 5.97	5.75 (0.20~28.00)
Health Assessment Questionnaire disability index, 0 to 3	0.90 ± 0.76	0.8125 (0~3)
Sharp/van der Heijde score at baseline	109.5 ± 101.1	77.5 (1~398)
Sharp/van der Heijde score at endpoint	112.7 ± 101.6	79.5 (2~401)
Annual change of Sharp/van der Heijde score	3.6 ± 7.9	1 (− 8~58)
Use of glucocorticoid	76 (44.7%)	
Use of methotrexate	141 (70.6%)	
Use of biologics	62 (36.5%)	
TNF inhibitors	40 (23.5%)	
Tocilizumab	12 (7.1%)	
Abatacept	10 (5.9%)	

Data representing the demographic characteristics of the 170 patients. Data are presented as means ± S.D. or n (percent) and median (range)

impairment represented by HAQ-DI indicated that sustained clinical remission contributed to functional remission of RA (Table 3). The radiographic progression rates of patients as assessed by DAS28–ESR, SDAI, CDAI, and Boolean-based remission criteria are illustrated in Table 4. The annual change in SHS and a cumulative probability plot showing the individual data for all patients are presented in Figs. 1, 2, 3, and 4. There were fewer radiological progressors in the complete sustained remission and nearly sustained remission groups than in the incomplete sustained remission and no remission groups, for all definitions of remission. The number of progressors was

Table 2 Proportions of patients who sustained clinical remission according to each criterion during follow-up period

	DAS28-ESR	CDAI	SDAI	Boolean-based
Mean (SD) maintain rate of remission, %	38.4 (38.3)	23.0 (31.5)	25.0 (32.7)	15.0 (25.7)
No. (%) of complete sustained remission	26 (15.3)	9 (5.3)	12 (7.1)	4 (2.4)
No. (%) of nearly sustained remission	39 (22.9)	29 (17.1)	27 (15.9)	18 (10.6)
No. (%) of incomplete sustained remission	43 (25.3)	42 (24.7)	47 (27.6)	36 (21.2)
No. (%) of none remission	62 (36.5)	90 (52.9)	84 (49.4)	112 (65.9)

Data represent the proportions of RA patients who sustained clinical remission according to each criterion during follow-up period. Complete sustained remission was defined as maintain rate of 100%. Nearly sustained remission was defined as maintain rate of 50% or more. Incomplete sustained remission was defined as maintain rate of less than 50%. None remission was defined as maintain rate of 0%. Boolean-based is one of the ACR/EULAR remission criteria
DAS28–ESR disease activity score based on 28 joint count and erythrocyte segmentation rate, *CDAI* clinical disease activity index, *SDAI* simplified disease activity index

Table 3 Functional disability of patients who sustained clinical remission according to each criterion during follow-up period

		DAS28-ESR	CDAI	SDAI	Boolean-based
Complete sustained remission	Mean (SD) HAQ-DI	0.37 (0.14)	0.36 (0.25)	0.43 (0.22)	0.22 (0.38)
	No. (%) of functional remission	20 (76.9)	7 (77.8)	9 (75.0)	4 (100)
Nearly sustained remission	Mean (SD) HAQ-DI	0.65 (0.12)	0.30 (0.13)	0.33 (0.14)	0.39 (0.18)
	No. (%) of functional remission	22 (56.4)	25 (86.2)	22 (81.5)	14 (77.8)
Incomplete sustained remission	Mean (SD) HAQ-DI	0.93 (0.12)	0.70 (0.12)	0.71 (0.11)	0.43 (0.12)
	No. (%) of functional remission	15 (34.9)	18 (42.9)	21 (44.7)	23 (63.9)
None remission	Mean (SD) HAQ-DI	1.26 (0.09)	1.24 (0.07)	1.26 (0.07)	1.15 (0.06)
	No. (%) of functional remission	14 (22.6)	21 (23.3)	19 (22.6)	30 (26.8)

Functional disability was assessed by HAQ-DI at endpoint. Complete sustained remission was defined as maintain rate of 100%. Nearly sustained remission was defined as maintain rate of 50% and more. Incomplete sustained remission was defined as maintain rate of less than 50%. None remission was defined as maintain rate of 0%. Functional remission was defined as HAQ-DI < 0.5
HAQ-DI health assessment questionnaire disability index

approximately equivalent in the complete and nearly sustained remission groups as assessed by all criteria, although no patients in either the complete or nearly sustained remission groups assessed by either SDAI or Boolean-based criteria were classified as RRP. To determine whether biological bDMARDs reduced radiological progression better than csDMARDs, we compared the annual change in SHS in the 62 patients treated with bDMARDs and the 108 patients treated with csDMARDs (Fig. 5). No instance of RRP was observed for patients treated with either bDMARDs or csDMARDs in the complete and nearly sustained remission groups as defined by the SDAI criteria. However, RRP was observed with both treatments in the groups with incomplete sustained or no remission defined by the SDAI criteria.

In conclusion, this study clearly demonstrated that sustained clinical remission contributes to reduced radiological progression in RA.

Bone and cartilage regeneration in rheumatology clinical practice

The results described above clearly show that not only achieving remission but also maintaining remission is crucial for preventing joint destruction. However, is it possible to achieve bone regeneration using any type of treatment? And if so, how?

Historically, it was the universal consensus in clinical rheumatology that joint destruction could not be reversed by any kind of treatment. In other words, once any part of the joint was destroyed, nothing could be done for the joint other than trying to prevent further destruction. This was the main reason why practitioners were eager to start aggressive treatment before any joint destruction was observed. This concept still holds mostly true in the current medical situation. However, even before the advent of highly effective treatments such as bDMARDs and targeted synthetic DMARDs (tsDMARDs), bone regeneration or healing was observed in a small proportion

Table 4 Radiographic progression of patients who sustained clinical remission according to each criterion during follow-up period

			DAS28-ESR	CDAI	SDAI	Boolean-based
Complete sustained remission	Annual change in SHS	Mean (SD)	2.2 (4.0)	1.7 (1.7)	1.3 (1.6)	2.4 (1.7)
		range	0–20	0–4	0–4	0–4
	No. (percent) of RRP		2 (7.7)	0 (0)	0 (0)	0 (0)
Nearly sustained remission	Annual change in SHS	Mean (SD)	2.7 (8.7)	1.7 (2.5)	1.6 (1.5)	1.3 (1.5)
		range	− 8–52	0–12	0–4	0–4
	No. (percent) of RRP		3 (7.7)	1 (3.4)	0 (0)	0 (0)
Incomplete sustained remission	Annual change in SHS	Mean (SD)	2.7 (3.9)	2.3 (8.2)	3.5 (8.6)	3.2 (9.0)
		range	− 2–14	− 8–52	− 8–52	− 2–52
	No. (percent) of RRP		9 (20.9)	4 (9.5)	9 (19.1)	3 (8.3)
None remission	Annual change in SHS	Mean (SD)	5.5 (10.3)	5.1 (9.1)	4.8 (9.1)	4.2 (8.3)
		range	− 6–58	− 6–58	− 6–58	− 8–58
	No. (percent) of RRP		20 (32.3)	29 (32.2)	25 (29.8)	31 (27.7)

Radiographic progression was assessed by annual change in Sharp/van der Heijde score (SHS) during follow-up period. RRP (rapid radiographic progression) was defined as 5 or more unit change in SHS per year. Complete sustained remission was defined as maintain rate of 100%. Nearly sustained remission was defined as maintain rate of 50% and more. Incomplete sustained remission was defined as maintain rate of less than 50%. None remission was defined as maintain rate of 0%

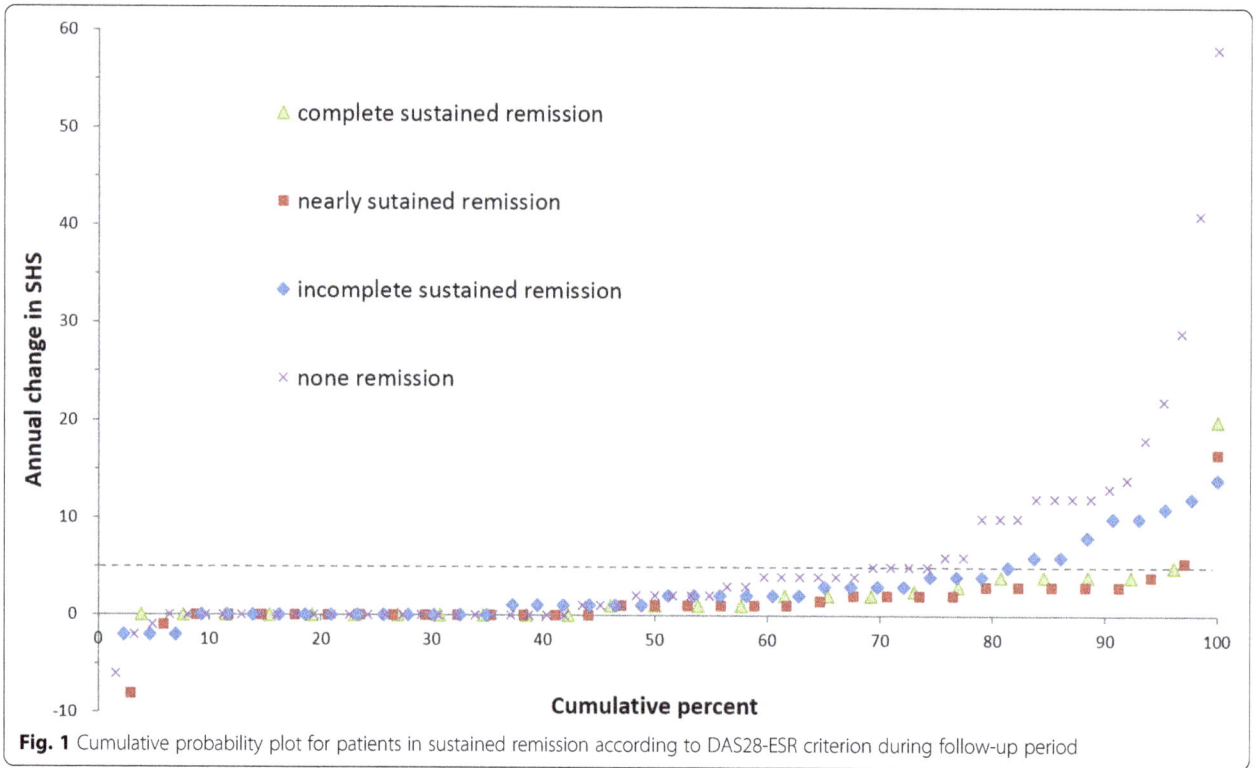

Fig. 1 Cumulative probability plot for patients in sustained remission according to DAS28-ESR criterion during follow-up period

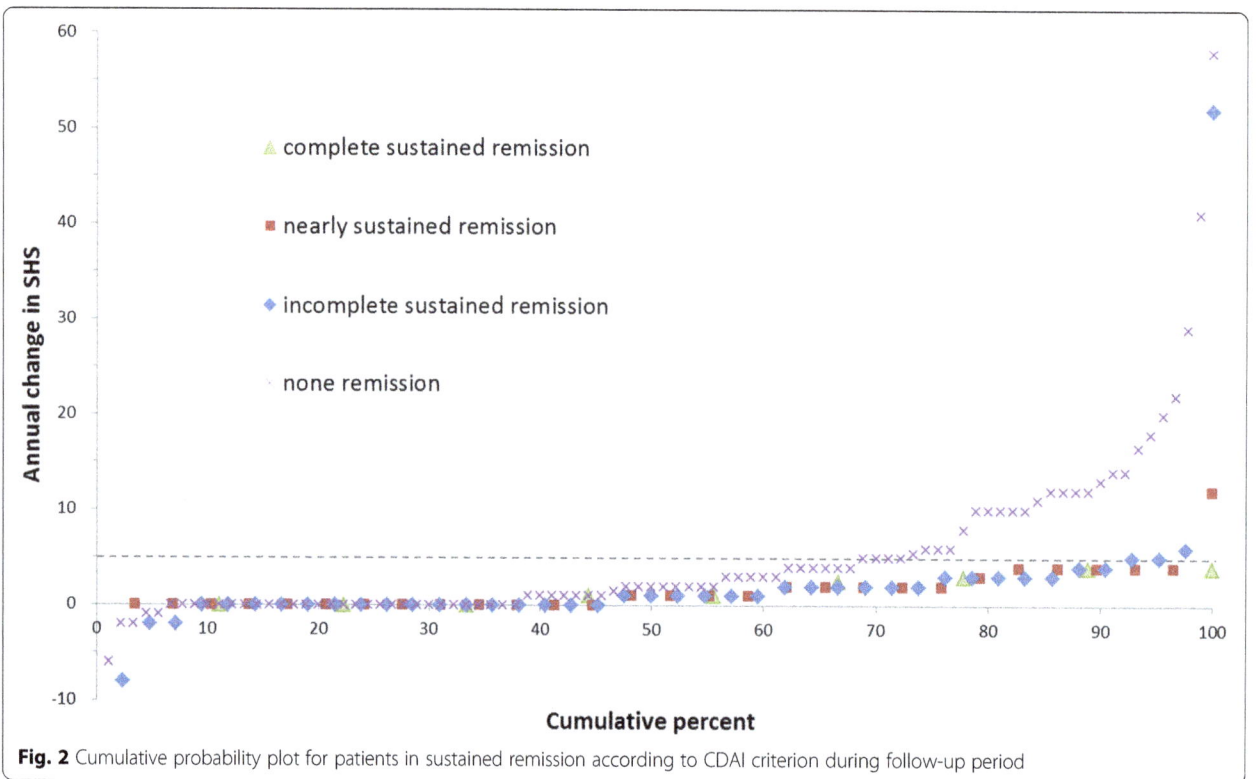

Fig. 2 Cumulative probability plot for patients in sustained remission according to CDAI criterion during follow-up period

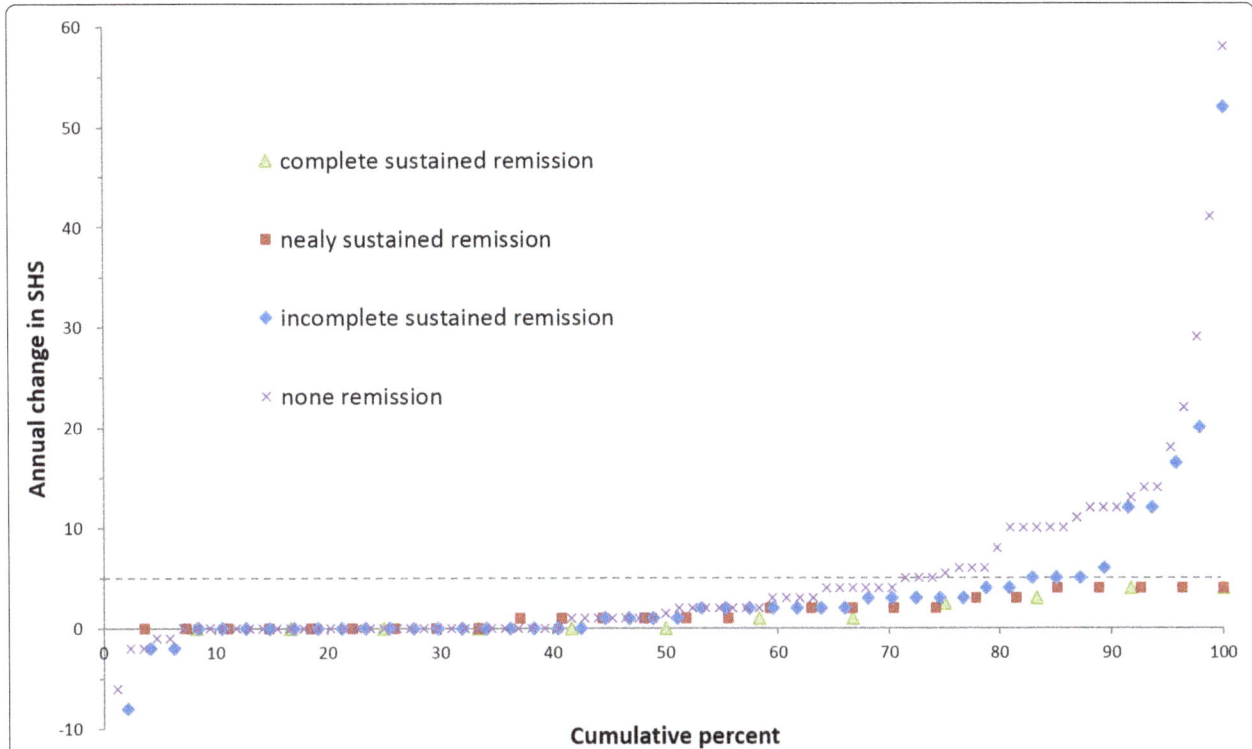

Fig. 3 Cumulative probability plot for patients in sustained remission according to SDAI criterion during follow-up period

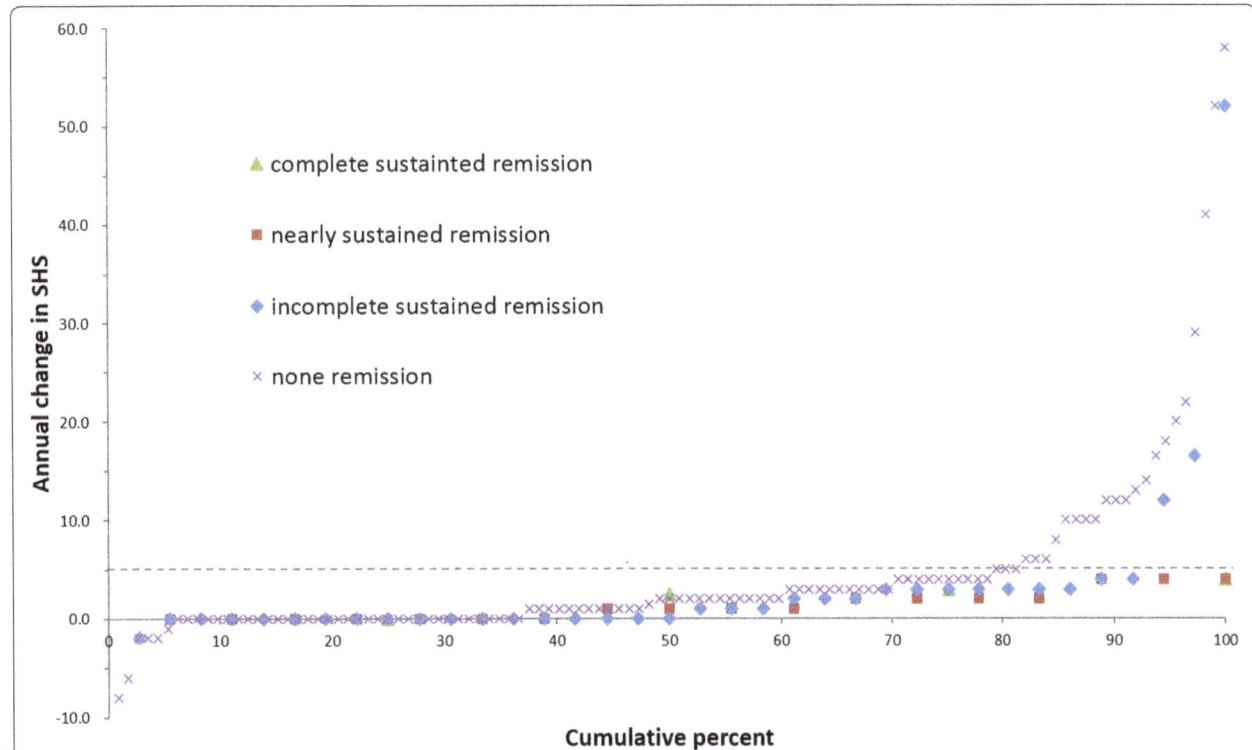

Fig. 4 Cumulative probability plot for patients in sustained remission according to Boolean based remission criterion during follow-up period

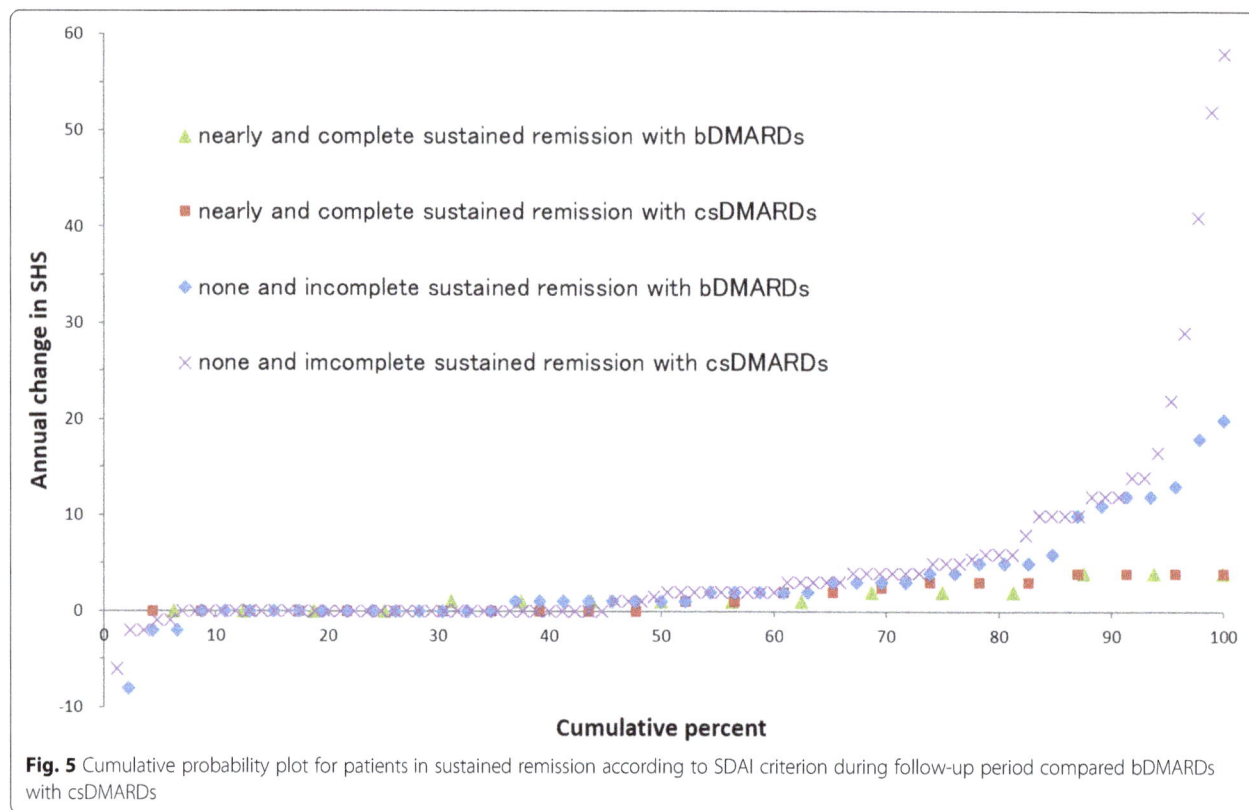

Fig. 5 Cumulative probability plot for patients in sustained remission according to SDAI criterion during follow-up period compared bDMARDs with csDMARDs

of RA patients. In a pioneering case report, Rau and Herborn described the healing of erosive changes in six RA patients who were treated with methotrexate and/or gold sodium thiomalate (GST) [26]. Although Rau and colleagues repeatedly reported such cases, it was still considered that such healing was very rare [26–28].

However, the dramatic results of treatment with bDMARDs have gradually changed the entire basis of the treatment strategy for RA and practitioners' frame of mind in terms of bone destruction and regeneration. The 2005 article by Ikari and Momohara clearly showed that methotrexate can induce bone regeneration [29], and many practitioners have seen such cases repeatedly in their routine clinical practice. Indeed, some of the first randomized controlled studies using bDMARDs reported negative average values for joint destruction after a certain period of treatment [30–32], which means that the majority of patients who used bDMARDs experienced bone regeneration in one way or another.

However, critics or doubters claimed that such regeneration was seen only in small joints such as the proximal interphalangeal, metacarpophalangeal, or metatarsophalangeal joints in the fingers or toes. Indeed, most case reports have shown bone regeneration only of small joints. However, Momohara's case report clearly showed that even a large joint (hip joint) can achieve cartilage regeneration, or at least the reappearance of the joint space, with

an effective treatment such as bDMARDs [33]. After this pioneering case report, clinical studies including a case series have described bone regeneration of large joints [34]. As a result, a Japanese research group has established a radiological change score called the ARASHI change score, which incorporates the improvements in bone quality, joint space narrowing, joint conformity, and the disappearance of bone erosion and joint surface destruction [35]. Unfortunately, it is still the case that joint regeneration in the large joints is relatively rare. Seki and Matsushita have shown that, once joint damage has been detected, damage in the ankle joint tends to be less progressive but joint destruction in the hip and knee joints is likely to progress even following a good response to anti-tumor necrosis factor alpha treatment [36–38]. Therefore, it remains largely unresolved whether a large joint can regenerate, and if so, how it regenerates. Other unresolved issues are the nature of the predictors of large-joint regeneration, and how we can intervene to stimulate regeneration or, at least, to prevent the progression of large-joint destruction.

Is it possible to induce joint regeneration by surgical management?

Most therapeutic strategies for prevention or regeneration of joint destruction are based on the use of effective medications. However, oral or intravenous medication has an effect on the whole body, i.e., it diffuses throughout the whole body and may therefore be less effective in a particular joint. One of the potent options for treating a particular joint is intra-articular injection. Indeed, several studies indicate that intra-articular injection of steroid is highly effective and comparable to bDMARDs for the alleviation of disease activity [39]. For example, a preliminary report showed that in osteoarthritis, intrajoint injection of bDMARDs can achieve a better response than injection of hyaluronan [40]. Moreover, a recent study showed that intra-articular glucocorticoids in combination with methotrexate can induce bone regeneration in some cases of RA, although this response is relatively rare [41]. Future investigations should determine which patients should receive intra-articular steroid injection and its optimal timing.

Another possible approach to this issue is surgical intervention. Joint regeneration, especially cartilage regeneration, has been widely investigated over the last three decades. We recently published a report of scaffoldless hyaline cartilaginous tissue derived from induced pluripotent stem cells [42]. However, despite committed, long-term efforts worldwide, clinically useful hyaline cartilage regeneration has not yet been achieved. To overcome this highly problematic threshold to achieving joint regeneration, the most plausible treatment strategy is to induce or assist the patient's own ability to regenerate bone and cartilage. In the case of inflammatory arthritis

such as RA, the reduction of synovitis or the surgical removal of inflammatory synovia is one plausible option. We have experienced one such case in the past.

The patient, a 21-year-old woman, presented to our hospital with pain and a soft tissue mass on her left fifth metatarsophalangeal joint. Radiographic and magnetic resonance imaging showed a tumor-like mass with destruction of the joint (Fig. 6a′, white arrow), which was reported as being suggestive of a benign tumor. At surgery, synovia-like tissues were observed that had migrated into the bare area of this joint. This lesion was successfully removed, and histological analysis confirmed synovitis, suspicious of RA. The patient gradually developed polyarticular synovitis, and methotrexate was started 3 years later. Surprisingly, bone repair of this joint was achieved 1 year after surgery and was maintained without recurrence of synovitis for more than 5 years (Fig. 6b′, c′, white arrows). In contrast, her left first metatarsophalangeal joint gradually developed destructive changes (Fig. 6a, b, white thick arrow), which led to surgical arthrodesis 3 years later (Fig. 6c, white thick arrow).

Some authors recommend surgical synovectomy for patients with RA who do not experience substantial pain relief in response to medications. By removing all synovial tissues, synovectomy can diminish local pain and swelling, but bone repair of damaged joints has not

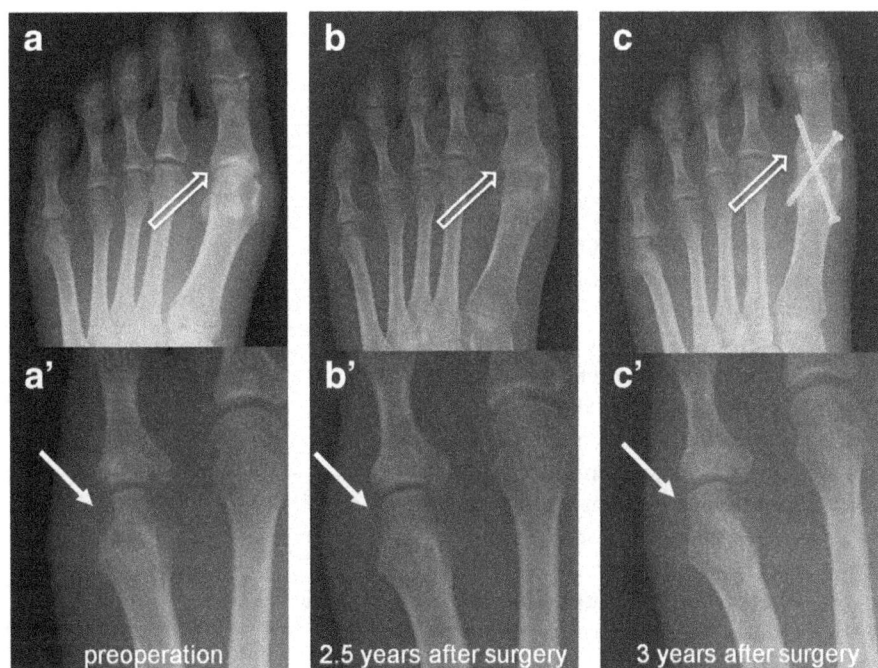

Fig. 6 a–c, a′–c′ Bone regeneration after synovectomy of the 5th metatarsophalangeal joint of the left foot. The left panel shows the preoperative radiograph of the left foot. Bone erosion was seen in the 5th metatarsal head. The middle panel shows the reappearance of the 5th metatarsal head 2.5 years after synovectomy of the joint. Joint space narrowing appeared at the 1st metatarsophalangeal joint. The right panel shows consolidation of the 5th metatarsal head. The 1st metatarsophalangeal joint was fixed

been expected. This case provides evidence that synovectomy can induce bone repair of a damaged joint in a patient with early RA. To the best of our knowledge, this is the very first report that synovectomy indeed stimulated joint regeneration. Pinder previously reported that synovectomy with drilling of areas of articular cartilage loss showed cartilage regeneration and relief of symptoms [43]. However, since then, no other report has shown similar results by any surgical procedures. The reason of his success may be that he probably conducted this procedure in patients with very low disease activity. But the regeneration potential of the joint should be paid with full attention even in RA patients in the current medication.

Also, the molecular mechanisms of how the regeneration occurs have been investigated and proposed, which has attracted huge attention from basic researchers. Several review articles recently summarized the proposed mechanism of bone remodeling in RA that proinflammatory cytokines such as TNF alpha stimulates the production of DKK-1 family and soluble frizzled related protein, suggesting that inhibition of such cytokines downregulates those proteins and revives bone formation processes [44, 45]. Wehmeyer et al. recently lay stress on the importance of stromal cells which release Wnt antagonists such as sclerostin and DKK-1 under inflammatory conditions [44, 46]. Taken together, blocking proinflammatory cytokines or removal of synovial tissues producing such cytokines can regain the balance of bone resorption and formation and can stimulate bone regeneration. Adding to the suppression of proinflammatory cytokines or cells, suppression of Wnt antagonists or stromal cells may be a potent therapeutic option in the future.

Future perspectives

In inflammatory arthritis, synovitis causes bone and cartilage destruction as described above. One of the most crucial requirements for regeneration of the destroyed joint is alleviation of synovitis. This can be achieved by use of adequate medication as soon as possible after the diagnosis of the disease. When the joint has the ability to regenerate the destroyed bone and/or articular cartilage, self-regeneration should occur after alleviation of the synovitis. However, regenerative medicine will have a crucial role in treatment when this ability is lost, or when the destruction is too severe to be overcome. Although it is still uncertain what kind of treatment options will be available in routine clinical practice, regenerative medicine should be able to rescue the damaged joint using potent cell therapies.

Conclusions

To prevent joint destruction in inflammatory arthritis such as RA, the universal consensus is to treat, to alleviate synovitis and to achieve clinical remission. Our study shows that maintaining remission is also crucial to prevent the progression of joint destruction. Although regeneration of the damaged joint has been considered to occur very rarely, accumulating evidence shows that it can actually occur in routine clinical practice after strong inhibition of synovitis with highly potent medications. Two potent options other than oral or intravenous medication for inducing joint regeneration in a particular joint would be intra-articular steroid injection and synovectomy. In the future, regenerative medicine could play a crucial role in inducing regeneration of damaged joints after synovitis is effectively inhibited when self-regeneration cannot overcome severe destruction.

Abbreviations
ACR: American College of Rheumatology; bDMARD: Biological DMARD; CDAI: Clinical disease activity index; csDMARD: Conventional synthetic DMARD; DAS28: Disease activity score involving a 28 joints; DAS44: Disease activity score based on 44 joints; DMARD: Disease-modifying anti-rheumatic drug; EGA: Global assessments of disease activity by evaluators; ESR: Erythrocyte sedimentation rate; EULAR: The European League Against Rheumatism; HAQ-DI: The Health Assessment Questionnaire disability index; KURAMA: The Kyoto University Rheumatoid Arthritis Management Alliance; PGA: Global assessments of disease activity by patients; RA: Rheumatoid arthritis; RF: Rheumatoid factor; RRP: Rapid radiographic progression; SDAI: Simplified disease activity index; SHS: Sharp/van der Heijde score; SJC28: Swollen joint count based on assessment of 28 joints; T2T: Treat to target; TJC28: Tender joint count based on assessment of 28 joints; tsDMARD: Targeted synthetic DMARD; VAS: Visual analogue scale

Acknowledgements
The authors thank Drs. Tsuneyo Mimori, Takao Fujii, Chicashi Terao, Noriyuki Yamakawa, Kohei Nishitani, Kosaku Murakami, and Hiroyuki Yoshitomi for their thoughtful discussion and technical assistance.

Authors' contributions
HI, MF, and SM contributed to the study conception and design. MF contributed to the analysis of the data. HI, MF, MH, and MT contributed to the acquisition of data. HI and MF contributed to the interpretation of the data. HI and MF drafted the article. HI, MF, MH, MT, SM revised the article and gave final approval. All authors read and approved the final manuscript.

Competing interests
The Department of Advanced Medicine for Rheumatic Diseases is supported by Nagahama City, Shiga, Japan, and four pharmaceutical companies (Mitsubishi Tanabe Pharma Co., Chugai Pharmaceutical Co. Ltd, UCB Japan Co. Ltd, and AYUMI Pharmaceutical Co.). KURAMA cohort study is supported by a grant from Daiichi Sankyo Co. Ltd. This study is conducted as investigator initiate study. HI has received a research grant and/or speaker fee from Bristol-Myers, Astellas, and Eli Lily. MH has received research grants from Astellas and Daiichi-Sankyo. MT has received research grants from Astellas, Abbvie, Pfizer, and Taisho-Toyama. MF and SM declared no conflicts of interest. The sponsors were not involved in the study design; in the collection, analysis, and interpretation of data; in the writing of this

manuscript; or in the decision to submit the article for publication. The authors, their immediate families, and any research foundations with which they are affiliated have not received any financial payments or other benefits from any commercial entity related to the subject of this article.

Author details

[1]The Department of Orthopaedic Surgery, Kyoto University Graduate School of Medicine, 54 Kawahara-cho, Shogoin, Sakyo, Kyoto 606-8507, Japan. [2]The Department of Advanced Medicine for Rheumatic Diseases, Kyoto University Graduate School of Medicine, Kyoto, Japan.

References

1. Terao C, Hashimoto M, Yamamoto K, Murakami K, Ohmura K, Nakashima R, et al. Three groups in the 28 joints for rheumatoid arthritis synovitis—analysis using more than 17,000 assessments in the KURAMA database. PLoS One. 2013;8(3):e59341.
2. Keystone EC, Haraoui B, Guerette B, Mozaffarian N, Liu S, Kavanaugh A. Clinical, functional, and radiographic implications of time to treatment response in patients with early rheumatoid arthritis: a posthoc analysis of the PREMIER study. J Rheumatol. 2014;41(2):235–43.
3. Scott DL, Pugner K, Kaarela K, Doyle DV, Woolf A, Holmes J, et al. The links between joint damage and disability in rheumatoid arthritis. Rheumatology (Oxford). 2000;39:122–32.
4. Welsing PM, Van Gestel AM, Swinkels HL, Kiemeney LA, Van Riel PL. The relationship between disease activity, joint destruction, and functional capacity over the course of rheumatoid arthritis. Arthritis Rheum. 2001;44:2009–17.
5. Sharp JT, Young DY, Bluhm GB, Brook A, Brower AC, Corbett M, Decker JL, Genant HK, Gofton JP, Goodman N, et al. How many joints in the hands and wrists should be included in a score of radiologic abnormalities used to assess rheumatoid arthritis? Arthritis Rheum. 1985;28(12):1326–35.
6. van der Heijde D. How to read radiographs according to the Sharp/van der Heijde method. J Rheumatol. 1999;26(3):743–5.
7. van der Heijde D, Dankert T, Nieman F, Rau R, Boers M. Reliability and sensitivity to change of a simplification of the Sharp/van der Heijde radiological assessment in rheumatoid arthritis. Rheumatology (Oxford). 1999;38(10):941–7.
8. Smolen JS, Aletaha D, Redlich K. The pathogenesis of rheumatoid arthritis: new insights from old clinical data? Nat Rev Rheumatol. 2012;8(4):235–43.
9. Smolen JS, Landewé R, Bijlsma J, Burmester G, Chatzidionysiou K, Dougados M, Nam J, Ramiro S, Voshaar M, van Vollenhoven R, Aletaha D, Aringer M, Boers M, Buckley CD, Buttgereit F, Bykerk V, Cardiel M, Combe B, Cutolo M, van Eijk-Hustings Y, Emery P, Finckh A, Gabay C, Gomez-Reino J, Gossec L, Gottenberg JE, Hazes JMW, Huizinga T, Jani M, Karateev D, Kouloumas M, Kvien T, Li Z, Mariette X, McInnes I, Mysler E, Nash P, Pavelka K, Poór G, Richez C, van Riel P, Rubbert-Roth A, Saag K, da Silva J, Stamm T, Takeuchi T, Westhovens R, de Wit M, van der Heijde D. EULAR recommendations for the management of rheumatoid arthritis with synthetic and biological disease-modifying antirheumatic drugs: 2016 update. Ann Rheum Dis. 2017;76(6):960–77.
10. Singh JA, Saag KG, Bridges SL Jr, Akl EA, Bannuru RR, Sullivan MC, Vaysbrot E, McNaughton C, Osani M, Shmerling RH, Curtis JR, Furst DE, Parks D, Kavanaugh A, O'Dell J, King C, Leong A, Matteson EL, Schousboe JT, Drevlow B, Ginsberg S, Grober J, St Clair EW, Tindall E, Miller AS, McAlindon T, American College of Rheumatology. 2015 American College of Rheumatology guideline for the treatment of rheumatoid arthritis. Arthritis Care Res (Hoboken). 2016;68(1):1–25.
11. van Steenbergen HW, da Silva JAP, Huizinga TWJ, van der Helm-van Mil AHM. Preventing progression from arthralgia to arthritis: targeting the right patients. Nat Rev Rheumatol. 2018;14(1):32–41.
12. van Nies JA, Tsonaka R, Gaujoux-Viala C, Fautrel B, van der Helm-van Mil AH. Evaluating relationships between symptom duration and persistence of rheumatoid arthritis: does a window of opportunity exist? Results on the Leiden early arthritis clinic and ESPOIR cohorts. Ann Rheum Dis. 2015;74(5):806–12.
13. Pinals RS, Masi AT, Larsen RA. Preliminary criteria for clinical remission in rheumatoid arthritis. Arthritis Rheum. 1981;24:1308–15.
14. Van der Heijde DMFM, van 't Hof MA, van Riel PLCM, Theunisse LM, Lubberts EW, van Leeuwen MA, van Rijswijk MH, van de LBA P. Judging disease activity in clinical practice in rheumatoid arthritis: first step in the development of a disease activity score. Ann Rheum Dis. 1990;49:916–20.
15. Prevoo ML, van 't Hof MA, Kuper HH, van Leeuwen MA, van de Putte LB, van Riel PL. Modified disease activity scores that include twenty-eight-joint counts: development and validation in a prospective longitudinal study of patients with rheumatoid arthritis. Arthritis Rheum. 1995;38:44–8.
16. Aletaha D, Nell VP, Stamm T, et al. Acute phase reactants add little to composite disease activity indices for rheumatoid arthritis: validation of a clinical activity score. Arthritis Res Ther. 2005;7:R796–806.
17. Aletaha D, Smolen JS. The simplified disease activity index (SDAI) and clinical disease activity index (CDAI) to monitor patients in standard clinical care. Best Pract Res Clin Rheumatol. 2007;21:663–75.
18. Felson DT, Smolen JS, Wells G, et al. American College of Rheumatology/European League against Rheumatism provisional definition of remission in rheumatoid arthritis for clinical trials. Ann Rheum Dis. 2011;70:404–13.
19. Smolen JS, Aletaha D, Bijlsma JW, Breedveld FC, Boumpas D, Burmester G, et al. Treating rheumatoid arthritis to target: recommendations of an international task force. Ann Rheum Dis. 2010;69:631–7.
20. Schipper LG, Vermeer M, Kuper HH, Hoekstra MO, Haagsma CJ, Broeder AA, et al. A tight control treatment strategy aiming for remission in early rheumatoid arthritis is more effective than usual care treatment in daily clinical practice: a study of two cohorts in the Dutch Rheumatoid Arthritis Monitoring registry. Ann Rheum Dis. 2012;71:845–50.
21. Vermeer M, Kuper HH, Hoekstra M, Haagsma CJ, Posthumus MD, Brus HL, et al. Implementation of a treat-to-target strategy in very early rheumatoid arthritis: results of the Dutch Rheumatoid Arthritis Monitoring remission induction cohort study. Arthritis Rheum. 2011;63:2865–72.
22. Ito H, Furu M, Matsuda S. What affects joint destruction in rheumatoid arthritis -effect of sustained remission ratio and biological disease modifying anti-rheumatic drugs. J Jpn Orthop Assoc. 2018;92(5):(in press). [in the Japanese].
23. Furu M, Hashimoto M, Ito H, Fujii T, Terao C, Yamakawa N, Yoshitomi H, Ogino H, Ishikawa M, Matsuda S, Mimori T. Discordance and accordance between patient's and physician's assessments in rheumatoid arthritis. Scand J Rheumatol. 2014;43(4):291–5.
24. Fries JF, Spitz P, Kraines RG, Holman HR. Measurement of patient outcome in arthritis. Arthritis Rheum. 1980;23:137–45.
25. van der Heijde D, Landewé R, van Vollenhoven R, et al. Level of radiographic damage and radiographic progression are determinants of physical function: a longitudinal analysis of the TEMPO trial. Ann Rheum Dis. 2008;67:1267–70.
26. Rau R, Herborn G. Healing phenomena of erosive changes in rheumatoid arthritis patients undergoing disease-modifying antirheumatic drug therapy. Arthritis Rheum. 1996;39(1):162–8.
27. Rau R, Wassenberg S, Herborn G, Perschel WT, Freitag G. Identification of radiologic healing phenomena in patients with rheumatoid arthritis. J Rheumatol. 2001;28(12):2608–15.
28. Wassenberg S, Rau R. Radiographic healing with sustained clinical remission in a patient with rheumatoid arthritis receiving methotrexate monotherapy. Arthritis Rheum. 2002;46(10):2804–7.
29. Ikari K, Momohara S. Images in clinical medicine. Bone changes in rheumatoid arthritis. N Engl J Med. 2005;353:e13.
30. Sharp JT, Van Der Heijde D, Boers M, Boonen A, Bruynesteyn K, Emery P, Genant HK, Herborn G, Jurik A, Lassere M, McQueen F, Østergaard M, Peterfy C, Rau R, Strand V, Wassenberg S, Weissman B, Subcommittee on Healing of Erosions of the OMERACT Imaging Committee. Repair of erosions in rheumatoid arthritis does occur. Results from 2 studies by the OMERACT Subcommittee on Healing of Erosions. J Rheumatol. 2003;30(5):1102–7.
31. Lipsky PE, van der Heijde DM, St Clair EW, Furst DE, Breedveld FC, Kalden JR, Smolen JS, Weisman M, Emery P, Feldmann M, Harriman GR, Maini RN; Anti-Tumor Necrosis Factor Trial in Rheumatoid Arthritis with Concomitant Therapy Study Group. Infliximab and methotrexate in the treatment of rheumatoid arthritis. Anti-Tumor Necrosis Factor Trial in Rheumatoid Arthritis with Concomitant Therapy Study Group. N Engl J Med 2000;343(22):1594-1602.
32. Klareskog L, van der Heijde D, de Jager JP, Gough A, Kalden J, Malaise M, Martín Mola E, Pavelka K, Sany J, Settas L, Wajdula J, Pedersen R, Fatenejad S, Sanda M, TEMPO (Trial of Etanercept and Methotrexate with Radiographic Patient Outcomes) study investigators. Therapeutic effect of the combination of etanercept and methotrexate compared with each

treatment alone in patients with rheumatoid arthritis: double-blind randomised controlled trial. Lancet. 2004;363(9410):675–81.

33. Momohara S, Tanaka E, Iwamoto T, Ikari K, Yamanaka H. Reparative radiological changes of a large joint after adalimumab for rheumatoid arthritis. Clin Rheumatol. 2011;30(4):591–2.

34. Kanbe K, Oh K, Chiba J, Inoue Y, Taguchi M, Yabuki A. Efficacy of golimumab for preventing large joint destruction in patients with rheumatoid arthritis as determined by the ARASHI score. Mod Rheumatol. 2017;27(6):938–45.

35. Kaneko A, Matsushita I, Kanbe K, Arai K, Kuga Y, Abe A, Matsumoto T, Nakagawa N, Nishida K. Development and validation of a new radiographic scoring system to evaluate bone and cartilage destruction and healing of large joints with rheumatoid arthritis: ARASHI (assessment of rheumatoid arthritis by scoring of large joint destruction and healing in radiographic imaging) study. Mod Rheumatol. 2013;23(6):1053–62.

36. Seki E, Matsushita I, Sugiyama E, Taki H, Shinoda K, Hounoki H, Motomura H, Kimura T. Radiographic progression in weight-bearing joints of patients with rheumatoid arthritis after TNF-blocking therapies. Clin Rheumatol. 2009;28(4):453–60.

37. Matsushita I, Motomura H, Seki E, Kimura T. Radiographic changes and factors associated with subsequent progression of damage in weight-bearing joints of patients with rheumatoid arthritis under TNF-blocking therapies-three-year observational study. Mod Rheumatol. 2017;27(4):570–5.

38. Nakajima A, Aoki Y, Sonobe M, Takahashi H, Saito M, Terayama K, Nakagawa K. Radiographic progression of large joint damage in patients with rheumatoid arthritis treated with biological disease-modifying anti-rheumatic drugs. Mod Rheumatol. 2016;26(4):517–21.

39. Axelsen MB, Eshed I, Hørslev-Petersen K, Stengaard-Pedersen K, Hetland ML, Møller J, Junker P, Pødenphant J, Schlemmer A, Ellingsen T, Ahlquist P, Lindegaard H, Linauskas A, Dam MY, Hansen I, Horn HC, Ammitzbøll CG, Jørgensen A, Krintel SB, Raun J, Krogh NS, Johansen JS, Østergaard M, OPERA study group. A treat-to-target strategy with methotrexate and intra-articular triamcinolone with or without adalimumab effectively reduces MRI synovitis, osteitis and tenosynovitis and halts structural damage progression in early rheumatoid arthritis: results from the OPERA randomised controlled trial. Ann Rheum Dis. 2015;74(5):867–75.

40. Ohtori S, Orita S, Yamauchi K, Eguchi Y, Ochiai N, Kishida S, Kuniyoshi K, Aoki Y, Nakamura J, Ishikawa T, Miyagi M, Kamoda H, Suzuki M, Kubota G, Sakuma Y, Oikawa Y, Inage K, Sainoh T, Sato J, Shiga Y, Abe K, Fujimoto K, Kanamoto H, Toyone T, Inoue G, Takahashi K. Efficacy of direct injection of etanercept into knee joints for pain in moderate and severe knee osteoarthritis. Yonsei Med J. 2015;56(5):1379–83.

41. Hørslev-Petersen K, Hetland ML, Ørnbjerg LM, Junker P, Pødenphant J, Ellingsen T, Ahlquist P, Lindegaard H, Linauskas A, Schlemmer A, Dam MY, Hansen I, Lottenburger T, Ammitzbøll CG, Jørgensen A, Krintel SB, Raun J, Johansen JS, Østergaard M, Stengaard-Pedersen K, OPERA Study-Group. Clinical and radiographic outcome of a treat-to-target strategy using methotrexate and intra-articularglucocorticoids with or without adalimumab induction: a 2-year investigator-initiated, double-blinded, randomised, controlled trial (OPERA). Ann Rheum Dis. 2016;75(9):1645–53.

42. Yamashita A, Morioka M, Yahara Y, Okada M, Kobayashi T, Kuriyama S, Matsuda S, Tsumaki N. Generation of scaffoldless hyaline cartilaginous tissue from human iPSCs. Stem Cell Rep. 2015;4(3):404–18.

43. Pinder I. Synovectomy with drilling of the rheumatoid knee. Proc R Soc Med. 1974;67(2):107–9.

44. Favero M, Giusti A, Geusens P, Goldring SR, Lems W, Schett G, Bianchi G. OsteoRheumatology: a new discipline? RMD Open. 2015;1(Suppl 1):e000083.

45. Goldring SR. Differential mechanisms of de-regulated bone formation in rheumatoid arthritis and spondyloarthritis. Rheumatology (Oxford). 2016; 55(suppl 2):ii56–60.

46. Wehmeyer C, Pap T, Buckley CD, Naylor AJ. The role of stromal cells in inflammatory bone loss. Clin Exp Immunol. 2017;189(1):1–11.

21

New application of anti-TLR monoclonal antibodies: detection, inhibition and protection

Ryutaro Fukui[1*], Yusuke Murakami[1,2] and Kensuke Miyake[1,3*]

Abstract

Monoclonal antibody (mAb) is an essential tool for the analysis in various fields of biology. In the field of innate immunology, mAbs have been established and used for the study of Toll-like receptors (TLRs), a family of pathogen sensors that induces cytokine production and activate immune responses. TLRs play the role as a frontline of protection against pathogens, whereas excessive activation of TLRs has been implicated in a variety of infectious diseases and inflammatory diseases. For example, TLR7 and TLR9 sense not only pathogen-derived nucleic acids, but also self-derived nucleic acids in noninfectious inflammatory diseases such as systemic lupus erythematosus (SLE) or hepatitis. Consequently, it is important to clarify the molecular mechanisms of TLRs for therapeutic intervention in these diseases. For analysis of the molecular mechanisms of TLRs, mAbs to nucleic acid-sensing TLRs were developed recently. These mAbs revealed that TLR7 and TLR9 are localized also in the plasma membrane, while TLR7 and TLR9 were thought to be localized in endosomes and lysosomes. Among these mAbs, antagonistic mAbs to TLR7 or TLR9 are able to inhibit in vitro responses to synthetic ligands. Furthermore, antagonistic mAbs mitigate inflammatory disorders caused by TLR7 or TLR9 in mice. These results suggest that antagonistic mAbs to nucleic acid-sensing TLRs are a promising tool for therapeutic intervention in inflammatory disorders caused by excessive activation of nucleic acid-sensing TLRs. Here, we summarize the molecular mechanisms of TLRs and recent progresses in the trials targeting TLRs with mAbs to control inflammatory diseases.

Keywords: Toll-like receptor, Monoclonal antibody, Inhibitory antibodies, Inflammation, Autoimmune

Background

Toll-like receptors (TLRs) recognize molecular patterns of pathogens and induce immune responses to protect host from pathogens. Although TLRs play important roles in the frontline of host defense, TLRs also recognize host-derived molecular patterns as a danger signal and lead to inflammation without infection. Given that the endogenous ligands of TLRs can be considered as metabolites, TLR responses to endogenous metabolites are likely to be under the homeostatic control [1]. Dysregulation of the interaction between TLRs and endogenous metabolites is thought to drive inflammation in a variety of diseases such as autoimmune diseases, metabolic syndrome, and heart

failure. Consequently, it is important to ask whether TLRs are targets for therapeutic intervention in these diseases.

To investigate the role of TLRs in a variety of diseases, mAbs to TLRs are of great importance. For example, the mAb to mouse TLR3, 7, and 9 have shown that endogenous these TLRs are expressed on the cell surface as well as in intracellular compartments. Furthermore, several mAbs to TLRs are able to intervene TLR responses. An anti-TLR7 mAb is able to inhibit TLR7 responses in vitro and mitigate TLR7-dependent inflammation in vivo [2, 3]. In this review, we describe the molecular mechanisms by which TLRs drive disease progression and our trials to control TLR-dependent inflammatory disorders by anti-TLR mAbs.

Overview of the molecular mechanisms of toll-like receptors

Toll-like receptors (TLRs) are a family of innate immune sensors, recognizing pathogen-associated molecular

* Correspondence: ryu-chan@ims.u-tokyo.ac.jp
[1]Division of Innate Immunity, Department of Microbiology and Immunology, The University of Tokyo, 4-6-1 Shirokanedai, Minato-ku, Tokyo 108-8639, Japan
Full list of author information is available at the end of the article

patterns (PAMPs) to activate immune response as a frontline of immune system [4–7]. TLR was found as a mammalian homolog of TOLL, the dorsoventral regulatory molecule of drosophila [8, 9]. The number of TLR varies with each species, for example, 10 TLRs are expressed in human whereas 12 TLRs are encoded in mice. Each TLR recognizes distinct PAMPs on the cell membrane of immune cells, and classified into two groups, depending on their ligands and cellular distribution. The cell surface TLRs, consisting of TLR1, TLR2, TLR4/MD-2, TLR5, and TLR6, recognize lipid or protein derived from bacteria (Fig. 1). The other group, consisting of TLR3, TLR7, TLR8, TLR9, and TLR13, respond to nucleic acids in endolysosome (Fig. 1).

All TLRs are categorized in type I transmembrane protein. TLRs recognize the ligands at the extracellular domain consisting of multiple leucine rich repeats to activate downstream signaling pathway via intracellular C-terminal region called Toll/interleukin-1 receptor (TIR) domain [10]. After the recognition of ligand, the conformation of TLR is changed and adapter proteins are recruited to the TIR domain [11–16]. Adapter proteins initiate the signal cascade to activate nuclear factor-kappa B (NF-κB) or interferon-regulatory factor (IRF), which promotes transcription of mRNA encoding cytokines/interferons [17–20].

PAMPs and DAMPs, recognized by TLRs

Although the main role for TLRs is the recognition of PAMPs to protect host from pathogens, TLRs also recognize host-derived molecules [21, 22]. These molecules are called damage/danger-associated molecular patterns (DAMPs), released from damaged or dead cells. DAMPs are recognized by innate immune sensors and induce inflammation to facilitate the clearance of damaged cells by phagocytes [23]. If the damage is not restored, DAMPs are continuously released and recognized by innate immune sensors. The cells expressing innate immune sensors strongly produce inflammatory cytokines, and the cytokines increase tissue damages, which in turn promote release of more DAMPs, and finally, a vicious circle is constructed among DAMPs, innate immune sensors and inflammation.

DAMPs are recognized by innate immune sensors because of the similarity of the structure to PAMPs. Recently, many types of DAMPs are found as endogenous ligands of TLRs [24, 25]. For example, TLR4/MD-2 recognizes bacteria-derived lipopolysaccharide (LPS) and host-derived fatty acids as PAMPs and DAMPs, respectively [26–28]. It is well known that fatty acid is a mediator of metabolic syndrome, and obesity is a condition where the response of TLR4/MD-2 is out of control. In obese adipose tissues, production of chemokines, such as monocyte chemoattractant protein-1 (MCP-1) is enhanced, and macrophages with C-C chemokine receptor type 2 (CCR2), the receptor of MCP-1, infiltrate into adipose tissues [29–31]. Infiltrated macrophages closely interact to adipocytes and strongly recognize saturated fatty acids released from adipocytes. As result, large amounts of cytokines are released from macrophages and vicious circle of inflammation is constructed by obesity.

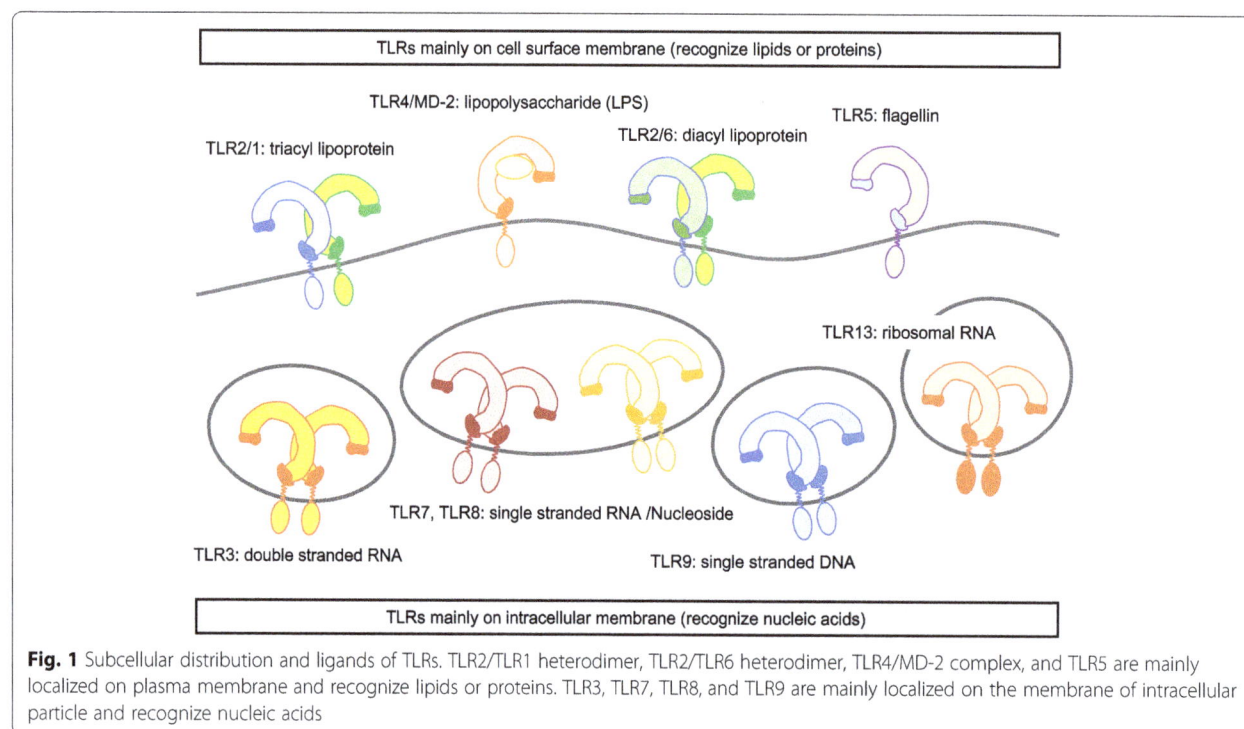

Fig. 1 Subcellular distribution and ligands of TLRs. TLR2/TLR1 heterodimer, TLR2/TLR6 heterodimer, TLR4/MD-2 complex, and TLR5 are mainly localized on plasma membrane and recognize lipids or proteins. TLR3, TLR7, TLR8, and TLR9 are mainly localized on the membrane of intracellular particle and recognize nucleic acids

DAMPs induce inflammation and diseases, but given that DAMPs are generated and released by metabolism, inflammation induced by DAMPs is a homeostatic responses. Excessive activation of innate immune sensors by DAMPs induces chronic inflammation and irreversible tissue damage. This concept is proposed as "homeostatic inflammation" [1, 32].

Controlling system of toll-like receptors

To avoid excessive homeostatic inflammation, there are multiple controlling systems for TLRs varying from gene transcription to protein degradation (Fig. 2). Especially, the responses of nucleic acid-sensing TLRs should be strictly controlled because the structure of nucleic acid is highly conserved between pathogens and hosts. TLR7, recognizing single-stranded RNA and guanosine analogs, is one of the well-known pathogenic factors of autoimmune disease model. For example, systemic lupus erythematosus (SLE)-like phenotype is spontaneously induced in BXSB^{Yaa} mice,

which harbor an additional copy of the *Tlr7* gene on Y chromosome (Table 1) [33–35]. *Tlr7* is originally encoded on the X chromosome, so that BXSB^{Yaa} mice express 2 copies of TLR7 and the response to endogenous TLR7 ligand is enhanced.

Not only the amount of TLR7, the controlling molecules of TLR7 is also important to avoid lethal inflammation [36]. Unc93 homolog B1 (UNC93B1) is one of the essential molecules for the function of nucleic acid-sensing TLRs. Furthermore, UNC93B1 balances the responses of nucleic acid-sensing TLRs [37]. UNC93B1 binds to TLRs in the ER and transport them to endolysosome where TLRs are matured by the proteolytic cleavage of the extracellular domain [38–40]. These function of UNC93B1 is abolished by the deletion or mutation of C-terminal region, while the deletion or mutation of N-terminal region collapse the balance of the responses between TLR7 and TLR9 [37, 41, 42]. In detail, the region around 34th aspartic acid (D34) is responsible for the regulation of the

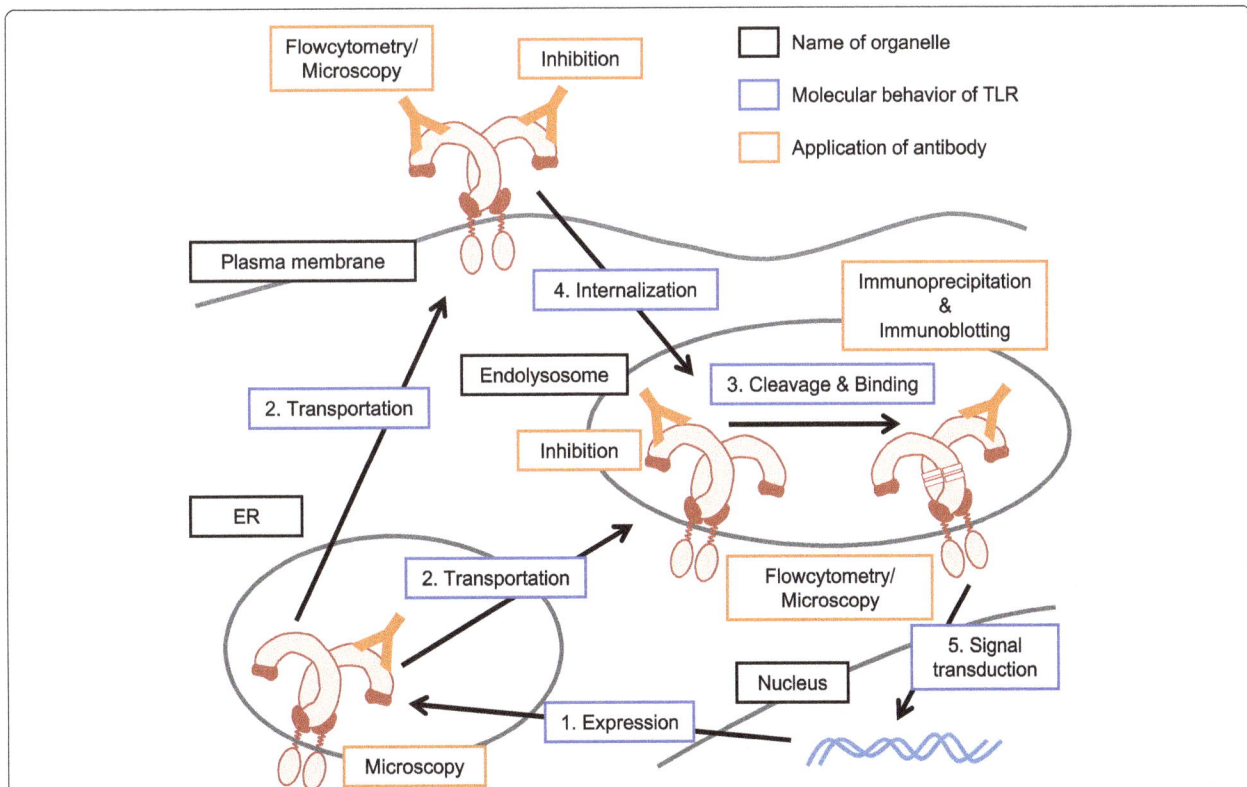

Fig. 2 Application of anti-TLR for the analysis of molecular mechanisms of TLR. Expressed TLRs are transported from ER to plasma membrane or endolysosome (1 and 2). In endolysosome, nucleic acid-sensing TLRs are cleaved and the N-terminal fragment binds to the C-terminal fragment (3). After the modification, TLR recognize ligand and signaling pathway is activated (5). TLRs on cell surface recognize ligand and activates signaling pathway. Some of them are internalized by the recognition of ligand or spontaneous trafficking (4). For the analysis of these molecular behaviors of TLR, monoclonal anti-TLR is well exploited. Amount and expression pattern among cell types are analyzed by flowcytometry. Subcellular distribution is observed by immunofluorescence microscopy. Alternatively, flowcytometry following the immunostaining with or without detergent is able to discriminate the distribution between cell surface and intracellular particle. Proteolytic cleavage and binding of nucleic acid-sensing TLR are detected by immunoprecipitation and immunoblotting. In addition to these application for detection, several antibodies have inhibitory effect on the response of TLRs. Words in black frames, blue frames, and orange frames are the name of organelle, the molecular behavior of TLR, and the application of anti-TLR, respectively

Table 1 Relation of TLRs with chronic inflammatory diseases

Disease	TLR	Roles for TLR on disease
Nonalcoholic steatohepatitis (NASH)	TLR4 TLR9	*TLR4* mRNA expression is increased in the liver of NASH patients [49]. TLR9 recognizes host-derived mitochondrial DNA and induces inflammation [47, 48].
Psoriasis	TLR7 TLR9	Antimicrobial peptide LL37, a factor of psoriasis, associates with self-derived DNA and stimulate TLR9 in pDCs [67]. Administration of imiquimod, a TLR7 ligand, induces psoriasis-like dermatitis via T cell activation with IL-17/IL-23 production [71] .
Systemic lupus erythematosus (SLE)	TLR7 TLR9	TLR7 and TLR9 contribute to the production of autoantibody in SLE model mouse [34, 35, 72]. Especially, TLR7 is thought as an inducer of the phenotype [34, 35, 73, 74]. Controversially, protective effect of TLR9 on SLE is also reported [73, 75, 76].
Celiac Disease	TLR7 TLR8	Suggestive association of the SNP on *TLR7* and *TLR8* with celiac disease is found by genome-wide association study (GWAS) [77].
Type 1 diabetes (T1D)	TLR4 TLR9	TLR4 expresses on β cells in islets and induces signaling by recognizing HMGB1 [78]. TLR9 contributes to the activation of T cells in NOD mice, a model of T1D [69, 79, 80].
Rheumatoid arthritis	TLR8 TLR9	Human TLR8 transgenic mice develop arthritis spontaneously [81]. Cathepsin K is required for the response of TLR9, and an inhibitor of Cathepsin K attenuates T_H17 polarization and arthritis [68].

responses of TLR7 and TLR9, so that the alanine mutation of the D34 (D34A mutation) enhances the response of TLR7 and declines the response of TLR9. The mice harboring D34A mutation on *Unc93b1* (D34A mice) suffer from systemic inflammation, such as hepatitis, thrombocytopenia, splenomegaly and nephritis, depending on the excessive response of TLR7 [43, 44].

These TLR7-dependent disease models might develop inflammation by recognizing endogenous TLR7 ligand, such as single-stranded RNA and guanosine analogs [45, 46]. Like TLR7, TLR9 recognizes endogenous DNA ligand and also contributes to the inflammatory disease (Table 1). TLR9 recognizes mitochondrial DNA (mtDNA) released from hepatocyte and drives nonalcoholic steatohepatitis (NASH) [47, 48]. NASH is a common liver diseases characterized by fatty liver, in which TLR9 plays a pathogenic role in driving inflammatory response by responding to mtDNA released from damaged hepatocytes [49].

Anti-TLR mAbs for the analysis of molecular mechanisms in TLRs

Given that TLRs contribute to the homeostatic inflammation and diseases, analysis of the molecular mechanisms of TLR is very important to develop therapeutic strategy. Monoclonal anti-TLRs have been established to detect endogenous TLRs from the early years of TLR research and many of new findings were brought. We also exploited mAbs for the studies of TLRs by establishing anti-murine TLR1, TLR2, TLR3, TLR4/MD-2, TLR5, TLR6, TLR7 and TLR9 (Table 2 and Fig. 2) [3, 50–54]. For example, anti-TLR4/MD-2 complex monoclonal antibody reveals the direct binding of LPS to TLR4/MD-2, which is confirmed by the analysis of crystal structure later [55–57].

Anti-TLR mAbs also reveal the subcellular distribution of TLRs. As shown in Fig. 1, it was believed that TLR1, TLR2, TLR4/MD-2, and TLR6 are localized on cell surface, and TLR3, TLR7, and TLR9 are localized on intracellular vesicles. It is true and important for TLRs to be

functional, but endogenous intracellular TLR1, TLR2, TLR4/−MD-2 and TLR6 were detected by flowcytometry analysis with mAbs [50, 58, 59], and intracellular nucleic acid-sensing TLRs were detected on plasma membrane [2, 52, 53, 60].

Another important application of mAb is immunoprecipitation for immunoblotting. Concentration by immunoprecipitation is required for detection of endogenous TLR because the amount of endogenous TLR is not enough to detect by the immunoblotting of whole cell lysate. Even if TLRs are overexpressed, non-tagged TLR or the fragments of TLR generated by proteolytic cleavage is detectable by anti-TLR mAbs. We found that TLR9 is cleaved in endolysosome and separated to N-terminal and C-terminal fragments by using anti-TLR9 mAb [53]. Previous reports suggested that the cleaved C-terminal region of TLR9 is functional with the cleaved N-terminal region serving as a negative regulator [61, 62]. We established two types of anti-TLR9 mAbs to

Table 2 Application of anti-monoclonal antibodies we established

TLR (mouse)	Name of clone	Application	Reference
TLR1	TR23	FC, IP	[50]
TLR2	CB225	FC, IP	[50]
TLR4/MD-2	MTS510 Sa15–21	FC, IP, BL (in vitro) FC, IP, BL (in vivo)	[54, 57, 64]
TLR6	C1N2	FC, IP	[50]
TLR5	ACT5	FC, IP	[51, 82]
TLR3	CaT3 PaT3	FC, IP FC, IP	[52]
TLR7	A94B10	FC, IP, IF, BL	[2, 3, 43]
TLR9	J15A7 B33A4 C34A1 NaR9	FC, IP, IF FC, IP FC, IP, IF FC, IP, IF, BL	[53, 66]

FC flowcytometry, *IP* immunoprecipitation, *IF* immunofluorescence microscopy, *BL* blocking

detect the both of fragments of TLR9; one clone is bound to N-terminal region and the other is bound to C-terminal region [53]. By using these mAbs, we clarified that the N-terminal region of TLR9 binds to the C-terminal region, and the binding is essential for the response of TLR9. Not only TLR9, the requirement of proteolytic cleavage and the binding of the fragments are also confirmed in TLR3 and TLR7 with monoclonal antibodies [3, 52, 63].

Inhibitory effect of anti-TLR mAbs

Among anti-TLR mAbs, several clones inhibit the response of cells to TLR ligand. For examples, mAbs to human TLR3 (clone TLR3.7), mouse TLR4/MD-2 (clone MTS510), mouse TLR7 (clone A94B10), and mouse TLR9 (clone NaR9) inhibit the response of target TLR [2, 43, 64, 65]. Interestingly, the responses of intracellular TLRs, such as TLR3, TLR7 and TLR9, are inhibited by the monoclonal antibody in culture medium. Although these TLRs are also localized on cell surface as described above, they recognize and signal nucleic acids in endolysosome. How do these inhibitory anti-TLR mAbs reach to intracellular TLRs?

In case of TLR7, a monoclonal anti-TLR7 "A94B10" binds to cell surface TLR7 and accumulated in endolysosomes as immune complex [2]. A part of the antibody uptake depends on Fc receptor, but the uptake of A94B10 remains without Fc receptor. Furthermore, the uptake of A94B10 by the cells from $Tlr7^{-/-}$ mice or UNC93B1 deficient mice is attenuated. Since UNC93B1 is essential for the cell surface localization of TLR7, inhibitory function of A94B10 might depend on cell surface TLR7.

A monoclonal anti-TLR9, clone "NaR9" also inhibits TLR9 responses. A94B10 inhibits the response of TLR7 in various types of cells, such as bone marrow-derived macrophages (BM-MCs), BM-conventional dendritic cells (BM-cDCs), BM-plasmacytoid DCs (BM-pDCs), and B cells, whereas NaR9 only inhibits the response of TLR9 in BM-MCs and BM-cDCs [66]. As a mechanism behind the difference between these two mAbs remains unclarified, NaR9 is internalized by BM-MCs and BM-cDCs but not by pDCs. Interaction between mAb and cell surface TLR7 or TLR9 and subsequent internalization are likely to be required for the inhibitory effect of these mAbs.

New application of anti-TLR mAbs for therapeutic intervention

If an inhibitory anti-TLR mAb is functional in vivo, the antibody is able to be applied to the treatment of inflammatory diseases induced by TLRs (Table 1). Among the antibodies mentioned above, an anti-TLR9 NaR9 rescues the mice from TLR9-dependent lethal experimental hepatitis [66]. Although the effect of NaR9 on the chronic inflammatory disease is unknown, pre-treatment of NaR9 significantly reduce the inflammatory cytokine production

and acute hepatitis induced by D-(+)-galactosamine and TLR9 ligand CpG-ODN. These results suggest that NaR9 is able to inhibit TLR9-dependent hepatitis. As TLR9 is suggested to drive inflammation in NASH, anti-TLR9 mAb may be promising for therapeutic intervention in NASH or other diseases such as psoriasis, rheumatoid arthritis, and type 1 diabetes (Table 1) [47, 67–69].

Anti-TLR4/MD-2 monoclonal antibody, Sa15–21 also rescues the mice from lethal experimental hepatitis induced by D-(+)-galactosamine and TLR4 ligand LPS [64]. Interestingly, Sa15–21 does not directly inhibit the response of TLR4/MD-2, on contrary, enhances the response of TLR4/MD-2 and increase the production of TNF-α. In fact, Sa15–21 induces antiapoptotic genes via TLR4/MD-2 with agonist effect and protects mice from lethal hepatitis.

For the treatment of inflammatory disease, an inhibitory anti-TLR7 monoclonal antibody, clone A94B10 is effective in the systemic inflammation caused by TLR7 hyper-response [2]. As mentioned above, the mice harboring the D34A mutation on UNC93B1 (D34A mice) suffer from severe inflammation with TLR7-dependent manner. The administration of A94B10 to D34A mice significantly attenuates the phenotypes, such as splenomegaly, thrombocytopenia, autoantibody production, and hepatitis with fibrosis of liver. It is important to distinguish whether the effect of antibody is therapeutic or prophylactic. Even if the administration of A94B10 was started when D34A mice had already developed thrombocytopenia, the anti-TLR7 mAb was still effective. These results suggest that anti-TLR7 is a promising candidate of therapeutic drug to cure TLR7-dependent autoimmune diseases, for examples, SLE or autoimmune hepatitis.

Conclusion

Homeostatic inflammation induced by TLRs is tightly related to health and disease. To investigate the molecular mechanisms of TLRs, monoclonal antibody is an essential tool for experiment. In these 2 decades, many researchers have revealed a variety of the molecular properties of TLRs with anti-TLR monoclonal antibodies. Moreover, the application of anti-TLR monoclonal antibody is expanding to therapeutic intervention. There is no evidence of the therapeutic effect of anti-TLR on the disease in human, however, TLR antagonist nucleic acids has already proceeded to clinical trial [70]. If the trial of nucleic acid medicine is successful, development of anti-human TLR mAbs will also be a promising way to control TLR-dependent diseases. Of course, the application of anti-TLR mAbs might compete nucleic acid medicine, but mAbs have advantages of higher specificity, lower off-target effect, and longer half-life comparing to nucleic acids. Not only for clinical application, anti-human TLR should be continuously established for the analysis of the molecular mechanism of human TLRs.

Abbreviations

BM-cDC: bone marrow-derived conventional dendritic cell; BM-MC: bone marrow-derived macrophage; BM-pDC: bone marrow-derived plasmacytoid dendritic cell; CCR2: C-C chemokine receptor type 2; D34A mutation: alanine mutant of 34th aspartic acid in UNC93B1; DAMPs: damage/danger-associated molecular patterns; IRF: interferon-regulatory factor; mAb: monoclonal antibody; MCP-1: monocyte chemoattractant protein-1; mtDNA: mitochondrial DNA; NASH: nonalcoholic steatohepatitis; NF-κB: nuclear factor-kappa B; PAMPs: pathogen-associated molecular patterns; SLE: systemic lupus erythematosus; TIR domain: Toll/IL-1 receptor domain; TLR: Toll-like receptor; UNC93B1: Unc93 homolog B1

Funding

This work was supported in part by a contract research fund from JSPS for Grant-in-Aid for Scientific Research (S), 16H06388; Grant-in-Aid for Exploratory Research, 17 K19548; from Takeda Science Foundation; from SENSHIN Medical Research Foundation.

Authors' contributions

RF wrote the manuscript. YM and KM revised manuscript. All authors read and approved the manuscript.

Competing interests

The authors declare that they have no competing interests.

Author details

[1]Division of Innate Immunity, Department of Microbiology and Immunology, The University of Tokyo, 4-6-1 Shirokanedai, Minato-ku, Tokyo 108-8639, Japan. [2]Department of Pharmacotherapy, Research Institute of Pharmaceutical Sciences, Musashino University, 1-1-20 Shin-machi, Nishitokyo-shi, Tokyo 202-8585, Japan. [3]Laboratory of Innate Immunity, Center for Experimental Medicine and Systems Biology, The Institute of Medical Science, The University of Tokyo, 4-6-1 Shirokanedai, Minato-ku, Tokyo 108-8639, Japan.

References

1. Miyake K, Kaisho T. Homeostatic inflammation in innate immunity. Curr Opin Immunol. 2014;30C:85–90.
2. Kanno A, Tanimura N, Ishizaki M, Ohko K, Motoi Y, Onji M, Fukui R, Shimozato T, Yamamoto K, Shibata T, et al. Targeting cell surface TLR7 for therapeutic intervention in autoimmune diseases. Nat Commun. 2015;6:6119.
3. Kanno A, Yamamoto C, Onji M, Fukui R, Saitoh S, Motoi Y, Shibata T, Matsumoto F, Muta T, Miyake K. Essential role for toll-like receptor 7 (TLR7)-unique cysteines in an intramolecular disulfide bond, proteolytic cleavage and RNA sensing. Int Immunol. 2013;25(7):413–22.
4. Akira S, Uematsu S, Takeuchi O. Pathogen recognition and innate immunity. Cell. 2006;124(4):783–801.
5. Takeda K, Akira S. Toll-like receptors in innate immunity. Int Immunol. 2005; 17(1):1–14.
6. Takeuchi O, Akira S. Pattern recognition receptors and inflammation. Cell. 2010;140(6):805–20.
7. Brubaker SW, Bonham KS, Zanoni I, Kagan JC. Innate immune pattern recognition: a cell biological perspective. Annu Rev Immunol. 2015;33:257–90.
8. Medzhitov R, Preston-Hurlburt P, Janeway CA Jr. A human homologue of the Drosophila toll protein signals activation of adaptive immunity. Nature. 1997;388(6640):394–7.
9. Lemaitre B, Nicolas E, Michaut L, Reichhart JM, Hoffmann JA. The dorsoventral regulatory gene cassette spatzle/toll/cactus controls the potent antifungal response in Drosophila adults. Cell. 1996;86(6):973–83.
10. Akira S, Takeda K. Toll-like receptor signalling. Nat Rev Immunol. 2004;4(7): 499–511.
11. Yamamoto M, Sato S, Hemmi H, Hoshino K, Kaisho T, Sanjo H, Takeuchi O, Sugiyama M, Okabe M, Takeda K, et al. Role of adaptor TRIF in the MyD88-independent toll-like receptor signaling pathway. Science. 2003;301(5633):640–3.
12. Yamamoto M, Sato S, Hemmi H, Sanjo H, Uematsu S, Kaisho T, Hoshino K, Takeuchi O, Kobayashi M, Fujita T, et al. Essential role for TIRAP in activation of the signalling cascade shared by TLR2 and TLR4. Nature. 2002;420(6913):324–9.
13. Yamamoto M, Sato S, Hemmi H, Uematsu S, Hoshino K, Kaisho T, Takeuchi O, Takeda K, Akira S. TRAM is specifically involved in the toll-like receptor 4-mediated MyD88-independent signaling pathway. Nat Immunol. 2003;4(11):1144–50.
14. Takeuchi O, Takeda K, Hoshino K, Adachi O, Ogawa T, Akira S. Cellular responses to bacterial cell wall components are mediated through MyD88-dependent signaling cascades. Int Immunol. 2000;12(1):113–7.
15. Oshiumi H, Matsumoto M, Funami K, Akazawa T, Seya T. TICAM-1, an adaptor molecule that participates in toll-like receptor 3-mediated interferon-beta induction. Nat Immunol. 2003;4(2):161–7.
16. Oshiumi H, Sasai M, Shida K, Fujita T, Matsumoto M, Seya T. TIR-containing adapter molecule (TICAM)-2, a bridging adapter recruiting to toll-like receptor 4 TICAM-1 that induces interferon-beta. J Biol Chem. 2003;278(50): 49751–62.
17. Zhang G, Ghosh S. Toll-like receptor-mediated NF-kappaB activation: a phylogenetically conserved paradigm in innate immunity. J Clin Invest. 2001;107(1):13–9.
18. Kawai T, Akira S. Signaling to NF-kappaB by toll-like receptors. Trends Mol Med. 2007;13(11):460–9.
19. Schoenemeyer A, Barnes BJ, Mancl ME, Latz E, Goutagny N, Pitha PM, Fitzgerald KA, Golenbock DT. The interferon regulatory factor, IRF5, is a central mediator of toll-like receptor 7 signaling. J Biol Chem. 2005;280(17): 17005–12.
20. Fitzgerald KA, Rowe DC, Barnes BJ, Caffrey DR, Visintin A, Latz E, Monks B, Pitha PM, Golenbock DT. LPS-TLR4 signaling to IRF-3/7 and NF-kappaB involves the toll adapters TRAM and TRIF. J Exp Med. 2003;198(7):1043–55.
21. Marshak-Rothstein A, Rifkin IR. Immunologically active autoantigens: the role of toll-like receptors in the development of chronic inflammatory disease. Annu Rev Immunol. 2007;25:419–41.
22. Chen GY, Nunez G. Sterile inflammation: sensing and reacting to damage. Nat Rev Immunol. 2010;10(12):826–37.
23. Schaefer L. Complexity of danger: the diverse nature of damage-associated molecular patterns. J Biol Chem. 2014;289(51):35237–45.
24. Alvarez K, Vasquez G. Damage-associated molecular patterns and their role as initiators of inflammatory and auto-immune signals in systemic lupus erythematosus. Int Rev Immunol. 2017;36(5):259–70.
25. Yu L, Wang L, Chen S. Endogenous toll-like receptor ligands and their biological significance. J Cell Mol Med. 2010;14(11):2592–603.
26. Suganami T, Mieda T, Itoh M, Shimoda Y, Kamei Y, Ogawa Y. Attenuation of obesity-induced adipose tissue inflammation in C3H/HeJ mice carrying a toll-like receptor 4 mutation. Biochem Biophys Res Commun. 2007;354(1):45–9.
27. Suganami T, Tanimoto-Koyama K, Nishida J, Itoh M, Yuan X, Mizuarai S, Kotani H, Yamaoka S, Miyake K, Aoe S, et al. Role of the toll-like receptor 4/NF-kappaB pathway in saturated fatty acid-induced inflammatory changes in the interaction between adipocytes and macrophages. Arterioscler Thromb Vasc Biol. 2007;27(1):84–91.
28. Wong SW, Kwon MJ, Choi AM, Kim HP, Nakahira K, Hwang DH. Fatty acids modulate toll-like receptor 4 activation through regulation of receptor dimerization and recruitment into lipid rafts in a reactive oxygen species-dependent manner. J Biol Chem. 2009;284(40):27384–92.
29. Ito A, Suganami T, Yamauchi A, Degawa-Yamauchi M, Tanaka M, Kouyama R, Kobayashi Y, Nitta N, Yasuda K, Hirata Y, et al. Role of CC chemokine receptor 2 in bone marrow cells in the recruitment of macrophages into obese adipose tissue. J Biol Chem. 2008;283(51):35715–23.
30. Kamei N, Tobe K, Suzuki R, Ohsugi M, Watanabe T, Kubota N, Ohtsuka-Kowatari N, Kumagai K, Sakamoto K, Kobayashi M, et al. Overexpression of monocyte chemoattractant protein-1 in adipose tissues causes macrophage recruitment and insulin resistance. J Biol Chem. 2006;281(36):26602–14.
31. Weisberg SP, Hunter D, Huber R, Lemieux J, Slaymaker S, Vaddi K, Charo I, Leibel RL, Ferrante AW Jr. CCR2 modulates inflammatory and metabolic effects of high-fat feeding. J Clin Invest. 2006;116(1):115–24.
32. Fukui R, Miyake K. Controlling systems of nucleic acid sensing-TLRs restrict homeostatic inflammation. Exp Cell Res. 2012;318(13):1461–6.
33. Fairhurst AM, Hwang SH, Wang A, Tian XH, Boudreaux C, Zhou XJ, Casco J, Li QZ, Connolly JE, Wakeland EK. Yaa autoimmune phenotypes are conferred by overexpression of TLR7. Eur J Immunol. 2008;38(7):1971–8.

34. Pisitkun P, Deane JA, Difilippantonio MJ, Tarasenko T, Satterthwaite AB, Bolland S. Autoreactive B cell responses to RNA-related antigens due to TLR7 gene duplication. Science. 2006;312(5780):1669–72.

35. Santiago-Raber ML, Kikuchi S, Borel P, Uematsu S, Akira S, Kotzin BL, Izui S. Evidence for genes in addition to Tlr7 in the Yaa translocation linked with acceleration of systemic lupus erythematosus. J Immunol. 2008;181(2):1556–62.

36. Lee CC, Avalos AM, Ploegh HL. Accessory molecules for toll-like receptors and their function. Nat Rev Immunol. 2012;12(3):168–79.

37. Tabeta K, Hoebe K, Janssen EM, Du X, Georgel P, Crozat K, Mudd S, Mann N, Sovath S, Goode J, et al. The Unc93b1 mutation 3d disrupts exogenous antigen presentation and signaling via toll-like receptors 3, 7 and 9. Nat Immunol. 2006;7(2):156–64.

38. Brinkmann MM, Spooner E, Hoebe K, Beutler B, Ploegh HL, Kim YM. The interaction between the ER membrane protein UNC93B and TLR3, 7, and 9 is crucial for TLR signaling. J Cell Biol. 2007;177(2):265–75.

39. Kim YM, Brinkmann MM, Paquet ME, Ploegh HL. UNC93B1 delivers nucleotide-sensing toll-like receptors to endolysosomes. Nature. 2008; 452(7184):234–8.

40. Lee BL, Moon JE, Shu JH, Yuan L, Newman ZR, Schekman R, Barton GM. UNC93B1 mediates differential trafficking of endosomal TLRs. elife. 2013;2: e00291.

41. Fukui R, Saitoh S, Matsumoto F, Kozuka-Hata H, Oyama M, Tabeta K, Beutler B, Miyake K. Unc93b1 biases toll-like receptor responses to nucleic acid in dendritic cells toward DNA- but against RNA-sensing. J Exp Med. 2009; 206(6):1339–50.

42. Casrouge A, Zhang SY, Eidenschenk C, Jouanguy E, Puel A, Yang K, Alcais A, Picard C, Mahfoufi N, Nicolas N, et al. Herpes simplex virus encephalitis in human UNC-93B deficiency. Science. 2006;314(5797):308–12.

43. Fukui R, Kanno A, Miyake K. Type I IFN contributes to the phenotype of Unc93b1D34A/D34A mice by regulating TLR7 expression in B cells and dendritic cells. J Immunol. 2016;196(1):416–27.

44. Fukui R, Saitoh S, Kanno A, Onji M, Shibata T, Ito A, Matsumoto M, Akira S, Yoshida N, Miyake K. Unc93B1 restricts systemic lethal inflammation by orchestrating toll-like receptor 7 and 9 trafficking. Immunity. 2011;35(1):69–81.

45. Shibata T, Ohto U, Nomura S, Kibata K, Motoi Y, Zhang Y, Murakami Y, Fukui R, Ishimoto T, Sano S, et al. Guanosine and its modified derivatives are endogenous ligands for TLR7. Int Immunol. 2016;28(5):211–22.

46. Zhang Z, Ohto U, Shibata T, Krayukhina E, Taoka M, Yamauchi Y, Tanji H, Isobe T, Uchiyama S, Miyake K, et al. Structural analysis reveals that toll-like receptor 7 is a dual receptor for guanosine and single-stranded RNA. Immunity. 2016;45(4):737–48.

47. Garcia-Martinez I, Santoro N, Chen Y, Hoque R, Ouyang X, Caprio S, Shlomchik MJ, Coffman RL, Candia A, Mehal WZ. Hepatocyte mitochondrial DNA drives nonalcoholic steatohepatitis by activation of TLR9. J Clin Invest. 2016;126(3):859–64.

48. Miura K, Kodama Y, Inokuchi S, Schnabl B, Aoyama T, Ohnishi H, Olefsky JM, Brenner DA, Seki E. Toll-like receptor 9 promotes steatohepatitis by induction of interleukin-1beta in mice. Gastroenterology. 2010;139(1):323–34. e327

49. Sharifnia T, Antoun J, Verriere TG, Suarez G, Wattacheril J, Wilson KT, Peek RM Jr, Abumrad NN, Flynn CR. Hepatic TLR4 signaling in obese NAFLD. Am J Physiol Gastrointest Liver Physiol. 2015;309(4):G270–8.

50. Motoi Y, Shibata T, Takahashi K, Kanno A, Murakami Y, Li X, Kasahara T, Miyake K. Lipopeptides are signaled by toll-like receptor 1, 2 and 6 in endolysosomes. Int Immunol. 2014;26(10):563–73.

51. Shibata T, Takemura N, Motoi Y, Goto Y, Karuppuchamy T, Izawa K, Li X, Akashi-Takamura S, Tanimura N, Kunisawa J, et al. PRAT4A-dependent expression of cell surface TLR5 on neutrophils, classical monocytes and dendritic cells. Int Immunol. 2012;24(10):613–23.

52. Murakami Y, Fukui R, Motoi Y, Kanno A, Shibata T, Tanimura N, Saitoh S, Miyake K. Roles of the cleaved N-terminal TLR3 fragment and cell surface TLR3 in double-stranded RNA sensing. J Immunol. 2014;193(10): 5208–17.

53. Onji M, Kanno A, Saitoh S, Fukui R, Motoi Y, Shibata T, Matsumoto F, Lamichhane A, Sato S, Kiyono H, et al. An essential role for the N-terminal fragment of toll-like receptor 9 in DNA sensing. Nat Commun. 2013;4:1949.

54. Akashi S, Shimazu R, Ogata H, Nagai Y, Takeda K, Kimoto M, Miyake K. Cutting edge: cell surface expression and lipopolysaccharide signaling via the toll-like receptor 4-MD-2 complex on mouse peritoneal macrophages. J Immunol. 2000;164(7):3471–5.

55. Ohto U, Fukase K, Miyake K, Satow Y. Crystal structures of human MD-2 and its complex with antiendotoxic lipid IVa. Science. 2007;316(5831):1632–4.

56. Park BS, Song DH, Kim HM, Choi BS, Lee H, Lee JO. The structural basis of lipopolysaccharide recognition by the TLR4-MD-2 complex. Nature. 2009; 458(7242):1191–5.

57. Akashi S, Saitoh S, Wakabayashi Y, Kikuchi T, Takamura N, Nagai Y, Kusumoto Y, Fukase K, Kusumoto S, Adachi Y, et al. Lipopolysaccharide interaction with cell surface toll-like receptor 4-MD-2: higher affinity than that with MD-2 or CD14. J Exp Med. 2003;198(7):1035–42.

58. Shibata T, Motoi Y, Tanimura N, Yamakawa N, Akashi-Takamura S, Miyake K. Intracellular TLR4/MD-2 in macrophages senses gram-negative bacteria and induces a unique set of LPS-dependent genes. Int Immunol. 2011;23(8):503–10.

59. Chan MP, Onji M, Fukui R, Kawane K, Shibata T, Saitoh S, Ohto U, Shimizu T, Barber GN, Miyake K. DNase II-dependent DNA digestion is required for DNA sensing by TLR9. Nat Commun. 2015;6:5853.

60. Pohar J, Pirher N, Bencina M, Mancek-Keber M, Jerala R. The role of UNC93B1 protein in surface localization of TLR3 receptor and in cell priming to nucleic acid agonists. J Biol Chem. 2013;288(1):442–54.

61. Park B, Brinkmann MM, Spooner E, Lee CC, Kim YM, Ploegh HL. Proteolytic cleavage in an endolysosomal compartment is required for activation of toll-like receptor 9. Nat Immunol. 2008;9(12):1407–14.

62. Ewald SE, Lee BL, Lau L, Wickliffe KE, Shi GP, Chapman HA, Barton GM. The ectodomain of toll-like receptor 9 is cleaved to generate a functional receptor. Nature. 2008;456(7222):658–62.

63. Toscano F, Estornes Y, Virard F, Garcia-Cattaneo A, Pierrot A, Vanbervliet B, Bonnin M, Ciancanelli MJ, Zhang SY, Funami K, et al. Cleaved/associated TLR3 represents the primary form of the signaling receptor. J Immunol. 2013;190(2):764–73.

64. Akashi-Takamura S, Furuta T, Takahashi K, Tanimura N, Kusumoto Y, Kobayashi T, Saitoh S, Adachi Y, Doi T, Miyake K. Agonistic antibody to TLR4/MD-2 protects mice from acute lethal hepatitis induced by TNF-alpha. J Immunol. 2006;176(7):4244–51.

65. Matsumoto M, Kikkawa S, Kohase M, Miyake K, Seya T. Establishment of a monoclonal antibody against human toll-like receptor 3 that blocks double-stranded RNA-mediated signaling. Biochem Biophys Res Commun. 2002; 293(5):1364–9.

66. Murakami Y, Fukui R, Motoi Y, Shibata T, Saitoh SI, Sato R, Miyake K. The protective effect of the anti-toll-like receptor 9 antibody against acute cytokine storm caused by immunostimulatory DNA. Sci Rep. 2017;7:44042.

67. Lande R, Gregorio J, Facchinetti V, Chatterjee B, Wang YH, Homey B, Cao W, Su B, Nestle FO, Zal T, et al. Plasmacytoid dendritic cells sense self-DNA coupled with antimicrobial peptide. Nature. 2007;449(7162):564–9.

68. Asagiri M, Hirai T, Kunigami T, Kamano S, Gober HJ, Okamoto K, Nishikawa K, Latz E, Golenbock DT, Aoki K, et al. Cathepsin K-dependent toll-like receptor 9 signaling revealed in experimental arthritis. Science. 2008; 319(5863):624–7.

69. Wong FS, Hu C, Zhang L, Du W, Alexopoulou L, Flavell RA, Wen L. The role of toll-like receptors 3 and 9 in the development of autoimmune diabetes in NOD mice. Ann N Y Acad Sci. 2008;1150:146–8.

70. Balak DM, van Doorn MB, Arbeit RD, Rijneveld R, Klaassen E, Sullivan T, Brevard J, Thio HB, Prens EP, Burggraaf J, et al. IMO-8400, a toll-like receptor 7, 8, and 9 antagonist, demonstrates clinical activity in a phase 2a, randomized, placebo-controlled trial in patients with moderate-to-severe plaque psoriasis. Clin Immunol. 2016;174:63–72.

71. van der Fits L, Mourits S, Voerman JS, Kant M, Boon L, Laman JD, Cornelissen F, Mus AM, Florencia E, Prens EP, et al. Imiquimod-induced psoriasis-like skin inflammation in mice is mediated via the IL-23/IL-17 axis. J Immunol. 2009;182(9):5836–45.

72. Christensen SR, Kashgarian M, Alexopoulou L, Flavell RA, Akira S, Shlomchik MJ. Toll-like receptor 9 controls anti-DNA autoantibody production in murine lupus. J Exp Med. 2005;202(2):321–31.

73. Christensen SR, Shupe J, Nickerson K, Kashgarian M, Flavell RA, Shlomchik MJ. Toll-like receptor 7 and TLR9 dictate autoantibody specificity and have opposing inflammatory and regulatory roles in a murine model of lupus. Immunity. 2006;25(3):417–28.

74. Deane JA, Pisitkun P, Barrett RS, Feigenbaum L, Town T, Ward JM, Flavell RA, Bolland S. Control of toll-like receptor 7 expression is essential to restrict autoimmunity and dendritic cell proliferation. Immunity. 2007;27(5):801–10.

75. Nickerson KM, Christensen SR, Cullen JL, Meng W, Luning Prak ET, Shlomchik MJ. TLR9 promotes tolerance by restricting survival of anergic anti-DNA B cells, yet is also required for their activation. J Immunol. 2013; 190(4):1447–56.

76. Nickerson KM, Christensen SR, Shupe J, Kashgarian M, Kim D, Elkon K, Shlomchik MJ. TLR9 regulates TLR7- and MyD88-dependent autoantibody production and disease in a murine model of lupus. J Immunol. 2010;184(4):1840–8.

77. Dubois PC, Trynka G, Franke L, Hunt KA, Romanos J, Curtotti A, Zhernakova A, Heap GA, Adany R, Aromaa A, et al. Multiple common variants for celiac disease influencing immune gene expression. Nat Genet. 2010;42(4):295–302.

78. Li M, Song L, Gao X, Chang W, Qin X. Toll-like receptor 4 on islet beta cells senses expression changes in high-mobility group box 1 and contributes to the initiation of type 1 diabetes. Exp Mol Med. 2012;44(4):260–7.

79. Tai N, Wong FS, Wen L. The role of the innate immune system in destruction of pancreatic beta cells in NOD mice and humans with type I diabetes. J Autoimmun. 2016;71:26–34.

80. Tai N, Wong FS, Wen L. TLR9 deficiency promotes CD73 expression in T cells and diabetes protection in nonobese diabetic mice. J Immunol. 2013; 191(6):2926–37.

81. Guiducci C, Gong M, Cepika AM, Xu Z, Tripodo C, Bennett L, Crain C, Quartier P, Cush JJ, Pascual V, et al. RNA recognition by human TLR8 can lead to autoimmune inflammation. J Exp Med. 2013;210(13):2903–19.

82. Huh JW, Shibata T, Hwang M, Kwon EH, Jang MS, Fukui R, Kanno A, Jung DJ, Jang MH, Miyake K, et al. UNC93B1 is essential for the plasma membrane localization and signaling of toll-like receptor 5. Proc Natl Acad Sci U S A. 2014;111(19):7072–7.

22

Introduction of vasculature in engineered three-dimensional tissue

Sachiko Sekiya and Tatsuya Shimizu[*]

Abstract

Background: With recent developments in tissue engineering technology, various three-dimensional tissues can be generated now. However, as the tissue thickness increases due to three-dimensionalization, it is difficult to increase the tissue scale without introduction of blood vessels.

Main text: Many methods for vasculature induction have been reported recently. In this review, we introduced several methods which are adjustable vascularization in three-dimensional tissues according to three steps. First, "selection" provides potents for engineered tissues with vascularization ability. Second, "assembly technology" is used to fabricate tissues as three-dimensional structures and simultaneously inner neo-vasculature. Third, a "perfusion" technique is used for maturation of blood vessels in three-dimensional tissues. In "selection", selection of cells and materials gives the ability to promote angiogenesis in three-dimensional tissues. During the cell assembly step, cell sheet engineering, nanofilm coating technology, and three-dimensional printing technology could be used to produce vascularized three-dimensional tissues. Perfusion techniques to perfuse blood or cell culture medium throughout three-dimensional tissues with a unified inlet and outlet could induce functional blood vessels within retransplantable three-dimensional tissues. Combination of each step technology allows simulation of perivascular microenvironments in target tissues and drive vascularization in three-dimensional tissues.

Conclusion: The biomimetic microenvironment of target tissues will induce adequate cell-cell interaction, distance, cell morphology, and function within tissues. It could be accelerated for vascularization within three-dimensional tissues and give us the functional tissues. Since vascularized three-dimensional tissues are highly functional, they are expected to contribute to the development of regenerative medicine and drug safety tests for drug discovery in the future.

Keywords: Induction vascularization, Selecting cells and material, Tissue engineering, Assemble, Perfusion, Three-dimensional tissues

Background

Tissue engineering (TE) technologies have been progressing recently. The development of these technologies has produced dramatic effects on cell transplantation therapy [1, 2]. Moreover, three-dimensional (3D) structures fabricated from cells express important functions and the differentiation capacity of stem cells in vitro. These 3D tissues will be also available as tools for safety tests on chemical substances or for drug discovery. Indeed, a reduction in the use of animals for laboratory experiments is required globally for the drug development process and other applications, from the perspective of

animal welfare. The use of animal-free technology to fabricate tissues will accelerate this reduction.

As the thickness of engineered 3D tissue increases, however, induction of inner vasculature is required in order to supply oxygen and nutrients, including fatty acids, and remove waste products. In typical two-dimensional (2D) cell culture conditions, the thickness of the cell population is approximately 20–30 μm, which is sufficient to allow diffusion of nutrients and oxygen. When the thickness of engineered tissues exceeds 100 μm, the oxygen and nutrients are difficult to diffuse to the inner side of the tissue [3]. Therefore, to resolve this thickness issue, introducing blood vessels into 3D engineered tissues has been studied, and various methodologies to achieve this have been established [4, 5].

* Correspondence: shimizu.tatsuya@twmu.ac.jp
Institute of Advanced Biomedical Engineering and Science, Tokyo Women's Medical University, 8-1 Kawada-cho, Shinjuku-ku, Tokyo 162-8666, Japan

For example, tissues exceeding 1 mm in thickness can be obtained in vivo when the 80-μm layered cell sheets are multistep-transplanted with a vascular linkage between each layered cell sheet [6]. Moreover, a perfusable system and micro-perfusable channel have recently been developed in vitro for 3D tissue vascularization. In this review, we will introduce the latest vessel induction strategies according to three steps: selecting cells and materials for vascularized 3D tissues, assembly selecting parts as vascularized 3D shapes, and promotion of vascularization, with perfusable culture (Fig. 1). Combination of these technologies will produce physiological mimic microenvironment in vivo and could drive vascularization for target engineered tissues. Such biomimetic microenvironments can approach the engineered tissues close to the ideal function and structure.

Selecting cells and materials for vascularization into 3D engineered tissues

During fabrication of 3D tissues from cells, it is necessary to induce the generation of blood vessels simultaneously. For conditioning vascularization microenvironments, we have to choose potent cells and materials including activating growth factor and promoting scaffold within 3D tissues (Fig. 2).

Cells constructing vasculature, endothelium-constructed endothelial cells (human umbilical vein endothelial cell: HUVEC, endothelial progenitor cell: EPC, and other kinds of endothelial cell: EC), and perivascular-constructed cells (mesenchymal stem cell: MSC and smooth muscle cell: SMC) could be considered as potent cells for vascularization within tissues. Selecting these cells is dependent on kinds of target tissue.

Simply coculturing cells is a technique to induce blood vessels within engineering of 3D tissues. Secreting cytokines and other factors, including cell adhesion factors and extracellular matrix (ECM), from cocultured cells

induce the neo-vasculature within 3D tissues. Previously, myocardial sheets with a vascular EC network structure could be fabricated by cultivation with vascular ECs and fetal left ventricle-derived cardiomyocytes [7]. The myocardial cell sheet contained not only ECs and myocardial cells but also fibroblasts and pericytes. This EC network containing myocardial tissue was able to promote blood circulation shortly, which guarantees the survival and growth of 3D tissues after transplantation in vivo [8]. Actually, the tricultured scaffold with ECs, myoblasts, and fibroblasts also induced vasculature within 3D tissues in vitro [9]. In contrast, the EC network can also observe during differentiation into hepatocytes from endoderm-differentiated induced pluripotent stem (iPS) cells by coculture [10] and renal tubular cells from iPS cells [11]. These EC networks within primitive tissues are probably similar to the primary vascular plexus during the embryonic period, which is associated with the supply of blood flow promptly into immature tissues during development. Thus, EC networks are considered as one better indicator of selecting cells for vascularized 3D tissues.

The EC network structure could be also induced by coculture with dermal fibroblasts, skeletal myoblasts, adipose-derived MSCs (ADMSCs), and bone marrow-derived MSCs (BMMSCs) [12–14]. In particular, MSCs could differentiate into vascular ECs [15], and pericytes could be also considered as adipose-derived MSCs [16]. Thus, MSCs have probably potents for promotion angiogenesis within the engineered 3D tissue. Notably, after transplantation, MSC-containing 3D tissues showed greater regeneration than that without MSCs by inducing macrophage infiltration [17]. Macrophage infiltration due to inflammation alters the EC network structure in vitro and promotes angiogenesis in vivo [18]. MSCs also exhibit immunomodulation after bone marrow transplantation [19]. This ability of MSCs to

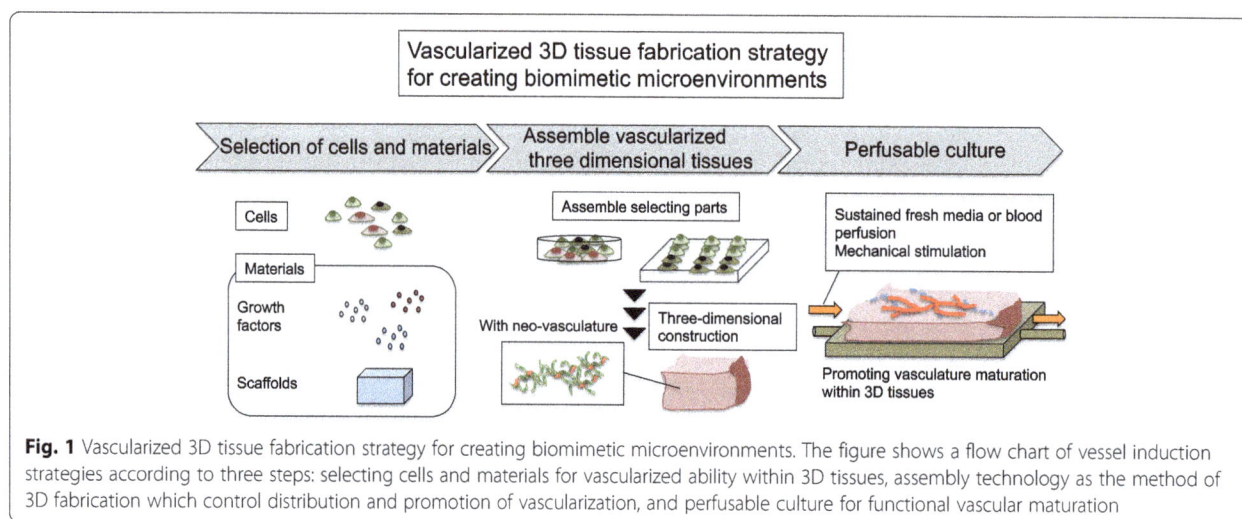

Fig. 1 Vascularized 3D tissue fabrication strategy for creating biomimetic microenvironments. The figure shows a flow chart of vessel induction strategies according to three steps: selecting cells and materials for vascularized ability within 3D tissues, assembly technology as the method of 3D fabrication which control distribution and promotion of vascularization, and perfusable culture for functional vascular maturation

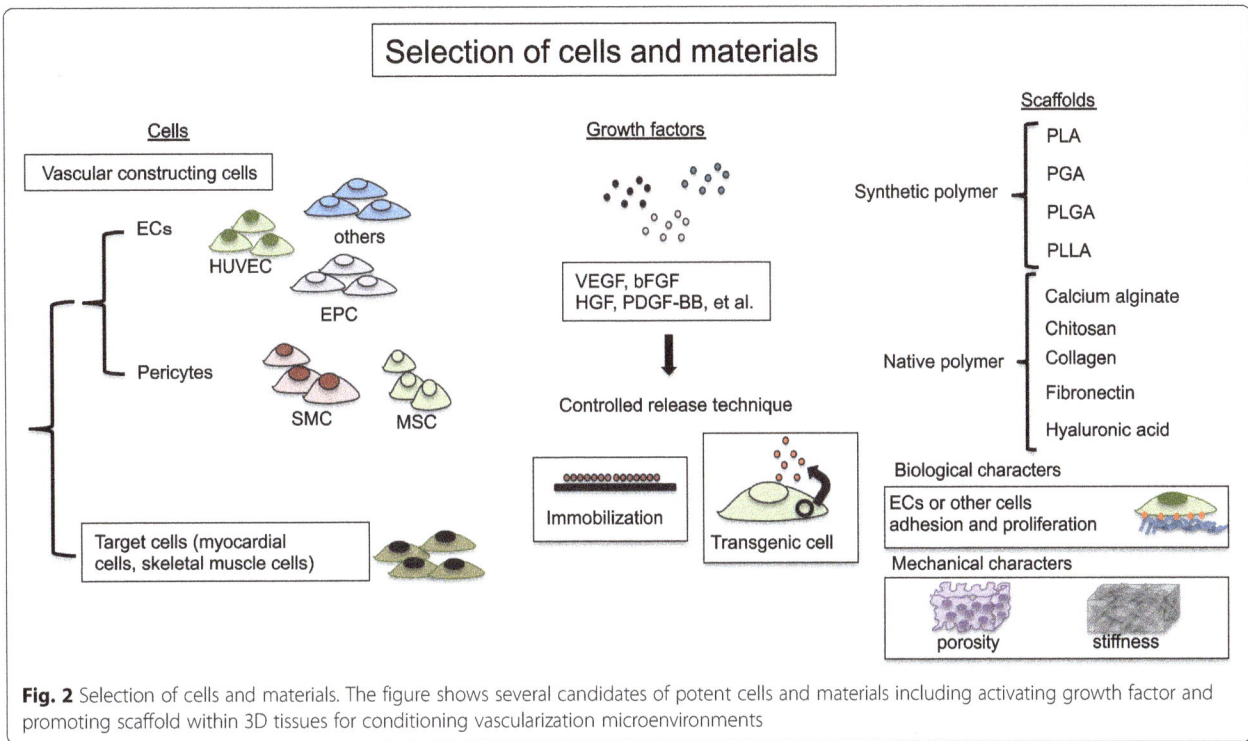

Fig. 2 Selection of cells and materials. The figure shows several candidates of potent cells and materials including activating growth factor and promoting scaffold within 3D tissues for conditioning vascularization microenvironments

affect inflammation may accelerate induction of vascularized 3D tissues in vivo.

Growth factor is also important for vascularization of 3D tissues. Culture medium containing growth factor is well known to induce vascularization in 3D tissues [20]. However, angiogenesis-promoting factors, vascular endothelial growth factor (VEGF), basic fibroblast growth factor (bFGF), hepatocyte growth factor (HGF), platelet-derived growth factor-BB (PDGF-BB), and angiopoietin-1 have common issues, quickly degradation and diffusion. To overcome these issues, we immobilized them with scaffolds [21] or co-cultured with VEGF transgenic cells [22]. It is also able to administrate sustained growth factors for local interested sites and cause gradients of growth factors [23]. It was reported that microvasculature is induced at the transplant position before transplantation via administration of a sustained-release VEGF or bFGF, to enhance vascularization of implanted 3D tissues [24]. Thus, the controlled release growth factors can be useful for vascularization within engineered 3D tissues.

Selecting scaffold materials (e.g., synthetic polymers and natural polymers) is also important for vascularization of 3D tissues [25]. Co-polymer of poly lactic acid (PLA) and poly glycolic acid (PGA) and poly-(L-lactide) (PLLA) and poly –(lactic-co-glycolic) acid (PLGA) are well known as synthetic biodegradable polymers for 3D tissue fabrication. Natural polymers, collagen, fibronectin, and hyaluronic acid are also well utilized for vascularization of 3D tissues.

Especially, extracellular matrix component could affect ECs adhesion and proliferation. These polymers could combine with each other for 3D tissue fabrication. In prior studies, well-vascularized 3D skeletal muscle tissues were fabricated in vivo with PLLA/PLGA scaffolds [26]. The EC network structures have been obtained within tri-cell cultured 3D tissues by adding fibrin to PLLA/PLGA scaffold during cultivation [27]. Moreover, mechanical characters (e.g., porous size and stiffness) of scaffold affected for vascularization ability within 3D tissues. The vascularization within the 3D tissue is probably controlled scaffold size, mechanical or chemical character optimization of the co-polymer biodegradation time [28]. Good selecting materials as scaffolds will mediate for vascularized 3D tissues.

Summarizing, suitable selective cells and materials are an important step for vascularization ability, EC-network formation, and vascular density inner 3D engineered tissues.

Assembly of cells into vascularized 3D engineered tissues: cell manipulation and scaffold shaping

Following selection step, cells and materials have to be arranged artificially or efficiently self-organization. Therefore, the assembly of cells and materials is another key point for fabrication of 3D tissues with vasculature (Fig. 3).

Recently, the thin coating of proteins on individual cell surfaces has been reported to facilitate the fabrication of 3D tissues without a scaffold in vitro [29]. The coated

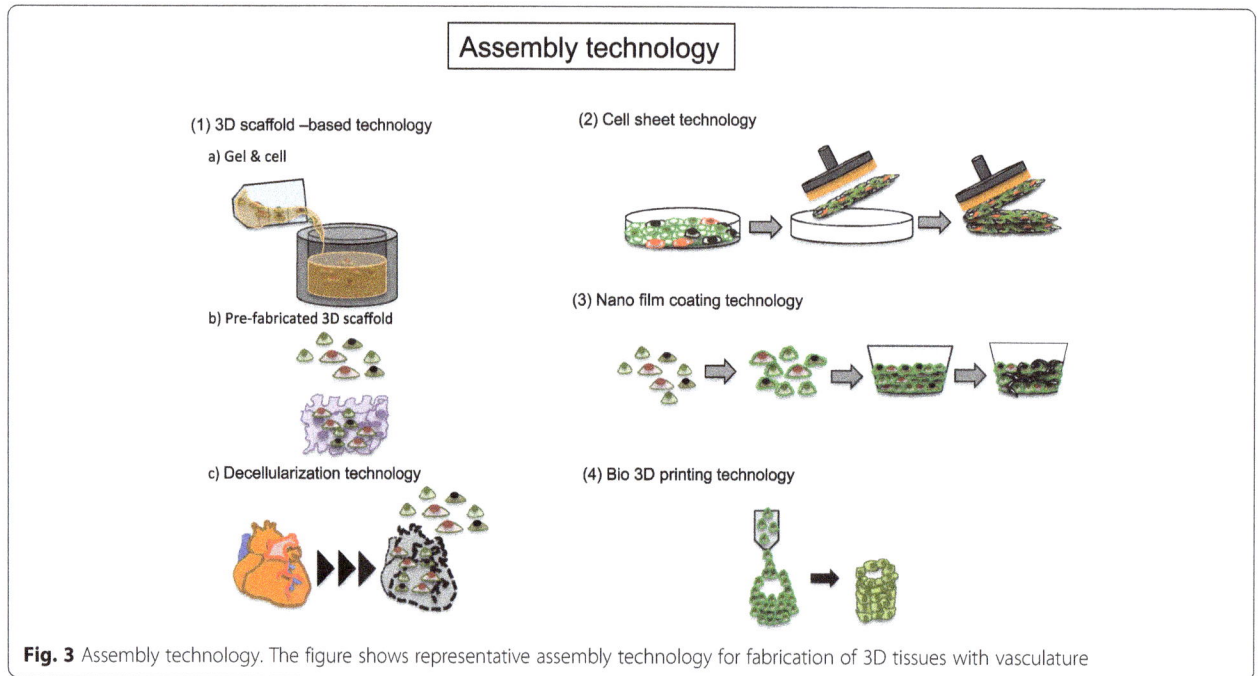

Fig. 3 Assembly technology. The figure shows representative assembly technology for fabrication of 3D tissues with vasculature

cells are cultured on a porous permeable membrane. After adhesion of the basic layer, the next layer of cells is cultured; this process is repeated to fabricate a 3D structure. Using this process, researchers have succeeded in constructing 3D tissues having an EC network structure by improving the cell-coating steps. Because nanofilm coating technology can be used to fabricate 3D tissues layer by layer, it cannot increase the thickness dynamically. In cell sheet technology, the thickness of a 3D tissue can be increased in units of several numbers of cell layers. Cell sheet technology uses cell culture dishes coated with the thermoresponsive polymer poly(N-isopropylacrylamide) (PIPAAM) with nanometer-level thickness [30]. These dishes allow cultured cells to be detached from the culture surface as cell sheets at a temperature of less than 32 °C. Simple ordinal cell culture methods with temperature-responsive culture dishes can be used to engineer 2D cell sheets under adequate temperature conditions. Preserved adhesive factors in fabricated 2D cell sheets are advantageous for readhesion during layering through adhesive factors released by the cells using the gelatin-gel stamp technique [31]. The stamp techniques allow several number of cell sheets layering for an hour. Fabricated 3D tissues with layered cell sheets can also be manipulated by highly intelligent tools [32].

As described above, prompt blood flow can be achieved in engineering of 3D tissues with cell sheet technology after transplantation because of preserved EC network during the fabrication of 3D tissues [7]. The network can be established as immature vessels in

transplanted 3D tissues within 24 h after transplantation. Even when only coculturing ECs and mesenchymal cells within Matrigel, at least 3 days are required to supply blood flow [33]. Thus, cell sheet technology can create dense 3D tissues with vascularization in vivo by exploiting the functions of the cells. In vitro EC networks and in vivo blood perfusion are achieved more quickly through cell sheet technology than scaffold or nanofilm coating technology (Table 1).

Additionally, vessels within tissues align and organize naturally into appropriate shapes and structures in vivo. Patterning techniques have been actively studied to create 2D shapes by micropatterning cell adhesive areas or nonadhesive areas on the surfaces of cell culture materials [34]. Microprinting of adhesive protein on the surface has also been achieved with polydimethylsiloxane (PDMS) micropatterning technology [35]. For lining cells in a specific direction, culture dishes having microgroove grids have also been studied [36]. These 2D patterning techniques could be combined with cell sheet layering methods to create precise 3D structures. However, patterning at the micrometer or nanometer level, i.e., smaller than the size of a cell (less than approximately 10 μm), tends to make cells disorganized within 3D cell-dense tissues. Moreover, 2D patterning structures can be modified easily by the surrounding cells. Compared with micropatterning technology, 3D bioprinting of cell-shaping scale is larger than micropatterning. Although a delicate pattern cannot be created, techniques that can control the amount of

Table 1 Comparison of EC-network assembly technologies. This table indicates the comparison of the period of EC network formation and connection to host blood circulation after transplantation among three assembly technologies, scaffold, and nanofilm coating and cell sheet technology

Technology	EC	EC network cultivation periods	Cocultured cells	Ratio of EC	Function as blood vessels checked in vivo	References
Scaffold (PLLA-PLGA)	HUVEC	3~7 days	Fibroblast Skeletal muscle cells	10~80%	Done (day 10)	[9, 26]
Nano film coating	HUVEC	3 day	Fibroblast, MSC, iPS, myocardial cells	9%	non	[29]
Cell sheet	Rat EC, HUVEC,	1 3 days	Fibroblast, SMC, myocardial cell	8~10%	Done (within 24 h)	[7, 8, 12]

Comparison of EC-network assembly technologies

blood vessels arranged in a 3D tissue are expected to be suitable for intentional blood vessel guidance into 3D tissues [37].

Native patterning and ECM could be used for tissue engineering with decellularized scaffold technique. Decellularized tissues are then recellularized with vascular ECs and perfused in vitro and in vivo. The kidneys of animals were decellularized and reseeded with human target cells [38]. Since the cell engraftment and infiltration of recellularization are affected by the decellularization protocol [39], further studies are needed to allow application of this technology.

These assembly methods have benefits and disadvantages (Table 2), and the appropriate method must be chosen based on the target tissue characteristics and applications. Because assembly technology will develop really day by day, we have to obtain information and arrange them adequately for target tissues.

Perfusion for maturation of vasculature within 3D tissues: fabrication perfusable basement for perfusion stimulation within vasculature within 3D tissues

Blood vessels function to transport blood throughout tissues and organs. During the embryonic stage, after vascularization, redundant vessels are remodeled [40]. Thus, if blood perfusion does not occur through vessel or EC networks, they should be removed as redundant vasculature. Researchers have used traditional approaches to perfuse 3D tissues, including transplantation

into animals to exploit biological circulation. In the selection of transplantation position, highly vascular sites, e.g., the kidney capsule, are usually chosen. However, engineered tissues have to be re-transplanted for therapeutic application. Accordingly, in the field of plastic surgery, the arteriovenous (AV) loop has been used to make a flap for promotion of vascularized 3D fabricated tissues [41, 42], allowing retransplantation into another site for maturation of 3D tissues by vascular anastomosis. Recently, vascular beds made from rat femoral tissues were perfused ex vivo, and 3D myocardial tissue was developed using cell sheet technology [43] (Fig. 4a).

In recent studies, microchannels within biodegradable scaffolds or ECM gel, such as collagen or fibrin, have been fabricated for perfusion into the channel. These microchannels have been employed in "body-on-a-chip" technology with PDMS microprocessing [44]. In our laboratory, a collagen gel microperfusable basement was vascularized by cell sheet technology [45]. Furthermore, microperfusable tubes were endothelialized with cells derived from cell sheets. Compared with the natural circulation system, these perfusable gel structures have no paracrine effects. By cocultivation with MSC inner scaffolds or ECM gel, it becomes possible to establish an effective perfusable basement for 3D tissue containing blood vessels without using animals. Microchannel fabricated by 3D printer with water-soluble polymer (poly vinyl alcohol: PVA) was also used as sacrificed template technique with embedding gelatin gel. The channel scale

Table 2 Assembly technology. The table shows several advantages and disadvantages of assembly technologies

Technology	Vascularization engineered 3D tissues	Advantage	Disadvantage	References
(1) 3D scaffold-based technology	Self-organization within scaffold or recellularization native vasculature ECM within decellularized tissues	Controlled selforganization with scaffold characters or native ECM and shape	With exogenous ECM or animal experiments	[38]
(2) Cell sheet technology	Self-organization within layered cell sheets	Without exogenous scaffolds	Specific manipulation	[31]
(3) Nanofilm coating technology	Self-organization within laded cells	Without specific equipment	Manipulation of 3D tissues to transplantation	[29]
(4) 3D printer technology	Vascular shaping with 3D printing	Fabrication free artificial shape	Patterning size limitation and degradation for long cultivation	[37]

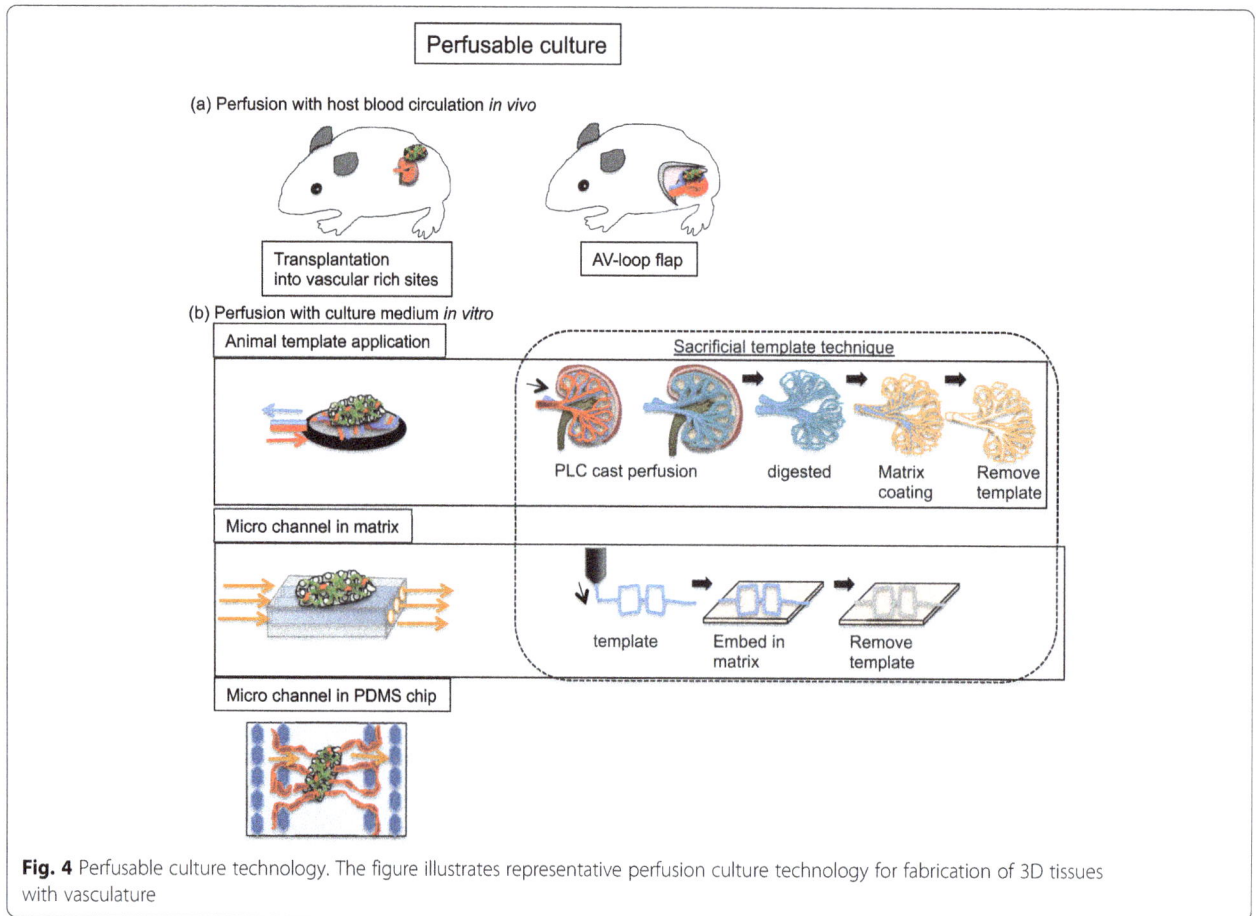

Fig. 4 Perfusable culture technology. The figure illustrates representative perfusion culture technology for fabrication of 3D tissues with vasculature

was more than 1 mm [46]. Perfusable vasculature under 100-μm diameter was also microfabricated by EC encapsulation with polymer by hydrodynamic shaping and photopolymerization. After embedded matrix, the microfabricated vessel could make branches from them [47]. More natural complex vasculature were tried to fabricate with perfusion poly caprolactone (PLC) cast into natural kidney vasculature. They digested kidney tissues without PLC cast and coated with collagen matrix. Finally, the PLC cast was removed as sacrificed template and remained complex structure of hollow collagen scaffolds (Fig. 4b animal material-applicated sacrificial template). They could be used as perfusable

microvasculature basement for engineered 3D tissues [48]. Perfusion stimulation causes biomechanics for maturation of vasculature within 3D tissues. However, perfusion medium has to be conditioned well. Especially, oxygen delivery carrier replaced to erythrocytes was important to maintain and maturate tissues [49]. Since these methodologies have also advantages and disadvantages (Table 3), we have to choose and combine these technologies according to suitable microenvironment for vascularization of target 3D tissues. In fact, vascularized cardiac cell tissues could be obtained in vivo and in vitro with perfusable cultivation [43, 45]. Moreover, 3D vascularized engineered tissues were reported to be obtained

Table 3 Perfusion culture technology. The table shows several advantages and disadvantages of perfusion culture technologies

	Technique	Advantage	Disadvantage	References
(a) Host blood circulation	Transplantation into rich vasculature sites	Without high technique and prompt vascularization	The size of transplantation tissues have limitation	[7, 8]
	AV-loop flap	Prompt vascularization and retransplantation with vascular anastomosis	Necessity of technique for anastomosis	[41, 42]
(b) Perfusion culture medium	Animal template application	Native vasculature can apply	Difficulty of maintaining animal template for long time in vitro	[43]
	Microchannel in matrix and on chip	Animal-free experiments	Necessity of promotion vascularization ability	[45]

with perfusion culture for 2 weeks in vitro [50, 51]. Thus, multistep vascularized tissue engineering is one of actualizing strategies for fabrication of functional vascularized 3D tissues.

Conclusion

In the fields of regenerative medicine and drug discovery, vascularized 3D tissues are needed for continued progress and the development of effective treatments. Key points for inducing vasculature within 3D tissues are selection of cells and materials, assembly methods, and perfusion techniques. In the past few decades, many technologies have been produced for generation of vascularized 3D tissues. Because there are numerous options for engineering 3D tissues, it is necessary to make an appropriate selection considering the specific target tissue. At the point to choose them, it is essential to understand suitable or native microenvironment for the target-tissue situation in vivo. The biomimetic microenvironment of target tissues will induce adequate cell-cell interaction, distance, cell morphology, and function within tissues. For fabrication of the microenvironment, multistep combination technologies might be a candidate of an actual strategy for vascularization within 3D tissues. It could progress for fabrication of vascularized 3D tissues and give us the generation functional tissues. We hope that these artificial tissue or organs will facilitate the development of effective treatment strategies for patients with intractable diseases in the future.

Abbreviations

2D: Two-dimensional; 3D: Three-dimensional; ADMSC: Adipose-derived MSC; AV: Arteriovenous; bFGF: Basic fibroblast growth factor; BMMSC: Bone marrow-derived MSC; EC: Endothelial cell; ECM: Extracellular matrix; EPC: Endothelial progenitor cell; HGF: Hepatocyte growth factor; HUVEC: Human umbilical vein endothelial cell; iPS: Induced pluripotent stem; MSC: Mesenchymal stem cell; PDGF-BB: Platelet-derived growth factor-BB; PDMS: Polydimethylsiloxane; PGA: Poly glycolic acid; PIPAAM: Poly(N-isopropylacrylamide); PLA: Poly lactic acid; PLC: Poly caprolactone; PLGA: Poly(lactide-co-glycolide); PLLA: Poly(L-lactide); PVA: Poly vinyl alcohol; SMC: Smooth muscle cell; TE: Tissue engineering; VEGF: Vascular endothelial growth factor

Acknowledgements
This work was supported by JSPS KAKENHI Grant Number JP17H02089.

Funding
This study was funded by Grants-in-Aid for Scientific Research (B).

Authors' contributions
SS drafted the original manuscript. ST gave final approval of the version to be published. All authors read and approved the final manuscript.

Competing interests
The corresponding author is a stakeholder of CellSeed Inc. The corresponding author received institutional research funds from CellSeed Inc.

References

1. Nishida K, Yamato M, Hayashida Y, Watanabe K, Yamamoto K, Adachi E, Nagai S, Kikuchi A, Maeda N, Watanabe H, Okano T, Tano Y. Corneal reconstruction with tissue-engineered cell sheets composed of autologous oral mucosal epithelium. N Engl J Med. 2004;351(12):1187–96.
2. Sawa Y, Miyagawa S. Cell sheet technology for heart failure. Curr Pharm Biotechnol. 2013;14(1):61–6.
3. Colton CK. Implantable biohybrid artificial organs. Cell Transplant. 1995;4(4):415–36.
4. Bersini S, Yazdi IK, Talo G, Shin SR, Moretti M, Khademhosseini A. Cell-microenvironment interactions and architectures in microvascular systems. Biotechnol Adv. 2016;34(6):1113–30.
5. Kim JJ, Hou L, Huang NF. Vascularization of three-dimensional engineered tissues for regenerative medicine applications. Acta Biomater. 2016;41:17–26.
6. Shimizu T, Sekine H, Yang J, Isoi Y, Yamato M, Kikuchi A, Kobayashi E, Okano T. Polysurgery of cell sheet grafts overcomes diffusion limits to produce thick, vascularized myocardial tissues. FASEB J. 2006;20(6):708–10.
7. Sekiya S, Shimizu T, Yamato M, Kikuchi A, Okano T. Bioengineered cardiac cell sheet grafts have intrinsic angiogenic potential. Biochem Biophys Res Commun. 2006;341(2):573–82.
8. Takeuchi R, Kuruma Y, Sekine H, Dobashi I, Yamato M, Umezu M, Shimizu T, Okano T. In vivo vascularization of cell sheets provided better long-term tissue survival than injection of cell suspension. J Tissue Eng Regen Med. 2016;10(8):700–10.
9. Levenberg S, Rouwkema J, Macdonald M, Garfein ES, Kohane DS, Darland DC, Marini R, van Blitterswijk CA, Mulligan RC, D'Amore PA, Langer R. Engineering vascularized skeletal muscle tissue. Nat Biotechnol. 2005;23(7):879–84.
10. Takebe T, Sekine K, Enomura M, Koike H, Kimura M, Ogaeri T, Zhang RR, Ueno Y, Zheng YW, Koike N, Aoyama S, Adachi Y, Taniguchi H. Vascularized and functional human liver from an iPSC-derived organ bud transplant. Nature. 2013;499(7459):481–4.
11. Takasato M, Er PX, Chiu HS, Maier B, Baillie GJ, Ferguson C, Parton RG, Wolvetang EJ, Roost MS, Lopes SM, Little MH. Kidney organoids from human iPS cells contain multiple lineages and model human nephrogenesis. Nature. 2016;536(7615):238.
12. Sekiya S, Muraoka M, Sasagawa T, Shimizu T, Yamato M, Okano T. Three-dimensional cell-dense constructs containing endothelial cell-networks are an effective tool for in vivo and in vitro vascular biology research. Microvasc Res. 2010;80(3):549–51.
13. Sasagawa T, Shimizu T, Sekiya S, Haraguchi Y, Yamato M, Sawa Y, Okano T. Design of prevascularized three-dimensional cell-dense tissues using a cell sheet stacking manipulation technology. Biomaterials. 2010;31(7):1646–54.
14. Sasagawa T, Shimizu T, Sekiya S, Yamato M, Okano T. Comparison of angiogenic potential between prevascular and non-prevascular layered adipose-derived stem cell-sheets in early post-transplanted period. J Biomed Mater Res A. 2014;102(2):358–65.
15. Ikhapoh IA, Pelham CJ, Agrawal DK. Atherogenic cytokines regulate VEGF-A-induced differentiation of bone marrow-derived mesenchymal stem cells into endothelial cells. Stem Cells Int. 2015;2015:498328.
16. Caplan AI, Correa D. The MSC: an injury drugstore. Cell Stem Cell. 2011;9(1):11–5.
17. Roh JD, Sawh-Martinez R, Brennan MP, Jay SM, Devine L, Rao DA, Yi T, Mirensky TL, Nalbandian A, Udelsman B, Hibino N, Shinoka T, Saltzman WM, Snyder E, Kyriakides TR, Pober JS, Breuer CK. Tissue-engineered vascular grafts transform into mature blood vessels via an inflammation-mediated process of vascular remodeling. Proc Natl Acad Sci U S A. 2010;107(10):4669–74.
18. Spiller KL, Anfang RR, Spiller KJ, Ng J, Nakazawa KR, Daulton JW, Vunjak-Novakovic G. The role of macrophage phenotype in vascularization of tissue engineering scaffolds. Biomaterials. 2014;35(15):4477–88.
19. Auletta JJ, Eid SK, Wuttisarnwattana P, Silva I, Metheny L, Keller MD, Guardia-Wolff R, Liu C, Wang F, Bowen T, Lee Z, Solchaga LA, Ganguly S, Tyler M, Wilson DL, Cooke KR. Human mesenchymal stromal cells attenuate graft-

versus-host disease and maintain graft-versus-leukemia activity following experimental allogeneic bone marrow transplantation. Stem Cells. 2015; 33(2):601–14.

20. Nomi M, Atala A, Coppi PD, Soker S. Principals of neovascularization for tissue engineering. Mol Asp Med. 2002;23(6):463–83.

21. Chiu LL, Radisic M. Scaffolds with covalently immobilized VEGF and Angiopoietin-1 for vascularization of engineered tissues. Biomaterials. 2010;31(2):226–41.

22. Liu B, Li X, Liang G, Liu X. VEGF expression in mesenchymal stem cells promotes bone formation of tissue-engineered bones. Mol Med Rep. 2011; 4(6):1121–6.

23. Tayalia P, Mooney DJ. Controlled growth factor delivery for tissue engineering. Adv Mater. 2009;21(32–33):3269–85.

24. Horikoshi-Ishihara H, Tobita M, Tajima S, Tanaka R, Oshita T, Tabata Y, Mizuno H. Coadministration of adipose-derived stem cells and control-released basic fibroblast growth factor facilitates angiogenesis in a murine ischemic hind limb model. J Vasc Surg. 2016;64(6):1825–1834 e1.

25. Langer R, Vacanti JP. Tissue engineering. Science. 1993;260(5110):920–6.

26. Lesman A, Koffler J, Atlas R, Blinder YJ, Kam Z, Levenberg S. Engineering vessel-like networks within multicellular fibrin-based constructs. Biomaterials. 2011;32(31):7856–69.

27. Lesman A, Gepstein L, Levenberg S. Cell tri-culture for cardiac vascularization. Methods Mol Biol. 2014;1181:131–7.

28. Kaushiva A, Turzhitsky VM, Darmoc M, Backman V, Ameer GA. A biodegradable vascularizing membrane: a feasibility study. Acta Biomater. 2007;3(5):631–42.

29. Amano Y, Nishiguchi A, Matsusaki M, Iseoka H, Miyagawa S, Sawa Y, Seo M, Yamaguchi T, Akashi M. Development of vascularized iPSC derived 3D-cardiomyocyte tissues by filtration layer-by-layer technique and their application for pharmaceutical assays. Acta Biomater. 2016;33:110–21.

30. Shimizu T. Cell sheet-based tissue engineering for fabricating 3-dimensional heart tissues. Circ J. 2014;78(11):2594–603.

31. Haraguchi Y, Shimizu T, Sasagawa T, Sekine H, Sakaguchi K, Kikuchi T, Sekine W, Sekiya S, Yamato M, Umezu M, Okano T. Fabrication of functional three-dimensional tissues by stacking cell sheets in vitro. Nat Protoc. 2012;7(5):850–8.

32. Tadakuma K, Tanaka N, Haraguchi Y, Higashimori M, Kaneko M, Shimizu T, Yamato M, Okano T. A device for the rapid transfer/transplantation of living cell sheets with the absence of cell damage. Biomaterials. 2013;34(36):9018–25.

33. Cheng G, Liao S, Kit Wong H, Lacorre DA, di Tomaso E, Au P, Fukumura D, Jain RK, Munn LL. Engineered blood vessel networks connect to host vasculature via wrapping-and-tapping anastomosis. Blood. 2011;118(17):4740–9.

34. Tsuda Y, Shimizu T, Yamato M, Kikuchi A, Sasagawa T, Sekiya S, Kobayashi J, Chen G, Okano T. Cellular control of tissue architectures using a three-dimensional tissue fabrication technique. Biomaterials. 2007;28(33):4939–46.

35. Tanaka N, Ota H, Fukumori K, Miyake J, Yamato M, Okano T. Micro-patterned cell-sheets fabricated with stamping-force-controlled micro-contact printing. Biomaterials. 2014;35(37):9802–10.

36. Zhou X, Hu J, Li J, Shi J, Chen Y. Patterning of two-level topographic cues for observation of competitive guidance of cell alignment. ACS Appl Mater Interfaces. 2012;4(8):3888–92.

37. Mir TA, Nakamura M. Three-dimensional bioprinting: toward the era of manufacturing human organs as spare parts for healthcare and medicine. Tissue Eng Part B Rev. 2017;23(3):245–56.

38. Song JJ, Guyette JP, Gilpin SE, Gonzalez G, Vacanti JP, Ott HC. Regeneration and experimental orthotopic transplantation of a bioengineered kidney. Nat Med. 2013;19(5):646–51.

39. Faulk DM, Carruthers CA, Warner HJ, Kramer CR, Reing JE, Zhang L, D'Amore A, Badylak SF. The effect of detergents on the basement membrane complex of a biologic scaffold material. Acta Biomater. 2014;10(1):183–93.

40. Lenard A, Daetwyler S, Betz C, Ellertsdottir E, Belting HG, Huisken J, Affolter M. Endothelial cell self-fusion during vascular pruning. PLoS Biol. 2015;13(4):e1002126.

41. Nau C, Henrich D, Seebach C, Schroder K, Fitzsimmons SJ, Hankel S, Barker JH, Marzi I, Frank J. Treatment of large bone defects with a vascularized periosteal flap in combination with biodegradable scaffold seeded with bone marrow-derived mononuclear cells: an experimental study in rats. Tissue Eng Part A. 2016;22(1–2):133–41.

42. Arkudas A, Beier JP, Pryymachuk G, Hoereth T, Bleiziffer O, Polykandriotis E, Hess A, Gulle H, Horch RE, Kneser U. Automatic quantitative micro-computed tomography evaluation of angiogenesis in an axially vascularized tissue-engineered bone construct. Tissue Eng Part C Methods. 2010;16(6):1503–14.

43. Sekine H, Shimizu T, Sakaguchi K, Dobashi I, Wada M, Yamato M, Kobayashi E, Umezu M, Okano T. In vitro fabrication of functional three-dimensional tissues with perfusable blood vessels. Nat Commun. 2013;4:1399.

44. Zhang B, Montgomery M, Chamberlain MD, Ogawa S, Korolj A, Pahnke A, Wells LA, Masse S, Kim J, Reis L, Momen A, Nunes SS, Wheeler AR, Nanthakumar K, Keller G, Sefton MV, Radisic M. Biodegradable scaffold with built-in vasculature for organ-on-a-chip engineering and direct surgical anastomosis. Nat Mater. 2016;15(6):669–78.

45. Sakaguchi K, Shimizu T, Horaguchi S, Sekine H, Yamato M, Umezu M, Okano T. In vitro engineering of vascularized tissue surrogates. Sci Rep. 2013;3:1316.

46. Li S, Liu YY, Liu LJ, Hu QX. A versatile method for fabricating tissue engineering scaffolds with a three-dimensional channel for prevasculature networks. ACS Appl Mater Interfaces. 2016;8(38):25096–103.

47. DiVito KA, Daniele MA, Roberts SA, Ligler FS, Adams AA. Microfabricated blood vessels undergo neoangiogenesis. Biomaterials. 2017;138:142–52.

48. Huling J, Ko IK, Atala A, Yoo JJ. Fabrication of biomimetic vascular scaffolds for 3D tissue constructs using vascular corrosion casts. Acta Biomater. 2016;32:190–7.

49. Seekell RP, Lock AT, Peng Y, Cole AR, Perry DA, Kheir JN, Polizzotti BD. Oxygen delivery using engineered microparticles. Proc Natl Acad Sci U S A. 2016;113(44):12380–5.

50. Nashimoto Y, Hayashi T, Kunita I, Nakamasu A, Torisawa YS, Nakayama M, Takigawa-Imamura H, Kotera H, Nishiyama K, Miura T, Yokokawa R. Integrating perfusable vascular networks with a three-dimensional tissue in a microfluidic device. Integr Biol (Camb). 2017;9(6):506–18.

51. Pagliari S, Tirella A, Ahluwalia A, Duim S, Goumans MJ, Aoyagi T, Forte G. A multistep procedure to prepare pre-vascularized cardiac tissue constructs using adult stem cells, dynamic cell cultures, and porous scaffolds. Front Physiol. 2014;5:210.

23

Endocannabinoids and related *N*-acylethanolamines: biological activities and metabolism

Kazuhito Tsuboi[1,2*], Toru Uyama[1], Yasuo Okamoto[2] and Natsuo Ueda[1]

Abstract

The plant *Cannabis sativa* contains cannabinoids represented by Δ^9-tetrahydrocannabinol, which exert psychoactivity and immunomodulation through cannabinoid CB1 and CB2 receptors, respectively, in animal tissues. Arachidonoylethanolamide (also referred to as anandamide) and 2-arachidonoylglycerol (2-AG) are well known as two major endogenous agonists of these receptors (termed "endocannabinoids") and show various cannabimimetic bioactivities. However, only 2-AG is a full agonist for CB1 and CB2 and mediates retrograde signals at the synapse, strongly suggesting that 2-AG is physiologically more important than anandamide. The metabolic pathways of these two endocannabinoids are completely different. 2-AG is mostly produced from inositol phospholipids via diacylglycerol by phospholipase C and diacylglycerol lipase and then degraded by monoacylglycerol lipase. On the other hand, anandamide is concomitantly produced with larger amounts of other *N*-acylethanolamines via *N*-acyl-phosphatidylethanolamines (NAPEs). Although this pathway consists of calcium-dependent *N*-acyltransferase and NAPE-hydrolyzing phospholipase D, recent studies revealed the involvement of several new enzymes. Quantitatively major *N*-acylethanolamines include palmitoylethanolamide and oleoylethanolamide, which do not bind to cannabinoid receptors but exert anti-inflammatory, analgesic, and anorexic effects through receptors such as peroxisome proliferator-activated receptor α. The biosynthesis of these non-endocannabinoid *N*-acylethanolamines rather than anandamide may be the primary significance of this pathway. Here, we provide an overview of the biological activities and metabolisms of endocannabinoids (2-AG and anandamide) and non-endocannabinoid *N*-acylethanolamines.

Keywords: Lipid mediator, Endocannabinoid, 2-Arachidonoylglycerol, Anandamide, *N*-Acylethanolamine, Metabolism, Phospholipid, Phospholipase

Background

Preparations of the plant *Cannabis sativa*, such as marijuana and hashish, have been used for recreational and medical purposes for thousands of years [1]. The oldest written description of medicinal cannabis dates back to around 2350 B.C., which was found on a stone from the pyramids in Egypt. Although their psychoactivities, including euphoria, hallucination, and analgesia, have been known for a long time, the purification of Δ^9-tetrahydrocannabinol (Δ^9-THC) as the major psychoactive

constituent, followed by the determination of its chemical structure, was not achieved until the 1960s [2] (Fig. 1). A large number of structurally related compounds were also isolated from cannabis and collectively referred to as cannabinoids. Synthetic analogs with more potent cannabimimetic activities were also developed and used to pharmacologically characterize a specific receptor for cannabinoids existing in rat brain crude membrane preparations [3]. The central-type CB1 cannabinoid receptor was then molecularly identified by its cDNA cloning in 1990 [4]. Subsequently, cDNA of the peripheral-type CB2 cannabinoid receptor was also found by using its sequence similarity to CB1 receptor [5]. In contrast to Δ^9-THC, cannabidiol, another major cannabinoid in cannabis, showing anti-inflammatory and anticonvulsive effects, was

* Correspondence: ktsuboi@med.kawasaki-m.ac.jp
[1]Department of Biochemistry, Kagawa University School of Medicine, 1750-1 Ikenobe, Miki, Kagawa 761-0793, Japan
[2]Department of Pharmacology, Kawasaki Medical School, 577 Matsushima, Kurashiki, Okayama 701-0192, Japan

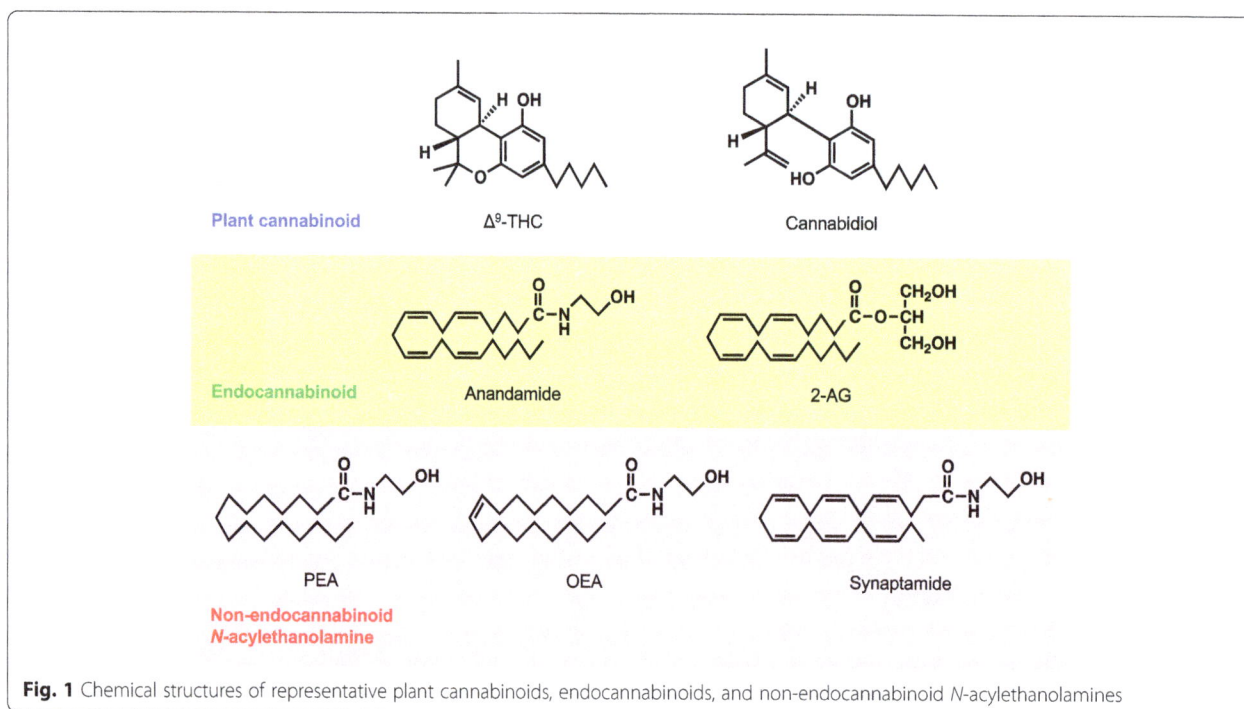

Fig. 1 Chemical structures of representative plant cannabinoids, endocannabinoids, and non-endocannabinoid N-acylethanolamines

almost inactive for cannabinoid receptors. Since cannabinoids are derived from the plant cannabis but not from mammals, animal tissues were expected to have endogenous counterparts capable of binding to cannabinoid receptors (later termed "endocannabinoids"). Arachidonoylethanolamide, the ethanolamide of arachidonic acid, was isolated as the first endocannabinoid from pig brain and named anandamide after "ananda," which means bliss in Sanskrit [6] (Fig. 1). Shortly after that, another derivative of arachidonic acid, 2-arachidonoylglycerol (2-AG), was also reported to show the same agonistic activity [7, 8]. It was surprising since 2-AG has been known for a long time simply as a common intermediate in the metabolisms of glycerophospholipids and triglyceride. Currently, 2-AG and anandamide are considered to be a full agonist and a partial agonist of cannabinoid receptors, respectively. Arachidonic acid is a polyunsaturated fatty acid (20:4) well known as the precursor of bioactive prostaglandins and other eicosanoids. Endocannabinoids are thus considered to be other members of arachidonic acid-related lipid mediators.

In addition to anandamide, ethanolamides of various long-chain fatty acids are also present in the body. These ethanolamides, including anandamide, are collectively referred to as N-acylethanolamines (Fig. 1). Ethanol-amides of saturated and monounsaturated fatty acids such as palmitic (16:0), stearic (18:0), and oleic acids (18:1) are much more abundant than anandamide in the body. These saturated and monounsaturated N-acylethanolamines do not bind to cannabinoid receptors, but they can activate peroxisome proliferator-activated receptor α (PPARα), a nuclear receptor, and other receptors, leading to the exertion of biological activities including anti-inflammation and appetite suppression. In this mini-review, we will outline the biological activities and metabolisms of endocannabinoids and related N-acylethanolamines and emphasize that 2-AG is physiologically more important than anandamide, which appears to be a minor component concomitantly produced with cannabinoid receptor-insensitive N-acylethanolamines.

Biological activities of endocannabinoids

CB1 and CB2 cannabinoid receptors are G protein-coupled receptors possessing seven transmembrane helices [4, 5]. When the primary structures of the two receptors from human are compared, 44% of the amino acid residues are identical over the entire length. In their transmembrane regions, the sequence identity increases to 68%. CB1 receptor exists in abundance at the presynaptic terminals in the various regions of the brain, including substantia nigra, striatum, hippocampus, and cerebral cortex, and negatively regulates the release of the neurotransmitters. CB1 is therefore the principal receptor mediating the psychoactivities of cannabis. CB1 receptor is also present in periphery such as adrenal gland, reproductive tissues, and immune cells at lower levels. On the other hand, CB2 receptor is mainly expressed in the immune system including the spleen, thymus, and lymph nodes and is involved in the immunomodulatory effects of cannabinoids. The expression levels of CB2 receptor in the human blood cells are in the following order: B cells > natural killer cells >> monocytes > polymorphonuclear neutrophil cells > CD8+ T cells > CD4+ T cells [9]. Activation of these receptors leads to a variety of cellular signal transduction such as a decrease in the cAMP level, an inhibition of N- and P/Q-type voltage-dependent Ca^{2+} channels, an opening of inwardly rectifying K^+ channels, and an activation of mitogen-activated protein kinases.

Anandamide and 2-AG exert a variety of bioactivities as cannabinoid receptor ligands, including the cannabinoid tetrad: analgesia, catalepsy, hypolocomotion, and hypothermia. They also cause bradycardia and reductions of blood and intraocular pressures. As mentioned above, anandamide is a partial agonist of CB1 receptor, while 2-AG is a full agonist of both CB1 and CB2 receptors. Furthermore, the tissue levels of 2-AG are generally hundreds to thousands of times higher than those of anandamide. Thus, 2-AG is recognized to be the true endogenous ligands of CB1 and CB2 receptors and is considered to play more important roles in vivo than anandamide [10]. However, when the anandamide-degrading enzyme, fatty acid amid hydrolase (FAAH), is pharmacologically inhibited or genetically deficient, the local concentration of anandamide would rise and could exert CB1-dependent activities. It is important that 2-AG mediates retrograde signals at the synapse [11]. 2-AG is synthesized at the postsynaptic neurons in response to the stimulus of neurotransmitters such as glutamic acid. The released 2-AG then binds to and activates presynaptic CB1 receptors and inhibits the further release of the neurotransmitter.

In addition to CB1 and CB2 receptors, pharmacological studies suggest the presence of non-CB1, non-CB2 receptors mediating the effects of cannabinoids. Although several proteins have been discussed as candidates for such potential "CB3" receptor, its existence is controversial and not yet established [12]. One of the candidates is GPR55, a G protein-coupled receptor. Δ^9-THC, a CB1/CB2 receptor agonist CP55940, anandamide, and 2-AG were reported to bind to GPR55 receptor overexpressed in human embryonic kidney HEK293s cells with nanomolar potencies, as analyzed with GTPγS binding experiments [13]. However, the pharmacological data of GPR55 gathered so far are conflicting and further analyses should be continued [14]. On the other hand, lysophosphatidylinositol, which is not a ligand of CB1 or CB2 receptor, was found to be the endogenous ligand of GPR55 [15]. Although this receptor can be activated by various molecular species of lysophosphatidylinositol having a different fatty acyl moiety at sn-1 or sn-2 position, 2-arachidonoyl-lysophosphatidylinositol is reported to be the most potent [16]. More recently, lysophosphatidylglucose was reported to be a more potent ligand of GPR55 and to mediate the correct guidance of nociceptive axons in the spinal cord [17]. Since anandamide also activates the transient receptor potential vanilloid type 1 (TRPV1) protein, a non-selective cation channel, anandamide is also regarded as one of endovanilloids [18]. However, its physiological significance as an endovanilloid is not fully elucidated.

Biological activities of non-endocannabinoid N-acylethanolamines

Not only anandamide but also several ethanolamides of polyunsaturated fatty acids possessing three or more double bonds, such as dihomo-γ-linolenic acid (C20:3 ω6), mead acid (C20:3 ω9), and adrenic acid (C22:4), bind to cannabinoid receptors [19, 20]. However, saturated and monounsaturated N-acylethanolamines do not show ligand activity for cannabinoid receptors. Instead, these non-endocannabinoid N-acylethanolamines exert biological activities through different receptors. Importantly, non-endocannabinoid N-acylethanolamines such as palmitoylethanolamide (PEA, C16:0 N-acylethanolamine), stearoylethanolamide (C18:0 N-acylethanolamine), oleoyl-ethanolamide (OEA, C18:1 N-acylethanolamine), and linoleoylethanolamide (C18:2 N-acylethanolamine) are much more abundant than anandamide in most animal tissues. Biosynthetic enzymes for N-acylethanolamines so far reported do not show selectivity for anandamide over other N-acylethanolamine species. Thus, anandamide could be concomitantly produced as a kind of by-product of non-endocannabinoid N-acylethanolamines.

PEA is a food component known for more than 60 years [21]. This molecule was isolated from soybean lecithin, egg yolk, and peanut meal and was shown to exert an anti-inflammatory activity in a local passive joint anaphylaxis assay in the guinea pig [22, 23]. Since then, PEA has been shown to have anti-inflammatory, analgesic, anti-epileptic, and neuroprotective actions [24, 25]. These actions are mediated at least in part by PPARα. Preclinical and clinical studies suggest that PEA is potentially useful in a wide range of therapeutic areas, including eczema, pain, and neurodegeneration [26]. In the USA and Europe, PEA is currently marketed as a nutraceutical, a food supplement, or a food for medical purposes, depending on the country, which is effective for chronic pain represented by neuropathic pain. PEA is also a constituent of cream marketed for dry, irritated, and reactive skin. Although it was reported that PEA could activate GPR55 [13], this agonist activity has not been fully elucidated.

OEA is known to have an anorexic activity in experimental animals [27]. Administration of OEA produces satiety and reduces body weight gain [28]. OEA binds with high affinity to PPARα, and these effects are not observed with PPARα-deficient mice, suggesting that the anorexic action of OEA is mediated by PPARα. Since OEA is proposed to be produced from the digested dietary fat in the enterocytes of small intestine [29], endogenous OEA may mediate the satiety after the intake of fatty food. Furthermore, the dysfunction of OEA signaling could contribute to overweight and obesity. Thus, analogs of OEA and the inhibitors of OEA-degrading enzymes, such as FAAH, could be expected as novel anti-obesity drugs. OEA is also reported to activate GPR119 in vitro [30]. This G protein-coupled receptor was expressed in the intestinal L-cells, which secrete glucagon-like peptide-1 (GLP-1), and intraileal administration of OEA to rats was found to increase plasma GLP-1 levels [31]. However, the anorexic action of OEA was observed even in GPR119-deficient mice [32], suggesting that GPR119 system is not essential for OEA-induced satiety. Although OEA was reported to be a weak agonist of TRPV1 [33], TRPV1-deficient mice also exhibit OEA-induced suppression of appetite [34]. On the other hand, TRPV1 is suggested to mediate the reducing effects of OEA on levodopa (L-DOPA)-induced dyskinesia [35]. Thus, the OEA-TRPV1 system might be an effective target for the treatment of L-DOPA-induced dyskinesias.

Docosahexaenoylethanolamide (C22:6 N-acylethanol-amine) is the ethanolamide of docosahexaenoic acid, one of major ω3 polyunsaturated fatty acids, and is referred to as synaptamide. At nanomolar concentrations, synaptamide promotes neurogenesis, neurite outgrowth, and synaptogenesis in developing neurons [36]. Recently, these actions were shown to be mediated by the activation of GPR110, which is also termed as adhesion G protein-coupled receptor F1 (ADGRF1) [37]. Although the physiological significance in the development of neurons and cognitive functions remains elusive, the synaptamide-GPR110 system could be a novel target for the treatment of neurodevelopmental diseases. Furthermore, the beneficial effects of docosahexaenoic acid on the central nervous system might be partly mediated by the generation of synaptamide.

Metabolism of endocannabinoid 2-arachidonoylglycerol

Although 2-AG is biosynthesized in multiple pathways, all the pathways start from sn-2 arachidonic acid-containing glycerophospholipids, which are abundant in cell membranes and therefore suitable as starting materials [10] (Fig. 2). The main precursors are inositol phospholipids with 2-arachidonoyl group such as 2-arachidonoyl-phosphatidylinositol 4,5-bisphosphate. The inositol phospholipids are hydrolyzed by phospholipase C to form 2-arachidonoyl-diacylglycerol, which is further deacylated by sn-1-specific diacylglycerol lipase (DAGL) to yield 2-AG (Fig. 2). Glycerophospholipids

other than inositol phospholipids, such as phosphatidic acid and phosphatidylcholine (PC), could also be hydrolyzed to 2-arachidonoyl-diacylglycerol [38–40]. Human DAGL has two isozymes, DAGLα and DAGLβ. Their cDNAs were cloned in 2003 [41]. In DAGLα-deficient mice, the retrograde suppression of synaptic transmission is lost with concomitant decreases in 2-AG levels of brain and spinal cord [42–44]. Thus, DAGLα is suggested to be the main biosynthetic enzyme of 2-AG in the central nervous system. While the role of DAGL in the hydrolysis of membrane phospholipid-derived sn-1,2-diacylglycerol species is well established, it was described that DAGL enzymes are unlikely to be involved in the degradation of rac-1,3- or sn-2,3-diacylglycerol that originates from lipolysis-driven triacylglycerol breakdown [45].

Alternatively, 2-arachidonoyl-phosphatidylinositol could be hydrolyzed at sn-1 position by an intracellular phospholipase A₁, DDHD domain containing 1, previously known as phosphatidic acid-preferring phospholipase A₁ [46] (Fig. 2). The formed 2-arachidonoyl-lysophosphatidylinositol is known as an endogenous agonist of GPR55 as described above and is further hydrolyzed to 2-AG by a phospholipase C-type enzyme. Furthermore, 2-AG could be produced by dephosphorylation of arachidonic acid-containing lysophosphatidic acid (LPA) [47]. These alternative pathways, which bypass 2-arachidonoyl-diacylglycerol and therefore do not involve DAGL, seemed to play a certain role in vivo since ~ 15% of 2-AG levels remained even in the cerebral cortex of DAGLα/β double-knockout mice, compared to those of wild-type mice [44].

The major degradative pathway of 2-AG is considered to be the hydrolysis to arachidonic acid and glycerol (Fig. 2). This reaction can be catalyzed by multiple enzymes, including monoacylglycerol lipase (MAGL), FAAH, α/β-hydrolase domain containing (ABHD) 6, and ABHD12. The relative contribution of these enzymes differs among tissues and cells. In mouse brain, MAGL is responsible for around 85% of the 2-AG-hydrolyzing activity in vitro [48]. cDNA of this enzyme was cloned from mouse adipocytes in 1997 [49]. MAGL hydrolyzes not only 2-AG but also other 2-monoacylglycerols and 1-monoacylglycerols. Pharmacological inhibition of MAGL in mice caused CB1-dependent symptoms including analgesia, hypothermia, and hypomotility, indicating the central role of this enzyme in the degradation of 2-AG in the brain [50]. Although MAGL-deficient mice exhibited increased 2-AG levels in the brain and spinal cord, no abnormalities in nociception, body temperature, or spontaneous locomotion were observed in MAGL-deficient mice [51, 52]. This apparent discrepancy is supposed to be due to the desensitization of CB1 receptor. Apart from the endocannabinoid system,

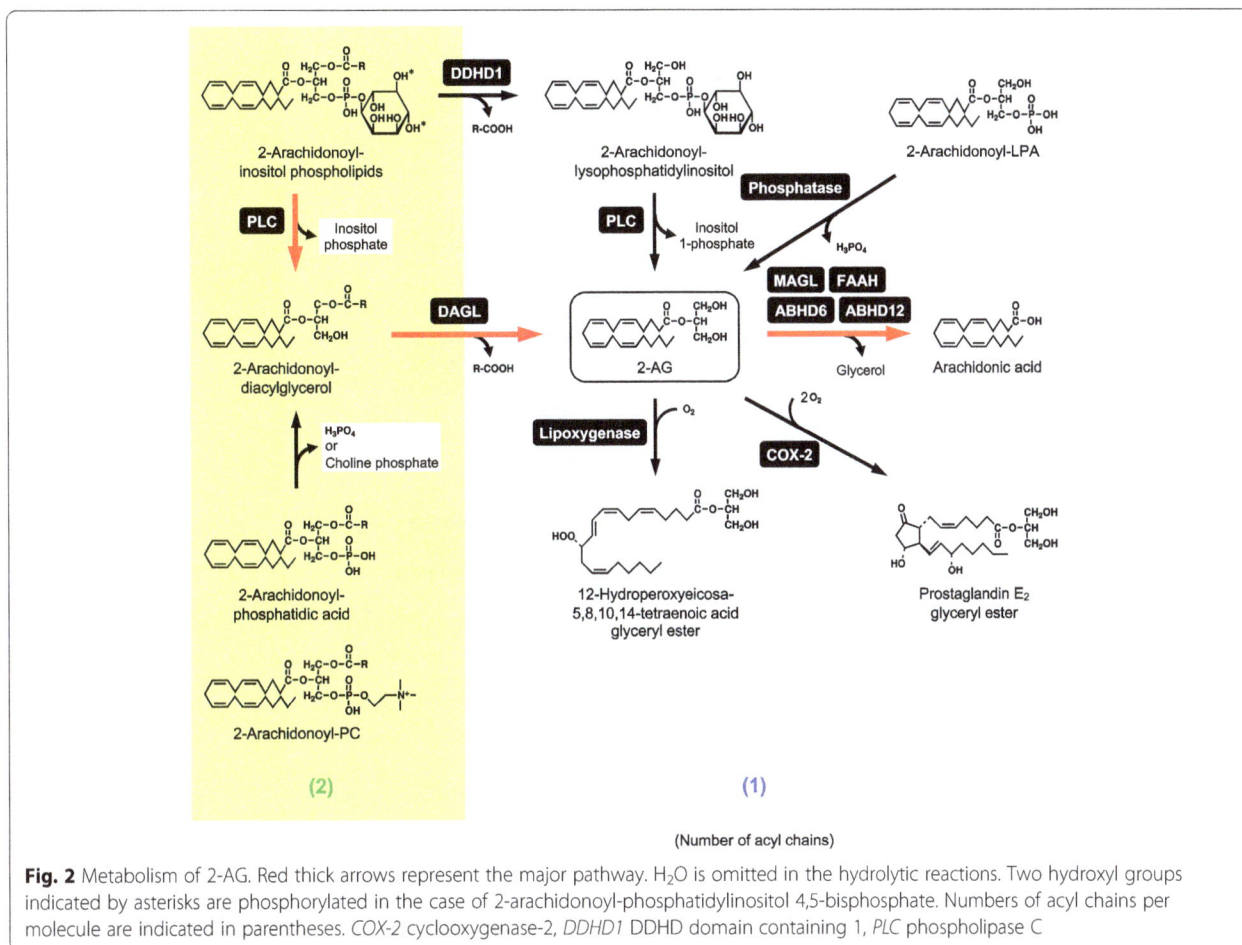

Fig. 2 Metabolism of 2-AG. Red thick arrows represent the major pathway. H₂O is omitted in the hydrolytic reactions. Two hydroxyl groups indicated by asterisks are phosphorylated in the case of 2-arachidonoyl-phosphatidylinositol 4,5-bisphosphate. Numbers of acyl chains per molecule are indicated in parentheses. *COX-2* cyclooxygenase-2, *DDHD1* DDHD domain containing 1, *PLC* phospholipase C

MAGL-dependent generation of arachidonic acid from 2-AG is also responsible for the production of prostaglandins that promote neuroinflammation and fever generation in the brain [53, 54].

FAAH plays the central role in the degradation of anandamide, another endocannabinoid, as described in the following section. FAAH also hydrolyzes 2-AG. However, the role of FAAH in 2-AG degradation in vivo is considered to be minor. In mouse microglia BV-2 cells, ABHD6 controls the accumulation of 2-AG, and knockdown of ABHD6 increases the efficacy with which 2-AG can stimulate CB2-mediated cell migration [55]. ABHD6 is also expressed postsynaptically in neurons, and the specific inhibitor of ABHD6 as well as MAGL inhibitors induces CB1-dependent long-term depression. As another metabolic route of 2-AG, the arachidonoyl moiety of 2-AG could be directly oxygenated by cyclooxygenase-2 and lipoxygenases to produce glycerol esters of prostaglandins and hydroperoxyeicosatetraenoic acids, respectively (Fig. 2). Glycerol esters of prostaglandins are reported to show biological activities including anti-inflammatory, pro-inflammatory, and hyperalgesic effects [56].

The pathway consisting of phospholipase C, DAGL, and MAGL has attracted attention due to the formation of two second messengers, diacylglycerol and inositol trisphosphate, and the release of free arachidonic acid from phospholipid, which may be utilized to generate eicosanoids. The major pathway for the biosynthesis and degradation of 2-AG completely agrees with this pathway, and this fact implies its multifunctionality of this pathway.

Metabolism of *N*-acylethanolamines

In animal tissues, a series of *N*-acylethanolamines including anandamide is biosynthesized through common metabolic pathways starting from glycerophospholipids (Fig. 3). The pathways are largely different from the aforementioned 2-AG metabolism. First, *sn*-1 acyl group of glycerophospholipids such as PC is transferred to the amino group of ethanolamine glycerophospholipids represented by phosphatidylethanolamine (PE). This *N*-acylation of PE results in the generation of *N*-acyl-PE (NAPE), which is a unique type of glycerophospholipid in that three fatty acyl chains exist per molecule. The responsible enzyme *N*-acyltransferase has been known

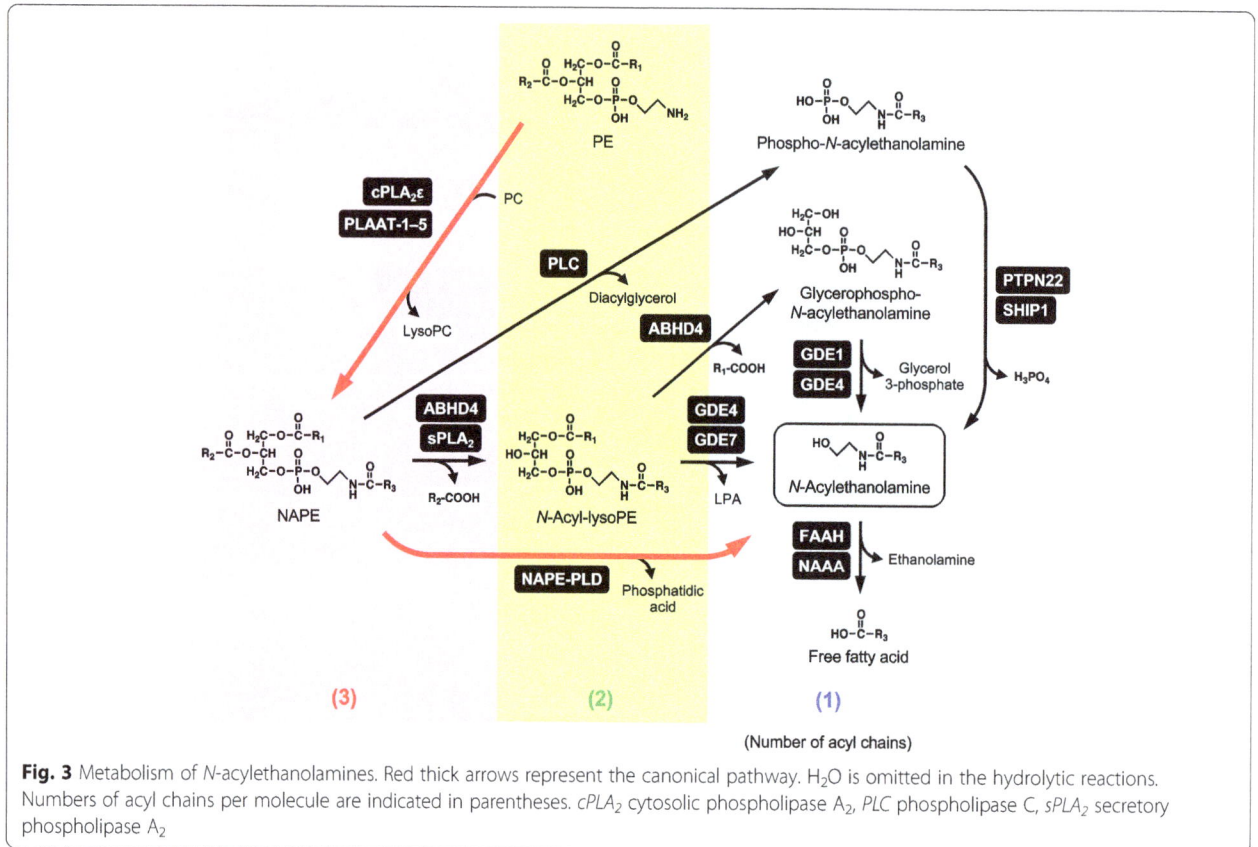

Fig. 3 Metabolism of *N*-acylethanolamines. Red thick arrows represent the canonical pathway. H₂O is omitted in the hydrolytic reactions. Numbers of acyl chains per molecule are indicated in parentheses. *cPLA₂* cytosolic phospholipase A₂, *PLC* phospholipase C, *sPLA₂* secretory phospholipase A₂

to be stimulated by Ca^{2+} since the 1980s [57–59] and called as Ca-dependent *N*-acyltransferase (Ca-NAT) to distinguish from Ca-independent enzymes discussed later. However, its molecular characterization was achieved only recently when mouse Ca-NAT was identified by an activity-based proteomic approach as isoform ε of cytosolic phospholipase A₂ (PLA2G4E) [60]. Our group then found that human ortholog has two isoforms, which are distinguished by the length and amino acid residues of their N-terminal sequences, and that both isoforms show Ca-NAT activity [61]. We also revealed that this Ca^{2+}-dependent activity is further enhanced by phosphatidylserine. In agreement with the fact that the *sn*-1 position of glycerophospholipids is mostly occupied by a saturated or monounsaturated fatty acid, the anandamide precursor *N*-arachidonoyl-PE is a minor component among various NAPEs with different *N*-acyl species. This may be the main reason why anandamide is a minor component of *N*-acylethanolamines.

Apart from Ca-NAT, we found that all of the five members of HRAS-like suppressor (HRASLS) family, HRASLS1–5, have Ca^{2+}-independent *N*-acyltransferase activities as well as phospholipase A₁/A₂ activities [62–67]. These family members were previously reported as tumor suppressor genes, negatively regulating the

oncogene *Ras*. On the basis of their enzyme activities, we proposed to rename them phospholipase A/acyltransferase (PLAAT)-1–5, respectively [66]. Among the members, PLAAT-1, PLAAT-2, and PLAAT-5 have relatively high *N*-acyltransferase activities over phospholipase A₁/A₂ activities [67, 68], suggesting their roles in the Ca^{2+}-independent generation of NAPE in vivo.

The formed NAPE is then hydrolyzed to release *N*-acylethanolamines by a phospholipase D (PLD)-type enzyme, NAPE-PLD (Fig. 3). Our group purified this enzyme from rat heart and cloned its cDNAs from human, mouse, and rat [69]. The enzyme specifically hydrolyzes NAPE, but not PE or PC. The primary structure of NAPE-PLD shows that this enzyme belongs to the metallo-β-lactamase family and has no sequence similarity with other PLDs, which typically hydrolyze PC to phosphatidic acid and choline. Thus, NAPE-PLD is distinct from other PLDs in both structure and catalytic function.

In addition to the one-step *N*-acylethanolamine-forming reaction catalyzed by NAPE-PLD, the presence of multi-step pathways via *N*-acyl-lysoPE was suggested using dog brain preparations in the 1980s [58] (Fig. 3). The cDNA cloning of NAPE-PLD enabled the generation of NAPE-PLD$^{-/-}$ mice, and three groups including ours independently established the mutant mice and confirmed the presence of the multi-step NAPE-PLD-independent pathways in brain and other mammalian tissues [70–73]. In these pathways, one O-acyl chain is first eliminated from NAPE, resulting in the formation of N-acyl-lysoPE. This reaction occurred in vitro by group IB, IIA, and V of secretory phospholipase A_2s [74]. N-Acyl-lysoPE can be further O-deacylated to glycerophospho-N-acylethanol-a-mine. ABHD4 was found to function as a hydrolase catalyzing these sequential O-deacylation reactions from NAPE to glycerophospho-N-acylethanolamine via N-acyl-lysoPE [75]. Glycerophospho-N-acylethanolamine is further hydrolyzed to form N-acylethanolamine by two members of the glycerophosphodiesterase (GDE) family, GDE1 [76] and GDE4 [77, 78]. Alternatively, N-acyl-ly-soPE can be directly converted to N-acyletha-nolamine by lysophospholipase D-type enzymes. In this reaction, LPA is also formed as another product. This lysophospholipase D-type reaction seems particularly important when the substrate N-acyl-lysoPE is "plasmalogen-type" containing a lipase-resistant alkenyl chain at sn-1 position of the gly-cerol backbone [71]. We found that GDE4 and GDE7 have this lysophospholipase D-type activity [77, 78]. Interest-ingly, the divalent cation requirement for the activity dif-fers among GDE members: GDE1 and GDE4 are Mg^{2+}-dependent while GDE7 is Ca^{2+}-dependent. In addition, an anandamide-forming pathway through phosphoanan-damide (anandamide phosphate) was previously suggested in the brain and macrophages. This pathway is composed of phospholipase C and phosphatase. Tyrosine phosphat-ase PTPN22 and inositol 5′-phosphatase SHIP1 were shown to have this phosphatase activity while the phospholipase C has not yet been identified [79, 80]. The reverse reaction of FAAH can synthesize anandamide from free arachidonic acid and ethanolamine in vitro [81, 82]. The analysis of FAAH-deficient mice suggests the in vivo production of anandamide through this route [83].

N-Acylethanolamines are degraded by the hydrolysis to free fatty acids and ethanolamine (Fig. 3). FAAH cata-lyzes this reaction, and this enzyme has been extensively studied since its cDNA cloning in 1996 [84]. FAAH is a membrane-bound serine hydrolase, belonging to the am-idase signature family. The catalytic activity is higher at neutral and alkaline pH. FAAH hydrolyzes various N-acylethanolamines with a higher reactivity toward anandamide. FAAH is ubiquitously present in various tissues with abundant expressions in the brain and liver, and FAAH-deficient mice exhibit increased tissue levels of various N-acylethanolamines including anandamide, suggesting the central role of this enzyme in the degrad-ation of N-acylethanolamines [85, 86]. Specific FAAH in-hibitors have been developed, and they are expected as novel therapeutic drugs against a variety of symptoms such as pain, depression, and anxiety. These beneficial effects are mostly considered to result from the

increased tissue levels of anandamide acting as an endo-cannabinoid. However, FAAH also hydrolyzes cannabin-oid receptor-insensitive N-acylethanolamines and other bioactive fatty acid amides such as oleamide and N-acyl-taurine. Thus, we should be careful in interpreting the molecular mechanisms of the phenotype caused by genetic and pharmacological depletion of FAAH. The dual inhibitors of FAAH and MAGL have also been developed, and they increase both anandamide and 2-AG levels to mimic the pharmacological activities of CB1 receptor agonist in vivo [87, 88]. FAAH-2, an isozyme having around 20% of amino acid sequence identity with FAAH (FAAH-1), is also present in pri-mates, but not in rodents [89], and this enzyme localizes on lipid droplets in cells [90].

N-Acylethanolamine-hydrolyzing acid amidase (NAAA) is a lysosomal enzyme hydrolyzing N-acyletha-nolamines only at acidic pH [91]. We cloned cDNA of this enzyme from rat lung in 2005 [92]. NAAA belongs to the cholylglycine hydrolase family and shows no sequence similarity with FAAH. Acid ceramidase is an-other lysosomal enzyme belonging to this family, which hydrolyzes ceramide under acidic conditions. NAAA and acid ceramidase have significant amino acid sequence similarity (33–34% identity), and their catalytic activities partially overlap each other: NAAA hydrolyzes ceramide at a low rate while acid ceramidase also has an N-acylethanolamine-hydrolyzing activity. NAAA is present in various tissues with abundant expression in macrophages and prostate [93, 94]. In contrast to the preference of FAAH to anandamide, the best substrate of NAAA in vitro is PEA. In consistence with the anti-inflammatory action of PEA, the administration of specific NAAA inhibitors suppresses inflammatory responses in rodent models with increased local PEA levels [95–99]. NAAA-deficient mice also show a strongly reduced inflammatory reaction, compared to wild-type animals [99]. Thus, NAAA inhibitors may have the therapeutic potential as novel anti-inflammatory drugs.

Conclusions

In this mini-review, we outlined the biological activities and metabolisms of two representative endocannabi-noids, 2-AG and anandamide, as well as cannabinoid receptor-insensitive N-acylethanolamines. Pharmaco-logical and biochemical analyses now reveal that 2-AG is a more important endocannabinoid than anandamide. The classical pathway composed of phospholipase C, DAGL, and MAGL attracts much attention again as the central pathway for the metabolism of 2-AG functioning as the major endocannabinoid. On the other hand, anan-damide is produced in a small amount along with PEA and OEA, which are cannabinoid receptor-insensitive, but quantitatively major bioactive *N*-acylethanolamines. The presence of Ca-NAT and NAPE-PLD, which appear to be exclusively responsible for the biosynthesis of *N*-acylethanolamines, strongly suggest the physiological importance of *N*-acylethanolamines and their precursors *N*-acyl-PEs. Thus, further studies on biological activities of various *N*-acylethanolamines are eagerly required, which include the development of specific enzyme inhibitors and analyses of gene-disrupted animals for the enzymes involved. As the research in this field progresses, the metabolic pathways have been found to be more complex than previously considered. Recently found enzymes, such as PLAAT and GDE family members, have not been fully elucidated and their roles in vivo must be clarified.

Abbreviations

2-AG: 2-Arachidonoylglycerol; ABHD: α/β-Hydrolase domain containing; Ca-NAT: Ca-dependent *N*-acyltransferase; DAGL: Diacylglycerol lipase; FAAH: Fatty acid amide hydrolase; GDE: Glycerophosphodiesterase; GLP-1: Glucagon-like peptide-1; HRASLS: HRAS-like suppressor; LPA: Lysophosphatidic acid; MAGL: Monoacylglycerol lipase; NAAA: *N*-Acylethanolamine-hydrolyzing acid amidase; NAPE: *N*-Acyl-phosphatidylethanolamine; OEA: Oleoylethanolamide; PC: Phosphatidylcholine; PE: Phosphatidylethanolamine; PEA: Palmitoylethanolamide; PLAAT: Phospholipase A/acyltransferase; PLD: Phospholipase D; PPARα: Peroxisome proliferator-activated receptor α; TRPV1: Transient receptor potential vanilloid type 1

Funding

KT was supported by the JSPS KAKENHI Grant Number JP17K01852 and Ryobi Teien Memory Foundation.

Authors' contributions

KT wrote the manuscript, and TU, YO, and NU improved it. All authors read and approved the final manuscript.

Competing interests

The authors declare that they have no competing interests.

References

1. Ligresti A, De Petrocellis L, Di Marzo V. From phytocannabinoids to cannabinoid receptors and endocannabinoids: pleiotropic physiological and pathological roles through complex pharmacology. Physiol Rev. 2016;96:1593–659.
2. Gaoni Y, Mechoulam R. Isolation, structure and partial synthesis of an active constituent of hashish. J Am Chem Soc. 1964;86:1646–7.
3. Devane WA, Dysarz FA, Johnson MR, Melvin LS, Howlett AC. Determination and characterization of a cannabinoid receptor in rat brain. Mol Pharmacol. 1988;34:605–13.
4. Matsuda LA, Lolait SJ, Brownstein MJ, Young AC, Bonner TI. Structure of a cannabinoid receptor and functional expression of the cloned cDNA. Nature. 1990;346:561–4.
5. Munro S, Thomas KL, Abu-Shaar M. Molecular characterization of a peripheral receptor for cannabinoids. Nature. 1993;365:61–5.

6. Devane WA, Hanus L, Breuer A, Pertwee RG, Stevenson LA, Griffin G, et al. Isolation and structure of a brain constituent that binds to the cannabinoid receptor. Science. 1992;258:1946–9.
7. Mechoulam R, Ben-Shabat S, Hanus L, Ligumsky M, Kaminski NE, Schatz AR, et al. Identification of an endogenous 2-monoglyceride, present in canine gut, that binds to cannabinoid receptors. Biochem Pharmacol. 1995;50:83–90.
8. Sugiura T, Kondo S, Sukagawa A, Nakane S, Shinoda A, Itoh K, et al. 2-Arachidonoylglycerol: a possible endogenous cannabinoid receptor ligand in brain. Biochem Biophys Res Commun. 1995;215:89–97.
9. Galiègue S, Mary S, Marchand J, Dussossoy D, Carrière D, Carayon P, et al. Expression of central and peripheral cannabinoid receptors in human immune tissues and leukocyte subpopulations. Eur J Biochem. 1995;232:54–61.
10. Sugiura T, Kishimoto S, Oka S, Gokoh M. Biochemistry, pharmacology and physiology of 2-arachidonoylglycerol, an endogenous cannabinoid receptor ligand. Prog Lipid Res. 2006;45:405–46.
11. Kano M, Ohno-Shosaku T, Hashimotodani Y, Uchigashima M, Watanabe M. Endocannabinoid-mediated control of synaptic transmission. Physiol Rev. 2009;89:309–80.
12. Pertwee RG, Howlett AC, Abood ME, Alexander SPH, Di Marzo V, Elphick MR, et al. International Union of Basic and Clinical Pharmacology. LXXIX. Cannabinoid receptors and their ligands: beyond CB$_1$ and CB$_2$. Pharmacol Rev. 2010;62:588–631.
13. Ryberg E, Larsson N, Sjögren S, Hjorth S, Hermansson N-O, Leonova J, et al. The orphan receptor GPR55 is a novel cannabinoid receptor. Br J Pharmacol. 2007;152:1092–101.
14. Sharir H, Abood ME. Pharmacological characterization of GPR55, a putative cannabinoid receptor. Pharmacol Ther. 2010;126:301–13.
15. Oka S, Nakajima K, Yamashita A, Kishimoto S, Sugiura T. Identification of GPR55 as a lysophosphatidylinositol receptor. Biochem Biophys Res Commun. 2007;362:928–34.
16. Oka S, Toshida T, Maruyama K, Nakajima K, Yamashita A, Sugiura T. 2-Arachidonoyl-*sn*-glycero-3-phosphoinositol: a possible natural ligand for GPR55. J Biochem. 2009;145:13–20.
17. Guy AT, Nagatsuka Y, Ooashi N, Inoue M, Nakata A, Greimel P, et al. Glycerophospholipid regulation of modality-specific sensory axon guidance in the spinal cord. Science. 2015;349:974–7.
18. van der Stelt M, Di Marzo V. Endovanilloids. Putative endogenous ligands of transient receptor potential vanilloid 1 channels. Eur J Biochem. 2004;271:1827–34.
19. Felder CC, Briley EM, Axelrod J, Simpson JT, Mackie K, Devane WA. Anandamide, an endogenous cannabimimetic eicosanoid, binds to the cloned human cannabinoid receptor and stimulates receptor-mediated signal transduction. Proc Natl Acad Sci U S A. 1993;90:7656–60.
20. Priller J, Briley EM, Mansouri J, Devane WA, Mackie K, Felder CC. Mead ethanolamide, a novel eicosanoid, is an agonist for the central (CB1) and peripheral (CB2) cannabinoid receptors. Mol Pharmacol. 1995;48:288–92.
21. Keppel Hesselink JM, de Boer T, Witkamp RF. Palmitoylethanolamide: a natural body-own anti-inflammatory agent, effective and safe against influenza and common cold. Int J Inflam. 2013;2013:151028.
22. Kuehl FA Jr, Jacob TA, Ganley OH, Ormond RE, Meisinger MAP. The identification of N-(2-hydroxyethyl)-palmitamide as a naturally occurring anti-inflammatory agent. J Am Chem Soc. 1957;79:5577–8.
23. Ganley OH, Graessle OE, Robinson HJ. Anti-inflammatory activity on compounds obtained from egg yolk, peanut oil, and soybean lecithin. J Lab Clin Med. 1958;51:709–14.
24. Mattace Raso G, Russo R, Calignano A, Meli R. Palmitoylethanolamide in CNS health and disease. Pharmacol Res. 2014;86:32–41.
25. Petrosino S, Di Marzo V. The pharmacology of palmitoylethanolamide and first data on the therapeutic efficacy of some of its new formulations. Br J Pharmacol. 2017;174:1349–65.
26. Gabrielsson L, Mattsson S, Fowler CJ. Palmitoylethanolamide for the treatment of pain: pharmacokinetics, safety and efficacy. Br J Clin Pharmacol. 2016;82:932–42.
27. Pavón FJ, Serrano A, Romero-Cuevas M, Alonso M, Rodríguez de Fonseca F. Oleoylethanolamide: a new player in peripheral control of energy metabolism. Therapeutic implications. Drug Discov Today Dis Mech. 2010;7:e175–83.

28. Fu J, Gaetani S, Oveisi F, Lo Verme J, Serrano A, Rodríguez de Fonseca F, et al. Oleylethanolamide regulates feeding and body weight through activation of the nuclear receptor PPAR-α. Nature. 2003;425:90–3.

29. Piomelli D. A fatty gut feeling. Trends Endocrinol Metab. 2013;24:332–41.

30. Overton HA, Babbs AJ, Doel SM, Fyfe MCT, Gardner LS, Griffin G, et al. Deorphanization of a G protein-coupled receptor for oleylethanolamide and its use in the discovery of small-molecule hypophagic agents. Cell Metab. 2006;3:167–75.

31. Lauffer LM, Iakoubov R, Brubaker PL. GPR119 is essential for oleylethanolamide-induced glucagon-like peptide-1 secretion from the intestinal enteroendocrine L-cell. Diabetes. 2009;58:1058–66.

32. Lan H, Vassileva G, Corona A, Liu L, Baker H, Golovko A, et al. GPR119 is required for physiological regulation of glucagon-like peptide-1 secretion but not for metabolic homeostasis. J Endocrinol. 2009;201:219–30.

33. Wang X, Miyares RL, Ahern GP. Oleylethanolamide excites vagal sensory neurones, induces visceral pain and reduces short-term food intake in mice via capsaicin receptor TRPV1. J Physiol. 2005;564:541–7.

34. Lo Verme J, Gaetani S, Fu J, Oveisi F, Burton K, Piomelli D. Regulation of food intake by oleylethanolamide. Cell Mol Life Sci. 2005;62:708–16.

35. González-Aparicio R, Moratalla R. Oleylethanolamide reduces L-DOPA-induced dyskinesia via TRPV1 receptor in a mouse model of Parkinson's disease. Neurobiol Dis. 2014;62:416–25.

36. Kim H-Y, Spector AA. N-Docosahexaenoylethanolamine: a neurotrophic and neuroprotective metabolite of docosahexaenoic acid. Mol Aspects Med. 2018. https://doi.org/10.1016/j.mam.2018.03.004.

37. Lee J-W, Huang BX, Kwon H, Rashid MA, Kharebava G, Desai A, et al. Orphan GPR110 (ADGRF1) targeted by N-docosahexaenoylethanolamine in development of neurons and cognitive function. Nat Commun. 2016;7:13123.

38. Bisogno T, Melck D, De Petrocellis L, Di Marzo V. Phosphatidic acid as the biosynthetic precursor of the endocannabinoid 2-arachidonoylglycerol in intact mouse neuroblastoma cells stimulated with ionomycin. J Neurochem. 1999;72:2113–9.

39. Carrier EJ, Kearn CS, Barkmeier AJ, Breese NM, Yang W, Nithipatikom K, et al. Cultured rat microglial cells synthesize the endocannabinoid 2-arachidonylglycerol, which increases proliferation via a CB$_2$ receptor-dependent mechanism. Mol Pharmacol. 2004;65:999–1007.

40. Oka S, Yanagimoto S, Ikeda S, Gokoh M, Kishimoto S, Waku K, et al. Evidence for the involvement of the cannabinoid CB2 receptor and its endogenous ligand 2-arachidonoylglycerol in 12-O-tetradecanoylphorbol-13-acetate-induced acute inflammation in mouse ear. J Biol Chem. 2005;280:18488–97.

41. Bisogno T, Howell F, Williams G, Minassi A, Cascio MG, Ligresti A, et al. Cloning of the first sn1-DAG lipases points to the spatial and temporal regulation of endocannabinoid signaling in the brain. J Cell Biol. 2003;163:463–8.

42. Gao Y, Vasilyev DV, Goncalves MB, Howell FV, Hobbs C, Reisenberg M, et al. Loss of retrograde endocannabinoid signaling and reduced adult neurogenesis in diacylglycerol lipase knock-out mice. J Neurosci. 2010;30:2017–24.

43. Tanimura A, Yamazaki M, Hashimotodani Y, Uchigashima M, Kawata S, Abe M, et al. The endocannabinoid 2-arachidonoylglycerol produced by diacylglycerol lipase a mediates retrograde suppression of synaptic transmission. Neuron. 2010;65:320–7.

44. Yoshino H, Miyamae T, Hansen G, Zambrowicz B, Flynn M, Pedicord D, et al. Postsynaptic diacylglycerol lipase mediates retrograde endocannabinoid suppression of inhibition in mouse prefrontal cortex. J Physiol. 2011;589:4857–84.

45. Eichmann TO, Lass A. DAG tales: the multiple faces of diacylglycerol–stereochemistry, metabolism, and signaling. Cell Mol Life Sci. 2015;72:3931–52.

46. Yamashita A, Kumazawa T, Koga H, Suzuki N, Oka S, Sugiura T. Generation of lysophosphatidylinositol by DDHD domain containing 1 (DDHD1): possible involvement of phospholipase D/phosphatidic acid in the activation of DDHD1. Biochim Biophys Acta. 1801;2010:711–20.

47. Nakane S, Oka S, Arai S, Waku K, Ishima Y, Tokumura A, et al. 2-Arachidonoyl-sn-glycero-3-phosphate, an arachidonic acid-containing lysophosphatidic acid: occurrence and rapid enzymatic conversion to 2-arachidonoyl-sn-glycerol, a cannabinoid receptor ligand, in rat brain. Arch Biochem Biophys. 2002;402:51–8.

48. Blankman JL, Simon GM, Cravatt BF. A comprehensive profile of brain enzymes that hydrolyze the endocannabinoid 2-arachidonoylglycerol. Chem Biol. 2007;14:1347–56.

49. Karlsson M, Contreras JA, Hellman U, Tornqvist H, Holm C. cDNA cloning, tissue distribution, and identification of the catalytic triad of monoglyceride lipase. Evolutionary relationship to esterases, lysophospholipases, and haloperoxidases. J Biol Chem. 1997;272:27218–23.

50. Long JZ, Li W, Booker L, Burston JJ, Kinsey SG, Schlosburg JE, et al. Selective blockade of 2-arachidonoylglycerol hydrolysis produces cannabinoid behavioral effects. Nat Chem Biol. 2009;5:37–44.

51. Schlosburg JE, Blankman JL, Long JZ, Nomura DK, Pan B, Kinsey SG, et al. Chronic monoacylglycerol lipase blockade causes functional antagonism of the endocannabinoid system. Nat Neurosci. 2010;13:1113–9.

52. Chanda PK, Gao Y, Mark L, Btesh J, Strassle BW, Lu P, et al. Monoacylglycerol lipase activity is a critical modulator of the tone and integrity of the endocannabinoid system. Mol Pharmacol. 2010;78:996–1003.

53. Nomura DK, Morrison BE, Blankman JL, Long JZ, Kinsey SG, Marcondes MCG, et al. Endocannabinoid hydrolysis generates brain prostaglandins that promote neuroinflammation. Science. 2011;334:809–13.

54. Kita Y, Yoshida K, Tokuoka SM, Hamano F, Yamazaki M, Sakimura K, et al. Fever is mediated by conversion of endocannabinoid 2-arachidonoylglycerol to prostaglandin E$_2$. PLOS ONE. 2015;e0133663:10.

55. Marrs WR, Blankman JL, Horne EA, Thomazeau A, Lin YH, Coy J, et al. The serine hydrolase ABHD6 controls the accumulation and efficacy of 2-AG at cannabinoid receptors. Nat Neurosci. 2010;13:951–7.

56. Alhouayek M, Muccioli GG. COX-2-derived endocannabinoid metabolites as novel inflammatory mediators. Trends Pharmacol Sci. 2014;35:284–92.

57. Natarajan V, Reddy PV, Schmid PC, Schmid HHO. N-acylation of ethanolamine phospholipids in canine myocardium. Biochim Biophys Acta. 1982;712:342–55.

58. Natarajan V, Schmid PC, Reddy PV, Zuzarte-Augustin ML, Schmid HHO. Biosynthesis of N-acylethanolamine phospholipids by dog brain preparations. J Neurochem. 1983;41:1303–12.

59. Schmid HHO, Schmid PC, Natarajan V. N-Acylated glycerophospholipids and their derivatives. Prog Lipid Res. 1990;29:1–43.

60. Ogura Y, Parsons WH, Kamat SS, Cravatt BF. A calcium-dependent acyltransferase that produces N-acyl phosphatidylethanolamines. Nat Chem Biol. 2016;12:669–71.

61. Hussain Z, Uyama T, Kawai K, Binte Mustafiz SS, Tsuboi K, Araki N, et al. Phosphatidylserine-stimulated production of N-acyl-phosphatidylethanolamines by Ca^{2+}-dependent N-acyltransferase. Biochim Biophys Acta. 1863;2018:493–502.

62. Jin X-H, Okamoto Y, Morishita J, Tsuboi K, Tonai T, Ueda N. Discovery and characterization of a Ca^{2+}-independent phosphatidylethanolamine N-acyltransferase generating the anandamide precursor and its congeners. J Biol Chem. 2007;282:3614–23.

63. Jin X-H, Uyama T, Wang J, Okamoto Y, Tonai T, Ueda N. cDNA cloning and characterization of human and mouse Ca^{2+}-independent phosphatidylethanolamine N-acyltransferases. Biochim Biophys Acta. 1791; 2009:32–8.

64. Uyama T, Morishita J, Jin X-H, Okamoto Y, Tsuboi K, Ueda N. The tumor suppressor gene H-Rev107 functions as a novel Ca^{2+}-independent cytosolic phospholipase A$_{1/2}$ of the thiol hydrolase type. J Lipid Res. 2009;50:685–93.

65. Uyama T, Jin X-H, Tsuboi K, Tonai T, Ueda N. Characterization of the human tumor suppressors TIG3 and HRASLS2 as phospholipid-metabolizing enzymes. Biochim Biophys Acta. 1791;2009:1114–24.

66. Shinohara N, Uyama T, Jin X-H, Tsuboi K, Tonai T, Houchi H, et al. Enzymological analysis of the tumor suppressor A-C1 reveals a novel group of phospholipid-metabolizing enzymes. J Lipid Res. 2011;52:1927–35.

67. Uyama T, Ikematsu N, Inoue M, Shinohara N, Jin X-H, Tsuboi K, et al. Generation of N-acylphosphatidylethanolamine by members of the phospholipase A/acyltransferase (PLA/AT) family. J Biol Chem. 2012;287:31905–19.

68. Uyama T, Inoue M, Okamoto Y, Shinohara N, Tai T, Tsuboi K, et al. Involvement of phospholipase A/acyltransferase-1 in N-acylphosphatidylethanolamine generation. Biochim Biophys Acta. 2013;1831:1690–701.

69. Okamoto Y, Morishita J, Tsuboi K, Tonai T, Ueda N. Molecular characterization of a phospholipase D generating anandamide and its congeners. J Biol Chem. 2004;279:5298–305.

70. Leung D, Saghatelian A, Simon GM, Cravatt BF. Inactivation of *N*-acyl phosphatidylethanolamine phospholipase D reveals multiple mechanisms for the biosynthesis of endocannabinoids. Biochemistry. 2006;45:4720–6.

71. Tsuboi K, Okamoto Y, Ikematsu N, Inoue M, Shimizu Y, Uyama T, et al. Enzymatic formation of *N*-acylethanolamines from *N*-acylethanolamine plasmalogen through *N*-acylphosphatidylethanolamine-hydrolyzing phospholipase D-dependent and -independent pathways. Biochim Biophys Acta. 2011;1811:565–77.

72. Leishman E, Mackie K, Luquet S, Bradshaw HB. Lipidomics profile of a NAPE-PLD KO mouse provides evidence of a broader role of this enzyme in lipid metabolism in the brain. Biochim Biophys Acta. 1861;2016:491–500.

73. Inoue M, Tsuboi K, Okamoto Y, Hidaka M, Uyama T, Tsutsumi T, et al. Peripheral tissue levels and molecular species compositions of *N*-acyl-phosphatidylethanolamine and its metabolites in mice lacking *N*-acyl-phosphatidylethanolamine-specific phospholipase D. J Biochem. 2017;162:449–58.

74. Sun Y-X, Tsuboi K, Okamoto Y, Tonai T, Murakami M, Kudo I, et al. Biosynthesis of anandamide and *N*-palmitoylethanolamine by sequential actions of phospholipase A₂ and lysophospholipase D. Biochem J. 2004;380:749–56.

75. Simon GM, Cravatt BF. Endocannabinoid biosynthesis proceeding through glycerophospho-*N*-acyl ethanolamine and a role for α/β-hydrolase 4 in this pathway. J Biol Chem. 2006;281:26465–72.

76. Simon GM, Cravatt BF. Anandamide biosynthesis catalyzed by the phosphodiesterase GDE1 and detection of glycerophospho-*N*-acyl ethanolamine precursors in mouse brain. J Biol Chem. 2008;283:9341–9.

77. Tsuboi K, Okamoto Y, Rahman IAS, Uyama T, Inoue T, Tokumura A, et al. Glycerophosphodiesterase GDE4 as a novel lysophospholipase D: a possible involvement in bioactive *N*-acylethanolamine biosynthesis. Biochim Biophys Acta. 2015;1851:537–48.

78. Rahman IAS, Tsuboi K, Hussain Z, Yamashita R, Okamoto Y, Uyama T, et al. Calcium-dependent generation of *N*-acylethanolamines and lysophosphatidic acids by glycerophosphodiesterase GDE7. Biochim Biophys Acta. 2016;1861:1881–92.

79. Liu J, Wang L, Harvey-White J, Osei-Hyiaman D, Razdan R, Gong Q, et al. A biosynthetic pathway for anandamide. Proc Natl Acad Sci U S A. 2006;103:13345–50.

80. Liu J, Wang L, Harvey-White J, Huang BX, Kim H-Y, Luquet S, et al. Multiple pathways involved in the biosynthesis of anandamide. Neuropharmacology. 2008;54:1–7.

81. Arreaza G, Devane WA, Omeir RL, Sajnani G, Kunz J, Cravatt BF, et al. The cloned rat hydrolytic enzyme responsible for the breakdown of anandamide also catalyzes its formation via the condensation of arachidonic acid and ethanolamine. Neurosci Lett. 1997;234:59–62.

82. Katayama K, Ueda N, Katoh I, Yamamoto S. Equilibrium in the hydrolysis and synthesis of cannabimimetic anandamide demonstrated by a purified enzyme. Biochim Biophys Acta. 1999;1440:205–14.

83. Patel S, Carrier EJ, Ho WSV, Rademacher DJ, Cunningham S, Reddy DS, et al. The postmortal accumulation of brain *N*-arachidonylethanolamine (anandamide) is dependent upon fatty acid amide hydrolase activity. J Lipid Res. 2005;46:342–9.

84. Cravatt BF, Giang DK, Mayfield SP, Boger DL, Lerner RA, Gilula NB. Molecular characterization of an enzyme that degrades neuromodulatory fatty-acid amides. Nature. 1996;384:83–7.

85. Cravatt BF, Demarest K, Patricelli MP, Bracey MH, Giang DK, Martin BR, et al. Supersensitivity to anandamide and enhanced endogenous cannabinoid signaling in mice lacking fatty acid amide hydrolase. Proc Natl Acad Sci U S A. 2001;98:9371–6.

86. Cravatt BF, Saghatelian A, Hawkins EG, Clement AB, Bracey MH, Lichtman AH. Functional disassociation of the central and peripheral fatty acid amide signaling systems. Proc Natl Acad Sci U S A. 2004;101:10821–6.

87. Nomura DK, Blankman JL, Simon GM, Fujioka K, Issa RS, Ward AM, et al. Activation of the endocannabinoid system by organophosphorus nerve agents. Nat Chem Biol. 2008;4:373–8.

88. Long JZ, Nomura DK, Vann RE, Walentiny DM, Booker L, Jin X, et al. Dual blockade of FAAH and MAGL identifies behavioral processes regulated by endocannabinoid crosstalk in vivo. Proc Natl Acad Sci U S A. 2009;106:20270–5.

89. Wei BQ, Mikkelsen TS, McKinney MK, Lander ES, Cravatt BF. A second fatty acid amide hydrolase with variable distribution among placental mammals. J Biol Chem. 2006;281:36569–78.

90. Kaczocha M, Glaser ST, Chae J, Brown DA, Deutsch DG. Lipid droplets are novel sites of *N*-acylethanolamine inactivation by fatty acid amide hydrolase-2. J Biol Chem. 2010;285:2796–806.

91. Tsuboi K, Takezaki N, Ueda N. The *N*-acylethanolamine-hydrolyzing acid amidase (NAAA). Chem Biodivers. 2007;4:1914–25.

92. Tsuboi K, Sun Y-X, Okamoto Y, Araki N, Tonai T, Ueda N. Molecular characterization of *N*-acylethanolamine-hydrolyzing acid amidase, a novel member of the choloylglycine hydrolase family with structural and functional similarity to acid ceramidase. J Biol Chem. 2005;280:11082–92.

93. Tsuboi K, Zhao L-Y, Okamoto Y, Araki N, Ueno M, Sakamoto H, et al. Predominant expression of lysosomal *N*-acylethanolamine-hydrolyzing acid amidase in macrophages revealed by immunochemical studies. Biochim Biophys Acta. 2007;1771:623–32.

94. Wang J, Zhao L-Y, Uyama T, Tsuboi K, Wu X-X, Kakehi Y, et al. Expression and secretion of *N*-acylethanolamine-hydrolysing acid amidase in human prostate cancer cells. J Biochem. 2008;144:685–90.

95. Solorzano C, Zhu C, Battista N, Astarita G, Lodola A, Rivara S, et al. Selective *N*-acylethanolamine-hydrolyzing acid amidase inhibition reveals a key role for endogenous palmitoylethanolamide in inflammation. Proc Natl Acad Sci U S A. 2009;106:20966–71.

96. Ribeiro A, Pontis S, Mengatto L, Armirotti A, Chiurchiù V, Capurro V, et al. A potent systemically active *N*-acylethanolamine acid amidase inhibitor that suppresses inflammation and human macrophage activation. ACS Chem Biol. 2015;10:1838–46.

97. Petrosino S, Ahmad A, Marcolongo G, Esposito E, Allarà M, Verde R, et al. Diacerein is a potent and selective inhibitor of palmitoylethanolamide inactivation with analgesic activity in a rat model of acute inflammatory pain. Pharmacol Res. 2015;91:9–14.

98. Bonezzi FT, Sasso O, Pontis S, Realini N, Romeo E, Ponzano S, et al. An important role for *N*-acylethanolamine acid amidase in the complete Freund's adjuvant rat model of arthritis. J Pharmacol Exp Ther. 2016;356:656–63.

99. Sasso O, Summa M, Armirotti A, Pontis S, De Mei C, Piomelli D. The N-acylethanolamine acid amidase inhibitor ARN077 suppresses inflammation and pruritus in a mouse model of allergic dermatitis. J Invest Dermatol. 2018;138:562–9.

24

Maintenance of memory-type pathogenic Th2 cells in the pathophysiology of chronic airway inflammation

Kiyoshi Hirahara[1*], Kenta Shinoda[1], Yusuke Endo[1], Tomomi Ichikawa[1] and Toshinori Nakayama[1,2]

Abstract

Background: Immunological memory is critical for long-standing protection against microorganisms; however, certain antigen-specific memory CD4[+] T helper (Th) cells drive immune-related pathology, including chronic allergic inflammation such as asthma. The IL-5-producing memory-type Tpath2 subset is important for the pathogenesis of chronic allergic inflammation. This memory-type pathogenic Th2 cell population (Tpath2) can be detected in various allergic inflammatory lesions. However, how these pathogenic populations are maintained at the local inflammatory site has remained unclear.

Methods: We performed a series of experiments using mice model for chronic airway inflammation. We also investigated the human samples from patients with eosinophilic chronic rhinosinusitis.

Results: We recently reported that inducible bronchus-associated lymphoid tissue (iBALT) was shaped during chronic inflammation in the lung. We also found that memory-type Tpath2 cells are maintained within iBALT. The maintenance of the Tpath2 cells within iBALT is supported by specific cell subpopulations within the lung. Furthermore, ectopic lymphoid structures consisting of memory CD4[+] T cells were found in nasal polyps of eosinophilic chronic rhinosinusitis patients, indicating that the persistence of inflammation is controlled by these structures.

Conclusion: Thus, the cell components that organize iBALT formation may be therapeutic targets for chronic allergic airway inflammation.

Keywords: Memory-type pathogenic Th2 cells, Interleukin-33, Inducible bronchus-associated lymphoid tissue (iBALT), Chronic inflammation

Background

Asthma is characterized by chronic airway inflammation, mucus hyperproduction, airway hyperresponsiveness, and variable airway obstruction. The pathophysiology of chronic airway inflammation involves in various types of immune cells such as CD4[+] T cells, B cells, innate lymphoid cells, and eosinophils. In particular, T helper (Th) 2 cells and type 2 innate lymphoid cells play central roles in the pathogenesis of allergic airway inflammation.

Recent studies have identified "epithelial cytokines" such as IL-25, IL-33, and TSLP as key modulators of type 2 immune responses. IL-33 is constitutively expressed on epithelial cells in mucosal barrier organs [1]. Chronic repeated exposure to various exogenous allergens or pathogens, such as tobacco smoke or inhaled irritant particles, prompts epithelial cells to release their stored IL-33, which is involved in chronic allergic inflammatory diseases such as asthma, eosinophilic chronic rhinosinusitis (ECRS), pollen allergy, and eosinophilic pneumonia. IL-33 was originally identified as a ligand for the ST2 receptor (also known as IL1RL1) [2]. Effector Th2 cells, regulatory T cells, mast cells, and ILC2s are known to be target cells of IL-33. We found that memory-type pathogenic Th2 (Tpath2) cells, which produce large amounts of IL-5, expressed high levels of ST2 [3, 4] (Fig. 1). The expression of ST2 on memory-type Tpath2 cells was higher than that on effector Th2 cells, which suggested that memory-type Tpath2 cells were novel targets of IL-33 in vivo.

* Correspondence: hiraharak@chiba-u.jp
[1]Department of Immunology, Graduate School of Medicine, Chiba University, 1-8-1 Inohana, Chuo-ku, Chiba-shi, Chiba 260-8670, Japan
Full list of author information is available at the end of the article

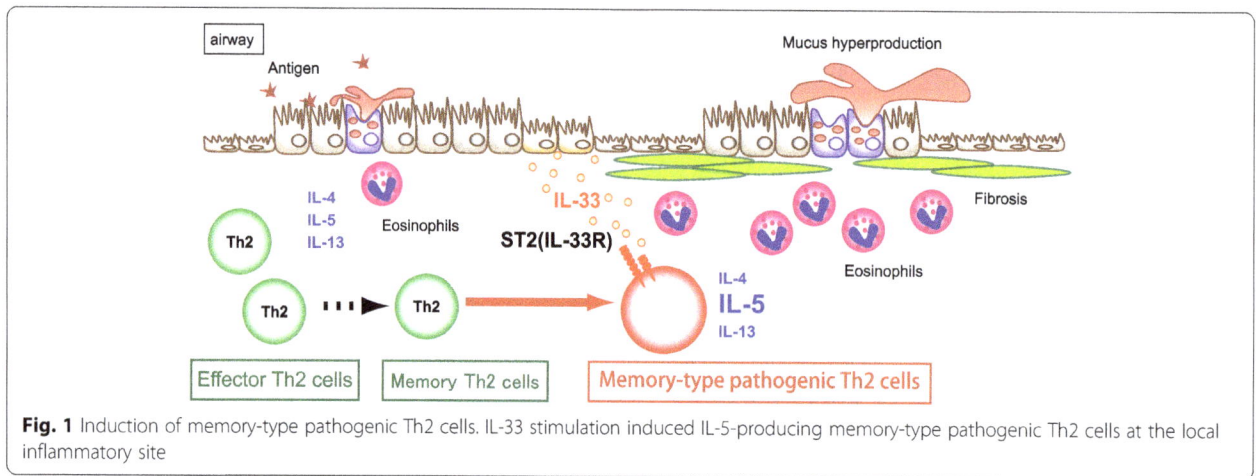

Fig. 1 Induction of memory-type pathogenic Th2 cells. IL-33 stimulation induced IL-5-producing memory-type pathogenic Th2 cells at the local inflammatory site

In humans, it has been shown that bronchus-associated lymphoid tissue (BALT) is shaped in the lung in response to inflammatory states caused by infectious organisms, smoking, and auto-immune diseases; under these conditions, this tissue known as inducible BALT (iBALT) [5, 6]. For example, patients with chronic obstructive pulmonary disease (COPD) showed ectopic lymphoid structures in the lungs [5]. However, whether or not iBALT is involved in the pathophysiology of chronic allergic diseases, such as asthma, and how memory-type T cells are maintained in the local inflammatory tissues has been unclear.

Results

To determine whether or not iBALT was induced in chronic allergic inflammation, we generated OVA-specific effector Th2 cells in vitro and then adoptively transferred them to syngeneic mice that were intra-nasally administered OVA twice. We analyzed these mice 42 days after the adoptive transfer. Hematoxylin and eosin (HE) staining of the mouse lungs showed that massive infiltration of inflammatory cells had been induced and persisted even 42 days after the intra-nasal administration of OVA (Fig. 2a). Immuno-histochemical staining showed the formation of iBALT structures containing donor-derived memory Th2 cells that were detected by KJ-1.26 (KJ1), which is a monoclonal antibody that recognizes OVA-specific TCR DO11.10, MHC class-ll-positive cells, B220-positive cells, CD11c-positive cells, stromal cells, and CD21-positive follicular dendritic cells (Fig. 2b). These results indicate that the iBALT detected in our experimental model was comparable to that noted in previous reports [6]. Notably, the memory Th2 cells showed greater accumulation in iBALT than in non-lymphoid areas (Fig. 2c).

We noted no difference in the number of memory Th2 cells in the spleen with and without intranasal administration of OVA. In sharp contrast, we observed a significant increase in the number of memory Th2 cells in the lung following the intranasal administration of OVA. These memory Th2 cells in the lung produced increased levels of IL-5 (Fig. 2d). Taken together, these findings show that the adoptive transfer of effector Th2 cells followed by the intra-nasal administration of OVA resulted in iBALT formation and the accumulation of memory-type Tpath2 cells in the lung.

We then assessed the patho-physiological role of memory-type Tpath2 cells maintained in iBALT. The OVA-induced airway inflammatory responses were assessed using the mice with iBALT formation. iBALT-induced mice showed enhanced infiltration of inflammatory cells in the BALF compared with the control animals. Consistent with this result, the airway hyperresponsiveness and mucus production were enhanced in the mice with iBALT. Thus, the memory-type Tpath2 cells in the mice with iBALT were involved in the pathogenicity of eosinophilic airway inflammation.

IL-7 is a key cytokine involved in the maintenance of T cells in vivo [7]. We therefore wanted to determine whether or not IL-7 was involved in the maintenance of memory Th2 cells in iBALT using IL-7 GFP knock-in mice (collaboration with Professor Ikuta in Kyoto University). We found that a main population of IL-7-producing cells was accumulated in iBALT in the lung (Fig. 2e). Within the iBALT, most memory Th2 cells were co-localized with IL-7-producing cells. When we analyzed the PECAM-1-positive endothelial cells, *Pdpn* and *Prox1*, which are specific markers for lymphatic endothelial cells, were highly expressed in the isolated PECAM1+IL-7-GFP+ cells. Interestingly, PECAM1+IL-7-GFP+ cells also expressed *Il33* mRNA. A FACS analysis revealed that the PECAM1+IL-7-GFP+ cells expressed Lyve-1 and podoplanin. Taken together, these results suggest that lymphatic endothelial cells in iBALT produce IL-7. We also found that PECAM1+IL-7-GFP+ cells showed high expression of Thy1. We generated *Il-7flox/*

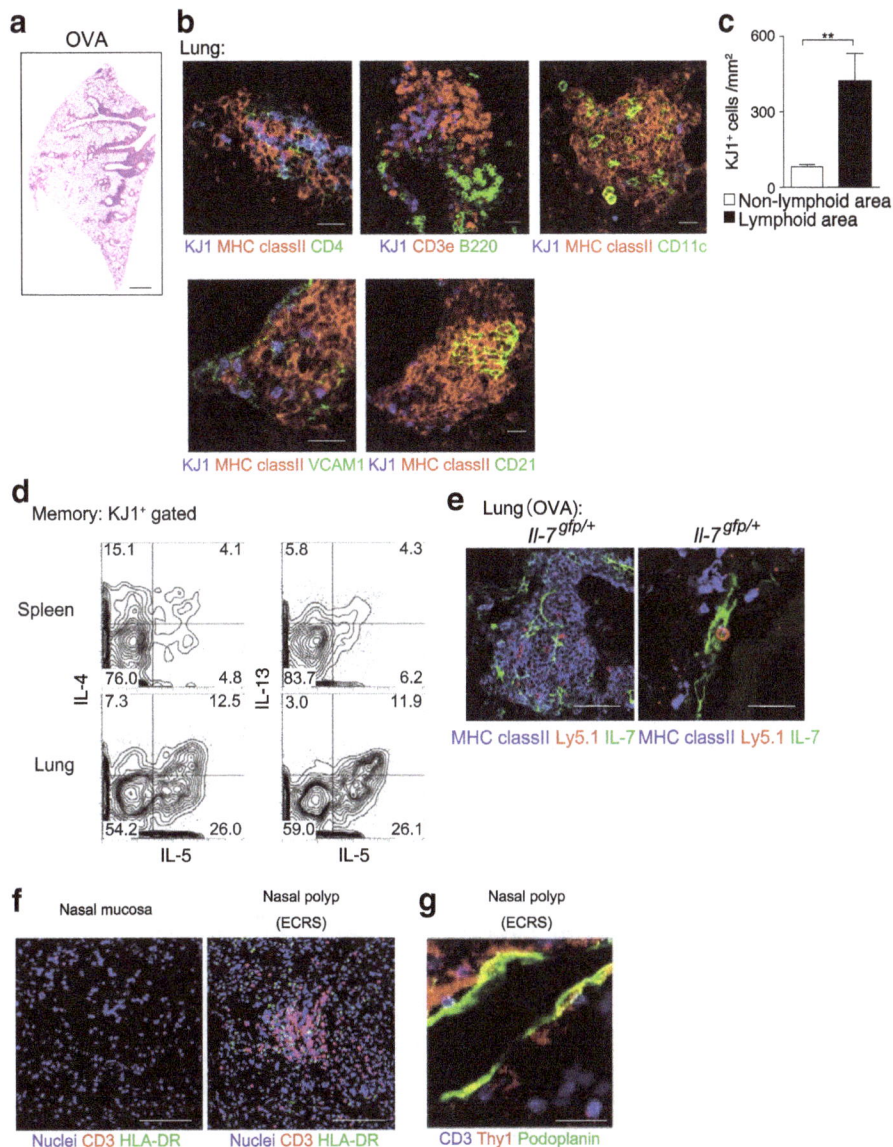

Fig. 2 iBALT is induced under conditions of chronic allergic inflammation in both mice and humans. **a** The intra-nasal administration of the antigen resulted in iBALT formation in the lungs of mice. **b** iBALT included memory Th2 cells, MHC-class II[+] cells, B220[+] cells, CD11c[+] cells, VCAM1[+] cells, and CD21[+] cells. **c** The memory Th2 cells showed greater accumulation in the lymphoid areas than in the non-lymphoid areas. **d** Memory Th2 cells in the lung produced more Th2 cytokines compared to those from memory Th2 cells in the spleen. **e** IL-7-producing cells and Ly5.1[+] memory Th2 cells were detected in mice iBALT. **f** Ectopic lymphoid structures were generated in the polyps of patients with ECRS. **g** Podoplanin-positive lymphatics were increased in the polyps of patients with ECRS. (*Shinoda* et al. *PNAS*(2016) Copyright (2016) National Academy of Sciences). KJ: OVA-specific T cell receptor

flox mice crossed with *Tie2*-Cre transgenic mice, in which the mouse endothelial-specific receptor tyrosine kinase (Tie2) promoter directs expression of Cre recombinase, to investigate the role of IL-7 produced by LECs. When iBALT was induced using *Il-7*^fl/fl*Tie2-Cre*+ Tg mice as hosts, iBALT formation was impaired in the lung of *Il-7*^fl/fl*Tie2-Cre*+ Tg mice. We also detected decreased numbers of memory Th2 cells in the lung. Taken together, these findings indicate that Thy1+IL-7+ lymphatic endothelial cells (LECs) support the memory Th2 cell survival in iBALT in vivo.

IL-5-producing Tpath2 cells have been detected in the PBMCs of patients with eosinophilic gastrointestinal disease [8]. However, whether or not Tpath2 cells are maintained in the local inflammatory tissue in humans has been unclear. ECRS is a chronic upper respiratory airway allergic disease characterized by the formation of nasal polyps and the infiltration of massive eosinophils in the polyps [9]. We analyzed local inflammatory tissues from the polyps of patients with ECRS. Very little T cell infiltration and few lymphoid structures were detected in the nasal mucosa of control subjects. However, in sharp contrast, the nasal polyps of patients with ECRS showed massive infiltration of CD3$^+$ T cells accompanied by elevated numbers of ectopic lymphoid structures (Fig. 2f). The majority of accumulated CD3$^+$ T cells were memory-type CD4$^+$ T cells, as they expressed CD4 together with CD45RO. Furthermore, podoplanin-positive lymphatics were increased in the nasal polyps of patients with ECRS compared to the control nasal mucosa (Fig. 2g). *IL7* and *IL33* were expressed more strongly in CD45$^-$PECAM1$^+$Thy1$^+$ cells than in CD45$^-$PECAM1$^+$Thy1$^-$ cells.

Discussion

Our research highlighted that Thy1$^+$IL-7$^+$ lymphatic endothelial cells (LECs) support memory Th2 cell survival in iBALT in the chronic inflamed lung from mice [10]. Moreover, we found that memory-type CD4$^+$ T cells and IL-7$^+$IL-33$^+$ LECs accumulated in polyps from ECRS patients. These results indicate that Thy1$^+$IL-7$^+$ LECs produce IL-33 and may confer the pathogenicity on Tpath2 cells. The major IL-7-producing cells in the iBALT are the LECs that are co-localized with memory Th2 cells in the lung. A set of experiments by using IL-7 conditional knockout mice (*Tie2*-Cre$^+$*Il-7*$^{fl/fl}$ mice) verified the importance of IL-7-production from LECs on the maintenance of memory Th2 cells in iBALT. Thus, these cells likely provide a survival niche for memory Th2 cells at local inflammatory sites in the airway. Further study is needed to investigate the contribution of IL-7 to T cell-mediated chronic inflammatory diseases such as steroid-resistant asthma.

Conclusion

In summary, our findings showed that the iBALT structure supports the Tpath2 cell survival in chronic airway inflammation. The cell components and or functional molecules that organize iBALT formation may be therapeutic targets for chronic allergic airway inflammation.

Abbreviations

BALF: Bronchoalveolar lavage fluid; COPD: Chronic obstructive pulmonary disease; iBALT: Inducible bronchus-associated lymphoid tissue; IL: Interleukin; ILC2s: Type 2 innate lymphoid cells; Tpath2 cells: Pathogenic Th2 cells

Acknowledgements

We would like to sincerely thank our collaborators, Professor Koichi Ikuta (Kyoto University) and Professor Yoshitaka Okamoto (Chiba University).

Authors' contributions

KH, KS, YE, TI, and TN prepared the manuscript and figures. All authors read and approved the final manuscript.

Competing interests

The authors declare that they have no competing interests.

Author details

[1]Department of Immunology, Graduate School of Medicine, Chiba University, 1-8-1 Inohana, Chuo-ku, Chiba-shi, Chiba 260-8670, Japan. [2]AMED-CREST, AMED, 1-8-1 Inohana Chuo-ku, Chiba 260-8670, Japan.

References

1. Pichery M, et al. Endogenous IL-33 is highly expressed in mouse epithelial barrier tissues, lymphoid organs, brain, embryos, and inflamed tissues: in situ analysis using a novel Il-33-LacZ gene trap reporter strain. J Immunol. 2012;188:3488–95. https://doi.org/10.4049/jimmunol.1101977.
2. Schmitz J, et al. IL-33, an interleukin-1-like cytokine that signals via the IL-1 receptor-related protein ST2 and induces T helper type 2-associated cytokines. Immunity. 2005;23:479–90. https://doi.org/10.1016/j.immuni.2005.09.015.
3. Endo Y, et al. The interleukin-33-p38 kinase axis confers memory T helper 2 cell pathogenicity in the airway. Immunity. 2015;42:294–308. https://doi.org/10.1016/j.immuni.2015.01.016.
4. Nakayama T, et al. Th2 cells in health and disease. Annu Rev Immunol. 2016; https://doi.org/10.1146/annurev-immunol-051116-052350.
5. Hogg JC, et al. The nature of small-airway obstruction in chronic obstructive pulmonary disease. N Engl J Med. 2004;350:2645–53. https://doi.org/10.1056/NEJMoa032158.
6. Rangel-Moreno J, et al. Inducible bronchus-associated lymphoid tissue (iBALT) in patients with pulmonary complications of rheumatoid arthritis. J Clin Invest. 2006;116:3183–94. https://doi.org/10.1172/JCI28756.
7. Mackall CL, Fry TJ, Gress RE. Harnessing the biology of IL-7 for therapeutic application. Nat Rev Immunol. 2011;11:330–42. https://doi.org/10.1038/nri2970.
8. Mitson-Salazar A, et al. Hematopoietic prostaglandin D synthase defines a proeosinophilic pathogenic effector human TH2 cell subpopulation with enhanced function. J Allergy Clin Immunol. 2016;137:907–918 e909. https://doi.org/10.1016/j.jaci.2015.08.007.
9. Hamilos DL. Drivers of chronic rhinosinusitis: inflammation versus infection. J Allergy Clin Immunol. 2015;136:1454–9. https://doi.org/10.1016/j.jaci.2015.10.011.
10. Shinoda K, et al. Thy1+IL-7+ lymphatic endothelial cells in iBALT provide a survival niche for memory T-helper cells in allergic airway inflammation. Proc Natl Acad Sci U S A. 2016;113:E2842–51. https://doi.org/10.1073/pnas.1512600113.

Myeloid-derived suppressor cells in non-neoplastic inflamed organs

Sho Sendo[1], Jun Saegusa[1,2] and Akio Morinobu[1*]

25

Myeloid-derived suppressor cells in non-neoplastic inflamed organs

Sho Sendo[1], Jun Saegusa[1,2] and Akio Morinobu[1*]

Abstract

Background: Myeloid-derived suppressor cells (MDSCs) are a highly heterogeneous population of immature myeloid cells with immunosuppressive function. Although their function in tumor-bearing conditions is well studied, less is known about the role of MDSCs in various organs under non-neoplastic inflammatory conditions.

Main body: MDSCs are divided into two subpopulations, G-MDSCs and M-MDSCs, and their distribution varies between organs. MDSCs negatively control inflammation in inflamed organs such as the lungs, joints, liver, kidneys, intestines, central nervous system (CNS), and eyes by suppressing T cells and myeloid cells. MDSCs also regulate fibrosis in the lungs, liver, and kidneys and help repair CNS injuries. MDSCs in organs are plastic and can differentiate into osteoclasts and tolerogenic dendritic cells according to the microenvironment under non-neoplastic inflammatory conditions.

Conclusion: This article summarizes recent findings about MDSCs under inflammatory conditions, especially with respect to their function and differentiation in specific organs.

Keywords: MDSC, Inflammation, T cell, Myeloid cell, Organ, Plasticity

Background

Myeloid-derived suppressor cells (MDSCs), which are best known for their role in tumor-bearing conditions, also mediate the resolution of inflammatory diseases. MDSCs can play conflicting roles in inflammation because the phenotypes and functions of this plastic, highly heterogeneous population depend largely on the local microenvironment. We here discuss the role of MDSCs under non-neoplastic inflammatory conditions, particularly in individual organs.

Main text

What are MDSCs?

MDSCs are a heterogeneous population of immature myeloid cells with immunosuppressive function. MDSCs were initially described in 1987 in a mouse model of lung cancer [1]. More recently, roles for MDSCs have been implicated in non-neoplastic inflammatory conditions such as infection, allergy, and autoimmune diseases [2, 3]. The major

populations of bone marrow-derived myeloid cells are neutrophils, monocytes, macrophages, and dendritic cells (DCs), which are differentiated from hematopoietic progenitor cells via granulocyte-macrophage progenitors (GMPs). MDSCs are also differentiated from the common progenitors especially under pathogenic conditions [4]. Strong but short activation signals coming from acute infection or trauma induce classic myeloid cell activation, e.g., neutrophil, monocyte/macrophage, and DC activation. On the other hand, weak but chronic activation signals from malignancies, chronic infections, and inflammatory diseases favor the development of MDSC [4].

MDSCs are classified as granulocytic (G)-MDSCs or monocytic (M)-MDSCs. G-MDSCs are morphologically similar to neutrophils, while M-MDSCs are morphologically similar to monocytes. These subtypes are distinguished from neutrophils or monocytes by their morphology, surface phenotype, and function (Table 1). In mice, MDSCs are phenotypically defined as $CD11b^+Gr1^+$ cells, which are further classified into G-MDSCs as $CD11b^+Ly6G^+Ly6C^{low}$ cells and M-MDSCs as $CD11b^+Ly6G^-Ly6C^{hi}$ cells [5]. In humans, markers for the entire MDSC population have not been clearly determined. Among peripheral blood mononuclear cells (PBMCs), the equivalent to G-MDSCs is

* Correspondence: morinobu@med.kobe-u.ac.jp
[1]Division of Rheumatology and Clinical Immunology, Department of Internal Medicine, Kobe University Graduate School of Medicine, 7-5-2 Kusunoki-cho, Chuo-ku, Kobe 650-0017, Japan
Full list of author information is available at the end of the article

Table 1 Comparisons of morphology, phenotype, and function between myeloid-derived cells

	Morphology	Surface phenotype	Immune suppression
Mouse			
Neutrophils	Round shape with a segmented nucleus	$CD11b^+Ly6G^{hi}Ly6C^{lo}$	−
Monocytes	Round shape with a indented nucleus	$CD11b^+Ly6G^-Ly6C^{hi}$	−
Macrophages	Round shape with pseudopodia	$CD11b^+F4/80^{hi}Ly6G^-Ly6C^{lo}$	−
Dendritic cells	Dendritic shape with polypodia	$CD11b^+CD11c^+Ly6G^-Ly6C^{-/lo}$ (classical)	−
		$CD11b^-CD11c^+Ly6G^-Ly6C^-$ (classical)	−
		$CD11b^-CD11c^{lo}Ly6G^-Ly6C^+PDCA\text{-}1^+$ (plasmacytoid)	−
Fibrocytes	Spindle shape	$CD11b^+CoII^+Ly6G^-Ly6C^+$	−
G-MDSCs	Round shape with a banded nucleus	$CD11b^+Ly6G^+Ly6C^{lo}$	+
M-MDSCs	Round shape with a indented nucleus	$CD11b^+Ly6G^-Ly6C^{hi}$	++
Human			
Neutrophils	Round shape with a segmented nucleus	$CD11b^+CD14^-CD15^+CD66b^+LOX\text{-}1^-$	−
Monocytes	Round shape with a indented nucleus	$CD14^+CD15^-CD16^-HLA\text{-}DR^+$ (classical)	−
		$CD14^+CD15^-CD16^+HLA\text{-}DR^+$ (intermediate)	−
		$CD14^-CD15^-CD16^+HLA\text{-}DR^+$ (non-classical)	−
Macrophages	Round shape with pseudopodia	$CD14^+CD15^-CD16^+CD80^+HLA\text{-}DR^+$ (M1)	−
		$CD11b^+CD14^+CD15^-CD206^+CD163^+HLA\text{-}DR^+$ (M2)	±
Dendritic cells	Dendritic shape with polypodia	$CD14^-CD16^-CD1C^+$ (classical)	−
		$CD14^-CD16^-CD141^+$ (classical)	−
		$CD14^-CD16^-CD303^+$ (plasmacytoid)	−
Fibrocytes	Spindle shape	$CD11b^+CoII^+CD13^+CD34^+CD45RO^+HLA\text{-}DR^+$	−
G-MDSCs	Round shape with a annular nucleus	$CD11b^+CD14^-CD15^+CD66b^+LOX\text{-}1^+$	+
M-MDSCs	Round shape with a indented nucleus	$CD14^+CD15^-HLA\text{-}DR^{-/lo}$	++

Abbreviations: *HLA* human leukocyte antigen, *Lox-1* lectin-type oxidized LDL receptor 1, *PDCA-1* plasmacytoid dendritic cell antigen-1

defined as $CD11b^+CD14^-CD15^+$ (or $CD66b^+$) cells, and that to M-MDSCs as $CD11b^+CD14^+HLA\text{-}DR^{-/low}CD15^-$ cells [6]. As it is difficult to phenotypically distinguish G-MDSCs from neutrophils, or M-MDSCs from monocytes, it is important to prove whether or not these cells have suppressive function. While G-MDSCs and M-MDSCs are differentiated from common progenitors, e.g., GMPs [4], only immature neutrophils and monocytes can be converted to G-MDSCs and M-MDSCs, respectively [7].

Macrophages are also known to be a highly heterogeneous population and M1/M2 subsets of macrophages are widely accepted [8]. Macrophages are differentiated from GMPs via monocyte-DC precursors and $Ly6C^{hi}$ monocytes [9]. Although M2 macrophages and M-MDSCs have a common origin and work as anti-inflammatory cells, these cells differ in several respects. For example, M-MDSCs express lower levels of MHC-II than M2 macrophages do, indicating that M-MDSCs are more immature populations. In addition, M-MDSCs, but not M2 macrophages, produce inducible nitric oxide synthase (iNOS), whereas arginase-I (Arg-I) is produced in both cell types [10].

MDSCs are thought to suppress immune function by depleting lymphocytes' nutrients, generating oxidative stress, and inducing regulatory T cells (Tregs) [11]. Signal transducer and activator of transcription (STAT), such as STAT1 and STAT3, is involved in regulating MDSC function. IFN-γ and interleukin (IL)-1β can trigger STAT1 signaling, leading to high levels of iNOS and Arg-I [12]. The resulting L-arginine depletion and nitric oxide (NO) production suppresses T cells. A lack of L-arginine decreases ζ-chain expression in the T cell receptor complex and arrests the proliferation of antigen-activated T cells [13]. On the other hand, NO production abolishes T cell function by inhibiting MHC-II expression and inducing T cell apoptosis [14]. Although both MDSC subsets can increase Arg-I levels, M-MDSCs produce higher levels of NO than do G-MDSCs [15]. T cell function is also regulated by modulating the CD3 ζ-chain expression, which is controlled by reactive oxygen species (ROS) production [16]. ROS are secreted primarily by G-MDSCs, and this secretion is upregulated by increased STAT-3 activation by IL-6, IL-10, and GM-CSF [11]. M-MDSCs, but not G-MDSCs, can promote Treg induction from purified

CD4$^+$ T cells [17], and Tregs suppress the activation and expansion of autoreactive T cells [18].

MDSC function in inflamed organs

This section describes the latest studies concerning the roles of MDSCs in individual organs, in both humans and mouse disease model systems (Table 2).

Lungs

Although the lungs were long considered to be sterile, they are constantly exposed to microbiota through inhalation or subclinical microaspiration. Far from being sterile, the lungs harbor an abundance of diverse interacting microbiota that regulate lung immunity and homeostasis [19]. In the healthy lung, two macrophage populations work to maintain lung homeostasis: alveolar macrophages and interstitial macrophages. A third population of monocyte-derived macrophages may be recruited during inflammatory responses [20]. MDSCs are critical for negatively regulating immune responses in inflammatory lung diseases.

Arora et al. and Deshane et al. demonstrated that MDSCs suppress the Th2-dominant allergic inflammation in a murine model of asthma [21, 22]. CD11b$^+$Gr1^{int}F4/80$^+$MDSC-like cells accumulate in the lung and suppress the lung DC-mediated reactivation of primed Th2 cells, which is mediated by IL-10 and Arg-1 [21]. The chemokine CCL2 recruits MDSCs into lung tissues in airway inflammation [23]. In humans, high numbers of CD11b$^+$CD14$^+$CD16$^-$HLA-DR$^-$ NO-producing myeloid-derived regulatory cells, which are phenotypically similar to MDSCs, were found in the airways of patients with asthma but not in patients with chronic obstructive pulmonary disease (COPD) or in healthy control subjects [24]. These cells suppressed the proliferation of activated autologous CD4$^+$T cells.

Patients with COPD have elevated levels of circulating-lineage HLA-DR$^-$CD33$^+$CD11b$^+$ MDSCs [25]. It was recently reported that collagen type 1$^+$CD45^{dim}CD34$^-$CD14$^-$CD15$^+$ MDSC-like fibrocytes are increased in the lungs and peripheral blood of COPD patients compared to control subjects [26]. The intensity of collagen type 1 staining, which marks MDSC-like fibrocytes, was positively associated with lung function; these cells appeared to play a role in air trapping, predominately in the upper lobes.

We recently reported that MDSCs are expanded in the lungs of SKG mice with interstitial lung disease (ILD) [27]. Other researchers demonstrated that CCR2$^+$ M-MDSCs inhibit collagen degradation and promote lung fibrosis by producing transforming growth factor-β1 (TGF-β1) [28].

The number of circulating activated MDSCs was found to be significantly increased in patients with pulmonary hypertension (PH) compared to control subjects, and was correlated with an increase in mean pulmonary artery pressure [29]. However, a direct mechanistic role for MDSCs in pulmonary hypertension and inflammation-associated vascular remodeling has yet to be defined.

Thus, MDSCs in the lungs appear to suppress inflammation in several diseases, including asthma, COPD, ILD, and PH. However, MDSCs may promote lung fibrosis under certain conditions.

Joints

A healthy joint has a thin synovial membrane and synovial fluid that does not contain leukocytes. Under arthritic conditions, leukocytes, including both innate and adaptive immune cells, infiltrate the joint cavity and cause proliferation of the synovium [30, 31]. The infiltrating leukocytes include macrophages, DCs, granulocytes, and lymphocytes. Leukocyte infiltration and the secretion of pro-inflammatory cytokines encourage pre-osteoclasts to mature into osteoclasts that erode the bone. The proliferating synovium secretes matrix metalloproteinases (MMPs) and collagenase, leading to the destruction of cartilage.

Egelston et al. identified MDSCs in the joints of mice with proteoglycan-induced arthritis, a model of rheumatoid arthritis (RA) [32]. G-MDSCs obtained from the synovial fluid suppressed DC maturation and T cell proliferation upon co-culture, primarily by producing NO and ROS (which are usually produced by G-MDSCs). Fujii et al. revealed that MDSCs play a crucial role in regulating mouse collagen-induced arthritis (CIA) [33, 34]. MDSCs from the spleens of arthritic mice suppressed the proliferation of CD4$^+$ T cells and their differentiation into Th17 cells in vitro. Moreover, the adoptive transfer of spleen-derived MDSCs reduced the severity of arthritis, and depleting MDSCs canceled this effect in vivo. Another report showed similar results in CIA and antigen-induced arthritis models [35]. Nishimura et al. found that tofacitinib, a JAK inhibitor, facilitates the expansion of MDSCs and ameliorates arthritis in SKG mice [36]. On the other hand, Zhang et al. reported that MDSCs are pro-inflammatory and aggravate arthritis in CIA [37]. However, although this group phenotypically defined CD11b$^+$Gr1$^+$ cells as MDSCs, the cells could not be distinguished from neutrophils or monocytes.

Little is known about MDSCs in human arthritis. Kurkó et al. reported that MDSCs were present in the synovial fluid (SF) of RA patients [38], and that while CD11b$^+$CD33$^+$HLADR$^{lo/-}$CD14$^-$CD15$^+$ G-MDSC-like cells were predominant, there was also a small CD11b$^+$CD33$^+$HLA-DR$^{lo/-}$CD14$^+$CD15$^-$ monocytic subset. The SF-MDSCs from RA patients significantly

Table 2 The roles of MDSCs in individual organs

Organ	Disease	Species	Surface phenotype	MDSC function	Reference
Lung	Asthma	Mouse (HDM)	CD11b+Gr1intF4/80+	Suppression of Th2 cell reactivation	[16]
	COPD	Human	CD11b+CD14+CD16−HLA-DR− (BAL)	NA	[19]
		Human	Lineage−HLA-DR−CD33+CD11b+ (peripheral blood)	NA	[20]
			Collagen type 1+CD45dimCD34−CD1−CD15+ (lung, peripheral blood)	NA	[21]
	Interstitial lung disease	Mouse (SKG)	CD11b+Gr1+ (lung)	Suppression of T cell proliferation	[22]
	Lung fibrosis	Mouse (silica)	CD11b+Ly6C+CCR2+ (lung)	Suppression of T cell proliferation, promotion of lung fibrosis by producing TGF-β1	[23]
	Pulmonary hypertension	Human	CD11b+CD33+MHC-II− (peripheral blood)	NA	[24]
Joint	Rheumatoid arthritis model	Mouse (PGIA)	CD11b+Ly6GhiLy6Cint/lo (synovial fluid)	Suppression of DC maturation and T cell proliferation	[27]
		Mouse (CIA)	CD11b+Gr1+ (spleen)	Suppression of T cell proliferation and Th17 cell differentiation, amelioration of arthritis	[28–30]
		Mouse (SKG)	CD11b+Gr1+ (spleen, BM)	Suppression of T cell proliferation, amelioration of arthritis	[31]
	Rheumatoid arthritis	Human	CD11b+CD33+HLA-DRlo/−CD14−CD15+ (synovial fluid)	NA	[33]
Liver	Immune-mediated hepatitis	Mouse (TGFb1−/−)	CD11b+Ly6GloLy6Chi	Suppression of CD4+ T cell proliferation	[42, 43]
		Mouse (Con A)	CD11b+Ly6G+Ly6Clo		
	Fulminant hepatitis	Mouse (D-Gal/LPS)	CD11b+Ly6GloLy6Chi	Suppression of CD4+ T cell proliferation and cytokine production	[44]
			CD11b+Ly6GhiLy6Cint		
	Liver fibrosis	Mouse (carbon tetrachloride)	CD11b+Ly6G−Ly6ChiF4/80+	Amelioration of fibrosis through inhibition of hepatic stellate cells	[45]
			CD11b+Ly6G+Ly6CloF4/80−		
		Mouse (bile duct ligation)	CD11b+Ly6C+		[46]
	HCV hepatitis	Human	CD11b+ HLA-DRlo CD33+ CD14+	Inhibition of T cell proliferation and IFN-γ production	[40, 41]
			CD11b+/lo HLA-DRlo/− CD33+ CD14+		
Kidney	AKI	Mouse (ischemia-reperfusion)	CD11b+Ly-6G+Ly-6C-low (kidney)	Attenuation of AKI via suppression of T cell infiltration, downregulation of pro-inflammatory cytokines	[50]
	FSGS	Mouse (doxorubicin)	CD11b+Gr1+ (peripheral blood, BM, spleen, kidney-draining lymph nodes, and kidney)	Attenuation of renal injury via inducing regulatory T cells	[51]
		Human	CD11b+HLA-DR−CD14−CD15+ (peripheral blood)	Suppression of T cell proliferation	[51]
	Kidney fibrosis	Mouse (adenine-enriched diet)	CD11b+Ly6G+ (kidney)	Suppression of T cell proliferation and kidney fibrosis	[46]
Intestine	IBD	Mouse (VILLIN-hemagglutinin)	CD11b+Gr1+ (spleen, intestine)	Suppression of CD8+ T cell proliferation via NO production	[54]
		Mouse (TNBS)	CD11b+Ly-6G+Ly-6C-lo (BM)	Attenuation of colitis via suppression of MPO activity and serum IL-6 levels	[55]
		Mouse (DSS)	CD11b+Gr1+ (spleen, BM)		[56]

Table 2 The roles of MDSCs in individual organs (Continued)

Organ	Disease	Species	Surface phenotype	MDSC function	Reference
		Human	CD14+HLA-DR−/lo (peripheral blood)	Attenuation of colitis via suppression macrophages in the lamina propria	[54]
CNS	Multiple sclerosis	Mouse (EAE)	CD11b+Ly-6Chi (peripheral blood, BM, spleen, and CNS)	Suppression of PBMC proliferation and IFN-γ production	[61]
		Mouse (EAE)	CD11b+Ly6G+ (peripheral lymphoid compartment, CNS)	Suppression of CD4 and CD8 T cell proliferation via NO production, Enhancement of T cell apoptosis and attenuation of EAE	[63]
		Mouse (EAE)		Attenuation of EAE via inhibition of encephalitogenic Th1 and Th17 immune responses.	[63]
		Human	HLA-DR−/loCD14−CD33+CD15+ (peripheral blood)	Suppression of autologous CD4+ T cell activation and proliferation	[63]
Eye	Spinal cord injury (SCI)	Mouse	CD11b+Ly6C+Ly6G− (spinal cord)	Promoting the repair process after SCI	[64]
	Stroke	Mouse	CD11b+Ly6C+MHC-IIlo (spleen)	Suppression of T cell proliferation	[65]
		Human	CD11b+CD33+HLA-DR− (peripheral blood)	NA	[65]
	Uveoretinitis	Mouse (EAU)	CD11b+Ly6G−Ly6C+ (peripheral blood, spleen, retina)	Suppression of T cell proliferation, attenuating uveoretinitis	[67, 68]
		Human (posterior uveitis)	HLA-DR−CD11b+CD33+ CD14+ (peripheral blood)	NA	[68]

Abbreviations: AKI acute kidney injury, BAL bronchoalveolar lavage, BM bone marrow, CIA collagen-induced arthritis, CNS central nervous system, COPD chronic obstructive pulmonary disease, D-Gal/LPS D-galactosamine/lipopolysaccharide, DSS dextran sulfate sodium, EAE experimental autoimmune encephalomyelitis, EAU experimental autoimmune uveoretinitis, FSGS focal segmental glomerulosclerosis, HCV hepatitis C virus, HDM house dust mite, ILD interstitial lung disease, MS multiple sclerosis, PGIA proteoglycan-induced arthritis, PH pulmonary hypertension, TGF-β transforming growth factor-β, TNBS 2,4,6-trinitrobenzenesulfonic acid

suppressed the anti-CD3/CD28 antibody-induced proliferation of autologous T cells.

These findings indicate that MDSCs, especially G-MDSCs, ameliorate arthritis by suppressing T cell proliferation and DC maturation in the joints.

Liver

The liver clears gut-derived microbial products from the blood, while functions as a metabolic organ. The unique microenvironments in the liver induce tolerogenic myeloid cells, including MDSCs, under conditions such as liver inflammation and fibrosis [39]. The recruitment and differentiation of MDSCs in the liver is promoted by mechanisms that depend on contact between various cell types and on soluble mediators. For example, hepatic stellate cells can induce MDSCs from myeloid cells in mice and humans [40]. The induction of MDSCs by hepatic stellate cells depends on CD44-mediated, direct cell–cell contact in humans [41], but on soluble factors such as IFN-γ or complement C3 in mice [42, 43]. Human mesenchymal stromal cells can also induce the expansion of MDSCs via hepatocyte growth factor and its receptor, c-Met [43]. IL-6 induces MDSCs to accumulate in the liver, where they protect mice from liver injury mediated by $CD8^+$ T cells [44].

The frequency of MDSCs is elevated in the peripheral blood of patients with chronic hepatitis C virus (HCV) infection [45, 46]. $CD11b^+HLA-DR^{low}CD14^+CD33^+$ MDSCs in the blood of patients with chronic HCV suppress T cells using arginase [45]. MDSCs also produce ROS, which inhibit T cell function in chronic HCV [46], and this might be one of the mechanisms by which HCV promotes persistent infection.

MDSCs are involved in the pathogenesis of a mouse model of autoimmune hepatitis. Th1 cell-mediated liver inflammation can induce MDSCs in BALB/c $Tgfb1^{-/-}$ mice, which develop an acute autoimmune liver injury [47]; IFN-γ production by $CD4^+$ T cells is necessary for inducing MDSCs in this model. MDSCs, especially M-MDSCs, were found to suppress $CD4^+$ T cell proliferation in this model via NO production, IFN-γ, and cell–cell contact. Zhang et al. also reported that MDSCs are involved in murine immunological hepatic injury [48]. Inhibiting mammalian target of rapamycin (mTOR) with rapamycin induced the recruitment of $CD11b^+Gr1^+Ly6C^{hi}$ MDSCs to the liver and protected against immunological hepatic injury. Downregulating the mTOR activity in MDSCs induced iNOS and NO, and the pharmacological inhibition of iNOS completely eliminated the recruitment of MDSCs.

MDSCs were elevated in the liver of a murine fulminant hepatitis model [49]; in this model, IL-25 induced MDSCs to accumulate in the liver, where they protected mice from acute hepatic damage induced by D-galactosamine and lipopolysaccharides.

Some studies indicate that MDSCs are involved in chronic liver injury and the development of liver fibrosis. Suh et al. reported that bone marrow-derived MDSCs ameliorated carbon tetrachloride-induced liver fibrosis in mice by producing IL-10 [50]. Activated hepatic stellate cells enhanced the MDSC expression of IL-10, which in turn suppressed the profibrotic function of activated hepatic stellate cells. Another study showed that M-MDSCs accumulated in the liver in the presence of inflammation and fibrosis in bile duct-ligated mice [51]. In addition, depleting MDSCs in the liver enhanced fibrosis markers, indicating that MDSCs play a protective role against organ fibrosis.

Thus, in the liver, MDSCs (especially M-MDSCs) prevent liver inflammation and fibrosis by suppressing immunogenic T cells.

Kidneys

The kidneys are frequently targeted by pathogenic immune responses against renal autoantigens or by local manifestations of systemic autoimmunity [52, 53]. Inflammation and immune system activation are important causal factors in the development of both acute and chronic renal disease [54]. Recent reports indicate that MDSCs are a key regulator for terminating excessive inflammation, but can also contribute to renal fibrosis.

MDSCs, especially G-MDSCs, ameliorate acute kidney injury (AKI). Rapamycin enhanced this protective effect by recruiting MDSCs, regulating MDSC induction, and strengthening the MDSC immunosuppressive activity in a mouse AKI model [55]. In mice fed an adenine-enriched diet, G-MDSCs were found to accumulate in the kidney during chronic kidney inflammation and fibrosis [51]. In addition, depleting MDSCs in the kidney enhanced fibrosis markers, indicating that MDSCs play a protective role against fibrosis. Li et al. reported that the efficacy of glucocorticoids in ameliorating focal segmental glomerulosclerosis (FSGS) depends on the MDSCs' capacity to expand [56]. After glucocorticoid treatment, the frequency of $CD11b^+HLA-DR^-CD14^-CD15^+$ MDSCs in peripheral blood was increased in patients with glucocorticoid-sensitive FSGS. In mice, glucocorticoid treatment increased the frequency of MDSCs in the peripheral blood, bone marrow, spleen, kidney-draining lymph nodes, and kidney. The induced MDSCs from glucocorticoid-treated mice were found to strongly suppress T cells, DCs, and macrophages but to induce regulatory T cells in the spleen, kidney-draining lymph nodes, and kidney.

Thus, MDSCs, especially G-MDSCs, suppress inflammation and fibrosis in the kidney by controlling the excessive expansion of effector T cells, DCs, and macrophages.

Intestine

The intestine, which is the largest immune organ, is continually exposed to antigens and immunomodulatory agents from the diet and from commensal microbiota [57]. An imbalance between effector T cells and regulatory cells in the intestine causes mucosal and systemic inflammation. Many studies report relationships between MDSCs and inflammatory bowel diseases (IBD) in humans and experimental mouse model systems [58]. In the first description of MDSC development in a murine IBD model, Haile et al. reported that MDSCs were induced in both the spleen and intestine and that they suppressed CD8$^+$ T cell proliferation ex vivo by producing NO [59]. The same study showed that the peripheral blood from IBD patients had an increased frequency of MDSCs, denoted as CD14$^+$HLA$^-$DR$^{-/low}$ cells. Su et al. showed that the adoptive transfer of bone marrow-derived G-MDSCs into mice with 2,4,6-trinitro-benzenesulfonic acid (TNBS)-induced colitis improved survival in the recipient mice and decreased injury scores, myeloperoxidase activities, and serum IL-6 levels [60]. Other researchers reported that the adoptive transfer of splenic MDSCs reduced inflammation and promoted mucosal healing in a dextran sulfate sodium (DSS)-induced colitis model [61]. MDSCs are induced by a strong variety factors such as granulocyte colony-stimulating factor (G-CSF), GM-CSF, TGF-β, and inflammatory cytokines. In addition to these factors, the antioxidant resveratrol, a naturally occurring polyphenol, induced Arg-1-expressing MDSCs in the colon of IL-10$^{-/-}$ mice [62].

These findings suggest that both M-MDSCs and G-MDSCs protect the intestines from excessive inflammation.

Central nervous system

The CNS has long been considered an immune-privileged site because the brain parenchyma, the interstitial fluid, and the cerebrospinal fluid (CSF) are isolated from the blood by two barriers, the blood–brain barrier (BBB) and the blood–CSF barrier (BCSFB). Despite these barriers, immune cells are detected in both the brain parenchyma and the CSF. Under pathological conditions, the integrity of the BBB and the BCSFB can be disturbed to allow the entry of inflammatory cells [63]. Recent studies have shown that, in the context of neuroimmunology, MDSCs are both powerful controllers of T cell activity and important modulatory agents for recovery from immunological insults [64].

Experimental autoimmune encephalomyelitis (EAE) is a commonly used mouse model of multiple sclerosis (MS), a T cell-mediated autoimmune inflammatory disease of the CNS [65]. Several recent studies report that MDSCs are involved in MS. Zhu et al. revealed that CD11b$^+$Ly6C^{hi} cells accumulated in the bone marrow, blood, spleen, and CNS of mice during the course of EAE and that

M-MDSCs isolated from the spleen suppressed the proliferation of CD4$^+$ T cells and CD8$^+$ T cells via NO production ex vivo [66]. Interestingly, the regulation of T cells by the CD11b$^+$Ly6C^{hi} cells was determined by the MDSCs' activation state and was plastic during the immune response [67]. IFN-γ, GM-CSF, TNF-α, and CD154 derived from the T cells activated the CD11b$^+$Ly6C^{hi} cells during their interactions. Activated CD11b$^+$Ly6C^{hi} cells suppressed T cells, but non-activated CD11b$^+$Ly6C^{hi} cells functioned as antigen-presenting cells (APCs). In EAE, the CD11b$^+$Ly6C^{hi} cells in the CNS were increasingly activated from disease onset to peak, and switched their function from antigen presentation to T cell suppression. Furthermore, the transfer of activated CD11b$^+$Ly6C^{hi} cells enhanced T cell apoptosis in the CNS and suppressed EAE. On the other hand, CD11b$^+$Ly6G$^+$ cells, which are G-MDSCs, accumulate abundantly within the peripheral lymphoid compartments and CNS of mice with EAE prior to remission of the disease [68]. Although the contribution of MDSCs to MS is less clear in humans, Ioannou et al. found significantly more G-MDSCs in the peripheral blood of MS patients at relapse than in the remission period or in control subjects [68]).

M-MDSCs are also critical in resolving acute inflammation and subsequently repairing the damaged tissue after spinal cord injury (SCI) in mice [69]. Furthermore, HMGB1-R AGE signaling promoted the expansion of CD11b$^+$Ly-6C$^+$MHC-II^{low} cells, which helped to resolve inflammation after a stroke in a murine ischemia model [70]. Interestingly, a similar increase in CD11b$^+$CD33$^+$HLA-DR$^-$ MDSCs was detected in the peripheral blood of stroke patients.

Collectively, both M-MDSCs and G-MDSCs contribute to the resolution of T cell-mediated CNS inflammation and the repair of CNS injury.

Eyes

In the eyes, local immune and inflammatory responses are limited, to preserve vision. This phenomenon, known as ocular immune privilege, is mediated by a combination of local and systemic mechanisms [71]. In addition, backup systems to resolve inflammation are needed if ocular immune privilege fails to work. MDSCs have recently emerged as an important cellular component in resolving eye inflammation [72]. Jeong et al. recently reported that HLA-DR$^+$CD11b$^+$CD33$^+$CD14$^+$ MDSCs in humans and CD11b$^+$Ly6G$^-$Ly6C$^+$ MDSCs in mice are markedly increased during and before the resolution phase of autoimmune uveoretinitis [73]. In experimental autoimmune uveoretinitis (EAU) mice during remission, the M-MDSCs were increased not only in the spleen and blood, but also in the retina. M-MDSCs isolated from EAU mice suppressed T cell proliferation in vitro, and the adoptive transfer of these cells accelerated the remission of auto-immune uveoretinitis in vivo.

These findings indicate that M-MDSCs serve as negative regulators to resolve eye inflammation.

MDSC plasticity

The plasticity of MDSCs has been discussed particularly in tumor models. MDSCs can differentiate into DCs, macrophages, and granulocytes. M-MDSCs from the spleen of EL-4 tumor-bearing mice differentiate into CD11b$^+$CD11c$^+$ DCs and CD11b$^+$F4/80$^+$ macrophages with GM-CSF stimulation in vitro [14]. CD11b$^+$Gr1$^+$ cells isolated from the spleens of tumor-bearing mice differentiate into CD11b$^+$Gr1$^+$F4/80$^+$ suppressor macrophages under the influence of tumor-derived factors in vitro [74]. Furthermore, CD11b$^+$Gr1$^+$ cells could differentiate into immunostimulatory DCs if cultured with Th1 cytokines, IL-3, and GM-CSF. Hypoxia elicited by hypoxia-inducible factor (HIF)-1α dramatically alters the function of MDSCs in the tumor microenvironment and redirects their differentiation toward tumor-associated macrophages (TAMs) [75]. G-MDSCs cultured in vitro for 24 h in the presence of GM-CSF resemble neutrophils in both phenotype and function [76]. Moreover, MDSCs isolated from a bone-tumor microenvironment differentiate into osteoclasts in the presence of macrophage colony-stimulating

factor (M-CSF) and receptor activator or NF-κB ligand (RANKL), and promote the destruction of bone in a mouse model of breast cancer metastasis to the bone [77].

Although little is known about the plasticity of MDSCs in non-neoplastic inflammatory conditions, recent reports demonstrate that they can differentiate into osteoclasts and tolerogenic DCs (tolDCs) (Fig. 1). Zhang et al. reported that MDSCs from the bone marrow of CIA mice can differentiate into tartrate-resistant acid phosphatase (TRAP)$^+$ osteoclasts by the stimulation of M-CSF and RANKL, which are capable of bone resorption in vitro and in vivo [78]. We recently showed that in the lungs of SKG mice, M-MDSCs differentiated into CD11b$^+$Gr1^{dim} tolerogenic DCs (CD11b$^+$Gr1^{dim} tolDCs), which suppressed the progression of ILD [27]. In that report, intraperitoneally injected zymosan induced ILD with various severity. The MDSC proportion were elevated in lungs with mild or moderate ILD, and the CD11b$^+$Gr1^{dim} tolDC population in particular was expanded in the lungs with severe ILD. Th17 cells and groups 1 and 3 innate lymphoid cells (ILC1s and ILC3s), which produced GM-CSF, were elevated in the lungs, and GM-CSF induced the M-MDSCs to differentiate into CD11b$^+$Gr1^{dim} tolDCs in vitro. CD11b$^+$Gr1^{dim} tolDCs suppressed T cell proliferation in vitro and suppressed the progression of ILD in vivo. Neutralizing TGF-β during the in vitro generation of

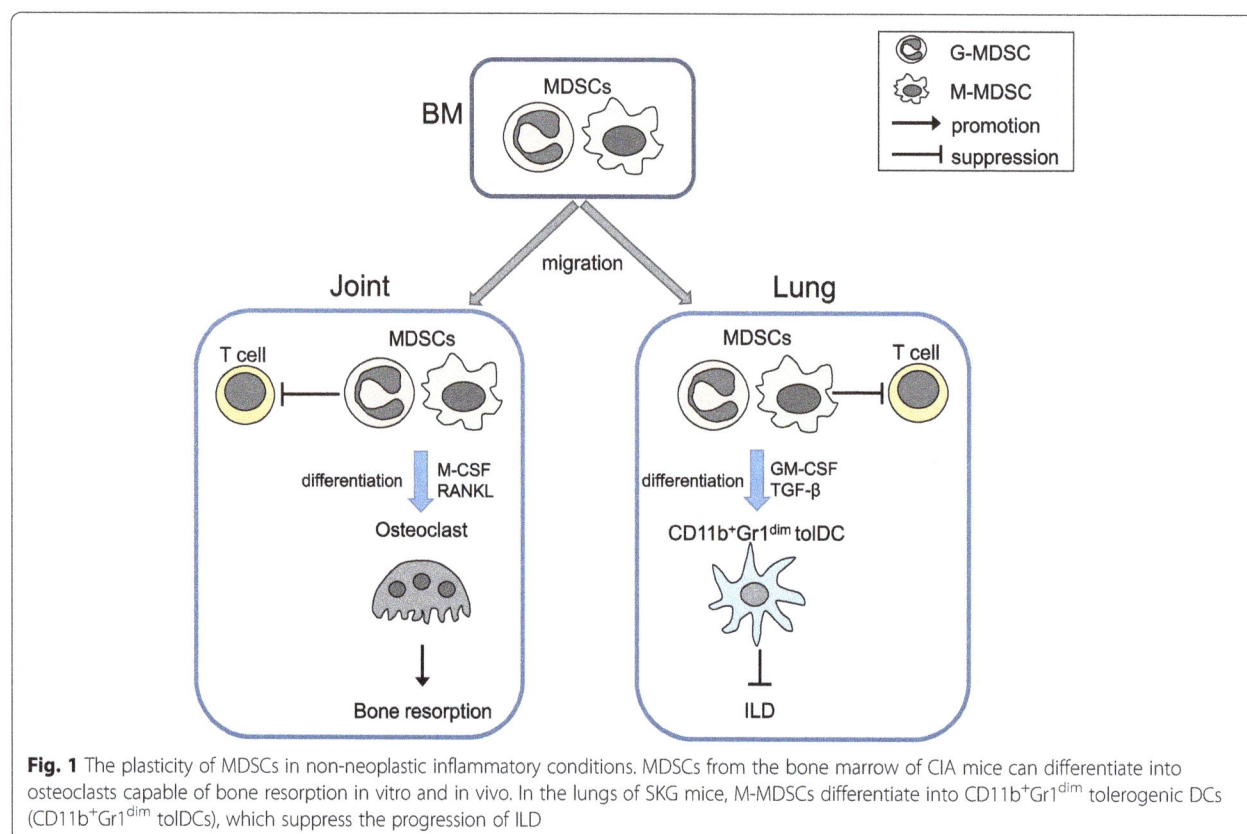

Fig. 1 The plasticity of MDSCs in non-neoplastic inflammatory conditions. MDSCs from the bone marrow of CIA mice can differentiate into osteoclasts capable of bone resorption in vitro and in vivo. In the lungs of SKG mice, M-MDSCs differentiate into CD11b$^+$Gr1^{dim} tolerogenic DCs (CD11b$^+$Gr1^{dim} tolDCs), which suppress the progression of ILD

CD11b$^+$Gr1^{dim} tolDCs partially canceled the cells' suppressive effect on T cell proliferation, indicating that TGF-β was critical for the tolerogenic nature of the CD11b$^+$Gr1^{dim} tolDCs. These results together suggested that MDSCs suppress pathogenic lymphocytes in the early stages of inflammation. When inflammation becomes severe, GM-CSF and TGF-β induce M-MDSCs to differentiate into CD11b$^+$Gr1^{dim} tolDCs, which further suppress lymphocytes to control excessive inflammation. Our report indicated that MDSCs can differentiate into unique tolDCs in the severely inflamed lung.

These reports indicate that MDSCs could differentiate into both pro-inflammatory and anti-inflammatory cells in the inflamed organs under pathogenic conditions.

Conclusions

MDSCs accumulate in inflamed organs. IL-6, the chemokine CCL2, rapamycin, and oxidizing agents recruit MDSCs from the bone marrow into the liver, lungs, kidneys, and intestines, respectively. On the other hand, hepatic stellate cells and mesenchymal stromal cells can induce MDSCs from myeloid cells in the liver. MDSCs negatively control inflammation by suppressing T cells and myeloid cells in inflamed organs. Moreover, they regulate fibrosis in the lungs, liver, and kidneys and may be involved in repairing CNS injuries. G-MDSCs act mostly in the joints, kidneys, intestines, and CNS, while M-MDSCs act in the lungs, liver, intestines, CNS, and eyes. MDSCs in organ microenvironments are plastic; MDSCs can differentiate into osteoclasts in the joints, and M-MDSCs can differentiate into tolDCs in the lungs. Further studies are required to characterize the behavior of MDSCs in various organs under non-neoplastic inflammatory conditions.

Abbreviations

AKI: Acute kidney injury; APC: Antigen-presenting cells; Arg-I: Arginase-I; BBB: Blood–brain barrier; BCSFB: Blood–CSF barrier; CIA: Collagen-induced arthritis; CNS: Central nervous system; COPD: Chronic obstructive pulmonary disease; CSF: Cerebrospinal fluid; DC: Dendritic cell; DSS: Dextran sulfate sodium; EAE: Experimental autoimmune encephalomyelitis; EAU: Experimental autoimmune uveoretinitis; FSGS: Focal segmental glomerulosclerosis; G-CSF: Granulocyte colony-stimulating factor; GM-CSF: Granulocyte macrophage colony-stimulating factor; HCV: Hepatitis C virus; HIF: Hypoxia-inducible factor; IBD: Inflammatory bowel diseases; IFN: Interferon; IL: Interleukin; ILC: Innate lymphoid cell; ILD: Interstitial lung disease; iNOS: Inducible nitric oxide synthase; M-CSF: Macrophage colony-stimulating factor; MDSC: Myeloid-derived suppressor cell; MMP: Matrix metalloproteinase; MS: Multiple sclerosis; mTOR: Mammalian target of rapamycin; NO: Nitric oxide; PBMC: Peripheral blood mononuclear cell; PH: Pulmonary hypertension; RA: Rheumatoid arthritis; RANKL: Receptor activator or NF-κB ligand; ROS: Reactive oxygen species; SCI: Spinal cord injury; SF: Synovial fluid; STAT: Signal transducer and activator of transcription; TAM: Tumor-associated macrophage; TGF-β: Transforming growth factor-β; TNBS: 2,4,6-Trinitrobenzenesulfonic acid; tolDC: Tolerogenic dendritic cell; TRAP: Tartrate-resistant acid phosphatase; Treg: Regulatory T cell

Acknowledgements
We are grateful to our colleagues and laboratory members for their helpful suggestions and experimental assistance.

Authors' contributions
SS drafted the manuscript. JS helped to draft the manuscript. AM gave the final approval of the version to be submitted and any revised version. All authors read and approved the final manuscript.

Competing interests
The authors declare that they have no competing interests.

Author details
[1]Division of Rheumatology and Clinical Immunology, Department of Internal Medicine, Kobe University Graduate School of Medicine, 7-5-2 Kusunoki-cho, Chuo-ku, Kobe 650-0017, Japan. [2]Division of Laboratory Medicine, Kobe University Graduate School of Medicine, 7-5-2 Kusunoki-cho, Chuo-ku, Kobe 650-0017, Japan.

References
1. Young MR, Newby M, Wepsic HT. Hematopoiesis and suppressor bone marrow cells in mice bearing large metastatic Lewis lung carcinoma tumors. Cancer Res. 1987;47(1):100–5.
2. Enioutina EY, Bareyan D, Daynes RA. A role for immature myeloid cells in immune senescence. J Immunol. 2011;186(2):697–707.
3. Cripps JG, Gorham JD. MDSC in autoimmunity. Int Immunopharmacol. 2011;11(7):789–93.
4. Veglia F, Perego M, Gabrilovich D. Myeloid-derived suppressor cells coming of age. Nat Immunol. 2018;19(2):108–19.
5. Youn JI, Gabrilovich DI. The biology of myeloid-derived suppressor cells: the blessing and the curse of morphological and functional heterogeneity. Eur J Immunol. 2010;40(11):2969–75.
6. Bronte V, Brandau S, Chen SH, Colombo MP, Frey AB, Greten TF, et al. Recommendations for myeloid-derived suppressor cell nomenclature and characterization standards. Nat Commun. 2016;7:12150.
7. Tcyganov E, Mastio J, Chen E, Gabrilovich DI. Plasticity of myeloid-derived suppressor cells in cancer. Curr Opin Immunol. 2018;51:76–82.
8. Mills CD, Kincaid K, Alt JM, Heilman MJ, Hill AM. M-1/M-2 macrophages and the Th1/Th2 paradigm. J Immunol. 2000;164(12):6166–73.
9. Udalova IA, Mantovani A, Feldmann M. Macrophage heterogeneity in the context of rheumatoid arthritis. Nat Rev Rheumatol. 2016;12(8):472–85.
10. Das A, Sinha M, Datta S, Abas M, Chaffee S, Sen CK, et al. Monocyte and macrophage plasticity in tissue repair and regeneration. Am J Pathol. 2015;185(10):2596–606.
11. Gabrilovich DI, Ostrand-Rosenberg S, Bronte V. Coordinated regulation of myeloid cells by tumours. Nat Rev Immunol. 2012;12(4):253–68.
12. Condamine T, Gabrilovich DI. Molecular mechanisms regulating myeloid-derived suppressor cell differentiation and function. Trends Immunol. 2011;32(1):19–25.
13. Rodriguez PC, Quiceno DG, Ochoa AC. L-arginine availability regulates T-lymphocyte cell-cycle progression. Blood. 2007;109(4):1568–73.
14. Harari O, Liao JK. Inhibition of MHC II gene transcription by nitric oxide and antioxidants. Curr Pharm Des. 2004;10(8):893–8.
15. Youn JI, Nagaraj S, Collazo M, Gabrilovich DI. Subsets of myeloid-derived suppressor cells in tumor-bearing mice. J Immunol. 2008;181(8):5791–802.
16. Otsuji M, Kimura Y, Aoe T, Okamoto Y, Saito T. Oxidative stress by tumor-derived macrophages suppresses the expression of CD3 zeta chain of T-cell receptor complex and antigen-specific T-cell responses. Proc Natl Acad Sci U S A. 1996;93(23):13119–24.
17. Pan PY, Ma G, Weber KJ, Ozao-Choy J, Wang G, Yin B, et al. Immune stimulatory receptor CD40 is required for T-cell suppression and T

regulatory cell activation mediated by myeloid-derived suppressor cells in cancer. Cancer Res. 2010;70(1):99–108.

18. Shevach EM. Regulatory T cells in autoimmmunity. Annu Rev Immunol. 2000;18:423–49.

19. O'Dwyer DN, Dickson RP, Moore BB. The lung microbiome, immunity, and the pathogenesis of chronic lung disease. J Immunol. 2016;196(12):4839–47.

20. Byrne AJ, Maher TM, Lloyd CM. Pulmonary macrophages: a new therapeutic pathway in fibrosing lung disease? Trends Mol Med. 2016;22(4):303–16.

21. Arora M, Poe SL, Oriss TB, Krishnamoorthy N, Yarlagadda M, Wenzel SE, et al. TLR4/MyD88-induced CD11b+Gr-1 int F4/80+ non-migratory myeloid cells suppress Th2 effector function in the lung. Mucosal Immunol. 2010;3(6):578–93.

22. Deshane J, Zmijewski JW, Luther R, Gaggar A, Deshane R, Lai JF, et al. Free radical-producing myeloid-derived regulatory cells: potent activators and suppressors of lung inflammation and airway hyperresponsiveness. Mucosal Immunol. 2011;4(5):503–18.

23. Song C, Yuan Y, Wang XM, Li D, Zhang GM, Huang B, et al. Passive transfer of tumour-derived MDSCs inhibits asthma-related airway inflammation. Scand J Immunol. 2014;79(2):98–104.

24. Deshane JS, Redden DT, Zeng M, Spell ML, Zmijewski JW, Anderson JT, et al. Subsets of airway myeloid-derived regulatory cells distinguish mild asthma from chronic obstructive pulmonary disease. J Allergy Clin Immunol. 2015; 135(2):413–24.

25. Scrimini S, Pons J, Agustí A, Soriano JB, Cosio BG, Torrecilla JA, et al. Differential effects of smoking and COPD upon circulating myeloid derived suppressor cells. Respir Med. 2013;107(12):1895–903.

26. Wright AK, Newby C, Hartley RA, Mistry V, Gupta S, Berair R, et al. Myeloid-derived suppressor cell-like fibrocytes are increased and associated with preserved lung function in chronic obstructive pulmonary disease. Allergy. 2017;72(4):645–55.

27. Sendo S, Saegusa J, Okano T, Takahashi S, Akashi K, Morinobu A. CD11b+Gr-1dim tolerogenic dendritic cell-like cells are expanded in interstitial lung disease in SKG mice. Arthritis Rheumatol. 2017;69(12):2314–27.

28. Lebrun A, Lo Re S, Chantry M, Izquierdo Carerra X, Uwambayinema F, Ricci D, et al. CCR2+ monocytic myeloid-derived suppressor cells (M-MDSCs) inhibit collagen degradation and promote lung fibrosis by producing transforming growth factor-β1. J Pathol. 2017;243(3):320–30.

29. Yeager ME, Nguyen CM, Belchenko DD, Colvin KL, Takatsuki S, Ivy DD, et al. Circulating myeloid-derived suppressor cells are increased and activated in pulmonary hypertension. Chest. 2012;141(4):944–52.

30. Tak PP, Smeets TJ, Daha MR, Kluin PM, Meijers KA, Brand R, et al. Analysis of the synovial cell infiltrate in early rheumatoid synovial tissue in relation to local disease activity. Arthritis Rheum. 1997;40(2):217–25.

31. Kraan MC, Reece RJ, Smeets TJ, Veale DJ, Emery P, Tak PP. Comparison of synovial tissues from the knee joints and the small joints of rheumatoid arthritis patients: implications for pathogenesis and evaluation of treatment. Arthritis Rheum. 2002;46(8):2034–8.

32. Egelston C, Kurkó J, Besenyei T, Tryniszewska B, Rauch TA, Glant TT, et al. Suppression of dendritic cell maturation and T cell proliferation by synovial fluid myeloid cells from mice with autoimmune arthritis. Arthritis Rheum. 2012;64(10):3179–88.

33. Fujii W, Ashihara E, Hirai H, Nagahara A, Kajitani N, Fujioka K, et al. Myeloid-derived suppressor cells play crucial roles in the regulation of mouse collagen-induced arthritis. J Immunol. 2013;191(3):1073–81.

34. Fujii W, Ashihara E, Kawahito W. Myeloid-derived suppressor cells in autoimmune diseases. Inflamm Regen. 2014;34(3):124–7.

35. Zhang L, Zhang Z, Zhang H, Wu M, Wang Y. Myeloid-derived suppressor cells protect mouse models from autoimmune arthritis via controlling inflammatory response. Inflammation. 2014;37(3):670–7.

36. Nishimura K, Saegusa J, Matsuki F, Akashi K, Kageyama G, Morinobu A. Tofacitinib facilitates the expansion of myeloid-derived suppressor cells and ameliorates arthritis in SKG mice. Arthritis Rheumatol. 2015;67(4):893–902.30.

37. Zhang H, Wang S, Huang Y, Wang H, Zhao J, Gaskin F, et al. Myeloid-derived suppressor cells are proinflammatory and regulate collagen-induced arthritis through manipulating Th17 cell differentiation. Clin Immunol. 2015; 157(2):175–86.

38. Kurkó J, Vida A, Glant TT, Scanzello CR, Katz RS, Nair A, et al. Identification of myeloid-derived suppressor cells in the synovial fluid of patients with rheumatoid arthritis: a pilot study. BMC Musculoskelet Disord. 2014;15:281.

39. Hammerich L, Tacke F. Emerging roles of myeloid derived suppressor cells in hepatic inflammation and fibrosis. World J Gastrointest Pathophysiol. 2015;6(3):43–50.

40. Höchst B, Schildberg FA, Sauerborn P, Gäbel YA, Gevensleben H, Goltz D, et al. Activated human hepatic stellate cells induce myeloid derived suppressor cells from peripheral blood monocytes in a CD44-dependent fashion. J Hepatol. 2013;59(3):528–35.

41. Chou HS, Hsieh CC, Yang HR, Wang L, Arakawa Y, Brown K, et al. Hepatic stellate cells regulate immune response by way of induction of myeloid suppressor cells in mice. Hepatology. 2011;53(3):1007–19.

42. Hsieh CC, Chou HS, Yang HR, Lin F, Bhatt S, Qin J, et al. The role of complement component 3 (C3) in differentiation of myeloid-derived suppressor cells. Blood. 2013;121(10):1760–8.

43. Yen BL, Yen ML, Hsu PJ, Liu KJ, Wang CJ, Bai CH, et al. Multipotent human mesenchymal stromal cells mediate expansion of myeloid-derived suppressor cells via hepatocyte growth factor/c-met and STAT3. Stem Cell Rep. 2013;1(2):139–51.

44. Cheng L, Wang J, Li X, Xing Q, Du P, Su L, et al. Interleukin-6 induces Gr-1 +CD11b+ myeloid cells to suppress CD8+ T cell-mediated liver injury in mice. PLoS One. 2011;6(3):e17631. https://doi.org/10.1371/journal.pone.0017631.

45. Cai W, Qin A, Guo P, Yan D, Hu F, Yang Q, et al. Clinical significance and functional studies of myeloid-derived suppressor cells in chronic hepatitis C patients. J Clin Immunol. 2013;33(4):798–808.

46. Tacke RS, Lee HC, Goh C, Courtney J, Polyak SJ, Rosen HR, et al. Myeloid suppressor cells induced by hepatitis C virus suppress T-cell responses through the production of reactive oxygen species. Hepatology. 2012;55(2): 343–53.

47. Cripps JG, Wang J, Maria A, Blumenthal I, Gorham JD. Type 1 T helper cells induce the accumulation of myeloid-derived suppressor cells in the inflamed Tgfb1 knockout mouse liver. Hepatology. 2010;52(4):1350–9.

48. Zhang Y, Bi Y, Yang H, Chen X, Liu H, Lu Y, et al. mTOR limits the recruitment of CD11b+Gr1+Ly6Chigh myeloid-derived suppressor cells in protecting against murine immunological hepatic injury. J Leukoc Biol. 2014;95(6):961–70.

49. Sarra M, Cupi ML, Bernardini R, Ronchetti G, Monteleone I, Ranalli M, et al. IL-25 prevents and cures fulminant hepatitis in mice through a myeloid-derived suppressor cell-dependent mechanism. Hepatology. 2013;58(4): 1436–50.

50. Suh YG, Kim JK, Byun JS, Yi HS, Lee YS, Eun HS, et al. CD11b(+) Gr1(+) bone marrow cells ameliorate liver fibrosis by producing interleukin-10 in mice. Hepatology. 2012;56(5):1902–12.

51. Höchst B, Mikulec J, Baccega T, Metzger C, Welz M, Peusquens J, et al. Differential induction of Ly6G and Ly6C positive myeloid derived suppressor cells in chronic kidney and liver inflammation and fibrosis. PLoS One. 2015; 10(3):e0119662. https://doi.org/10.1371/journal.pone.0119662.

52. Beck LH Jr, Bonegio RG, Lambeau G, Beck DM, Powell DW, Cummins TD, et al. M-type phospholipase A2 receptor as target antigen in idiopathic membranous nephropathy. N Engl J Med. 2009;361(1):11–21.

53. Kurts C, Panzer U, Anders HJ, Rees AJ. The immune system and kidney disease: basic concepts and clinical implications. Nat Rev Immunol. 2013; 13(10):738–53.

54. Imig JD, Ryan MJ. Immune and inflammatory role in renal disease. Compr Physiol. 2013;3(2):957–76.

55. Zhang C, Wang S, Li J, Zhang W, Zheng L, Yang C, et al. The mTOR signal regulates myeloid-derived suppressor cells differentiation and immunosuppressive function in acute kidney injury. Cell Death Dis. 2017;8(3):e2695.

56. Li L, Zhang T, Diao W, Jin F, Shi L, Meng J, et al. Role of myeloid-derived suppressor cells in glucocorticoid-mediated amelioration of FSGS. J Am Soc Nephrol. 2015;26(9):2183–97.

57. Mowat AM, Agace WW. Regional specialization within the intestinal immune system. Nat Rev Immunol. 2014;14(10):667–85.

58. Ostanin DV, Bhattacharya D. Myeloid-derived suppressor cells in the inflammatory bowel diseases. Inflamm Bowel Dis. 2013;19(11):2468–77.

59. Haile LA, von Wasielewski R, Gamrekelashvili J, Krüger C, Bachmann O, Westendorf AM, et al. Myeloid-derived suppressor cells in inflammatory bowel disease: a new immunoregulatory pathway. Gastroenterology. 2008; 135(3):871–81. e1–5

60. Su H, Cong X, Liu YL. Transplantation of granulocytic myeloid-derived suppressor cells (G-MDSCs) could reduce colitis in experimental murine models. J Dig Dis. 2013;14(5):251–8.

61. Zhang R, Ito S, Nishio N, Cheng Z, Suzuki H, Isobe KI. Dextran sulphate sodium increases splenic Gr1(+)CD11b(+) cells which accelerate recovery from colitis following intravenous transplantation. Clin Exp Immunol. 2011; 164(3):417–27.

62. Singh UP, Singh NP, Singh B, Hofseth LJ, Taub DD, Price RL, et al. Role of resveratrol-induced CD11b(+) Gr-1(+) myeloid derived suppressor cells (MDSCs) in the reduction of CXCR3(+) T cells and amelioration of chronic colitis in IL-10(−/−) mice. Brain Behav Immun. 2012;26(1):72–82.

63. Poli A, Kmiecik J, Domingues O, Hentges F, Bléry M, Chekenya M, et al. NK cells in central nervous system disorders. J Immunol. 2013;190(11):5355–62.

64. Melero-Jerez C, Ortega MC, Moliné-Velázquez V, Clemente D. Myeloid derived suppressor cells in inflammatory conditions of the central nervous system. Biochim Biophys Acta. 2016;1862(3):368–80.

65. Roder J, Hickey WF. Mouse models, immunology, multiple sclerosis and myelination. Nat Genet. 1996;12(1):6–8.

66. Zhu B, Bando Y, Xiao S, Yang K, Anderson AC, Kuchroo VK, et al. CD11b+Ly-6C(hi) suppressive monocytes in experimental autoimmune encephalomyelitis. J Immunol. 2007;179(8):5228–37.

67. Zhu B, Kennedy JK, Wang Y, Sandoval-Garcia C, Cao L, Xiao S, et al. Plasticity of Ly-6C(hi) myeloid cells in T cell regulation. J Immunol. 2011;187(5):2418–32.

68. Ioannou M, Alissafi T, Lazaridis I, Deraos G, Matsoukas J, Gravanis A, et al. Crucial role of granulocytic myeloid-derived suppressor cells in the regulation of central nervous system autoimmune disease. J Immunol. 2012;188(3):1136–46.

69. Saiwai H, Kumamaru H, Ohkawa Y, Kubota K, Kobayakawa K, Yamada H, et al. Ly6C+ Ly6G- Myeloid-derived suppressor cells play a critical role in the resolution of acute inflammation and the subsequent tissue repair process after spinal cord injury. J Neurochem. 2013;125(1):74–88.

70. Liesz A, Dalpke A, Mracsko E, Antoine DJ, Roth S, Zhou W, et al. DAMP signaling is a key pathway inducing immune modulation after brain injury. J Neurosci. 2015;35(2):583–98.

71. Zhou R, Caspi RR. Ocular immune privilege. F1000 Biol Rep. 2010;2. https://doi.org/10.3410/B2-3.

72. Kerr EC, Raveney BJ, Copland DA, Dick AD, Nicholson LB. Analysis of retinal cellular infiltrate in experimental autoimmune uveoretinitis reveals multiple regulatory cell populations. J Autoimmun. 2008;31(4):354–61.

73. Jeong HJ, Lee HJ, Ko JH, Cho BJ, Park SY, Park JW, et al. Myeloid-derived suppressor cells mediate inflammation resolution in humans and mice with autoimmune uveoretinitis. J Immunol. 2018;200(4):1306–15.

74. Narita Y, Wakita D, Ohkur T, Chamoto K, Nishimura T. Potential differentiation of tumor bearing mouse CD11b+Gr-1+ immature myeloid cells into both suppressor macrophages and immunostimulatory dendritic cells. Biomed Res. 2009;30(1):7–15.

75. Corzo CA, Condamine T, Lu L, Cotter MJ, Youn JI, Cheng P, et al. HIF-1α regulates function and differentiation of myeloid-derived suppressor cells in the tumor microenvironment. J Exp Med. 2010;207(11):2439–53.

76. Youn JI, Collazo M, Shalova IN, Biswas SK, Gabrilovich DI. Characterization of the nature of granulocytic myeloid-derived suppressor cells in tumor-bearing mice. J Leukoc Biol. 2012;91(1):167–81.

77. Sawant A, Deshane J, Jules J, Lee CM, Harris BA, Feng X, et al. Myeloid-derived suppressor cells function as novel osteoclast progenitors enhancing bone loss in breast cancer. Cancer Res. 2013;73(2):672–82.

78. Zhang H, Huang Y, Wang S, Fu R, Guo C, Wang H, et al. Myeloid-derived suppressor cells contribute to bone erosion in collagen-induced arthritis by differentiating to osteoclasts. J Autoimmun. 2015;65:82–9.

26

Deterioration in saliva quality in patients with Sjögren's syndrome: impact of decrease in salivary epidermal growth factor on the severity of intraoral manifestations

Naoto Azuma[1*], Yoshinori Katada[2] and Hajime Sano[1]

Abstract

Background: Sjögren's syndrome (SS) is a chronic inflammatory autoimmune disease characterized by lymphocytic infiltration of the exocrine glands, especially the salivary and lacrimal glands. As a result of salivary gland dysfunction, most patients with SS have xerostomia related to a reduced salivary flow rate. In addition to the discomfort due to xerostomia, dry mouth can cause various intraoral manifestations such as refractory stomatitis, ulcer, and atrophic changes in the oral mucosa and tongue, and the patient's quality of life (QoL) is severely impaired. These manifestations are believed to be caused mainly by a decrease in the clearance in the oral cavity owing to hyposalivation. However, because saliva has several beneficial physiological effects on the intraoral environment, qualitative changes in sialochemistry should also be considered a cause of the refractory intraoral manifestations in SS.

Main text: Salivary epidermal growth factor (EGF) is considered an important cytoprotective factor against injuries. It contributes to wound healing in the oral cavity and to maintenance of mucosal integrity in the oral cavity and gastrointestinal tract. We evaluated changes in salivary EGF levels and assessed the association between salivary EGF levels and the severity of intraoral manifestations in patients with SS. The following novel findings were obtained: (1) salivary EGF levels in SS patients were significantly lower than those in non-SS patients; (2) salivary EGF levels as well as the salivary flow rate decreased with the progression of SS; (3) with prolonged SS disease duration, salivary EGF levels decreased more rapidly than the salivary flow rate; and (4) decreases in salivary EGF levels significantly correlated with exacerbation of the oral health-related QoL in patients with SS.

Conclusions: The deterioration in saliva quality as well as lower intraoral clearance by hyposalivation could play a role in the pathogenesis of refractory intraoral manifestations in patients with SS. Our findings suggest a new target for therapeutic intervention for SS.

Keywords: Dry mouth, Epidermal growth factor, Intraoral manifestation, Oral mucosal involvement, Quality of life, Saliva, Saliva quality, Sjögren's syndrome, Xerostomia

Background

Sjögren's syndrome (SS) is a chronic inflammatory auto-immune disease characterized by lymphocytic infiltration of the exocrine glands, especially the salivary and lacrimal glands. As a result of salivary gland dysfunction, most patients with SS have xerostomia caused by a reduced salivary

flow rate. In addition to the discomfort, xerostomia can cause various intraoral manifestations, for example, dental caries and oral mucosal involvements, such as refractory stomatitis, oral ulcers, and atrophic changes in the oral mucosa and lingual papilla. In the chronic form, these manifestations can severely impair a patient's quality of life (QoL) [1]. The intraoral manifestations in patients with SS are believed to be caused mainly by decreased clearance in the oral cavity owing to hyposalivation. However, because saliva has several beneficial physiological effects on the intraoral environment,

* Correspondence: naoazuuh@hyo-med.ac.jp
[1]Division of Rheumatology, Department of Internal Medicine, Hyogo College of Medicine, 1-1 Mukogawa-cho, Nishinomiya, Hyogo 663-8501, Japan
Full list of author information is available at the end of the article

such as lubrication, maintenance of mucosal integrity, and antimicrobial activity [2], qualitative changes in its composition should also be considered as a cause of the refractory intraoral manifestations in SS.

Epidermal growth factor (EGF), which accelerates incisor eruption and eyelid opening in newborn animals, was first isolated from mouse submandibular glands [3]. EGF is a polypeptide comprising 53 amino acids (molecular weight, 6.045 kDa) that promotes the growth of various tissues in several species [4]. In humans, EGF is produced by the salivary glands and duodenal Brunner's glands [5]. The main source of EGF in the oral cavity is the parotid glands [4, 6]; however, salivary EGF has been found to be secreted not only from the parotid and submandibular glands but also from the sublingual or minor salivary glands [4, 6, 7]. EGF binding to the EGF receptor stimulates the activity of intracellular kinase cascades, producing signals that consequently alter gene regulation, which leads to cell proliferation and anti-apoptogenic survival [8, 9]. Salivary EGF is considered an important cytoprotective factor against injuries, and it contributes to wound healing and maintenance of mucosal integrity in the oral cavity [10, 11] and in the gastrointestinal tract [12]. Although the detailed mechanisms by which EGF secretion into the saliva is controlled are not yet known, several studies have found that salivary EGF levels are significantly decreased in patients with intraoral inflammatory lesions, such as aphthous stomatitis [4, 13] and peritonsillar abscess [4]. In addition, patients with oral mucositis induced by radiation therapy for head and neck carcinoma were also found to have markedly low salivary EGF levels [14, 15]. These findings suggested that low salivary EGF levels reduce the capacity of the oral mucosa to heal after injury and maintain its physiological integrity.

To the best of our knowledge, no study conducted to date has measured salivary EGF levels in patients with SS. Thus, we evaluated changes in salivary EGF levels in patients with SS and assessed the association between salivary EGF levels and the severity of intraoral manifestations in SS [16, 17].

Assessment of the association between salivary EGF and SS

Methods
Selection of patients

To assess changes in the salivary EGF levels in patients with SS Forty patients with SS (27 primary SS, 13 secondary SS) participated in this study. All patients (SS group) fulfilled the revised Japanese criteria for the diagnosis of SS proposed by the Japanese Ministry of Health and Welfare (1999) [18] and the American-European Consensus Group classification criteria for SS (2002) [19]. Twenty-three individuals without SS, including healthy individuals and those with rheumatoid arthritis,

polymyalgia rheumatica, dermatomyositis, bronchial asthma, systemic lupus erythematosus, adult-onset Still's disease, relapsing polychondritis, synovitis-acne-pustulosis-hyperostosis-osteitis (SAPHO) syndrome, and eosinophilia, were recruited as controls (non-SS group). The non-SS group patients could not be diagnosed with SS and salivary gland dysfunction on the basis of their clinical symptoms, physical findings, and laboratory findings through the clinical course. The exclusion criteria consisted of factors that are known to affect the intraoral environment or saliva secretion and salivary EGF levels and were as follows: current smoking; chronic alcohol use; ongoing dental treatment; recurrent oral mucositis due to conditions other than SS; treatment with antiparkinson drugs or psychiatric drugs such as antidepressants, anti-anxiety agents, and antipsychotic agents; severe diabetes mellitus; severe reflux esophagitis; past history of head and neck carcinoma; previous radiation therapy to the head and neck region; and previous chemotherapy for cancer.

To assess changes in the salivary EGF levels at 3-year follow-up in the same patients with SS Twenty-three patients with SS (14 primary SS, nine secondary SS) and 14 individuals without SS serving as controls (non-SS group) who participated in the above study and were subsequently followed up for 3 years were enrolled in this study.

These studies were approved by the ethics committee of the Hyogo College of Medicine (no. 758). All subjects provided written informed consent to participate in the study.

Saliva collection and quantification of salivary EGF

Whole stimulated saliva was collected after the subjects chewed gum (Free Zone Gum Hi-Mint®; Lotte, Tokyo, Japan) for 10 min and expectorated into graduated centrifuge tubes. All samples were similarly collected at approximately the same time before breakfast in the morning, with fasting, because salivary EGF concentrations show apparent changes related to food intake [4]. The final saliva volume was measured, and EGF levels in the supernatants obtained by centrifuging the saliva samples were measured using a commercial enzyme-linked immunosorbent assay kit (Quantikine®; R&D System, Minneapolis, MN, USA). Total salivary EGF output (pg/10 min) was calculated by multiplying salivary EGF concentration (pg/ml) by saliva volume (ml/10 min) [15].

Quantitative assessment of intraoral manifestations

At the time of saliva collection, subjective intraoral manifestations were assessed using the short Japanese version of the Oral Health Impact Profile (OHIP) [20, 21], which is a self-administered questionnaire. The OHIP is one of the most widely used instruments to measure oral health-related QoL (OHRQoL). The OHIP-14 consists of 14 questions designed to measure the frequency of problems associated with the teeth, mouth, or dentures. The questions have seven aspects: functional limitation, physical pain, psychological discomfort, physical disability, psychological disability, social disability, and handicap. The answers to the questions were given using a 5-point scale ranging from 0 to 4 (0, never; 1, hardly ever; 2, occasionally; 3, fairly often; and 4, very often). The unweighted scores were subsequently combined to obtain a single summary score with a possible range of 0–56, with a high score indicating more frequent problems, that is, poorer OHRQoL. It has been demonstrated by Stewart et al. that in patients with SS, lower salivary flow rates are significantly associated with poorer oral health, as assessed using the OHIP-14 summary score [1].

Statistical analysis

Results are expressed as mean ± standard deviation. The Mann-Whitney U test, chi-square test, Fisher's exact test, or Wilcoxon signed-rank test was used as appropriate to compare differences between groups. The correlations were examined using the Spearman's rank correlation coefficient. A p value < 0.05 was considered statistically significant.

Results
Assessment of changes in the salivary EGF levels in patients with SS

Comparison of the clinical data in patients with and without SS The characteristics of the study groups are presented in Table 1. No significant differences in age and sex were observed between the groups. The mean disease duration of SS was 5.6 years. The salivary flow rate in the SS group (7.8 ± 4.4 mL/10 min) was significantly lower than that in the non-SS group (16.9 ± 5.9 mL/10 min) (p < 0.0001). The OHIP-14 score in the SS group (11.3 ± 9.4) was significantly higher than that in the non-SS group (7.1 ± 7.6) (p = 0.037). Thus, the OHRQoL of SS patients was poorer than non-SS patients.

Comparison of salivary EGF levels in patients with and without SS The salivary EGF output in the SS group (9237.6 ± 8447.0 pg/10 min) was significantly lower than that in the non-SS group (13,296.9 ± 7907.1 pg/10 min) (p = 0.033) (Table 1). Because the clinical background varied widely among the SS patients, the SS group was divided into two groups according to two clinical factors.

Disease duration The SS group was divided into the long- and the short-duration groups by disease duration. The cut-off level was provisionally set at 5.6 years based on the mean disease duration of the entire SS group (≥ 5.6 years: long-duration group [n = 11], < 5.6 years: short-duration group [n = 13]). The OHIP-14 score in the long-duration SS group (13.9 ± 10.8) was significantly higher than that in the non-SS group (7.1 ± 7.6) (p < 0.05), but the score did not differ significantly between the short-duration SS group and the non-SS group. With regard to the salivary flow rate, the rate was significantly lower in the long-duration SS group (4.7 ± 2.4 mL/10 min) than in the short-duration SS group (9.1 ± 5.7 mL/10 min) and the non-SS group (16.9 ± 5.9 mL/10 min) (p < 0.05 and p < 0.0001, respectively). The rate in the short-duration SS group was also significantly lower than that in the non-SS group (p < 0.001) (Table 2). Furthermore, the salivary EGF output in the long-duration SS group (4087.2 ± 4356.7 pg/10 min) was significantly lower than that in the short-duration SS group (13,881.3 ± 10,480.2 pg/10 min) and the non-SS group (13,296.9 ± 7907.1 pg/10 min) (p < 0.01 and p < 0.001, respectively). However, no significant difference was found in the salivary EGF output in the short-duration SS group compared to that in the non-SS group (Fig. 1a).

Oral health-related quality of life (OHIP-14 score) The SS group was stratified according to the OHIP-14 score into the severe intraoral manifestations group and the mild group. When one point out of four was given for all 14 questions, the total OHIP-14 score was 14.

Table 1 Clinical characteristics of the study groups

	SS (n = 40)	Non-SS (n = 23)	p value
Age (years)	55.4 ± 13.2	56.1 ± 17.4	0.425
Sex (male/female, number)	3:37	5:18	0.129
Disease duration (years)	5.6 ± 3.7 (n = 24)	–	–
Salivary flow rate (mL/10 min)	7.8 ± 4.4	16.9 ± 5.9	< 0.0001
OHIP-14 score (out of 56)	11.3 ± 9.4 (n = 35)	7.1 ± 7.6	0.037
Salivary EGF output (pg/10 min)	9237.6 ± 8447.0	13,296.9 ± 7907.1	0.033

Mean ± SD

SS Sjögren's syndrome, *OHIP-14* Oral Health Impact Profile-14

Table 2 Clinical characteristics of the SS and non-SS groups. Classification of the SS group by disease duration

	SS: long duration (≥ 5.6 years) (n = 11)	SS: short duration (< 5.6 years) (n = 13)	Non-SS (n = 23)
Disease duration (years)	9.2 ± 1.8*	2.6 ± 1.3	–
Age (years)	63.9 ± 5.9**	53.2 ± 13.0	56.1 ± 17.4
OHIP-14 score (out of 56)	13.9 ± 10.8†	8.6 ± 6.6 (n = 11)	7.1 ± 7.6
Salivary flow rate (mL/10 min)	4.7 ± 2.4***, †††	9.1 ± 5.7††	16.9 ± 5.9

*p < 0.0001 versus the short duration (< 5.6 years) group, **p < 0.01 versus the short duration (< 5.6 years) group, ***p < 0.05 versus the short duration (< 5.6 years) group, †p < 0.05 versus the non-SS group, ††p < 0.001 versus the non-SS group, †††p < 0.0001 versus the non-SS group

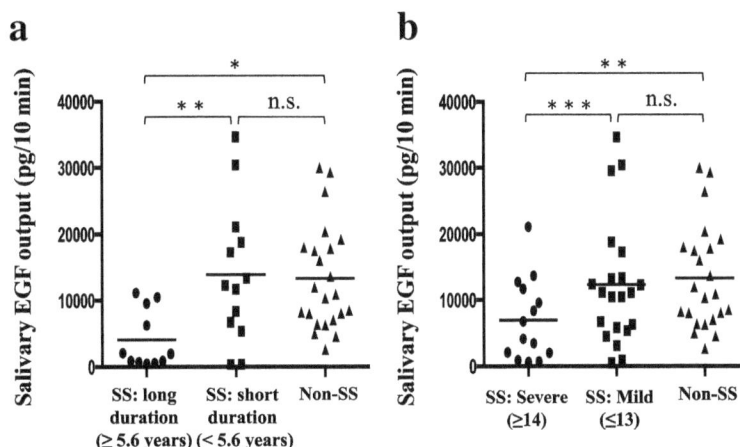

Fig. 1 Salivary epidermal growth factor (EGF) levels of the Sjögren's syndrome (SS) and non-SS groups. **a** The SS group was divided into the long-duration group and short-duration groups depending on disease duration, and salivary EGF output levels were compared between these groups and the non-SS group. **b** The SS group was divided into the severe and mild groups according to the severity of intraoral manifestations determined using the Oral Health Impact Profile (OHIP)-14 score, and salivary EGF output levels were compared between these groups and the non-SS group. Statistical differences were assessed using the Mann–Whitney U test. *$p < 0.001$, **$p < 0.01$, ***$p < 0.05$; n.s., not significant

Therefore, the cutoff level was provisionally set at 14 points (≥ 14: severe group [$n = 14$], ≤ 13: mild group [$n = 21$]). In the severe SS group, the disease duration was longer and the salivary flow rate was lower than that in the mild SS group, but neither showed a significant difference (Table 3). The salivary EGF output in the severe SS group (6965.8 ± 6161.1 pg/10 min) was significantly lower than that in the mild SS group ($12,275.7 \pm 9420.0$ pg/10 min) and the non-SS group ($13,296.9 \pm 7907.1$ pg/10 min) ($p < 0.05$ and $p < 0.01$, respectively). In contrast, the salivary EGF output did not differ significantly between the mild SS group and the non-SS group (Fig. 1b).

Correlation analysis The correlation between salivary flow rate and salivary EGF output was evaluated in 13 SS patients, excluding those under medical treatment that might have affected salivary flow rate (e.g., muscarinic M3 receptor agonist, corticosteroids, and immunosuppressants). The salivary flow rate was found to be significantly correlated with salivary EGF output ($r_s = 0.824$, $p = 0.0005$) (Fig. 2a). In SS patients whose disease duration could be confirmed ($n = 24$), the disease duration was found to be significantly and inversely correlated with salivary EGF output ($r_s = -0.484$, $p = 0.008$) (Fig. 2b). A similar analysis was also conducted in 10 SS patients excluding those under the abovementioned medical treatments to test the correlation between the OHIP-14 score and salivary EGF output. The OHIP-14 score was significantly and inversely correlated with salivary EGF output ($r_s = -0.721$, $p = 0.012$) (Fig. 2c).

Assessment of changes in the salivary EGF levels within 3-year follow-up in the same patients with SS

Comparison of clinical data at baseline and at re-evaluation in patients with and without SS No significant differences in age and sex were observed between the SS group (mean age, 59.5 ± 12.7 years, 21 women and two men) and the non-SS group (59.9 ± 15.2 years, 10 women and four men) ($p = 0.468$ and $p = 0.173$, respectively). The mean SS disease duration at baseline (initial evaluation) was 5.5 years.

In the SS group, there were no significant differences in the number of patients treated with a muscarinic M3 receptor agonist (pilocarpine or cevimeline) and corticosteroids or immunosuppressants at baseline (12/23 [52%] and 6/23 [26%], respectively) and at re-evaluation (14/23 [61%] and 8/23 [35%], respectively) ($p = 0.766$ and $p = 0.749$, respectively). The OHIP-14 score at re-evaluation (12.6 ± 9.2) was significantly higher than that at baseline (10.2 ± 8.8) ($p = 0.040$), indicating a significant exacerbation of the

Table 3 Clinical characteristics of the SS and non-SS groups. Classification of the SS group by oral health-related quality of life (OHIP-14 score)

	SS: severe (≥ 14) ($n = 14$)	SS: mild (≤ 13) ($n = 21$)	Non-SS ($n = 23$)
Age (years)	61.5 ± 10.4*	52.7 ± 14.0	56.1 ± 17.4
Disease duration (years)	7.2 ± 3.7 ($n = 9$)	4.9 ± 3.6 ($n = 13$)	–
Salivary flow rate (mL/10 min)	$6.9 \pm 4.2^{\dagger}$	$9.3 \pm 4.4^{\dagger}$	16.9 ± 5.9

Mean ± SD

SS Sjögren's syndrome, OHIP-14 Oral Health Impact Profile-14

*$p < 0.05$ versus the mild (≤ 13) group, $^{\dagger}p < 0.0001$ versus the non-SS group

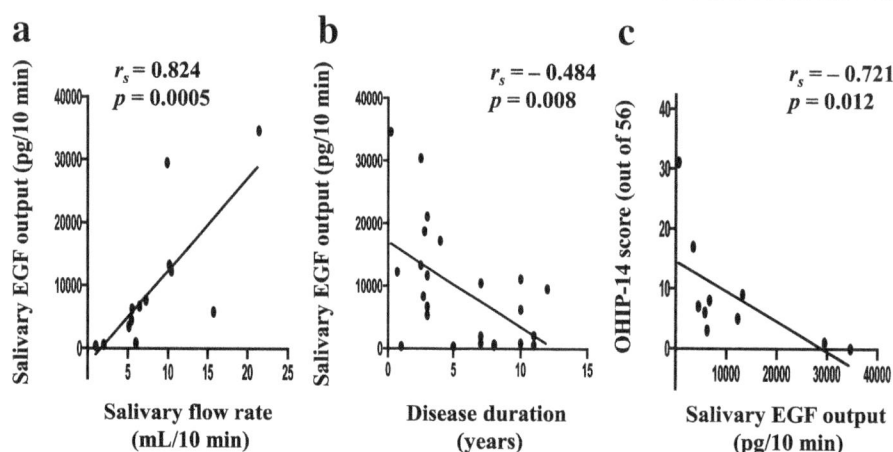

Fig. 2 Correlations between different factors and salivary epidermal growth factor (EGF) output in the Sjögren's syndrome (SS) group. **a** Correlation of salivary flow rate with salivary EGF output ($n = 13$). **b** Correlation of disease duration with salivary EGF output ($n = 24$). **c** Correlation of the Oral Health Impact Profile (OHIP)-14 score with salivary EGF output ($n = 10$). Correlations were assessed using Spearman's rank correlation coefficient

OHRQoL. No significant differences were observed in the salivary flow rate at baseline (8.1 ± 5.3 mL/10 min) and at re-evaluation (7.4 ± 5.1 mL/10 min) ($p = 0.149$). However, the salivary EGF output at re-evaluation (8352.8 ± 7813.3 pg/10 min) was significantly lower than that at baseline ($10,158.4 \pm 9820.9$ pg/10 min) ($p = 0.032$) (Table 4 (a)).

In the non-SS group, no significant differences were observed in the OHIP-14 score, salivary flow rate, and salivary EGF output at baseline (9.1 ± 6.8, 16.8 ± 6.7 mL/10 min, and $13,623.1 \pm 9546.2$ pg/10 min, respectively) and at re-evaluation (10.7 ± 9.4, 16.7 ± 6.0 mL/10 min, and $11,904.9 \pm 6995.4$ pg/10 min, respectively) ($p = 0.169$, $p = 0.628$, and $p = 0.184$, respectively) (Table 4 (b)).

Table 4 Clinical characteristics at baseline (initial evaluation) and at re-evaluation 3 years later

	Baseline (initial evaluation)	3 years later (re-evaluation)	p value
(a) SS group ($n = 23$)			
OHIP-14 score (out of 56)	10.2 ± 8.8 ($n = 22$)	12.6 ± 9.2 ($n = 22$)	0.040
Salivary flow rate (mL/10 min)	8.1 ± 5.3	7.4 ± 5.1	0.149
Salivary EGF output (pg/10 min)	$10,158.4 \pm 9820.9$	8352.8 ± 7813.3	0.032
(b) Non-SS group ($n = 14$)			
OHIP-14 score (out of 56)	9.1 ± 6.8	10.7 ± 9.4	0.169
Salivary flow rate (mL/10 min)	16.8 ± 6.7	16.7 ± 6.0	0.628
Salivary EGF output (pg/10 min)	$13,623.1 \pm 9546.2$	$11,904.9 \pm 6995.4$	0.184

Mean ± SD

SS Sjögren's syndrome, OHIP-14 Oral Health Impact Profile-14

Changes in salivary flow rate and EGF output according to disease duration and oral health-related quality of life The clinical background varied widely among the SS patients in the present study; thus, the SS group was subdivided into two groups depending on two clinical factors.

Disease duration The SS group was divided into short- and long-disease duration subgroups. The cutoff level was provisionally set at 5 years at the starting point based on the mean disease duration of the entire SS group (≤ 5 years: short-duration group [$n = 7$], ≥ 6 years: long-duration group [$n = 6$]). In the short-duration group, no significant differences were observed in the salivary flow rate and salivary EGF output between baseline (10.5 ± 7.0 mL/10 min and $15,646.9 \pm 12,986.2$ pg/10 min, respectively) and re-evaluation levels (9.4 ± 5.4 mL/10 min and $13,187.6 \pm 9902.1$ pg/10 min, respectively) (Fig. 3a). In contrast, in the long-duration group, although the salivary flow rate did not differ significantly between baseline (3.6 ± 1.4 mL/10 min) and re-evaluation levels (3.3 ± 1.6 mL/10 min), the salivary EGF output at re-evaluation (1640.9 ± 1774.8 pg/10 min) was significantly lower than that at baseline (3652.4 ± 4211.2 pg/10 min) ($p < 0.05$) (Fig. 3b).

Oral health-related quality of life (OHIP-14 score) The SS group was subdivided on the basis of the magnitude of changes in the OHIP-14 scores after 3 years into the non-exacerbation group (the score decreased or was unchanged in 3 years; $n = 8$) and the exacerbation group (the score increased in 3 years; $n = 14$). In the non-exacerbation group, the salivary flow rate and the salivary EGF output did not significantly differ between baseline (9.0 ± 6.3 mL/10 min and $12,448.0 \pm 12,727.1$ pg/10 min, respectively) and re-evaluation values (9.0 ± 5.9 mL/10 min

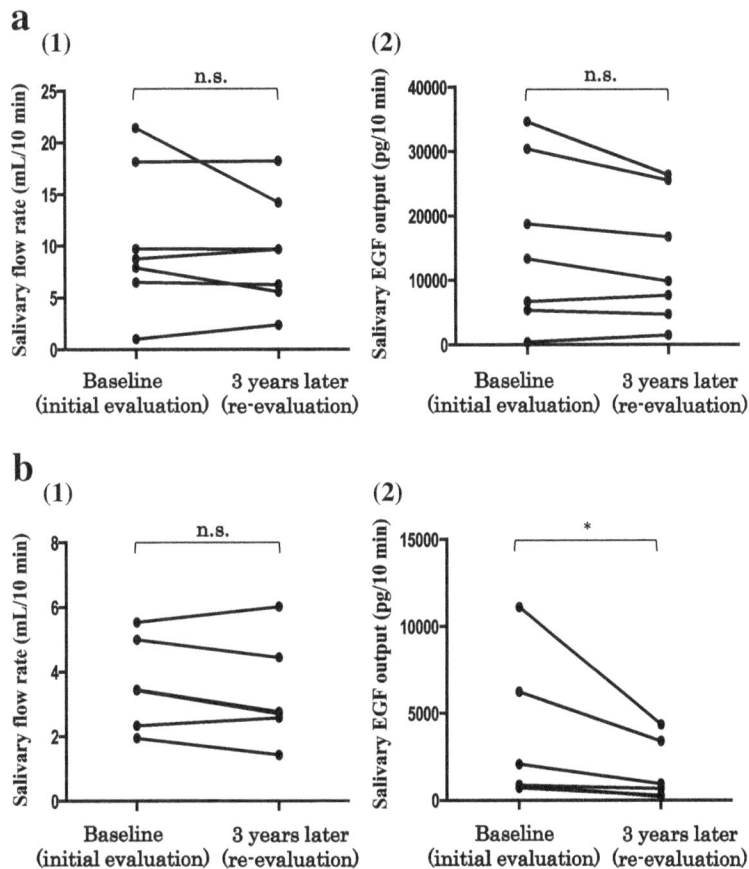

Fig. 3 Changes in the salivary flow rate and salivary epidermal growth factor (EGF) output according to the disease duration. **a** Short-duration Sjögren's syndrome (SS) group. **b** Long-duration SS group. (1) Changes in the salivary flow rate. (2) Changes in the salivary EGF output. Statistical analysis was performed using the Wilcoxon signed-rank test. *$p < 0.05$; n.s., not significant

and $10{,}310.9 \pm 9565.9$ pg/10 min, respectively) (Fig. 4a). In contrast, in the exacerbation group, both the salivary flow rate and the salivary EGF output at re-evaluation (6.8 ± 4.6 mL/10 min and 7724.2 ± 6901.4 pg/10 min, respectively) were significantly lower than at baseline (8.0 ± 4.6 mL/10 min and 9548.6 ± 8063.6 pg/10 min, respectively) ($p < 0.05$ in both cases) (Fig. 4b).

Decrease in salivary EGF levels: deterioration in saliva quality and intraoral manifestations in SS

The following novel results were obtained in the present study: (1) salivary EGF output in SS patients was significantly lower than that in non-SS patients. (2) In SS patients, with prolonged disease duration, in addition to the progressive reduction in the salivary flow rate, the salivary EGF output also decreased. The salivary EGF output correlated with the salivary flow rate and showed an inverse correlation with disease duration. (3) In cases of prolonged SS disease duration, the salivary EGF output in SS patients decreased more rapidly than the salivary flow rate in a short period of time. (4) The decrease in salivary EGF output as well as the salivary

flow rate was closely associated with poor OHRQoL in SS patients. Koski et al. [22] reported that EGF expression diminished in the labial salivary glands of patients with SS and concluded that the continuous lymphocytic inflammation in SS affected not only the salivary flow rates but also the EGF production in the salivary glands. However, our reports are the first to demonstrate the association between SS and salivary EGF levels.

Hutson et al. [23] showed that wound healing of the skin was enhanced by licking, that is, by transfer of saliva to the wound. Subsequent reports have suggested that EGF synthesized in the salivary glands and secreted into the saliva is involved in wound healing inside and outside the oral cavity. In animal models, oral wound healing was delayed significantly after removal of the submandibular glands, which are the major source of salivary EGF in rodents, and oral administration or topical application of EGF was found to restore the rate of wound healing [10, 11]. Fujisawa et al. [11] reported that topical EGF application promoted proliferation of fibroblasts and keratinocytes and accelerated the healing of gingival ulcers. These findings suggest that salivary

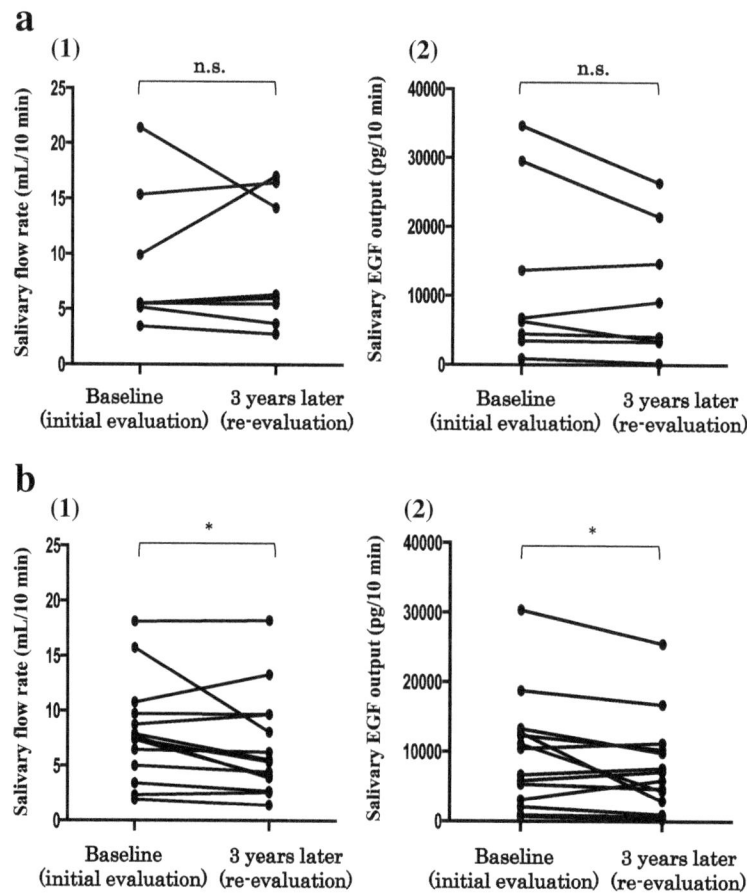

Fig. 4 Changes in the salivary flow rate and salivary epidermal growth factor (EGF) output according to the extent of changes in the Oral Health Impact Profile (OHIP)-14 score at 3-year re-evaluation. **a** Patient group in which the OHIP-14 score decreased or did not change (non-exacerbation group). **b** Patient group in which the OHIP-14 score increased (exacerbation group). (1) Changes in the salivary flow rate. (2) Changes in the salivary EGF output. Statistical analysis was performed using the Wilcoxon signed-rank test. *$p < 0.05$; n.s., not significant

EGF is involved in repair mechanisms that lead to wound healing and maintenance of the integrity of the mucosa of the oral cavity.

Several studies have demonstrated an association between intraoral inflammatory diseases and changes in salivary EGF levels. Salivary EGF concentrations were found to be significantly lower in patients with aphthous stomatitis [4, 13] or peritonsillar abscess [4] and decreased even after healing and in the absence of these lesions [4, 13]. In patients with radiation-induced oral mucositis, salivary EGF levels were significantly lower and inversely correlated with the severity of oral mucositis [14, 15]. The authors of the above reports all speculated that low salivary EGF levels reduced the capacity of the oral mucosa to heal and maintain physiologic integrity, thereby increasing susceptibility to intraoral inflammatory lesions [4, 13–15].

Patients with SS frequently develop refractory intraoral inflammatory lesions, such as oral mucositis and glossitis. In the present study, the comparisons between various subgroups of SS patients showed a close association between lower salivary EGF levels and poorer OHRQoL in patients with SS. This finding indicated that decreased salivary EGF levels, that is, deterioration in saliva quality accompanied by lower intraoral clearance owing to hyposalivation, could play a role in the pathogenesis of refractory intraoral manifestations and reduced OHRQoL. Moreover, in the present study, the OHRQoL and salivary EGF output but not the salivary flow rate decreased significantly in the same patients with SS only 3 years after the initial evaluation. Such findings were not observed in patients without SS. This decrease was especially striking in SS patients with long disease duration and progressive exacerbation of the OHRQoL. These findings strongly support the association between intraoral manifestations and decreased salivary EGF levels in SS and suggest that salivary EGF output decreases rapidly within a short period of time and progressive worsening of the OHRQoL depends on this rapid decrease in salivary EGF output when the SS disease duration becomes prolonged.

Topical EGF supplementation: a novel target for the therapeutic intervention of SS?

The currently accepted treatment for xerostomia in SS consists of maintaining good oral hygiene (e.g., mouthwash), using saliva substitutes (e.g., artificial saliva), and utilizing salivary stimulation (e.g., muscarinic M3 receptor agonists). The main purpose of these agents is to compensate for the reduced or inadequate supply of water via the natural saliva. Unfortunately, a substantial number of SS patients with refractory intraoral manifestations suffer from poor OHRQoL despite these treatments, especially in cases with long disease duration and declining residual salivary gland function. The findings of the present study and previous reports suggest that improving the quality of saliva by EGF supplementation into the oral cavity in combination with conventional treatments may promote mucosal healing, reduce the severity of intraoral manifestations, and ameliorate the OHRQoL in patients with SS. In previous studies using oral epithelial cell lines, the cell migration response [24] and the wound-closure effects [25] of EGF have been demonstrated. Girdler et al. [26] investigated the effect of an EGF mouthwash on oral ulceration in patients undergoing cancer chemotherapy. Although the rate of healing of established ulcers in patients who received EGF mouthwash and placebo did not differ, a delay in the onset and a smaller mean area of ulceration were noticed in the EGF mouthwash group. Patients develop oral mucosal manifestations rapidly in a few days after the initiation of chemotherapy. In SS, the progression of oral mucosal manifestations is not rapid compared with that as a consequence of chemotherapy. Considering the difference between the pathological mechanisms of both, we expect that topical EGF application will be more effective for SS patients than for patients undergoing chemotherapy. In addition, the EGF concentration was found to be decreased in the tear fluid of patients with SS [27, 28]. Tsubota et al. [29] reported that corneal epithelial damage decreased significantly after the initiation of treatment with autologous serum eye drops containing EGF, vitamin A, and transforming growth factor-β. These results strongly indicate that topical EGF application in the treatment of oral mucosal manifestations in patients with SS has not only an improving effect by EGF supplementation in patients with prolonged disease duration but also a prophylactic effect in patients with short disease duration. We expect that topical EGF application that can adhere to wounds longer than mouthwash (e.g., in the form of gel formulation) may lead to better results. However, the concentration and frequency of EGF administration remain to be elucidated. Excess EGF stimulates the proliferation and differentiation of malignant cells [30].

Conclusions

A decrease in salivary flow rates and salivary EGF output appears with the progression of SS. The deterioration in saliva quality as well as lower intraoral clearance by hyposalivation could contribute to the progression of the intraoral manifestations. We believe that our findings may lead to the development of novel effective therapies for SS.

Abbreviations
EGF: Epidermal growth factor; OHIP: Oral Health Impact Profile; OHRQoL: Oral health-related quality of life; QoL: Quality of life; SS: Sjögren's syndrome

Acknowledgements
The authors would like to express sincere appreciation to Prof. Hideyuki Okano for providing the opportunity to write this review article, to Sachie Kitano for the technical assistance, and to Dr. Aki Nishioka, Dr. Masahiro Sekiguchi, Dr. Masayasu Kitano, Dr. Naoaki Hashimoto, Dr. Kiyoshi Matsui, and Dr. Tsuyoshi Iwasaki for the data collection and useful comments.

Funding
This work was partly supported by a Grant-in-Aid for Scientific Research from the Japanese Ministry of Education, Culture, Sports, Science and Technology (MEXT KAKENHI Grant Number: 22791820) and grants for intractable disease from the Japanese Ministry of Health, Labour, and Welfare.

Authors' contributions
NA designed the study and wrote the manuscript. YK and HS contributed to the analysis and interpretation of the data and critically reviewed the manuscript. All authors read and approved the final version of the manuscript.

Authors' information
NA is a Lecturer at the Division of Rheumatology, Department of Internal Medicine, Hyogo College of Medicine, 1-1 Mukogawa-cho, Nishinomiya, Hyogo 663-8501, Japan. YK is a Director at the Division of General Medicine, Department of Internal Medicine, Sakai City Medical Center, 1-1-1 Ebaraji-cho, Nishi-ku, Sakai 593-8304, Japan. HS is a Professor and Chairman at the Division of Rheumatology, Department of Internal Medicine, Hyogo College of Medicine, 1-1 Mukogawa-cho, Nishinomiya, Hyogo 663-8501, Japan.

Competing interests
NA and YK declare that they have no competing interests. HS has received consulting fees, lecture fees, and/or honoraria from Mitsubishi Tanabe Pharma, Chugai Pharmaceutical, Astellas Pharma, and Kissei Pharmaceutical and has received research grants from Chugai Pharmaceutical and Astellas Pharma.

Author details
[1]Division of Rheumatology, Department of Internal Medicine, Hyogo College of Medicine, 1-1 Mukogawa-cho, Nishinomiya, Hyogo 663-8501, Japan. [2]Division of General Medicine, Department of Internal Medicine, Sakai City Medical Center, 1-1-1 Ebaraji-cho, Nishi-ku, Sakai 593-8304, Japan.

References

1. Stewart CM, Berg KM, Cha S, Reeves WH. Salivary dysfunction and quality of life in Sjögren syndrome: a critical oral-systemic connection. J Am Dent Assoc. 2008;139:291–9.
2. Zelles T, Purushotham KR, Macauley SP, Oxford GE, Humphreys-Beher MG. Saliva and growth factors: the fountain of youth resides in us all. J Dent Res. 1995;74:1826–32.
3. Cohen S. Isolation of a mouse submaxillary gland protein accelerating incisor eruption and eyelid opening in the new-born animal. J Biol Chem. 1962;237:1555–62.
4. Ino M, Ushiro K, Ino C, Yamashita T, Kumazawa T. Kinetics of epidermal growth factor in saliva. Acta Otolaryngol Suppl. 1993;500:126–30.
5. Heitz PU, Kasper M, van Noorden S, Polak JM, Gregory H, Pearse AG. Immunohistochemical localisation of urogastrone to human duodenal and submandibular glands. Gut. 1978;19:408–13.
6. Thesleff I, Viinikka L, Saxén L, Lehtonen E, Perheentupa J. The parotid gland is the main source of human salivary epidermal growth factor. Life Sci. 1988;43:13–8.
7. Ino M, Ushiro K, Ino C, Yamashita T, Kumazawa T, Takahashi T. Epidermal growth factor in salivary glands—epidermal growth factor and its receptor in human salivary glands—. Jibirinsho. 1992;85:805–14. (in Japanese).
8. Scaltriti M, Baselga J. The epidermal growth factor receptor pathway: a model for targeted therapy. Clin Cancer Res. 2006;12:5268–72.
9. Nakamura H, Kawakami A, Ida H, Koji T, Eguchi K. EGF activates PI3K-Akt and NF-κB via distinct pathways in salivary epithelial cells in Sjögren's syndrome. Rheumatol Int. 2007;28:127–36.
10. Noguchi S, Ohba Y, Oka T. Effect of salivary epidermal growth factor on wound healing of tongue in mice. Am J Phys. 1991;260(4 Pt 1):E620–5.
11. Fujisawa K, Miyamoto Y, Nagayama M. Basic fibroblast growth factor and epidermal growth factor reverse impaired ulcer healing of the rabbit oral mucosa. J Oral Pathol Med. 2003;32:358–66.
12. Playford RJ. Peptides and gastrointestinal mucosal integrity. Gut. 1995; 37:595–7.
13. Adişen E, Aral A, Aybay C, Gürer MA. Salivary epidermal growth factor levels in Behçet's disease and recurrent aphthous stomatitis. Dermatology. 2008; 217:235–40.
14. Dumbrigue HB, Sandow PL, Nguyen KH, Humphreys-Beher MG. Salivary epidermal growth factor levels decrease in patients receiving radiation therapy to the head and neck. Oral Surg Oral Med Oral Pathol Oral Radiol Endod. 2000;89:710–6.
15. Epstein JB, Gorsky M, Guglietta A, Le N, Sonis ST. The correlation between epidermal growth factor levels in saliva and the severity of oral mucositis during oropharyngeal radiation therapy. Cancer. 2000;89:2258–65.
16. Azuma N, Katada Y, Kitano S, Sekiguchi M, Kitano M, Nishioka A, et al. Correlation between salivary epidermal growth factor levels and refractory intraoral manifestations in patients with Sjögren's syndrome. Mod Rheumatol. 2014;24:626–32.
17. Azuma N, Katada Y, Kitano S, Sekiguchi M, Kitano M, Nishioka A, et al. Rapid decrease in salivary epidermal growth factor levels in patients with Sjögren's syndrome: a 3-year follow-up study. Mod Rheumatol. 2015;25:876–82.
18. Fujibayashi T, Sugai S, Miyasaka N, Hayashi Y, Tsubota K. Revised Japanese criteria for Sjögren's syndrome (1999): availability and validity. Mod Rheumatol. 2004;14:425–34.
19. Vitali C, Bombardieri S, Jonsson R, Moutsopoulos HM, Alexander EL, Carsons SE, et al. European study group on classification criteria for Sjögren's syndrome. Classification criteria for Sjögren's syndrome: a revised version of the European criteria proposed by the American-European Consensus Group. Ann Rheum Dis. 2002;61:554–8.
20. Slade GD. Derivation and validation of a short-form oral health impact profile. Community Dent Oral Epidemiol. 1997;25:284–90.
21. Yamazaki M, Inukai M, Baba K, John MT. Japanese version of the Oral Health Impact Profile (OHIP-J). J Oral Rehabil. 2007;34:159–68.
22. Koski H, Konttinen YT, Hietanen J, Tervo T, Malmöstrom M. Epidermal growth factor, transforming growth factor-alpha, and epidermal growth factor receptor in labial salivary glands in Sjögren's syndrome. J Rheumatol. 1997;24:1930–5.
23. Hutson JM, Niall M, Evans D, Fowler R. Effect of salivary glands on wound contraction in mice. Nature. 1979;279:793–5.
24. Royce LS, Baum BJ. Physiologic levels of salivary epidermal growth factor stimulate migration of an oral epithelial cell line. Biochim Biophys Acta. 1991;1092:401–3.
25. Oudhoff MJ, Bolscher JG, Nazmi K, Kalay H, van't Hof W, Amerongen AV, et al. Histatins are the major wound-closure stimulating factors in human saliva as identified in a cell culture assay. FASEB J. 2008;22:3805–12.
26. Girdler NM, McGurk M, Aqual S, Prince M. The effect of epidermal growth factor mouthwash on cytotoxic-induced oral ulceration. A phase I clinical trial. Am J Clin Oncol. 1995;18:403–6.
27. Pflugfelder SC, Jones D, Ji Z, Afonso A, Monroy D. Altered cytokine balance in the tear fluid and conjunctiva of patients with Sjögren's syndrome keratoconjunctivitis sicca. Curr Eye Res. 1999;19:201–11.
28. Ohashi Y, Ishida R, Kojima T, Goto E, Matsumoto Y, Watanabe K, et al. Abnormal protein profiles in tears with dry eye syndrome. Am J Ophthalmol. 2003;136:291–9.
29. Tsubota K, Goto E, Fujita H, Ono M, Inoue H, Saito I, et al. Treatment of dry eye by autologous serum application in Sjögren's syndrome. Br J Ophthalmol. 1999;83:390–5.
30. Tokunaga A, Onda M, Okuda T, Teramoto T, Fujita I, Mizutani T, et al. Clinical significance of epidermal growth factor (EGF), EGF receptor, and c-erbB-s in human gastric cancer. Cancer. 1995;75(6 Suppl):1418–25.

27

Cell transfer technology for tissue engineering

Keiko Akazawa[1], Kengo Iwasaki[2*], Mizuki Nagata[1], Naoki Yokoyama[3], Hirohito Ayame[3], Kazumasa Yamaki[3], Yuichi Tanaka[3], Izumi Honda[4], Chikako Morioka[5], Tsuyoshi Kimura[4], Motohiro Komaki[2], Akio Kishida[6], Yuichi Izumi[1] and Ikuo Morita[7]

Abstract: We recently developed novel cell transplantation method "cell transfer technology" utilizing photolithography. Using this method, we can transfer ex vivo expanded cells onto scaffold material in desired patterns, like printing of pictures and letters on a paper. We have investigated the possibility of this novel method for cell-based therapy using several disease models. We first transferred endothelial cells in capillary-like patterns on amnion. The transplantation of the endothelial cell-transferred amnion enhanced the reperfusion in mouse ischemic limb model. The fusion of transplanted capillary with host vessel networks was also observed. The osteoblast- and periodontal ligament stem cell-transferred amnion were next transplanted in bone and periodontal defects models. After healing period, both transplantations improved the regeneration of bone and periodontal tissues, respectively. This method was further applicable to transfer of multiple cell types and the transplantation of osteoblasts and periodontal ligament stem cell-transferred amnion resulted in the improved bone regeneration compared with single cell type transplantation. These data suggested the therapeutic potential of the technology in cell-based therapies for reperfusion of ischemic limb and regeneration of bone and periodontal tissues. Cell transfer technology is applicable to wide range of regenerative medicine in the future.

Keywords: Cell-based therapy, Cell transfer, Cell transplantation, Regeneration

Background

Recent progress in tissue engineering made it possible to treat various diseases using ex vivo expanded cells [1]. The possibility of the cell-based therapy for many diseases has been widely studied. The selection of cell culture methods, which facilitate therapeutic effect of the cells, and methods of transplantation, which include the ideal carrier for the local transplantation, are essential considerations in cell-based therapy [2]. We have developed novel cell transplantation method "cell transfer technology," utilizing photolithography, which is often used for micropatterning formation in semiconductor manufacturing and printing [3]. This technology allows us to transfer cultured cells onto scaffold material, like pictures and letters printed on a paper. We have investigated the possibility of this novel method for cell-based therapy using several disease models. In this review, we

outline the cell therapies that we have reported so far using the cell transfer technique.

Cell transfer using photolithography

Photolithography is a word with a prefix "photo" meaning light to "lithography," which is originated from lithograph. Literally, among various lithographic methods, photolithography uses the pattern made by light for document copy. Due to its precision, reproducibility, and mass productivity, photolithography is widely used in the precision machinery industry and printing. Photolithography consists mainly of two steps, namely the depiction of desired pattern on the substrate and "transfer" of the pattern to the product surface.

We have developed "cell transfer technology" that enables transfer of cultured cells onto the surface of transplantation scaffold. Figure 1 shows a schematic diagram of the cell transfer process by cell transfer technology. First, we made thin layer of tetraethyleneglycol (TEG) or polyethyleneglycol (PEG) on glass substrate. Next, we applied photomask on TEG/PEG layer and it was

* Correspondence: k-iwasaki.peri@tmd.ac.jp
[2]Department of Nanomedicine (DNP), Graduate School of Medical and Dental Sciences, Tokyo Medical and Dental University (TMDU), 1-5-45 Yushima, Bunkyo-ku, Tokyo 113-8510, Japan
Full list of author information is available at the end of the article

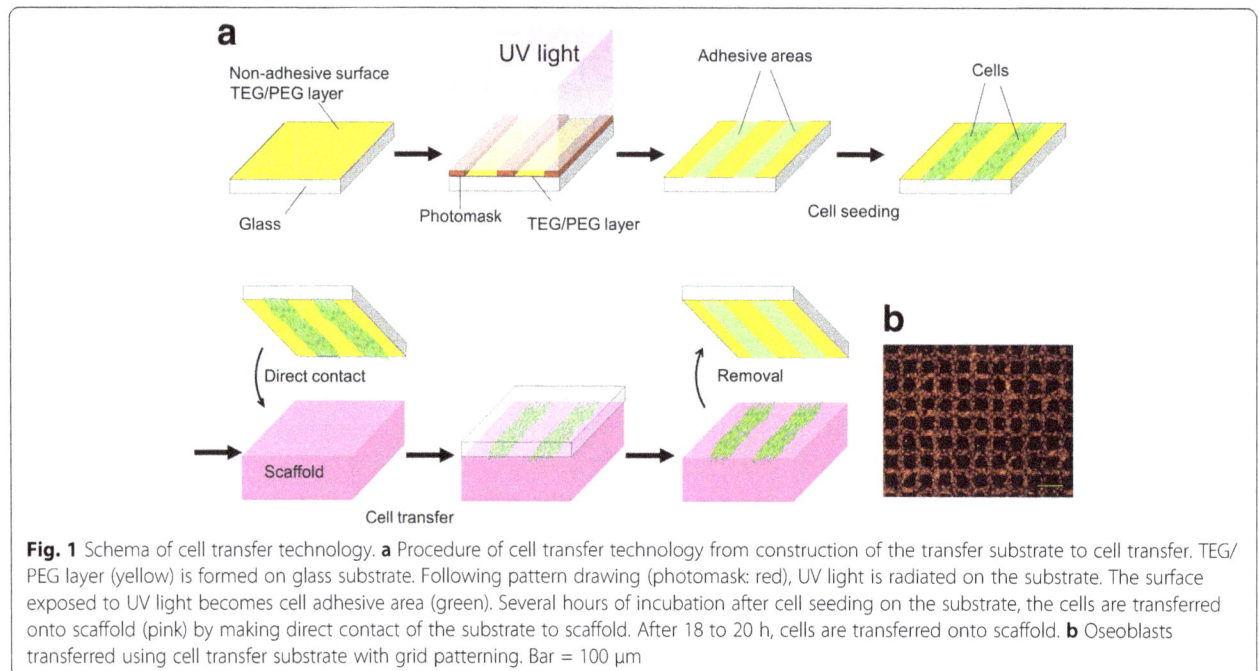

Fig. 1 Schema of cell transfer technology. **a** Procedure of cell transfer technology from construction of the transfer substrate to cell transfer. TEG/PEG layer (yellow) is formed on glass substrate. Following pattern drawing (photomask: red), UV light is radiated on the substrate. The surface exposed to UV light becomes cell adhesive area (green). Several hours of incubation after cell seeding on the substrate, the cells are transferred onto scaffold (pink) by making direct contact of the substrate to scaffold. After 18 to 20 h, cells are transferred onto scaffold. **b** Oseoblasts transferred using cell transfer substrate with grid patterning. Bar = 100 μm

exposed to ultraviolet light. Ultraviolet irradiation partially collapses TEG/PEG chain and made the difference in the length of remaining TEG/PEG chain between photo-masked and non-masked surface. The remaining length of TEG/PEG appears as the difference between hydrophilicity and hydrophobicity of the substrate surface. This difference is involved in the strength of cell adhesion to the substrate surface (Fig. 2). Area with disrupted TEG/PEG is cell adhesive and area with preserved TEG/PEG by photomasking is non-adhesive.

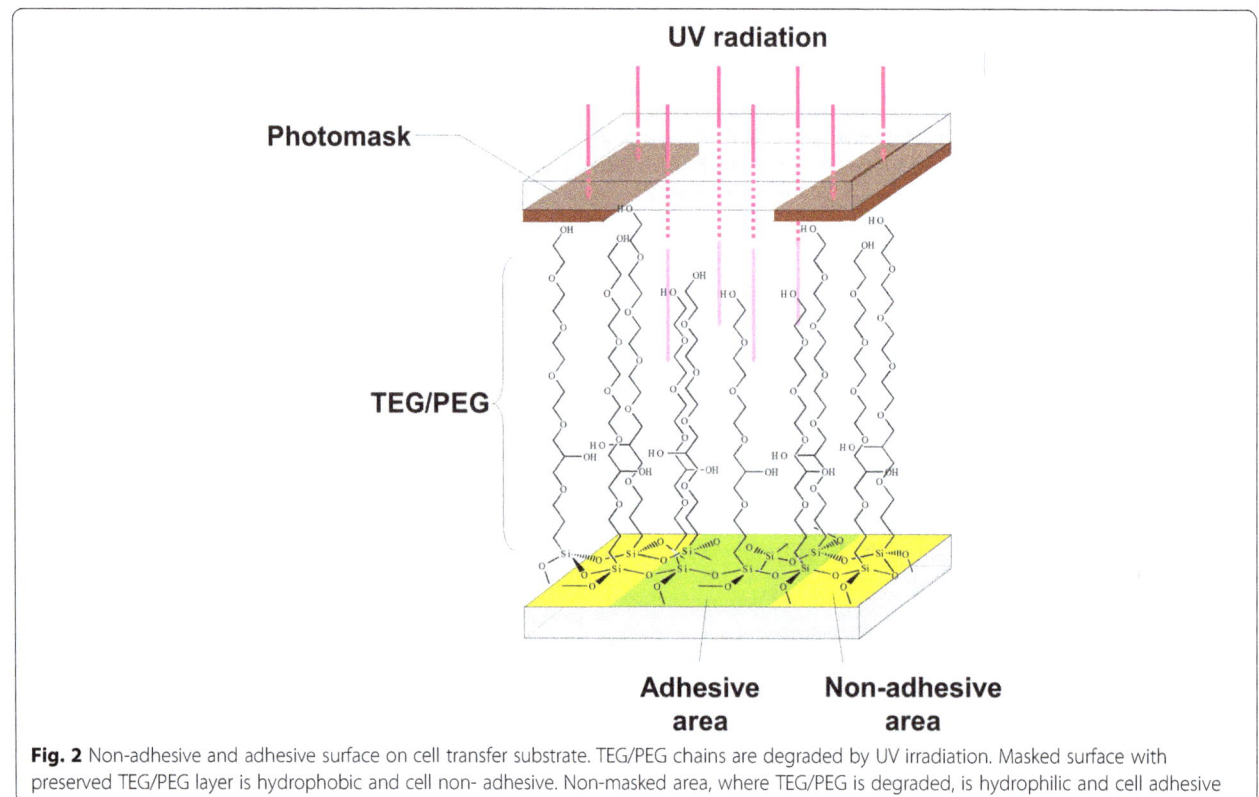

Fig. 2 Non-adhesive and adhesive surface on cell transfer substrate. TEG/PEG chains are degraded by UV irradiation. Masked surface with preserved TEG/PEG layer is hydrophobic and cell non-adhesive. Non-masked area, where TEG/PEG is degraded, is hydrophilic and cell adhesive

Using this difference in hydrophilicity/hydrophilicity, it is possible to stick cells on substrate according to various patterns made by photomasking. Figure 1b demonstrates PKH26-labeled osteoblasts adhered to substrate with grid-like patterning. After adhesion of cells onto substrate, the substrate was placed onto scaffold material making direct contact of the cell surface to scaffold. Eighteen to 24 h later, cells were transferred onto scaffold upon removal of the substrate. The transfer substrate was easily removed from scaffold without any disturbance to the cells. In this step, the strength of substrate-cell adhesion must be less than that between carrier and cells. This can be controlled by the strength and duration of the UV irradiation on TEG/PEG surface after masking. The degradation rate of PEG/TEG can be optimized to maximize the cell transfer efficiency. After removal of the transfer substrate from the scaffold, cells were transferred onto the scaffold surface and were then ready for transplantation.

For surface coating of the transfer substrate, we first coated glass the plate with fluoroalkyl silane (FAS). However, because of the lower stability of patterning on the substrate, FAS was replaced with PEG/TEG. We observed longer stability of patterns made with PEG/TEG on the substrate compared with those made with FAS. The time needed for cell transfer was also found to be shorter for PEG/TEG substrate than that with FAS.

Amnion as a scaffold

Using cell transfer technology, ex vivo expanded cells were transferred to scaffold materials including hydrogels. Among these, we have used amnion, a part of amniotic membrane, as a scaffold material for cell transfer because of its elasticity, flexibility, and high success rate of cell transfer. Amniotic membrane is the biological membrane forming amniotic sac, which keeps and protects amniotic fluid and embryo inside [4]. Amniotic membrane could be obtained at the time of delivery; however, it is discarded in general. The membrane is composed of amnion and chorion [5]. Amnion is the inner layer of the amniotic membrane. Amnion has been used to treat dermal burns and ulceration, necrosis, and severe inflammation of eyes as dressing material, taking advantage of its anti-microbial and anti-fibrosis property [6, 7]. We isolated amnion from egg membrane by the removal of chorion, and cell components were removed from amnion by high-hydrostatic pressure treatment [8, 9]. The resulting decellurized amnion was used for cell transfer. Considering clinical applications, further evaluations are needed to determine the safety of the membrane in humans.

Almost 100% of cells on transfer substrate were successfully transferred onto amnion after several hours of incubation. Amnion is great scaffold material for cell

transfer, as to facilitate high transfer efficiency. Moreover, the most prominent characteristics of amnion upon cell transfer is the stability of transferred cells on the membrane [10, 11]. The transferred cells on amnion are firmly adhered to amnion surface, and this makes it possible to deform and trim the membrane with surgical instruments [10, 11]. This unique characteristic allows easy and reliable cell transplantation.

Patterned and layered cell transfer

One of the notable features of photolithography is precise transfer of substances according to the fine pattering drawn on substrate. Taking advantage of this unique characteristic of photolithography, we are able to transfer cells in any desired patterns onto scaffold. We made patterns resembling to capillaries on glass substrate and tried to make capillaries by tissue engineering approach. We seeded bovine carotid artery endothelial cells (BCAECs) on transfer substrate with capillary-like pattering and transfer them onto amnion [12]. BCAECs, transferred onto amnion, showed capillary-like structure, and it was also revealed in electron microscopy that the capillary was consisted of vessel wall by BCAECs and lumen inside. We transplanted the BCAEC-transferred amnion into mouse auricle and found that the capillary was kept its structure until 5 days after transplantation. In vivo imaging demonstrated that the capillary functioned in host mouse ear. It is thus conceivable that mimicking the anatomical structure of target tissue, prior to transplantation, may favor the results of cell transplantation. Microvasculature is one good example of this type of cell transplantation.

On the other hand, we can also fabricate cell transfer substrate with whole cell adhesive characteristics. With this substrate, cells are transferred onto amnion in layer structure. In case of cell transplantation requires cell numbers, not positioning, this sheet-like cell transplantation material is useful. We succeeded in transfer of cells and fabricating cell sheet-like materials using various cell types such as fibroblasts, mesenchymal stem cells (MSC), osteoblasts, and endothelial cells [10–13]. Approximately, 5×10^5 cells/cm^2 were transferred onto an amnion using the cell transfer technology. Furthermore, we transferred two different cell types in overlapping two layers using cell transfer technology and named it "double cell transfer" [11]. For this double cell transfer, we cultured two cell types on transfer substrate and transfer them through single transfer process. This method was applicable to three different cell types and triple cell layers were successfully fabricated. This multiple cell transfer may enable unique cell transplantation considering three-dimensional cell structure and cell-cell communication.

Various cell patterning and cell sheet formation methods have been reported. For cell patterning, two modalities have been mainly studied. One is to utilize the specificity of cell adhesion to the extracellular matrix for cell placement, and this can form sharp edge of patterns [14, 15]. However, it is difficult to form patterns using more than two types of cells using this method. The other method involves the use of "force" to locate cells, including magnetic, electrokinetic, and fluidic forces [16–18]. These methods allow manipulation of large cell numbers, but some of them need labeling of cells and may affect cell viability. The use of temperature responsive polymers has been studied and reported for cell sheet formation [19]. Cell sheets made through this method are too fragile to directly manipulate with surgical instruments. Our method generates a cell sheet by transferring a single cell layer onto a scaffold surface and endows physical strength that achieves stable cell transplantation.

Cell transplantation using cell transfer technology in animal models

Ischemic vascular disease

Ischemic vascular diseases, including myocardial infarction, cerebral infarction, and peripheral arterial embolism, develop by the absence of blood flow due to blockage of the artery and veins [20, 21]. Arterial bypass graft surgery or percutaneous endovascular angioplasty has been performed to restore blood flow for these diseases [22, 23]. Recently, many studies have reported that ischemic conditions were improved by the injection or transplantation of various types of cultured cells including bone marrow-derived mononuclear cells, hematopoietic stem cells, vascular endothelial cells, and endothelial progenitor cells [24, 25]. We fabricated endothelial cell-transferred amnion using transfer substrate with capillary patterning and examined its possibility for the treatment of ischemic diseases by transplanting it into limb ischemia mouse model (Fig. 3) [12]. Reperfusion of ischemic limb was observed after the transplantation of endothelial cell-transferred amnion in laser doppler blood flow and necrosis of the lower limb and gait disturbance were improved. Transplanted capillary fused with the host vascular networks and functioned 5 days after the transplantation. This capillary transplantation is an intermediate method between conventional bypass surgery and cell transplantation and could be new therapeutic option for ischemic disease. To make more stable transplantable capillary, some modifications have been under investigation such as formation of endothelial cell capillary with mural cells.

Bone defect

For bone defects caused by tumor resection and fracture, various treatment strategies have been investigated

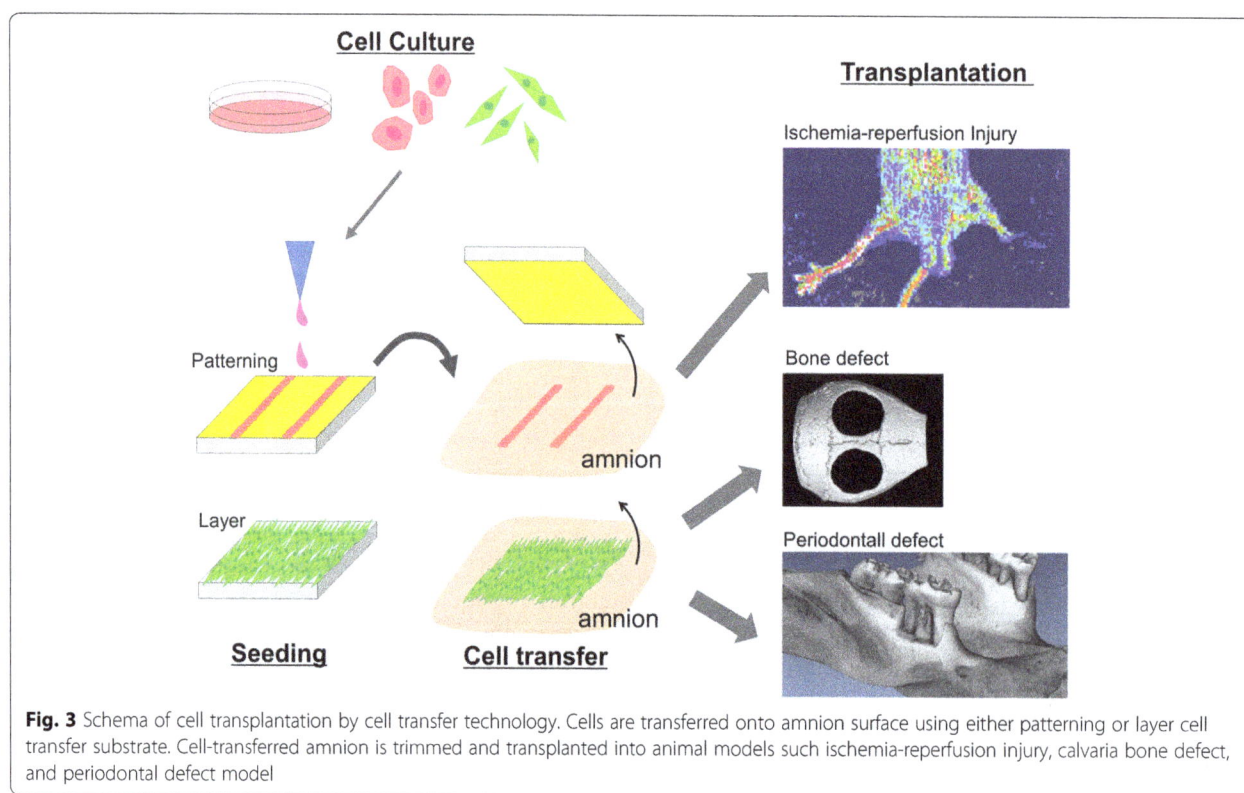

Fig. 3 Schema of cell transplantation by cell transfer technology. Cells are transferred onto amnion surface using either patterning or layer cell transfer substrate. Cell-transferred amnion is trimmed and transplanted into animal models such ischemia-reperfusion injury, calvaria bone defect, and periodontal defect model

including local application of growth factor with bone-forming activity such as bone morphogenetic proteins and transplantation of autologous or allogeanic bone graft and artificial bone substitute materials such as hydroxyapatite and beta-tricalcium phosphate [26, 27]. Recently, the therapeutic potential of cell transplantation was proposed for bone defect and regeneration of bone defect have been reported by the transplantation of MSC and osteoblasts [28, 29]. We made transfer substrate with entire cell adhesive surface and transferred mouse osteoblasts (Kusa-A1) onto amnion (Fig. 3) [13]. Mouse calvaria bony defect was created, and the osteoblast-transferred amnion was placed to cover the defect. Approximately, 7.8×10^4 cells were transplanted per defect. After 5 weeks, complete closure of bone defect was observed in osteoblast-transplanted defect while control defect did not show the healing. Compared with other test groups including injection of osteoblast, only amnion transplantation, and no treatment, significant bone regeneration was found in osteoblast-transferred amnion defects. Transplanted osteoblasts were found around newly formed bone 5 weeks post operation, and it is suggested that those osteoblasts are directly involved in the regeneration of bone. The firm adhesion of osteoblasts to amnion may contribute to the longer cell retention in bone defects and the prominent bone regeneration observed in osteoblast-amnion transplantation compared with that in cell injection. These results suggested the therapeutic potential of osteoblast-transferred amnion for the treatment of bone defect. We also observed the improvement in bone healing by transplanting double cell-transferred amnion, made using osteoblasts and MSC from periodontal ligament (periodontal ligament stem cells, PDLSC) [11]. We transferred human primary osteoblasts and PDLSC onto amnion to form osteoblast-PDLSC layers on the membrane and transplanted them into mouse calvarial bone defect model. Eight weeks after the transplantation, we observed the enhanced bone regeneration in osteoblast-PDLSC transplanted defects compared with single cell transplanted (osteoblasts or PDLSC alone) defects. These results suggested the clinical feasibility of cell transfer technology in bone regeneration.

Periodontal defect

Periodontal disease is characterized by the chronic inflammation and destruction of tooth supporting tissues including bone, periodontal ligament, and cementum mainly due to infection of gram-negative bacteria [30]. Conventional periodontal treatments consisted of mechanical removal of bacterial factors, and it leads to reduction of inflammation and stability of disease status [31]. However, reconstruction of tooth supporting tissues, lost by the disease progression, was hardly observed. Although several regenerative approaches have been applied clinically, sufficient regeneration has not yet been achieved. Recently, it has been

demonstrated that cell transplantation is effective in regeneration of periodontal tissues, including bone, periodontal ligament, and cementum, using bone marrow-derived MSC, adipose-derived MSC, PDLSC, and periosteum-derived cells [32]. We made periodontal defect model by removing bone, cementum, and periodontal ligament in rat maxillary molar and transplanted cells using cell transfer technology (Fig. 3) [10]. As a cell type for transplantation, we selected PDLSC because they have been shown to possess the differentiation capacity into various linages of cells such as osteoblast, adipocyte, chondrocyte, and cementoblast [33]. We examined the regenerative potential of PDLSC-transferred amnion (PDLSC-amnion) by transplanting it into surgically created periodontal defect and compared with the defect transplanted with amnion alone. After 4 weeks of healing period, enhanced periodontal tissue regeneration was observed in PDLSC-amnion transplanted defects. Newly regenerated cementum, periodontal ligament, and bone were observed in histological sections. These results suggested that transplantation of PDLSC-amnion could be a novel periodontal regenerative therapy.

Conclusion

We developed novel cell transplantation method "cell transfer technology" using photolithography technique. By transplanting cell transferred-amnion made by the method, we have demonstrated the therapeutic potential of the material in cell-based treatment including reperfusion of ischemic limb and regeneration of bone and periodontal tissues. Forming a fine patterning by cultured cell is the most unique characteristics of cell transfer technique. In this regard, capillary patterning grafting is taking full advantage of this technology. However, the cell transplantation, which requires cell patterning, might be rather limited. Therefore, cell sheet-like amnion, which we used for bone and periodontal defects, maybe widely applicable for tissue regeneration. Depending on the target tissue to be regenerated, we can select patterned or non-patterned cell transfer substrate. We also found that the transferred cells are firmly and stably adhered on amnion and withstand against the deformation and movement of the membrane by surgical manipulations. Additionally, the flexibility of amnion enables us to transplant cultured cell in direct contact with defects or tissue surface, which is vital importance in certain regenerative cases. Taking these advantages and unique features, cell transfer technology is applicable to wide range of regenerative medicine in the future.

Abbreviations
BCAEC: Bovine carotid artery endothelial cell; MSC: Mesenchymal stem cells; PDLSC: Periodontal ligament stem cells; PEG: Polyethyleneglycol; TEG: Tetraethyleneglycol

Acknowledgements
The authors would like to thank all our laboratory members for their helpful and constructive comments to this study.

Funding
This work is supported by the JSPS KAKENHI Grant Numbers 15K11381, 15K11342, and 15K11380.

Authors' contributions
KA, KI, MN, and MK performed the research. IH and CM contributed collection of amniotic membrane. YT, NY, HA, and KY fabricated cell transfer base. TK, AK, and KA contributed decellularization of amnion. KA, KI, and IM wrote the manuscript. All authors read and approved the content of the manuscript.

Competing interests
The authors declare that they have no competing interests.

Author details
[1]Department of Periodontology, Graduate School of Medical and Dental Sciences, Tokyo Medical and Dental University (TMDU), 1-5-45 Yushima, Bunkyo-ku, Tokyo 113-8510, Japan. [2]Department of Nanomedicine (DNP), Graduate School of Medical and Dental Sciences, Tokyo Medical and Dental University (TMDU), 1-5-45 Yushima, Bunkyo-ku, Tokyo 113-8510, Japan. [3]Life Science Laboratory, Research and Development Center, Dai Nippon Printing Co., Ltd., 1-1-1 Kaga-cho, Shinjuku-ku, Tokyo 162-8001, Japan. [4]Department of Comprehensive Reproductive Medicine, Graduate School of Medical and Dental Science, Tokyo Medical and Dental University, 1-5-45 Yushima, Bunkyo-ku, Tokyo 113-8510, Japan. [5]Department of Pediatrics and Developmental Biology, Graduate School of Medical and Dental Science, Tokyo Medical and Dental University (TMDU), 1-5-45 Yushima, Bunkyo-ku, Tokyo 113-8510, Japan. [6]Department of Material-based Medical Engineering, Institute of Biomaterials and Bioengineering, Tokyo Medical and Dental University (TMDU), 2-3-10, Kanda-Surugadai, Chiyoda-ku, Tokyo 101-0062, Japan. [7]Department of Cellular Physiological Chemistry, Graduate School of Medical and Dental Sciences, Tokyo Medical and Dental University (TMDU), 1-5-45 Yushima, Bunkyo-ku, Tokyo 113-8510, Japan.

References
1. Langer R, Vacanti JP. Tissue engineering. Science. 1993;260:920–6.
2. Howard D, Buttery LD, Shakesheff KM, Roberts SJ. Tissue engineering: strategies, stem cells and scaffolds. J Anat. 2008;213:66–72.
3. Kobayashi A, Miyake H, Hattori H, Kuwana R, Hiruma Y, Nakahama K, Ichinose S, Ota M, Nakamura M, Takeda S, Morita I. In vitro formation of capillary networks using optical lithographic techniques. Biochem Biophys Res Commun. 2007;358:692–7.
4. Niknejad H, Peirovi H, Jorjani M, Ahmadiani A, Ghanavi J, Seifalian AM. Properties of the amniotic membrane for potential use in tissue engineering. Eur Cell Mater. 2008;15:88–99.
5. Toda A, Okabe M, Yoshida T, Nikaido T. The potential of amniotic membrane/amnion-derived cells for regeneration of various tissues. J Pharmacol Sci. 2007;105:215–28.
6. Lo V, Pope E. Amniotic membrane use in dermatology. Int J Dermatol. 2009; 48:935–40.
7. Altan-Yaycioglu R, Akova YA, Oto S. Amniotic membrane transplantation for treatment of symblepharon in a patient with recessive dystrophic epidermolysis bullosa. Cornea. 2006;25:971–3.
8. Fujisato T, Minatoya K, Yamazaki S, Meng Y, Niwaya K, Kishida A, Nakatani T, Kitamura S. Preparation and recellularization of tissue engineered

9. Wilshaw SP, Kearney JN, Fisher J, Ingham E. Production of an acellular amniotic membrane matrix for use in tissue engineering. Tissue Eng. 2006;12:2117–29.
10. Iwasaki K, Komaki M, Yokoyama N, Tanaka Y, Taki A, Honda I, Kimura Y, Takeda M, Akazawa K, Oda S, Izumi Y, Morita I. Tissue Eng Part A. 2014;20:693–704.
11. Akazawa K, Iwasaki K, Nagata M, Yokoyama N, Ayame H, Yamaki K, Tanaka Y, Honda I, Morioka C, Kimura T, Komaki M, Kishida A, Izumi Y, Morita I. Sci Rep. 2016;6:33286.
12. Akahori T, Kobayashi A, Komaki M, Hattori H, Nakahama K, Ichinose S, Abe M, Takeda S, Morita I. Implantation of capillary structure engineered by optical lithography improves hind limb ischemia in mice. Tissue Eng Part A. 2010;16:953–9.
13. Tsugawa J, Komaki M, Yoshida T, Nakahama K, Amagasa T, Morita I. Cell-printing and transfer technology applications for bone defects in mice. J Tissue Eng Regen Med. 2011;5:695–703.
14. Fukuda J, Khademhosseini A, Yeh J, Eng G, Cheng J, Farokhzad OC, Langer R. Micropatterned cell co-cultures using layer-by-layer deposition of extracellular matrix components. Biomaterials. 2006;27:1479–86.
15. Zhang S, Yan L, Altman M, Lässle M, Nugent H, Frankel F, Lauffenburger DA, Whitesides GM, Rich A. Biological surface engineering: a simple system for cell pattern formation. Biomaterials. 1999;20:1213–20.
16. Chiu DT, Jeon NL, Huang S, Kane RS, Wargo CJ, Choi IS, Ingber DE, Whitesides GM. Patterned deposition of cells and proteins onto surfaces by using three-dimensional microfluidic systems. Proc Natl Acad Sci U S A. 2000;97:2408–13.
17. Ozkan M, Pisanic T, Scheel J, Barlow C, Esener S, Bhatia SN. Electro-optical platform for the manipulation of live cells. Langmuir. 2003;19:1532–8.
18. Chiou PY, Ohta AT, Wu MC. Massively parallel manipulation of single cells and microparticles using optical images. Nature. 2005;436:370–2.
19. Elloumi-Hannachi I, Yamato M, Okano T. Cell sheet engineering: a unique nanotechnology for scaffold-free tissue reconstruction with clinical applications in regenerative medicine. J Intern Med. 2010;267:54–70.
20. Schaller B, Graf R. Cerebral ischemia and reperfusion: the pathophysiologic concept as a basis for clinical therapy. J Cereb Blood Flow Metab. 2004;24:351–71.
21. Shimokawa H, Yasuda S. Myocardial ischemia: current concepts and future perspectives. J Cardiol. 2008;52:67–78.
22. Ferket BS, Spronk S, Colkesen EB, Hunink MG. Systematic review of guidelines on peripheral artery disease screening. Am J Med. 2012;125:198–208.
23. Allemang MT, Rajani RR, Nelson PR, Hingorani A, Kashyap VS. Prescribing patterns of antiplatelet agents are highly variable after lower extremity endovascular procedures. Ann Vasc Surg. 2013;27:62–7.
24. Aranguren XL, Verfaillie CM, Luttun A. Emerging hurdles in stem cell therapy for peripheral vascular disease. J Mol Med. 2009;87:3–16.
25. Sieveking DP, Ng MK. Cell therapies for therapeutic angiogenesis: back to the bench. Vasc Med. 2009;14:153–66.
26. Dimitriou R, Jones E, McGonagle D, Giannoudis PV. Bone regeneration: current concepts and future directions. BMC Med. 2011;9:66.
27. McAllister BS, Haghighat K. Bone augmentation techniques. J Periodontol. 2007;78:377–94.
28. Colnot C. Skeletal cell fate decisions within periosteum and bone marrow during bone regeneration. J Bone Miner Res. 2009;24:274–82.
29. Akahane M, Nakamura A, Ohgushi H, Shigematsu H, Dohi Y, Takakura Y. Osteogenic matrix sheet-cell transplantation using osteoblastic cell sheet resulted in bone formation without scaffold at an ectopic site. J Tissue Eng Regen Med. 2008;2:196–201.
30. Pihlstrom BL, Michalowicz BS, Johnson NW. Periodontal diseases. Lancet. 2005;366:1809–20.
31. Graziani F, Karapetsa D, Alonso B, Herrera D. Nonsurgical and surgical treatment of periodontitis: how many options for one disease? Periodontol 2000. 2017;75:152–88.
32. Ishikawa I, Iwata T, Washio K, Okano T, Nagasawa T, Iwasaki K, Ando T. Cell sheet engineering and other novel cell-based approaches to periodontal regeneration. Periodontol 2000. 2009;51:220–38.
33. Seo BM, Miura M, Gronthos S, Bartold PM, Batouli S, Brahim J, Young M, Robey PG, Wang CY, Shi S. Investigation of multipotent postnatal stem cells from human periodontal ligament. Lancet. 2004;364:149–55.

28

Transcriptome analysis of peripheral blood from patients with rheumatoid arthritis

Shuji Sumitomo[1], Yasuo Nagafuchi[1], Yumi Tsuchida[1], Haruka Tsuchiya[1], Mineto Ota[1], Kazuyoshi Ishigaki[2], Akari Suzuki[3], Yuta Kochi[3], Keishi Fujio[1*] and Kazuhiko Yamamoto[4]

Abstract

In the era of precision medicine, transcriptome analysis of whole gene expression is an essential technology. While DNA microarray has a limited dynamic range and a problem of background hybridization, RNA sequencing (RNA-seq) has a broader dynamic range and a lower background signal that increase the sensitivity and reproducibility. While transcriptome analyses in rheumatoid arthritis (RA) have generally focused on whole peripheral blood mononuclear cells (PBMC), analyses of detailed cell subsets have an increased need for understanding the pathophysiology of disease because the involvement of CD4+ T cells in the pathogenesis of RA has been established. Transcriptome analysis of detailed CD4+ T cell subsets or neutrophils shed new light on the pathophysiology of RA. There are several analyses about the effect of biological treatment. Many studies report the association between type I interferon signature gene expression and response to therapy.

Keywords: Rheumatoid arthritis, Transcriptome analysis, RNA sequencing (RNA-seq)

Background

Rheumatoid arthritis (RA) is an autoimmune disease characterized by chronic inflammatory synovitis and progressive disability. Environmental factors including smoking [1] and periodontitis, epigenetic modification, and susceptibility genes [2] generate self-proteins with a citrulline residue by post-translational modification. Breakdown of immunological tolerance to citrullinated self-proteins is considered to be an important feature of RA pathogenesis [3]. This anticitrulline response can be detected in T cell and B cell compartments and is probably initiated in secondary lymphoid tissues or bone marrow. Thereafter, synovitis occurs when leukocytes infiltrate the synovial compartment [4]. Synovium is the principal target of inflammation in RA, and the resident fibroblast-like synoviocytes (FLSs) are implicated in the pathogenesis of synovitis [5].

There is much interest in transcriptome analysis as a mechanism for predicting RA pathogenesis and effect of treatment. Gene expression profiling is a quantitative measurement of messenger RNA levels for thousands of genes at once, to create a global picture of cellular function and contribute to the era of stratified medicine [6]. DNA microarrays have been used to drive genetic analyses for more than two decades. However, microarrays have limited dynamic range that often prevents accurate assessment of low signal intensities, and suffer from the problem of background hybridization. Such limitations are largely absent in RNA sequencing (RNA-seq), a next-generation sequencing (NGS) method largely used for the genome-wide measurement of RNA abundance. Compared with microarrays, RNA-seq has several advantages, such as low background signal, a broader dynamic range, increased sensitivity, and high reproducibility [7].

Transcriptome analyses in RA generally focused on whole peripheral blood mononuclear cells (PBMC) [8, 9]. However, the importance of cell-type specificity is becoming increasingly apparent in gene expression work. Cell-type specificity would be missed in whole blood samples, especially when investigating low abundance genes. Moreover, dynamic variations in leukocyte subsets may confound the interpretation of results [6].

* Correspondence: kfujio-tky@umin.ac.jp
[1]Department of Allergy and Rheumatology, Graduate School of Medicine, the University of Tokyo, 7-3-1 Hongo, Bunkyo-ku, Tokyo 113-8655, Japan
Full list of author information is available at the end of the article

Transcriptome analyses also contribute to the understandings of the effect of treatment. For example, transcriptome analysis revealed that type I interferon (IFN) signature genes were particularly associated with clinical response to bDMARDs including TNF-α inhibitor [10], tocilizumab [8], and rituximab [9]. In the analysis of the effect of treatment, samples must be taken at the same time points and from the same source in order to lead biologically meaningful comparative transcriptome analyses. Moreover, longitudinal studies may yield more relevant answers compared to cross-sectional studies.

In this review, we discuss the transcriptome analysis of various cell subsets in PBMC of RA and analysis about the effect of biological treatment.

Main text
CD4+ T cells
The involvement of CD4+ T cells in the pathogenesis of RA has been established based on the fact that HLA-DRB1 genotype is by far the strongest genetic risk factor for RA [2]. Moreover, RA genetic risk loci preferentially map to enhancers and promoters active in CD4+ T cell subpopulations [11]. We conducted expression quantitative trait loci (eQTL) analysis on five subsets of immune cells (CD4+ T cells, CD8+ T cells, B cells, natural killer (NK) cells, and monocytes) and unfractionated peripheral blood from 105 healthy Japanese volunteers. We developed a three-step analytical pipeline comprising (i) prediction of individual gene expression using our eQTL database and public epigenomic data, (ii) gene-level association analysis, and (iii) prediction of cell-specific pathway activity by integrating the direction of eQTL effects. By applying this pipeline to RA GWAS data sets, the tumor necrosis factor (TNF) pathway was predicted to be significantly activated, specifically in CD4+ T cells [12].

Ye et al. examined the whole-genome transcription profile of CD4+ T cells in RA compared with healthy individuals using microarray analysis [13]. They reported that CD4+ T cells from patients with RA have abnormal functional networks in STAT3 signaling and Wnt signaling. Their results also suggested that the aberrant expression of several zinc finger transcription factors (ZEB1, ZNF292, and ZNF644) may be potential pathogenic factors for RA.

CD4+ T cell subsets
There are few reports for detailed transcriptome analysis of CD4+ T cell subsets in RA. Although contributions of Th17 cells [14], regulatory T cells (Treg) [15], and follicular helper T cells (Tfh) [16] have been reported, the actual modifications of CD4+ T cells in RA have not been elucidated. We performed RNA-seq of seven CD4+ T cell subsets (naive, Th1, Th17, Th1/17, nonTh1/17, Tfh, and Treg) of peripheral blood taken from RA patients and healthy controls (HC) [17]). We found that

several pathways including GTPase-associated signaling and apoptosis signaling were upregulated in RA as previously reported [18, 19]. Weighted gene co-expression network analysis (WGCNA) [20] identified a gene module that consisted of 227 genes and was correlated with DAS28-CRP. The most highly connected 30 genes of this module included ZAP70 and JAK3, and pathway analysis of this module revealed dysregulation of the TCR signaling pathway network.

Co-stimulatory molecules
Abatacept is a fusion protein composed of the Fc region of immunoglobulin and the extracellular domain of CTLA-4 that inhibits T cell activation by blocking co-stimulation [21]. We performed RNA-seq of seven CD4+ T cell subsets (naive, Th1, Th17, Th1/17, nonTh1/17, Tfh, and Treg) of peripheral blood taken from RA patients before and 6 months after abatacept treatment [17]. Overview of expression pattern of RA revealed that administration of abatacept exerts a large shift toward the expression pattern of healthy control. Knowledge-based pathway analysis revealed the upregulation of activation-related pathways in RA that was substantially ameliorated by abatacept. We found that dysregulated TCR signaling pathways in RA were detected in RA through CD4+ T cell subsets and ameliorated by abatacept treatment.

B cells
Rituximab is monoclonal anti-CD20 antibody and used to treat RA and B cell non-Hodgkin's lymphoma although RA treatment has not been approved in Japan. Sellam et al. performed microarray of whole peripheral blood samples of RA patients before and 24 weeks after treatment of rituximab [9]. They detected signature 143 genes for response featured upregulation of inflammatory genes centered on NF-kB, including IL33 and STAT5A, and downregulation of the IFN pathway. This signature accurately identifies patients with RA who will not respond to rituximab therapy. Raterman et al. also performed microarray of whole peripheral blood samples and found that the baseline expression of type I IFN response genes (LY6E, HERC5, IFI44L, ISG15, MxA, MxB, EPSTI1, and RSAD2) could be useful as a predictive biomarker for non-response to rituximab in RA [22]. Relationship between the type I IFN signature and the response to rituximab in RA had been reported by others [23, 24].

Neutrophils
Wright et al. performed RNA-Seq of RA neutrophils to identify pre-therapy gene expression signatures that correlate with disease activity or response to TNF inhibitor (TNFi) therapy [10]. Pathway analysis predicted activation of IFN signaling in RA neutrophils, identifying 178 IFN-response genes regulated by IFN-α, IFN-β, or IFN-γ.

Patients could be categorized as IFN-high or IFN-low. Patients in the IFN-high group achieved a better response to TNFi therapy than patients in the IFN-low group. IFN-response genes are significantly upregulated in RA neutrophils compared with healthy controls. Higher IFN-response gene expression in RA neutrophils correlates with a good response to TNFi therapy.

Proinflammatory cytokines

Koczan et al. performed microarray of PBMC of RA patients before the first application of the TNFα blocker etanercept as well as after 72 h [25]. Early downregulation of expression levels was associated with good clinical responses. Informative gene sets include genes (NFKBIA, CCL4, IL8, IL1B, TNFAIP3, PDE4B, PPP1R15A, and ADM) involved in different pathways and cellular processes such as TNFα signaling via NFκB; Van Baarsen et al. performed microarray of PBMC of RA patients before and 1 month after infliximab treatment [26]. While the change in IFN response genes was unrelated to baseline expression levels, treatment-induced increase of IFN response gene activity was associated with poor clinical response to infliximab treatment.

Sanayama et al. performed genome-wide DNA microarray of PBMC of RA patients before and after treatment with an anti-IL-6 receptor antibody, tocilizumab [8]. They found that three type I IFN response genes (IFI6, MX2, and OASL) and MT1G was significantly different between nonresponders and responders. MT1G encodes metallothionein-1G, a member of the metallothionein (MT) proteins that are involved in protection against oxidative stress and inflammatory responses. The MT-1 promoter contains a STAT binding site, and the gene expression of MT-1 is directly upregulated by IL-6. They suggested that type I IFN signaling and metallothioneins are involved in the pathophysiology of RA. Saito et al. performed microarray of CD4$^+$ T cells before and after treatment with tocilizumab [27]. They found that ARID-5A was downregulated by tocilizumab therapy. ARID-5A was a lineage-specific attenuator of Th17 cell differentiation and might be involved in the pathogenesis of RA.

Future perspective

While we have reviewed transcriptome analysis of peripheral blood from RA patients, there are several reports of specimens other than peripheral blood, mainly synovial tissue [28] and FLS [29]. Dennis et al. revealed that baseline synovial myeloid, but not lymphoid, gene signature expression was higher in patients with good compared with poor clinical response to anti-TNFα therapy [28]. Galligans et al. analyzed gene expression of FLS obtained from RA and osteoarthritis (OA), and identified 34 genes specific to RA and OA FLS, and 8 genes correlated with RA disease activity. Epigenetic evaluation of FLS has also been extensively studied [30], and recently, Ai et al. reported comprehensive epigenetic landscape of RA FLS including histone modifications (H3K27ac, H3K4me1, H3K4me3, H3K36me3, H3K27me3, and H3K9me3), open chromatin, RNA expression, and whole-genome DNA methylation [31].

There are several reports concerning the effect of treatments other than biologic treatment on gene expression. Blits et al. investigated peripheral blood cells from methotrexate (MTX)-naïve and MTX-treated RA patients as well as from healthy controls. Concurrent with an immune activation gene signature, a significant upregulation of folate metabolizing enzymes (g-glutamyl hydrolase, dihydrofolate reductase), and MTX/folate efflux transporters (ABCC2 and ABCC5) was observed in MTX-naïve RA patients. Strikingly, MTX treatment normalized such differential gene expression levels to those observed in healthy controls [32]. Moreover, there is a report about effect of JAK inhibitor tofacitinib on gene expression of RA FLS [33]. Tofacitinib reduces matrix metalloproteinase (MMP)-1 and MMP-3 and IFN-regulated chemokines CCL2, CXCL10, and CXCL13 expression.

Type I IFNs are cytokines that regulate antiviral immune responses. Upregulation of type I IFN signature genes in RA [8, 10], and its relationship with therapeutic reactivity [8, 10, 23, 24] has been reported. The relationship between the type I IFN signature and the humoral autoimmune response in RA was analyzed in a number of previous studies. The presence of an IFN signature was associated with the persistence of ACPA after TNF blockade [26]. It has been hypothesized that patients with high activity of type I IFN may respond better to TNF blockade because of the anti-inflammatory effects of their disease-associated high levels of IFNβ. Alternatively, patients with an IFN high signature may have an overall higher level of inflammatory activity than do patients with an IFN low signature and may respond better to TNF blockade because of the higher TNFα activity.

Okada et al. described that comprehensive genetic study sheds light on fundamental genes, pathways, and cell types that contribute to RA pathogenesis and provides important information for drug discovery [2]. On the other hand, merely gene expression analysis has a limitation for precision treatment for RA, for example, upregulation of type I IFN signature gene were detected commonly in autoimmune disease including RA, systemic lupus erythematosus [34], dermatomyositis [35], and systemic sclerosis [36]. It is necessary to increase the number of patients for analysis and to integrate more precise clinical information, genomic and epigenetic data, and gene expression data of various cell subsets. Recently, data of 1424 early RA patients from two consortia were combined to carry out a genome-wide study of response to MTX. The strongest evidence for association was with rs168201 in NRG3, and some support was also seen for association with ZMIZ1, previously highlighted in a study of response to MTX in juvenile idiopathic arthritis [37].

Conclusion

In the era of precision medicine, transcriptome analysis of whole gene expression is an essential technology. Analyses of detailed cell subsets should have an increased need for understanding the pathophysiology of disease. Careful and extensive consideration of study design is necessary for successful gene expression studies because gene expression is dependent on stages of the disease, time course of treatment, type of tissue, and cell types. While testing peripheral blood has been a standard transcriptome analysis of RA patients, it would be better to test synovial tissue, as this is the site of inflammation. The disadvantage of synovial tissue approach is that arthroplasty and blind needle biopsy had not been widely available, although the use of arthroscopic and ultrasonographic technologies has improved the reliability of synovial biopsies. Researchers will need to carefully consider the advantages of using peripheral blood samples to investigate.

Abbreviations

DAS28-CRP: Disease activity score- CRP; eQTL: Expression quantitative trait loci; FLS: Fibroblast-like synoviocyte; GWAS: Genome-wide association study; IFN: Interferon; MTX: Methotrexate; NGS: Next-generation sequencing; OA: Osteoarthritis; PBMC: Peripheral blood mononuclear cell; RA: Rheumatoid arthritis; RNA-seq: RNA sequencing; TCR: T cell receptor; Tfh: Follicular helper T cells; TNF: Tumor necrosis factor; Treg: Regulatory T cells; WGCNA: Weighted gene co-expression network analysis

Authors' contributions

SS collected the entire literature and made the draft of the review. YN, YT, HT, MO, KI, AS, YK, and KY contributed to summarize literature and analyze and interpret our research results. KF revised the manuscript and gave final approval of the version to be published. All authors read and approved the final manuscript.

Competing interests

S.S. received honoraria from AbbVie, Eisai, Chugai, Takeda, Bristol-Myers Squibb, Astrazeneca and UCB. K.F. received speaking fees and/or honoraria from Astellas, Bristol-Myers Squibb, Daiichi-Sankyo, MitsubishiTanabe, Pfizer, Santen, Takeda, Chugai, Eisai, Taisho Toyama, UCB, and Janssen. K.Y. received speaking fees and/or honoraria from AbbVie, Astellas, Bristol-Myers Squibb, Daiichi-Sankyo, MitsubishiTanabe, Pfizer, Sanofi, Santen, Takeda, Teijin, Boehringer Ingelheim, Chugai, Eisai, Ono, Taisho Toyama, UCB, ImmunoFuture, Asahi Kasei, and Janssen. All other authors declare no competing financial interests.

Author details

[1]Department of Allergy and Rheumatology, Graduate School of Medicine, the University of Tokyo, 7-3-1 Hongo, Bunkyo-ku, Tokyo 113-8655, Japan.

[2]Laboratory for Statistical Analysis, Center for Integrative Medical Sciences, the Institute of Physical and Chemical Research (RIKEN), 1-7-22 Suehirocho, Tsurumi-ku, Yokohama City, Kanagawa 230-0045, Japan. [3]Laboratory for Autoimmune Diseases, Center for Integrative Medical Sciences, the Institute of Physical and Chemical Research (RIKEN), 1-7-22 Suehirocho, Tsurumi-ku, Yokohama City, Kanagawa 230-0045, Japan. [4]Center for Integrative Medical Sciences, the Institute of Physical and Chemical Research (RIKEN), 1-7-22 Suehirocho, Tsurumi-ku, Yokohama City, Kanagawa 230-0045, Japan.

References

1. Mahdi H, Fisher BA, Kallberg H, Plant D, Malmstrom V, Ronnelid J, et al. Specific interaction between genotype, smoking and autoimmunity to citrullinated alpha-enolase in the etiology of rheumatoid arthritis. Nat Genet. 2009;41:1319–24.
2. Okada Y, Wu D, Trynka G, Raj T, Terao C, Ikari K, et al. Genetics of rheumatoid arthritis contributes to biology and drug discovery. Nature. 2014;506:376–81.
3. Trouw LA, Rispens T, Toes REM. Beyond citrullination: other post-translational protein modifications in rheumatoid arthritis. Nat Rev Rheumatol. 2017;13:331–9.
4. Malmstrom V, Catrina AI, Klareskog L. The immunopathogenesis of seropositive rheumatoid arthritis: from triggering to targeting. Nat Rev Immunol. 2017;17:60–75.
5. Orr C, Vieira-Sousa E, Boyle DL, Buch MH, Buckley CD, Canete JD, et al. Synovial tissue research: a state-of-the-art review. Nat Rev Rheumatol. 2017;13:463–75.
6. Smith SL, Plant D, Eyre S, Barton A. The potential use of expression profiling: implications for predicting treatment response in rheumatoid arthritis. Ann Rheum Dis. 2013;72:1118–24.
7. Giannopoulou EG, Elemento O, Ivashkiv LB. Use of RNA sequencing to evaluate rheumatic disease patients. Arthritis Res Ther. 2015;17:167.
8. Sanayama Y, Ikeda K, Saito Y, Kagami S, Yamagata M, Furuta S, et al. Prediction of therapeutic responses to tocilizumab in patients with rheumatoid arthritis: biomarkers identified by analysis of gene expression in peripheral blood mononuclear cells using genome-wide DNA microarray. Arthritis Rheumatol. 2014;66:1421–31.
9. Sellam J, Marion-Thore S, Dumont F, Jacques S, Garchon HJ, Rouanet S, et al. Use of whole-blood transcriptomic profiling to highlight several pathophysiologic pathways associated with response to rituximab in patients with rheumatoid arthritis: data from a randomized, controlled, open-label trial. Arthritis Rheumatol. 2014;66:2015–25.
10. Wright HL, Thomas HB, Moots RJ, Edwards SW. Interferon gene expression signature in rheumatoid arthritis neutrophils correlates with a good response to TNFi therapy. Rheumatology (Oxford). 2015; 54:188–93.
11. Farh KK, Marson A, Zhu J, Kleinewietfeld M, Housley WJ, Beik S, et al. Genetic and epigenetic fine mapping of causal autoimmune disease variants. Nature. 2015;518:337–43.
12. Ishigaki K, Kochi Y, Suzuki A, Tsuchida Y, Tsuchiya H, Sumitomo S, et al. Polygenic burdens on cell-specific pathways underlie the risk of rheumatoid arthritis. Nat Genet. 2017;49:1120–5.
13. Ye H, Zhang J, Wang J, Gao Y, Du Y, Li C, et al. CD4 T-cell transcriptome analysis reveals aberrant regulation of STAT3 and Wnt signaling pathways in rheumatoid arthritis: evidence from a case-control study. Arthritis Res Ther. 2015;17:76.
14. Shen H, Goodall JC, Hill Gaston JS. Frequency and phenotype of peripheral blood Th17 cells in ankylosing spondylitis and rheumatoid arthritis. Arthritis Rheum. 2009;60:1647–56.
15. Esensten JH, Wofsy D, Bluestone JA. Regulatory T cells as therapeutic targets in rheumatoid arthritis. Nat Rev Rheumatol. 2009;5:560–5.
16. He J, Tsai LM, Leong YA, Hu X, Ma CS, Chevalier N, et al. Circulating precursor CCR7(lo)PD-1(hi) CXCR5(+) CD4(+) T cells indicate Tfh cell activity and promote antibody responses upon antigen reexposure. Immunity. 2013;39:770–81.
17. Sumitomo S, Nagafuchi Y, Tsuchida Y, Tsuchiya H, Ota M, Ishigaki K, et al. A gene module associated with dysregulated TCR signaling pathways in CD4(+) T cell subsets in rheumatoid arthritis. J Autoimmun. 2018;89:21–9.

19. Bremer E, Abdulahad WH, de Bruyn M, Samplonius DF, Kallenberg CG, Armbrust W, et al. Selective elimination of pathogenic synovial fluid T-cells from rheumatoid arthritis and juvenile idiopathic arthritis by targeted activation of Fas-apoptotic signaling. Immunol Lett. 2011;138:161–8.

20. Langfelder P, Horvath S. WGCNA: an R package for weighted correlation network analysis. BMC Bioinf. 2008;9:559.

21. Kremer JM, Westhovens R, Leon M, Di Giorgio E, Alten R, Steinfeld S, et al. Treatment of rheumatoid arthritis by selective inhibition of T-cell activation with fusion protein CTLA4Ig. N Engl J Med. 2003;349:1907–15.

22. Raterman HG, Vosslamber S, de Ridder S, Nurmohamed MT, Lems WF, Boers M, et al. The interferon type I signature towards prediction of non-response to rituximab in rheumatoid arthritis patients. Arthritis Res Ther. 2012;14:R95.

23. Vosslamber S, Raterman HG, van der Pouw Kraan TC, Schreurs MW, von Blomberg BM, Nurmohamed MT, et al. Pharmacological induction of interferon type I activity following treatment with rituximab determines clinical response in rheumatoid arthritis. Ann Rheum Dis. 2011;70:1153–9.

24. Thurlings RM, Boumans M, Tekstra J, van Roon JA, Vos K, van Westing DM, et al. Relationship between the type I interferon signature and the response to rituximab in rheumatoid arthritis patients. Arthritis Rheum. 2010;62:3607–14.

25. Koczan D, Drynda S, Hecker M, Drynda A, Guthke R, Kekow J, et al. Molecular discrimination of responders and nonresponders to anti-TNF alpha therapy in rheumatoid arthritis by etanercept. Arthritis Res Ther. 2008;10:R50.

26. van Baarsen LG, Wijbrandts CA, Rustenburg F, Cantaert T, van der Pouw Kraan TC, Baeten DL, et al. Regulation of IFN response gene activity during infliximab treatment in rheumatoid arthritis is associated with clinical response to treatment. Arthritis Res Ther. 2010;12:R11.

27. Saito Y, Kagami S, Sanayama Y, Ikeda K, Suto A, Kashiwakuma D, et al. AT-rich-interactive domain-containing protein 5A functions as a negative regulator of retinoic acid receptor-related orphan nuclear receptor gammat-induced Th17 cell differentiation. Arthritis Rheumatol. 2014;66:1185–94.

28. Dennis G Jr, Holweg CT, Kummerfeld SK, Choy DF, Setiadi AF, Hackney JA, et al. Synovial phenotypes in rheumatoid arthritis correlate with response to biologic therapeutics. Arthritis Res Ther. 2014;16:R90.

29. Galligan CL, Baig E, Bykerk V, Keystone EC, Fish EN. Distinctive gene expression signatures in rheumatoid arthritis synovial tissue fibroblast cells: correlates with disease activity. Genes Immun. 2007;8:480–91.

30. Nakano K, Whitaker JW, Boyle DL, Wang W, Firestein GS. DNA methylome signature in rheumatoid arthritis. Ann Rheum Dis. 2013;72:110–7.

31. Ai R, Laragione T, Hammaker D, Boyle DL, Wildberg A, Maeshima K, et al. Comprehensive epigenetic landscape of rheumatoid arthritis fibroblast-like synoviocytes. Nat Commun. 2018;9:1921.

32. Blits M, Jansen G, Assaraf YG, van de Wiel MA, Lems WF, Nurmohamed MT, et al. Methotrexate normalizes up-regulated folate pathway genes in rheumatoid arthritis. Arthritis Rheum. 2013;65:2791–802.

33. Boyle DL, Soma K, Hodge J, Kavanaugh A, Mandel D, Mease P, et al. The JAK inhibitor tofacitinib suppresses synovial JAK1-STAT signalling in rheumatoid arthritis. Ann Rheum Dis. 2015;74:1311–6.

34. Crow MK. Type I interferon in systemic lupus erythematosus. Curr Top Microbiol Immunol. 2007;316:359–86.

35. Bilgic H, Ytterberg SR, Amin S, McNallan KT, Wilson JC, Koeuth T, et al. Interleukin-6 and type I interferon-regulated genes and chemokines mark disease activity in dermatomyositis. Arthritis Rheum. 2009;60:3436–46.

36. Bos CL, van Baarsen LG, Timmer TC, Overbeek MJ, Basoski NM, Rustenburg F, et al. Molecular subtypes of systemic sclerosis in association with anti-centromere antibodies and digital ulcers. Genes Immun. 2009;10:210–8.

37. Taylor JC, Bongartz T, Massey J, Mifsud B, Spiliopoulou A, Scott IC, et al. Genome-wide association study of response to methotrexate in early rheumatoid arthritis patients. Pharmacogenomics J. 2018. https://doi.org/10.1038/s41397-018-0025-5. [Epub ahead of print].

29

Maintenance of intestinal homeostasis by mucosal barriers

Ryu Okumura[1,2,3] and Kiyoshi Takeda[1,2,3]*

Abstract

Background: The intestine is inhabited by a tremendous number of microorganisms, which provide many benefits to nutrition, metabolism and immunity. Mucosal barriers by intestinal epithelial cells make it possible to maintain the symbiotic relationship between the gut microbiota and the host by separating them. Recent evidence indicates that mucosal barrier dysfunction contributes to the development of inflammatory bowel disease (IBD). In this review, we focus on the mechanisms by which mucosal barriers maintain gut homeostasis.

Main text: Gut mucosal barriers are classified into chemical and physical barriers. Chemical barriers, including antimicrobial peptides (AMPs), are chemical agents that attack invading microorganisms, and physical barriers, including the mucus layer and the cell junction, are walls that physically repel invading microorganisms. These barriers, which are ingeniously modulated by gut microbiota and host immune cells, spatially segregate gut microbiota and the host immunity to avoid unnecessary immune responses to gut commensal microbes. Therefore, mucosal barrier dysfunction allows gut bacteria to invade gut mucosa, inducing excessive immune responses of the host immune cells, which result in intestinal inflammation.

Conclusion: Gut mucosal barriers constructed by intestinal epithelial cells maintain gut homeostasis by segregating gut microbiota and host immune cells. Impaired mucosal barrier function contributes to the development of IBD. However, the mechanism by which the mucosal barrier is regulated by gut microbiota remains unclear. Thus, it should be further elucidated in the future to develop a novel therapeutic approach to IBD by targeting the mucosal barrier.

Keywords: Mucosal barrier, Gut microbiota, Intestinal epithelial cells, Inflammatory bowel disease

Background

The mammalian intestine is a special place for microorganisms, where a high abundance of nutrients derived from foods are present and an aerobic condition is maintained. Therefore, tremendous numbers of microorganisms mainly composed of aerobic bacteria grow and inhabit the intestine. The intestinal microorganisms including bacteria, fungi and viruses form an ecological community termed the gut microbiota, which does not only reside in the gut but also provide many benefits to nutrition, metabolism and immunity. Short-chain fatty acid (SCFA), which is a gut microbial metabolite produced from dietary fibers, is used as an energy source of the host. In addition, SCFA

contributes to the modulation of mucosal immunity by enhancing mucus production and promoting regulatory T cell (T_{reg}) development [1–3]. Moreover, gut bacteria synthesize several kinds of vitamins including vitamin B and vitamin K, which are critical for sugar and fat metabolism and maintenance of hemostatic function. Thus, gut microbiota forms a win-win relationship with the host.

However, mammalian immune cells such as macrophages and neutrophils are programmed to attack invading extraneous organisms. Gut microbes are no exception and can be targeted by host immune cells. Accordingly, there is a barrier system—mucosal barrier—for separating gut microbiota and the host immunity to avoid an unfavorable interaction between the two. Mucosal barrier impairment allows gut microbes to easily enter the mucosa, which induce intestinal inflammation as a consequence of the host's excessive immune responses to gut microbes.

Inflammatory bowel diseases (IBD) such as Crohn's disease (CD) and ulcerative colitis (UC) involve choric

* Correspondence: ktakeda@ongene.med.osaka-u.ac.jp
[1]Department of Microbiology and Immunology, Graduate School of Medicine, Osaka University, Osaka 565-0871, Japan
[2]WPI Immunology Frontier Research Center, Osaka University, Osaka 565-0871, Japan
Full list of author information is available at the end of the article

intestinal inflammation in humans. Recent evidence based on the combination of the human genome-wide association study (GWAS) and genetically modified mouse studies have revealed that intestinal barrier dysfunction is one cause of IBD [4]. In addition, reduced production of mucosal barrier components such as mucus and antimicrobial peptides is observed in the intestine of some IBD patients. These findings indicate that the mucosal barrier is indispensable for maintaining the gut environment and preventing intestinal inflammation.

In this review, we discuss the mechanisms of the gut mucosal barrier constructed by IECs and the regulation of intestinal inflammation by the mucosal barrier.

Mucosal barriers formed by intestinal epithelial cells

IECs at the surface of the gut mucosa absorb nutrients and water from ingested foods. They also play important roles in generating various types of barriers to protect mucosa from commensal microbes and invading pathogenic microorganisms (Fig. 1). These barriers have two subtypes, chemical and physical barriers.

Chemical barrier

Chemical barriers consist of antimicrobial peptides (AMPs), the regenerating islet-derived 3 (Reg3) family of proteins, lysozyme and secretory phospholipase A2. All of these are mainly involved in the segregation of gut bacteria and IECs in the small intestine [5, 6]. Paneth cells play a crucial role in the mucosal barrier of the small intestine by producing a large number of antimicrobials [7].

AMPs are basic amino acid-rich cationic small proteins, which are evolutionarily conserved in a wide range of organisms. They include the defensin family of proteins and cathelicidins, both of which bind to the negatively charged microbial cell membrane and induce disruption of membrane integrity by forming a pore-like structure [8]. Defensin family proteins are classified into α-, β- and θ-defensins, among which α-defensin (also referred to as cryptdins in mice) is most highly expressed in Paneth cells and mainly protects against infection by Gram-positive and Gram-negative bacteria. Pro-cryptdin is converted into mature-cryptdin by matrix metalloproteinase-7 (MMP-7) in mice. Therefore, MMP-7-deficient mice lack mature-cryptdin, resulting in high susceptibility to *Salmonella typhimurium* infection [9]. Moreover, mature α-defensin deficiency is associated with alteration of the gut microbiota: a decrease of Bacteroidetes and an increase in Firmicutes [10]. These results demonstrate that AMPs largely contribute to the homeostatic state of the gut environment by regulating pathogenic bacteria [11].

The Reg3 family proteins are C-type lectins, which exert an antibacterial effect on Gram-positive bacteria by binding to the bacterial membrane and forming a hexameric membrane-permeabilizing oligomeric pore [12]. In mice lacking Reg3γ, increased bacterial colonization on the epithelial surface of the small intestine was observed, indicating that Reg3γ is indispensable to the spatial separation of the intestinal bacteria and intestinal epithelia of the small intestine [6, 12, 13].

Physical barriers

Chemical barriers are major players in the segregation of gut microbiota and the small intestinal epithelia. However,

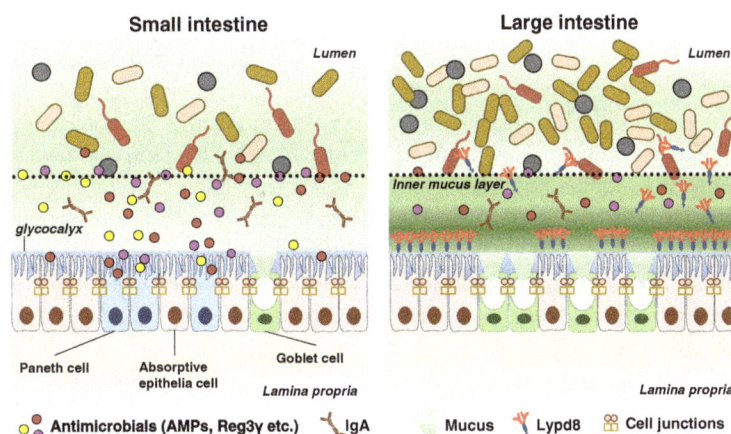

Fig. 1 Mucosal barriers in the gut. Chemical barriers including AMPs and Reg3γ secreted by Paneth cells mainly contribute to the separation between intestinal bacteria and IECs in the small intestine. By contrast, in the large intestine where a tremendous number of bacteria exist, intestinal bacteria and IECs are largely segregated by physical barriers such as the inner mucus layer composed of polymerized MUC2 mucin. Lypd8, a highly glycosylated GPI-anchored protein expressed on IECs, inhibits the bacterial invasion of the inner mucus layer by binding to intestinal bacteria, especially flagellated bacteria. AMP: antimicrobial peptide

in the large intestine, where there is nothing resembling Paneth cells that secrete antimicrobials, physical barriers mainly contribute to spatial segregation of gut microbiota and intestinal epithelia. Physical barriers consist of the mucus layer covering the intestinal mucosa, the glycocalyx on the microvilli of absorptive IECs, and the cell junctions firmly linking IECs. These barriers physically inhibit the microbial invasion of the mucosa.

Mucus is a viscous fluid secreted by goblet cells. It is enriched in mucin glycoproteins that form large net-like polymers [14]. In the large intestine, where tremendous numbers of intestinal bacteria exist compared with the small intestine, the number of goblet cells is much higher and the large intestinal epithelia are covered by a thick two-layered mucus layer: the outer loose and the inner firm mucus layer [15]. These two mucus layers are constructed of goblet cell-secreted Mucin2 (MUC2) protein, which is a highly O-glycosylated protein, forming large net-like structures. The inner mucus layer is stratified and anchored to the intestinal epithelia, which does not allow gut bacteria to easily penetrate into the inner mucus layer and thereby keeps the inner mucus layer free of bacteria [15]. The inner mucus layer is converted into the outer mucus layer by the proteolytic processing of polymerized MUC2 by the host or gut bacteria. The outer mucus layer is inhabited by numerous bacteria, some of which use polysaccharides of MUC2 as an energy source; therefore, the absence of dietary fiber, a major energy source of intestinal bacteria, leads to the expansion of mucin-degrading species, resulting in the increase of inner mucus degradation [16].

Regarding the mechanism by which the inner mucus layer is free of gut bacteria, various antimicrobial molecules such as immunoglobulin A (IgA) and the defensin family of proteins transported or produced by IECs may be involved in protecting against bacterial invasion of the inner mucus layer [17]. Although higher numbers of bacteria exist in the large intestine, the expression level of antimicrobial molecules in the large intestine is not higher than that in the small intestine, indicating that there is another mechanism to inhibit gut microbial invasion of the large intestinal epithelia without killing bacteria.

Ly6/Plaur domain containing 8 (Lypd8) is a highly glycosylated GPI-anchored protein highly and selectively expressed on the mucosal surface of the large intestine. A recent study demonstrated that many intestinal bacteria, including *Escherichia* spp. and *Proteus* spp., invaded the inner mucus layer in Lypd8-deficient mice [18]. In addition, it was revealed that Lypd8 inhibited bacterial motility of flagellated bacteria such as *Escherichia coli* and *Proteus mirabilis* through binding to their flagella, thereby inhibiting their bacterial invasion of the colonic epithelia. These results indicate that Lypd8 contributes to the segregation of intestinal bacteria and the large intestinal epithelia [18].

As mentioned above, Muc2 and Lypd8 are highly glycosylated. Glycans of the physical barrier-related proteins are critical for maintaining their barrier function. In mice lacking the O-glycan core structure of the MUC2 protein, bacterial invasion of the colonic mucosa was observed [19]. With removal of N-glycans from Lypd8, the inhibitory effect of Lypd8 against bacterial attachment on Caco-2 cells was severely reduced [18]. Furthermore, mice devoid of Fut2, which mediates the transfer of fucoses to the terminal galactose on glycans in cell-surface glycoproteins, are highly susceptible to pathogenic bacteria infection [20, 21]. The glycocalyx, a meshwork of carbohydrate moieties of glycolipids or glycoproteins including transmembrane mucins, blocks bacterial invasion into the intestinal tissue as a second wall followed by the mucus layer. These findings indicate that glycans of barrier-related proteins generated by IECs are vital for physical barrier function.

For intestinal bacteria passing through the mucus layer and glycocalyx by evading various kinds of antimicrobial molecules from the host, cell junctions, including the tight and adhesion junctions linking epithelial cells, are the final wall to physically hamper the invasion into the intestinal tissue through the paracellular pathway. Hence, the perturbed gut integrity and permeability caused by disruption of the cell junction of IECs leads to microbial translocation, and the consequent leakage of bacteria or their metabolites into the gut tissue can induce a chronic or acute inflammatory response in the intestine [22, 23].

Regulation of mucosal barrier function by gut microbiota and immune cells

Mucosal barrier function is regulated by various signals from gut microbiota and host immune cells. IECs express a variety of pattern recognition receptors, including Toll-like receptors (TLRs) and nucleotide-binding oligomerization domain-containing proteins (NODs) to directly sense bacterial components. The production of antimicrobial molecules by IECs is controlled by TLR4/MyD88 signaling and NOD2 signaling driven by gut microorganisms [5, 6, 24]. In mice deficient in NOD2 sensing muramyl dipeptides, which are conserved structures in bacterial peptidoglycans, the expression of defensins is substantially reduced, resulting in high susceptibility to *Listeria monocytogenes* infection [24]. Moreover, mice lacking MyD88 in IECs show the decreased production of AMPs, Reg3γ and mucus by IECs, and eventually they become highly susceptible to experimental colitis and enteric bacterial infection [25, 26]. In addition, recent studies demonstrated that NOD-like receptor family pyrin domain containing 6 (NLRP6), a member of the NOD-like receptor family of pattern recognition receptors, is necessary for mucus granule exocytosis from goblet cells [27].

Metabolites from gut bacteria also directly enhance the mucosal barrier function of IECs. Mucus secretion from goblet cells is upregulated by butyrate, one of the SCFAs provided by gut bacteria [28]. Recent evidence revealed that the expression of cell junction-associated molecules such as occludins and claudins in IECs is enhanced by indole, a metabolite of dietary tryptophan from commensal bacteria possessing tryptophanase, via Pregnane X receptor (PXR) stimulation [29, 30].

The mucosal barrier function of IECs is also enhanced by cytokines from immune cells activated by gut commensal bacteria or pathogenic bacteria. Segmented filamentous bacteria (SFB) is a type of commensal bacteria found in the mouse or rat intestine. The attachment of SFB to IECs strongly promotes Th17 cell differentiation in the lamina propria by inducing serum amyloid A (SAA) production by IECs [31, 32]. In addition, SFB facilitates type3 innate lymphoid cells (ILC3) to produce Interleukin (IL)-22 in an IL-23 receptor-dependent manner. In the case of Citrobacter rodentium infection associated with enteritis, a potent Th17 cell-mediated response is induced [32]. IL-17 and IL-22 produced by Th17 cells or ILC3 upregulate the secretion of AMPs and Reg3 family proteins by IECs, and induce the fucosylation of cell membrane proteins on IECs of the small intestine, which work to regulate commensal and pathogenic bacteria [20, 33]. When parasite infection occurs, tuft cells, taste-chemosensory epithelial cells, produce IL-25 which activates ILC2 to secrete IL-13. This induces Th2 responses, resulting in an enhancement of mucin production and goblet cell differentiation [34–36].

In mucosal injury, IL-6 derived from intraepithelial lymphocytes enhances intestinal epithelial cell proliferation and contributes to healing from mucosal injury [37]. Moreover, activated macrophages differentiated from monocytes recruited to the mucosal wound site trigger the colonic epithelial progenitor niche with direct cell-cell contact to promote epithelial regeneration, which helps to recover the mucosal barrier [38]. Th2 cytokines, such as IL-5 and IL-13, promote colonic wound healing by inducing the alternative activation of macrophages, which contributes to epithelial cell proliferation [39]. Conversely, other pro-inflammatory cytokines, such as tumor necrosis factor (TNF)-α and interferon (IFN)-γ, inhibit epithelial cell proliferation through the suppression of β-catenin/T cell factor signaling [40]. Mucosal barrier function of IECs are maintained by intestinal microbiota and immune cell-derived cytokines (Fig. 2).

Intestinal inflammation induced by the dysfunction of mucosal barriers

IBD is a group of chronic inflammatory states of the digestive tract, characterized by CD and UC. The incidence and prevalence of IBD are increasing around the world, suggesting that the elucidation of the pathogenesis of IBD is an emergent matter to be solved [41]. Recent remarkable advances of sequencing technology make it possible to identify various IBD susceptibility genes and the gut microbial composition of IBD patients. Accumulated evidence strongly indicates that both gut environmental factors including gut microbiota and host immune dysregulation associated with a genetic predisposition contribute to the occurrence and development of IBD [42]. IECs, which are present between gut microbiota and the host immunity, play an important role in the segregation of both factors by generating mucosal barriers to avoid excessive immune response to gut microbiota, which results in intestinal inflammation. Indeed, GWAS using next generation sequencing technology identified various IBD susceptibility genes including the mucosal barrier-related genes FUT2, MUC19 and NOD2 [43–46]. Additionally, the decreased production of mucosal barrier-related molecules, such as AMPs and mucins, is observed in the intestines of IBD patients [4].

To investigate the roles of mucosal barriers in preventing intestinal inflammation, many studies using genetically modified mice with mucosal barrier impairment have been conducted. Mice devoid of Muc2 show the disappearance of the inner mucus layer and develop spontaneous colitis resulting from the bacterial invasion of the colonic mucosa [15, 47]. The deficiency of cooperation of core 1 synthase (C1galt), which synthesizes the major constituent of the O-glycan core structure of the MUC2 protein, conduces to the disrupted mucus constitution and allows bacteria to invade the inner mucus layer, resulting in spontaneous colitis [19]. Abrogation of IEC fucosylation is associated with intestinal dysbiosis and leads to high susceptibility to intestinal inflammation. [48, 49] In mice deficient in Lypd8, a highly N-glycosylated protein expressed on IECs, the invasion of the colonic mucosa by a large number of flagellated bacteria such as Proteus spp. and Escherichia spp. causes high susceptibility to dextran sulfate sodium (DSS)-induced intestinal inflammation [18]. The absence of NLRP6 in IECs impairs mucus secretion from goblet cells, consequently leading to the disappearance of the bacteria-free zone just above the colonic epithelia. This is accompanied with high sensitivity to DSS-induced or bacterial pathogen-induced colitis [27, 50]. Interestingly, wild-type mice cohoused with NLRP6-deficient mice show high susceptibility to DSS-induced intestinal inflammation, indicating colitogenic dysbiosis of NLRP6-deficient mice is transmissible to normal mice [50]. The dysfunction of cell junctions also causes intestinal inflammation. Intestinal deletion of Claudin-7, which is a critical component of the tight junctions of IECs, enhances the paracellular flux of a bacterial product and consequently causes spontaneous colitis in mice [23]. In

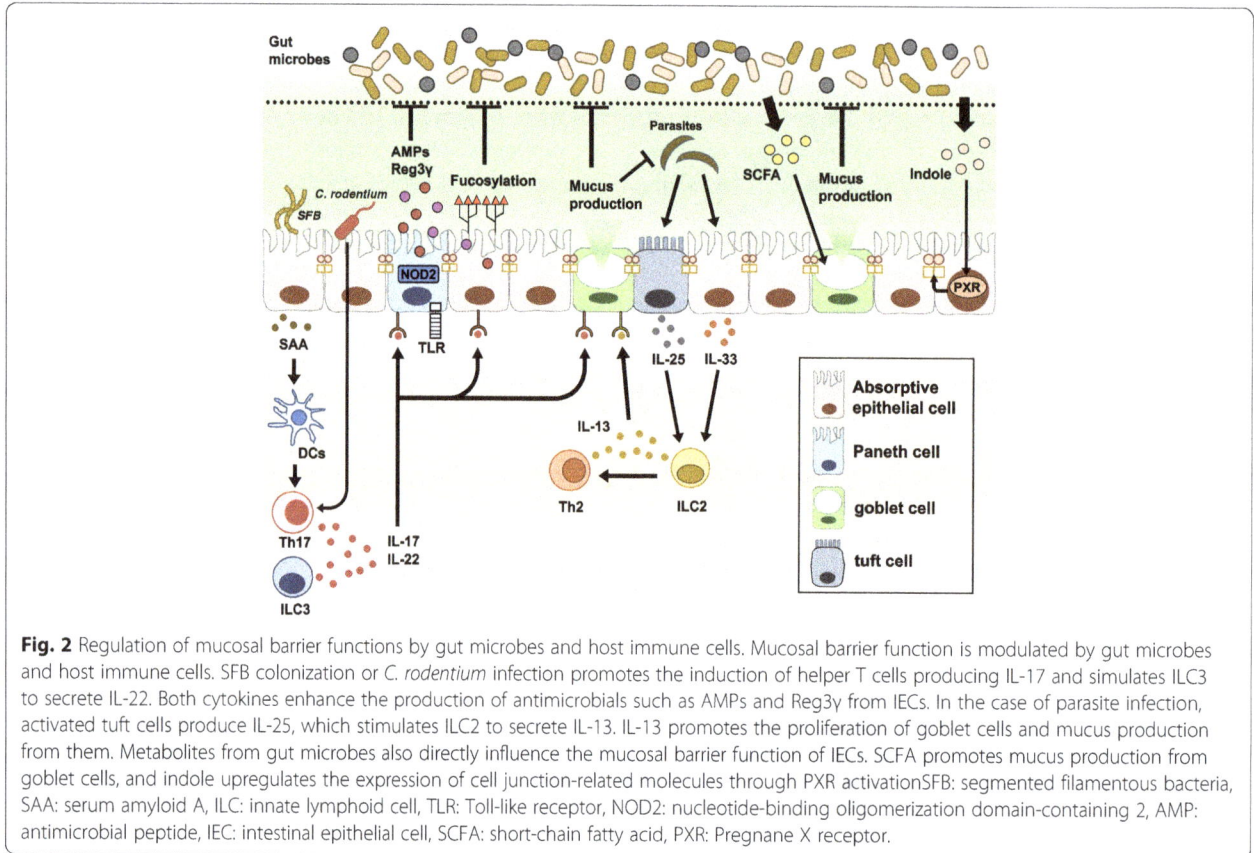

Fig. 2 Regulation of mucosal barrier functions by gut microbes and host immune cells. Mucosal barrier function is modulated by gut microbes and host immune cells. SFB colonization or *C. rodentium* infection promotes the induction of helper T cells producing IL-17 and simulates ILC3 to secrete IL-22. Both cytokines enhance the production of antimicrobials such as AMPs and Reg3γ from IECs. In the case of parasite infection, activated tuft cells produce IL-25, which stimulates ILC2 to secrete IL-13. IL-13 promotes the proliferation of goblet cells and mucus production from them. Metabolites from gut microbes also directly influence the mucosal barrier function of IECs. SCFA promotes mucus production from goblet cells, and indole upregulates the expression of cell junction-related molecules through PXR activationSFB: segmented filamentous bacteria, SAA: serum amyloid A, ILC: innate lymphoid cell, TLR: Toll-like receptor, NOD2: nucleotide-binding oligomerization domain-containing 2, AMP: antimicrobial peptide, IEC: intestinal epithelial cell, SCFA: short-chain fatty acid, PXR: Pregnane X receptor.

addition, in the absence of RING finger protein (RNF) 186, which acts as an E3 ligase to mediate polyubiquitination of its substrates, the sensitivity to intestinal inflammation is elevated because of the high permeability of small organic molecule and enhanced endoplasmic reticulum (ER) stress in IECs [51].

The impairment of chemical barriers also causes high susceptibility to intestinal inflammation. Mice devoid of IL-22 which enhances the production of antimicrobials by IECs also show high sensitivity to DSS colitis, indicating IL-22 from T cells is protective against intestinal inflammation [52]. Moreover, intestinal epithelial cell-specific inhibition of nuclear factor (NF)-κB through the conditional ablation of NEMO, an IκB kinase subunit essential for NF-κB activation, causes chronic intestinal inflammation in mice because of bacterial translocation into the colonic mucosa due to the reduced production of antimicrobial peptides [53]. Mice deficient in the *Nod2* gene, which is a susceptibility gene for human CD, do not show spontaneous intestinal inflammation but show severe Th1-driven granulomatous inflammation of the ileum induced by *Helicobacter hepaticus* because of the decreased expression of AMPs by Paneth cells [54–56]. The deficiency of multi-drug resistance protein 1 (MDR1), a xenobiotic transporter, leads to

chronic colitis because of the increased permeability of IECs [57]. Deficiency in adaptor protein (AP)-1B, which mediates the sorting of membrane proteins, induced the reduced expression of antimicrobial proteins and the impaired secretion of IgA, leading to chronic colitis with an enhanced Th17 response [58].

As described above, many human and mouse studies have demonstrated that intestinal barrier dysfunction is clearly implicated in the development of intestinal inflammation, indicating that the segregation of gut microbiota and host immunity by the mucosal barriers is critically involved in maintaining gut homeostasis (Fig. 3).

Conclusions

IECs generate various kinds of mucosal barriers to segregate gut microbiota and gut immune cells to prevent excessive immune responses leading to intestinal inflammation. Accordingly, a defect in mucosal barrier function promotes the development of intestinal inflammation such as IBD. There are three major players involved in the pathogenesis of IBD. These include gut microbes in the lumen, immune cells in the lamina propria and IECs between the two. Regarding therapies for IBD, there are several immunosuppressive agents such as mesalazine, steroids and infliximab. Recently, fecal transplantation has been developed to

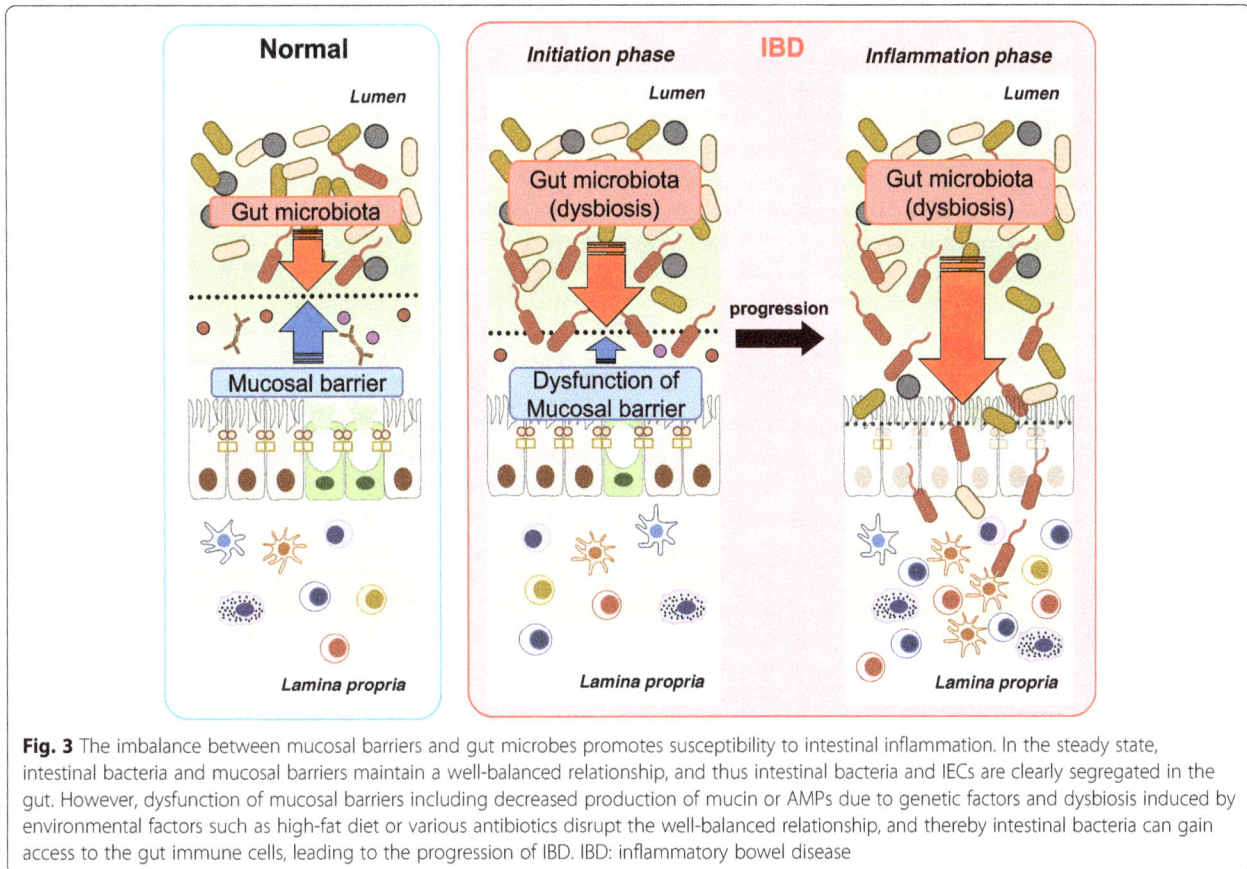

Fig. 3 The imbalance between mucosal barriers and gut microbes promotes susceptibility to intestinal inflammation. In the steady state, intestinal bacteria and mucosal barriers maintain a well-balanced relationship, and thus intestinal bacteria and IECs are clearly segregated in the gut. However, dysfunction of mucosal barriers including decreased production of mucin or AMPs due to genetic factors and dysbiosis induced by environmental factors such as high-fat diet or various antibiotics disrupt the well-balanced relationship, and thereby intestinal bacteria can gain access to the gut immune cells, leading to the progression of IBD. IBD: inflammatory bowel disease

improve the gut environment. However, extremely few therapies targeting the mucosal barrier function of IECs exist. The therapies for intractable IBD are limited, and several different immunosuppressive therapies are required, each having at least a few side effects. Further clarification of the mechanisms regulating the gut mucosal barrier system will certainly shed light on the development of novel therapeutic approaches for IBD.

Abbreviations
AMP: Antimicrobial peptide; AP: Adaptor protein; C1galt: Cooperation of core 1 synthase; CD: Crohn's disease; DSS: Dextran sulfate sodium; ER: Endoplasmic reticulum; GWAS: Genome-wide association study; IBD: Inflammatory bowel disease; IEC: Intestinal epithelial cell; IFN: Interferon; IgA: Immunoglobulin A; IL: Interleukin; ILC: Innate lymphoid cell; Lypd8: Ly6/Plaur domain containing 8; MDR: Multi-drug resistance protein; MMP-7: Matrix metalloproteinase-7; NEMO: Inhibitor of nuclear factor kappa B kinase subunit gamma; NF: Nuclear factor; NLRP6: NOD-like receptor family pyrin domain containing 6; NOD2: Nucleotide-binding oligomerization domain-containing protein 2; PXR: Pregnane X receptor; Reg3: Regenerating islet-derived 3; RNF: RING finger protein; SAA: Serum amyloid A; SCFA: Short-chain fatty acid; SFB: Segmented filamentous bacteria; TLR: Toll-like receptor; TNF: Tumor necrosis factor; T_{reg}: Regulatory T cell; UC: Ulcerative colitis

Acknowledgements
We thank T. Kondo, and Y. Magota for their technical assistance, and C. Hidaka for secretarial assistance.

Funding
Not applicable.

Authors' contributions
RO. drafted the original manuscript. KT. revised the manuscript and gave final approval of the version to be published. All authors read and approved the manuscript.

Competing interests
The authors declare that they have no competing financial interests.

Author details
[1]Department of Microbiology and Immunology, Graduate School of Medicine, Osaka University, Osaka 565-0871, Japan. [2]WPI Immunology Frontier Research Center, Osaka University, Osaka 565-0871, Japan. [3]Core Research for Evolutional Science and Technology, Japan Agency for Medical Research and Development, Tokyo 100-0004, Japan.

References
1.   Gaudier E, Jarry A, Blottiere HM, de Coppet P, Buisine MP, Aubert JP, Laboisse C, Cherbut C, Hoebler C. Butyrate specifically modulates MUC gene expression in intestinal epithelial goblet cells deprived of glucose. Am J Physiol Gastrointest Liver Physiol. 2004;287(6):G1168–74.

2. Furusawa Y, Obata Y, Fukuda S, Endo TA, Nakato G, Takahashi D, Nakanishi Y, Uetake C, Kato K, Kato T, et al. Commensal microbe-derived butyrate induces the differentiation of colonic regulatory T cells. Nature. 2013; 504(7480):446–50.

3. Shimotoyodome A, Meguro S, Hase T, Tokimitsu I, Sakata T. Short chain fatty acids but not lactate or succinate stimulate mucus release in the rat colon. Comp Biochem Physiol A Mol Integr Physiol. 2000;125(4):525–31.

4. Jager S, Stange EF, Wehkamp J. Inflammatory bowel disease: an impaired barrier disease. Langenbeck's Arch Surg. 2013;398(1):1–12.

5. Ayabe T, Satchell DP, Wilson CL, Parks WC, Selsted ME, Ouellette AJ. Secretion of microbicidal alpha-defensins by intestinal Paneth cells in response to bacteria. Nat Immunol. 2000;1(2):113–8.

6. Vaishnava S, Yamamoto M, Severson KM, Ruhn KA, Yu X, Koren O, Ley R, Wakeland EK, Hooper LV. The antibacterial lectin RegIIIgamma promotes the spatial segregation of microbiota and host in the intestine. Science. 2011; 334(6053):255–8.

7. Salzman NH, Underwood MA, Bevins CL. Paneth cells, defensins, and the commensal microbiota: a hypothesis on intimate interplay at the intestinal mucosa. Semin Immunol. 2007;19(2):70–83.

8. Brogden KA. Antimicrobial peptides: pore formers or metabolic inhibitors in bacteria? Nat Rev Microbiol. 2005;3(3):238–50.

9. Wilson CL, Ouellette AJ, Satchell DP, Ayabe T, Lopez-Boado YS, Stratman JL, Hultgren SJ, Matrisian LM, Parks WC. Regulation of intestinal alpha-defensin activation by the metalloproteinase matrilysin in innate host defense. Science. 1999;286(5437):113–7.

10. Salzman NH, Hung K, Haribhai D, Chu H, Karlsson-Sjoberg J, Amir E, Teggatz P, Barman M, Hayward M, Eastwood D, et al. Enteric defensins are essential regulators of intestinal microbial ecology. Nat Immunol. 2010;11(1):76–83.

11. Salzman NH, Bevins CL. Dysbiosis–a consequence of Paneth cell dysfunction. Semin Immunol. 2013;25(5):334–41.

12. Mukherjee S, Zheng H, Derebe MG, Callenberg KM, Partch CL, Rollins D, Propheter DC, Rizo J, Grabe M, Jiang QX, et al. Antibacterial membrane attack by a pore-forming intestinal C-type lectin. Nature. 2014;505(7481):103–7.

13. Cash HL, Whitham CV, Behrendt CL, Hooper LV. Symbiotic bacteria direct expression of an intestinal bactericidal lectin. Science. 2006;313(5790):1126–30.

14. Rodriguez-Pineiro AM, Bergstrom JH, Ermund A, Gustafsson JK, Schutte A, Johansson ME, Hansson GC. Studies of mucus in mouse stomach, small intestine, and colon. II. Gastrointestinal mucus proteome reveals Muc2 and Muc5ac accompanied by a set of core proteins. Am J Physiol Gastrointest Liver Physiol. 2013;305(5):G348–56.

15. Johansson ME, Phillipson M, Petersson J, Velcich A, Holm L, Hansson GC. The inner of the two Muc2 mucin-dependent mucus layers in colon is devoid of bacteria. Proc Natl Acad Sci U S A. 2008;105(39):15064–9.

16. Desai MS, Seekatz AM, Koropatkin NM, Kamada N, Hickey CA, Wolter M, Pudlo NA, Kitamoto S, Terrapon N, Muller A, et al. A dietary Fiber-deprived gut microbiota degrades the colonic mucus barrier and enhances pathogen susceptibility. Cell. 2016;167(5):1339–53. e1321

17. Maynard CL, Elson CO, Hatton RD, Weaver CT. Reciprocal interactions of the intestinal microbiota and immune system. Nature. 2012;489(7415):231–41.

18. Okumura R, Kurakawa T, Nakano T, Kayama H, Kinoshita M, Motooka D, Gotoh K, Kimura T, Kamiyama N, Kusu T, et al. Lypd8 promotes the segregation of flagellated microbiota and colonic epithelia. Nature. 2016; 532(7597):117–21.

19. Fu J, Wei B, Wen T, Johansson ME, Liu X, Bradford E, Thomsson KA, McGee S, Mansour L, Tong M, et al. Loss of intestinal core 1-derived O-glycans causes spontaneous colitis in mice. J Clin Invest. 2011;121(4):1657–66.

20. Goto Y, Obata T, Kunisawa J, Sato S, Ivanov II, Lamichhane A, Takeyama N, Kamioka M, Sakamoto M, Matsuki S, et al. Innate lymphoid cells regulate intestinal epithelial cell glycosylation. Science. 2014;345(6202):1254009.

21. Pham TA, Clare S, Goulding D, Arasteh JM, Stares MD, Browne HP, Keane JA, Page AJ, Kumasaka N, Kane L, et al. Epithelial IL-22RA1-mediated fucosylation promotes intestinal colonization resistance to an opportunistic pathogen. Cell Host Microbe. 2014;16(4):504–16.

22. Nagpal R, Yadav H. Bacterial translocation from the gut to the distant organs: an overview. Ann Nutr Metab. 2017;71(Suppl 1):11–6.

23. Tanaka H, Takechi M, Kiyonari H, Shioi G, Tamura A, Tsukita S. Intestinal deletion of Claudin-7 enhances paracellular organic solute flux and initiates colonic inflammation in mice. Gut. 2015;64(10):1529–38.

24. Kobayashi KS, Chamaillard M, Ogura Y, Henegariu O, Inohara N, Nunez G, Flavell RA. Nod2-dependent regulation of innate and adaptive immunity in the intestinal tract. Science. 2005;307(5710):731–4.

25. Frantz AL, Rogier EW, Weber CR, Shen L, Cohen DA, Fenton LA, Bruno ME, Kaetzel CS. Targeted deletion of MyD88 in intestinal epithelial cells results in compromised antibacterial immunity associated with downregulation of polymeric immunoglobulin receptor, mucin-2, and antibacterial peptides. Mucosal Immunol. 2012;5(5):501–12.

26. Bhinder G, Stahl M, Sham HP, Crowley SM, Morampudi V, Dalwadi U, Ma C, Jacobson K, Vallance BA. Intestinal epithelium-specific MyD88 signaling impacts host susceptibility to infectious colitis by promoting protective goblet cell and antimicrobial responses. Infect Immun. 2014;82(9):3753–63.

27. Wlodarska M, Thaiss CA, Nowarski R, Henao-Mejia J, Zhang JP, Brown EM, Frankel G, Levy M, Katz MN, Philbrick WM, et al. NLRP6 inflammasome orchestrates the colonic host-microbial interface by regulating goblet cell mucus secretion. Cell. 2014;156(5):1045–59.

28. Burger-van Paassen N, Vincent A, Puiman PJ, van der Sluis M, Bouma J, Boehm G, van Goudoever JB, van Seuningen I, Renes IB. The regulation of intestinal mucin MUC2 expression by short-chain fatty acids: implications for epithelial protection. Biochem J. 2009;420(2):211–9.

29. Shimada Y, Kinoshita M, Harada K, Mizutani M, Masahata K, Kayama H, Takeda K. Commensal bacteria-dependent indole production enhances epithelial barrier function in the colon. PLoS One. 2013; 8(11):e80604.

30. Venkatesh M, Mukherjee S, Wang H, Li H, Sun K, Benechet AP, Qiu Z, Maher L, Redinbo MR, Phillips RS, et al. Symbiotic bacterial metabolites regulate gastrointestinal barrier function via the xenobiotic sensor PXR and toll-like receptor 4. Immunity. 2014;41(2):296–310.

31. Ivanov II, Atarashi K, Manel N, Brodie EL, Shima T, Karaoz U, Wei D, Goldfarb KC, Santee CA, Lynch SV, et al. Induction of intestinal Th17 cells by segmented filamentous bacteria. Cell. 2009;139(3):485–98.

32. Atarashi K, Tanoue T, Ando M, Kamada N, Nagano Y, Narushima S, Suda W, Imaoka A, Setoyama H, Nagamori T, et al. Th17 cell induction by adhesion of microbes to intestinal epithelial cells. Cell. 2015;163(2):367–80.

33. Liang SC, Tan XY, Luxenberg DP, Karim R, Dunussi-Joannopoulos K, Collins M, Fouser LA. Interleukin (IL)-22 and IL-17 are coexpressed by Th17 cells and cooperatively enhance expression of antimicrobial peptides. J Exp Med. 2006;203(10):2271–9.

34. Gerbe F, Sidot E, Smyth DJ, Ohmoto M, Matsumoto I, Dardalhon V, Cesses P, Garnier L, Pouzolles M, Brulin B, et al. Intestinal epithelial tuft cells initiate type 2 mucosal immunity to helminth parasites. Nature. 2016;529(7585):226–30.

35. Howitt MR, Lavoie S, Michaud M, Blum AM, Tran SV, Weinstock JV, Gallini CA, Redding K, Margolskee RF, Osborne LC, et al. Tuft cells, taste-chemosensory cells, orchestrate parasite type 2 immunity in the gut. Science. 2016;351(6279):1329–33.

36. von Moltke J, Ji M, Liang HE, Locksley RM. Tuft-cell-derived IL-25 regulates an intestinal ILC2-epithelial response circuit. Nature. 2016;529(7585):221–5.

37. Kuhn KA, Manieri NA, Liu TC, Stappenbeck TS. IL-6 stimulates intestinal epithelial proliferation and repair after injury. PLoS One. 2014;9(12):e114195.

38. Pull SL, Doherty JM, Mills JC, Gordon JI, Stappenbeck TS. Activated macrophages are an adaptive element of the colonic epithelial progenitor niche necessary for regenerative responses to injury. Proc Natl Acad Sci U S A. 2005;102(1):99–104.

39. Seno H, Miyoshi H, Brown SL, Geske MJ, Colonna M, Stappenbeck TS. Efficient colonic mucosal wound repair requires Trem2 signaling. Proc Natl Acad Sci U S A. 2009;106(1):256–61.

40. Capaldo CT, Beeman N, Hilgarth RS, Nava P, Louis NA, Naschberger E, Sturzl M, Parkos CA, Nusrat A. IFN-gamma and TNF-alpha-induced GBP-1 inhibits epithelial cell proliferation through suppression of beta-catenin/TCF signaling. Mucosal Immunol. 2012;5(6):681–90.

41. Molodecky NA, Soon IS, Rabi DM, Ghali WA, Ferris M, Chernoff G, Benchimol EI, Panaccione R, Ghosh S, Barkema HW, et al. Increasing incidence and prevalence of the inflammatory bowel diseases with time, based on systematic review. Gastroenterology. 2012;142(1):46–54. e42; quiz e30

42. Goto Y, Kurashima Y, Kiyono H. The gut microbiota and inflammatory bowel disease. Curr Opin Rheumatol. 2015;27(4):388–96.

43. Anderson CA, Boucher G, Lees CW, Franke A, D'Amato M, Taylor KD, Lee JC, Goyette P, Imielinski M, Latiano A, et al. Meta-analysis identifies 29 additional ulcerative colitis risk loci, increasing the number of confirmed associations to 47. Nat Genet. 2011;43(3):246–52.

44. Franke A, McGovern DP, Barrett JC, Wang K, Radford-Smith GL, Ahmad T, Lees CW, Balschun T, Lee J, Roberts R, et al. Genome-wide meta-analysis

increases to 71 the number of confirmed Crohn's disease susceptibility loci. Nat Genet. 2010;42(12):1118–25.

45. Jostins L, Ripke S, Weersma RK, Duerr RH, McGovern DP, Hui KY, Lee JC, Schumm LP, Sharma Y, Anderson CA, et al. Host-microbe interactions have shaped the genetic architecture of inflammatory bowel disease. Nature. 2012;491(7422):119–24.

46. Liu JZ, van Sommeren S, Huang H, Ng SC, Alberts R, Takahashi A, Ripke S, Lee JC, Jostins L, Shah T, et al. Association analyses identify 38 susceptibility loci for inflammatory bowel disease and highlight shared genetic risk across populations. Nat Genet. 2015;47(9):979–86.

47. Van der Sluis M, De Koning BA, De Bruijn AC, Velcich A, Meijerink JP, Van Goudoever JB, Buller HA, Dekker J, Van Seuningen I, Renes IB, et al. Muc2-deficient mice spontaneously develop colitis, indicating that MUC2 is critical for colonic protection. Gastroenterology. 2006;131(1):117–29.

48. Pickard JM, Maurice CF, Kinnebrew MA, Abt MC, Schenten D, Golovkina TV, Bogatyrev SR, Ismagilov RF, Pamer EG, Turnbaugh PJ, et al. Rapid fucosylation of intestinal epithelium sustains host-commensal symbiosis in sickness. Nature. 2014;514(7524):638–41.

49. Wang Y, Huang D, Chen KY, Cui M, Wang W, Huang X, Awadellah A, Li Q, Friedman A, Xin WW, et al. Fucosylation deficiency in mice leads to colitis and adenocarcinoma. Gastroenterology. 2017;152(1):193–205.

50. Elinav E, Strowig T, Kau AL, Henao-Mejia J, Thaiss CA, Booth CJ, Peaper DR, Bertin J, Eisenbarth SC, Gordon JI, et al. NLRP6 inflammasome regulates colonic microbial ecology and risk for colitis. Cell. 2011;145(5):745–57.

51. Fujimoto K, Kinoshita M, Tanaka H, Okuzaki D, Shimada Y, Kayama H, Okumura R, Furuta Y, Narazaki M, Tamura A, et al. Regulation of intestinal homeostasis by the ulcerative colitis-associated gene RNF186. Mucosal Immunol. 2017;10(2):446–59.

52. Zenewicz LA, Yancopoulos GD, Valenzuela DM, Murphy AJ, Stevens S, Flavell RA. Innate and adaptive interleukin-22 protects mice from inflammatory bowel disease. Immunity. 2008;29(6):947–57.

53. Nenci A, Becker C, Wullaert A, Gareus R, van Loo G, Danese S, Huth M, Nikolaev A, Neufert C, Madison B, et al. Epithelial NEMO links innate immunity to chronic intestinal inflammation. Nature. 2007;446(7135):557–61.

54. Hugot JP, Chamaillard M, Zouali H, Lesage S, Cezard JP, Belaiche J, Almer S, Tysk C, O'Morain CA, Gassull M, et al. Association of NOD2 leucine-rich repeat variants with susceptibility to Crohn's disease. Nature. 2001;411(6837):599–603.

55. Biswas A, Liu YJ, Hao L, Mizoguchi A, Salzman NH, Bevins CL, Kobayashi KS. Induction and rescue of Nod2-dependent Th1-driven granulomatous inflammation of the ileum. Proc Natl Acad Sci U S A. 2010;107(33):14739–44.

56. Ogura Y, Bonen DK, Inohara N, Nicolae DL, Chen FF, Ramos R, Britton H, Moran T, Karaliuskas R, Duerr RH, et al. A frameshift mutation in NOD2 associated with susceptibility to Crohn's disease. Nature. 2001;411(6837):603–6.

57. Resta-Lenert S, Smitham J, Barrett KE. Epithelial dysfunction associated with the development of colitis in conventionally housed mdr1a–/– mice. Am J Physiol Gastrointest Liver Physiol. 2005;289(1):G153–62.

58. Takahashi D, Hase K, Kimura S, Nakatsu F, Ohmae M, Mandai Y, Sato T, Date Y, Ebisawa M, Kato T, et al. The epithelia-specific membrane trafficking factor AP-1B controls gut immune homeostasis in mice. Gastroenterology. 2011;141(2):621–32.

Permissions

All chapters in this book were first published in I&R, by BioMed Central; hereby published with permission under the Creative Commons Attribution License or equivalent. Every chapter published in this book has been scrutinized by our experts. Their significance has been extensively debated. The topics covered herein carry significant findings which will fuel the growth of the discipline. They may even be implemented as practical applications or may be referred to as a beginning point for another development.

The contributors of this book come from diverse backgrounds, making this book a truly international effort. This book will bring forth new frontiers with its revolutionizing research information and detailed analysis of the nascent developments around the world.

We would like to thank all the contributing authors for lending their expertise to make the book truly unique. They have played a crucial role in the development of this book. Without their invaluable contributions this book wouldn't have been possible. They have made vital efforts to compile up to date information on the varied aspects of this subject to make this book a valuable addition to the collection of many professionals and students.

This book was conceptualized with the vision of imparting up-to-date information and advanced data in this field. To ensure the same, a matchless editorial board was set up. Every individual on the board went through rigorous rounds of assessment to prove their worth. After which they invested a large part of their time researching and compiling the most relevant data for our readers.

The editorial board has been involved in producing this book since its inception. They have spent rigorous hours researching and exploring the diverse topics which have resulted in the successful publishing of this book. They have passed on their knowledge of decades through this book. To expedite this challenging task, the publisher supported the team at every step. A small team of assistant editors was also appointed to further simplify the editing procedure and attain best results for the readers.

Apart from the editorial board, the designing team has also invested a significant amount of their time in understanding the subject and creating the most relevant covers. They scrutinized every image to scout for the most suitable representation of the subject and create an appropriate cover for the book.

The publishing team has been an ardent support to the editorial, designing and production team. Their endless efforts to recruit the best for this project, has resulted in the accomplishment of this book. They are a veteran in the field of academics and their pool of knowledge is as vast as their experience in printing. Their expertise and guidance has proved useful at every step. Their uncompromising quality standards have made this book an exceptional effort. Their encouragement from time to time has been an inspiration for everyone.

The publisher and the editorial board hope that this book will prove to be a valuable piece of knowledge for researchers, students, practitioners and scholars across the globe.

List of Contributors

Takehiro Kamo
Department of Cardiovascular Medicine, Graduate School of Medicine, The University of Tokyo, 7-3-1 Hongo, Bunkyo-ku, Tokyo 113-8655, Japan

Hiroshi Akazawa and Issei Komuro
Department of Cardiovascular Medicine, Graduate School of Medicine, The University of Tokyo, 7-3-1 Hongo, Bunkyo-ku, Tokyo 113-8655, Japan
AMED-CREST, Japan Agency for Medical Research and Development, Chiyoda-ku, Tokyo 100-0004, Japan

Jun-ichi Suzuki
Department of Advanced Clinical Science and Therapeutics, Graduate School of Medicine, The University of Tokyo, Bunkyo-ku, Tokyo 113-8655, Japan

Atsunori Tsuchiya, Yuichi Kojima, Shunzo Ikarashi, Satoshi Seino, Yusuke Watanabe, Yuzo Kawata and Shuji Terai
Division of Gastroenterology and Hepatology, Graduate School of Medical and Dental Science, Niigata University, 1-757 Asahimachi-dori, Chuo-ku, Niigata 951-8510, Japan

Sumito Ogawa, Mitsutaka Yakabe and Masahiro Akishita
Department of Geriatric Medicine, Graduate School of Medicine, The University of Tokyo, Bunkyo-ku, Tokyo 113-8655, Japan

Seitaro Fujishima
Center for General Medicine Education, Keio University School of Medicine, Tokyo, Japan

Sachiko Ono and Gyohei Egawa
Department of Dermatology, Kyoto University Graduate School of Medicine, 54 Shogoin-Kawahara, Sakyo, Kyoto 606-8507, Japan

Kenji Kabashima
Department of Dermatology, Kyoto University Graduate School of Medicine, 54 Shogoin-Kawahara, Sakyo, Kyoto 606-8507, Japan
Singapore Immunology Network (SIgN) and Institute of Medical Biology, Agency for Science, Technology and Research (A*STAR), Biopolis, Singapore
PRESTO, Japan Science and Technology Agency, Saitama, Japan

Yuko Nitahara-Kasahara and Takashi Okada
Department of Biochemistry and Molecular Biology, Nippon Medical School, Bunkyo-ku, Tokyo, Japan
Department of Molecular Therapy, National Institute of Neuroscience, National Center of Neurology and Psychiatry, Kodaira, Tokyo, Japan

Shin'ichi Takeda
Department of Molecular Therapy, National Institute of Neuroscience, National Center of Neurology and Psychiatry, Kodaira, Tokyo, Japan

Hironori Hara, Norifumi Takeda and Issei Komuro
Department of Cardiovascular Medicine, The University of Tokyo Hospital, 7-3-1 Hongo, Bunkyo-ku, Tokyo 113-8655, Japan

Yusuke Yamamoto and Takahiro Ochiya
Division of Molecular and Cellular Medicine, National Cancer Center Research Institute, 5-1-1, Tsukiji, Chuo-ku, Tokyo 104-0045, Japan

Yuki Sato
Medical Innovation Center, TMK project, Graduate School of Medicine, Kyoto University, Kyoto, Japan
Department of Nephrology, Graduate School of Medicine, Kyoto University, Kyoto, Japan

Motoko Yanagita
Department of Nephrology, Graduate School of Medicine, Kyoto University, Kyoto, Japan

Atsuhiro Kanda and Susumu Ishida
Laboratory of Ocular Cell Biology and Visual Science, Department of Ophthalmology, Hokkaido University Graduate School of Medicine, N-15, W-7, Kita-ku, Sapporo, Hokkaido 060-8638, Japan

Toshio Imai and Nobuyuki Yasuda
KAN Research Institute, Inc., 6-8-2 Minatojima-minamimachi Chuo-ku, Kobe, Hyogo 650-0047, Japan

Tadayoshi Karasawa and Masafumi Takahashi
Division of Inflammation Research, Center for Molecular Medicine, Jichi Medical University, 3311-1 Yakushiji, Shimotsuke, Tochigi 329-0498, Japan

Hiroyuki Yamakawa
Department of Clinical and Molecular Cardiovascular Research, Keio University School of Medicine, Shinjuku-ku, Tokyo, Japan

Department of Cardiology, Keio University School of Medicine, 35 Shinanomachi, Shinjuku-ku, Tokyo 160-8582, Japan

Mitsuhiro Yamada, Naoya Fujino and Masakazu Ichinose
Department of Respiratory Medicine, Graduate School of Medicine, Tohoku University, 1-1 Seiryo-machi, Aoba-ku, Sendai 980-8574, Japan

Pornkawee Charoenlarp, Arun Kumar Rajendran and Sachiko Iseki
Section of Molecular Craniofacial Embryology, Tokyo Medical and Dental University Graduate School of Medical and Dental Sciences, 1-5-45 Yushima, Bunkyo-ku, Tokyo 113-8549, Japan

Goro Katsuumi and Tohru Minamino
Department of Cardiovascular Biology and Medicine, Niigata University Graduate School of Medical and Dental Sciences, 1-757 Asahimachidori, Chuo-ku, Niigata 951-8510, Japan

Ippei Shimizu and Yohko Yoshida
Department of Cardiovascular Biology and Medicine, Niigata University Graduate School of Medical and Dental Sciences, 1-757 Asahimachidori, Chuo-ku, Niigata 951-8510, Japan
Division of Molecular Aging and Cell Biology, Niigata University Graduate School of Medical and Dental Sciences, 1-757 Asahimachidori, Chuo-ku, Niigata 951-8510, Japan

Sandesh Panthi
Otago School of Biomedical Sciences, University of Otago, Otago, New Zealand

Kripa Gautam
China Medical University, Shenyang, People's Republic of China

Naohiro Toda, Motoko Yanagita and Hideki Yokoi
Department of Nephrology, Graduate School of Medicine, Kyoto University, 54 Shogoin Kawahara-cho, Sakyo-ku, Kyoto 606-8507, Japan

Masashi Mukoyama
Department of Nephrology, Kumamoto University Graduate School of Medical Sciences, Kumamoto, Japan

Chiao-Ching Hsu, Ryu Okumura and Kiyoshi Takeda
Department of Microbiology and Immunology, Graduate School of Medicine, Osaka University, Osaka 565-8871, Japan
WPI Immunology Frontier Research Center, Osaka University, Osaka 565-8871, Japan

Core Research for Evolutional Science and Technology, Japan Agency for Medical Research and Development, Tokyo 100-0004, Japan

Hiromu Ito, Furu Moritoshi and Shuichi Matsuda
The Department of Orthopaedic Surgery, Kyoto University Graduate School of Medicine, 54 Kawahara-cho, Shogoin, Sakyo, Kyoto 606-8507, Japan

Motomu Hashimoto and Masao Tanaka
The Department of Advanced Medicine for Rheumatic Diseases, Kyoto University Graduate School of Medicine, Kyoto, Japan

Ryutaro Fukui
Division of Innate Immunity, Department of Microbiology and Immunology, The University of Tokyo, 4-6-1 Shirokanedai, Minato-ku, Tokyo 108-8639, Japan

Yusuke Murakami
Division of Innate Immunity, Department of Microbiology and Immunology, The University of Tokyo, 4-6-1 Shirokanedai, Minato-ku, Tokyo 108-8639, Japan
Department of Pharmacotherapy, Research Institute of Pharmaceutical Sciences, Musashino University, 1-1-20 Shin-machi, Nishitokyo shi, Tokyo 202-8585, Japan

Kensuke Miyake
Division of Innate Immunity, Department of Microbiology and Immunology, The University of Tokyo, 4-6-1 Shirokanedai, Minato-ku, Tokyo 108-8639, Japan
Laboratory of Innate Immunity, Center for Experimental Medicine and Systems Biology, The Institute of Medical Science, The University of Tokyo, 4-6-1 Shirokanedai, Minato-ku, Tokyo 108-8639, Japan

Sachiko Sekiya and Tatsuya Shimizu
Institute of Advanced Biomedical Engineering and Science, Tokyo Women's Medical University, 8-1 Kawada-cho, Shinjuku-ku, Tokyo 162-8666, Japan

Toru Uyama and Natsuo Ueda
Department of Biochemistry, Kagawa University School of Medicine, 1750-1 Ikenobe, Miki, Kagawa 761-0793, Japan

Kazuhito Tsuboi
Department of Biochemistry, Kagawa University School of Medicine, 1750-1 Ikenobe, Miki, Kagawa 761-0793, Japan
Department of Pharmacology, Kawasaki Medical School, 577 Matsushima, Kurashiki, Okayama 701-0192, Japan

Yasuo Okamoto
Department of Pharmacology, Kawasaki Medical School, 577 Matsushima, Kurashiki, Okayama 701-0192, Japan

Kiyoshi Hirahara, Kenta Shinoda, Yusuke Endo and Tomomi Ichikawa
Department of Immunology, Graduate School of Medicine, Chiba University, 1-8-1 Inohana, Chuo-ku, Chiba-shi, Chiba 260-8670, Japan

Toshinori Nakayama
Department of Immunology, Graduate School of Medicine, Chiba University, 1-8-1 Inohana, Chuo-ku, Chiba-shi, Chiba 260-8670, Japan
AMED-CREST, AMED, 1-8-1 Inohana Chuo-ku, Chiba 260-8670, Japan

Sho Sendo and Akio Morinobu
Division of Rheumatology and Clinical Immunology, Department of Internal Medicine, Kobe University Graduate School of Medicine, 7-5-2 Kusunoki-cho, Chuo-ku, Kobe 650-0017, Japan

Jun Saegusa
Division of Rheumatology and Clinical Immunology, Department of Internal Medicine, Kobe University Graduate School of Medicine, 7-5-2 Kusunoki-cho, Chuo-ku, Kobe 650-0017, Japan
Division of Laboratory Medicine, Kobe University Graduate School of Medicine, 7-5-2 Kusunoki-cho, Chuo-ku, Kobe 650-0017, Japan

Naoto Azuma and Hajime Sano
Division of Rheumatology, Department of Internal Medicine, Hyogo College of Medicine, 1-1 Mukogawa-cho, Nishinomiya, Hyogo 663-8501, Japan

Yoshinori Katada
Division of General Medicine, Department of Internal Medicine, Sakai City Medical Center, 1-1-1 Ebaraji-cho, Nishi-ku, Sakai 593-8304, Japan

Keiko Akazawa, Mizuki Nagata and Yuichi Izumi
Department of Periodontology, Graduate School of Medical and Dental Sciences, Tokyo Medical and Dental University (TMDU), 1-5-45 Yushima, Bunkyo-ku, Tokyo 113-8510, Japan

Kengo Iwasaki and Motohiro Komaki
Department of Nanomedicine (DNP), Graduate School of Medical and Dental Sciences, Tokyo Medical and Dental University (TMDU), 1-5-45 Yushima, Bunkyo-ku, Tokyo 113-8510, Japan

Naoki Yokoyama, Hirohito Ayame, Kazumasa Yamaki and Yuichi Tanaka
Life Science Laboratory, Research and Development Center, Dai Nippon Printing Co., Ltd., 1-1-1 Kaga-cho, Shinjuku-ku, Tokyo 162-8001, Japan

Izumi Honda and Tsuyoshi Kimura
Department of Comprehensive Reproductive Medicine, Graduate School of Medical and Dental Science, Tokyo Medical and Dental University, 1-5-45 Yushima, Bunkyo-ku, Tokyo 113-8510, Japan

Chikako Morioka
Department of Pediatrics and Developmental Biology, Graduate School of Medical and Dental Science, Tokyo Medical and Dental University (TMDU), 1-5-45 Yushima, Bunkyo ku, Tokyo 113-8510, Japan

Akio Kishida
Department of Material-based Medical Engineering, Institute of Biomaterials and Bioengineering, Tokyo Medical and Dental University (TMDU), 2-3-10, Kanda Surugadai, Chiyoda-ku, Tokyo 101-0062, Japan

Ikuo Morita
Department of Cellular Physiological Chemistry, Graduate School of Medical and Dental Sciences, Tokyo Medical and Dental University (TMDU), 1-5-45 Yushima, Bunkyo-ku, Tokyo 113-8510, Japan

Shuji Sumitomo, Yasuo Nagafuchi, Yumi Tsuchida, Haruka Tsuchiya, Mineto Ota and Keishi Fujio
Department of Allergy and Rheumatology, Graduate School of Medicine, the University of Tokyo, 7-3-1 Hongo, Bunkyo-ku, Tokyo 113-8655, Japan

Kazuyoshi Ishigaki
Laboratory for Statistical Analysis, Center for Integrative Medical Sciences, the Institute of Physical and Chemical Research (RIKEN), 1-7-22 Suehirocho, Tsurumi-ku, Yokohama City, Kanagawa 230-0045, Japan

Akari Suzuki and Yuta Kochi
Laboratory for Autoimmune Diseases, Center for Integrative Medical Sciences, the Institute of Physical and Chemical Research (RIKEN), 1-7-22 Suehirocho, Tsurumi-ku, Yokohama City, Kanagawa 230-0045, Japan

Kazuhiko Yamamoto
Center for Integrative Medical Sciences, the Institute of Physical and Chemical Research (RIKEN), 1-7-22 Suehirocho, Tsurumi-ku, Yokohama City, Kanagawa 230-0045, Japan

Ryu Okumura and Kiyoshi Takeda
Department of Microbiology and Immunology, Graduate School of Medicine, Osaka University, Osaka 565-0871, Japan

WPI Immunology Frontier Research Center, Osaka University, Osaka 565-0871, Japan
Core Research for Evolutional Science and Technology, Japan Agency for Medical Research and Development, Tokyo 100-0004, Japan

Index

www.ingramcontent.com/pod-product-compliance
Lightning Source LLC
Chambersburg PA
CBHW080524200326

41458CB00012B/4325